an atlas of

ANATOMY
BASIC TO
RADIOLOGY

Volume 2

ISADORE MESCHAN, M.A., M.D.

Professor and Director of the Department of Radiology
at the Bowman Gray School of Medicine of Wake Forest University,
Winston-Salem, North Carolina; Consultant, Walter Reed Army
Hospital; Chairman, Committee on Radiology, National Research
Council, National Academy of Sciences, 1974–1976

1975 · *W. B. SAUNDERS COMPANY* · *Philadelphia* · *London* · *Toronto*

L FFH

W. B. Saunders Company: West Washington Square
Philadelphia, PA 19105

12 Dyott Street
London, WC1A 1DB

833 Oxford Street
Toronto, Ontario M8Z 5T9, Canada

Library of Congress Cataloging in Publication Data

Meschan, Isadore.

An atlas of anatomy basic to radiology.

Includes indexes.

1. Anatomy, Human—Atlases.   I. Title. [DNLM: 1. Radiography—Atlases.   2. Technology, Radiologic—Atlases.
   WN17 M578ab]

QM25.M47   611′.0022′2   73–89936

ISBN 0–7216–6310–9

Anatomy Basic to Radiology

Single Volume ISBN 0-7216-6310-9

Volume 1 ISBN 0-7216-6308-7

Volume 2 ISBN 0-7216-6309-5

Last digit is the print number: 9   8   7   6   5   4   3   2   1

PREFACE

Among the basic sciences of medicine fundamental to the practice of radiology, the most important is anatomy. In the past I have addressed myself to the anatomic interpretation of normal radiographs, first in the two editions of the *Atlas of Normal Radiographic Anatomy,* and thereafter in an abbreviated version of this, *Radiographic Positioning and Related Anatomy.* Although no attempt was made to include the innumerable variations of normal anatomy, attention was given to changes with growth and development.

In the present text, I have tried to cover the gross anatomy basic to radiologic interpretation in considerably greater depth and from much wider and broader perspectives, recognizing that the radiograph is a two-dimensional representation of all tissues in the coronal and sagittal planes. Vascular anatomy has been added in considerable detail, as have neuroanatomy, the intricacies of the skull, and correlated sagittal and coronal sections of the chest and abdomen. In essence, this is a new text.

The study of anatomy has unique applications to all branches of medicine. It has been my purpose in this text, however, to extract those basic features from the science of anatomy that are especially pertinent to the practice of radiology. It is my hope that the student or practitioner of radiology will find this text of special advantage, since I have culled not only the conventional textbooks of anatomy for this purpose, but also the wider expanse of scientific literature.

Needless to say, on a subject so broad, decisions must be made as to omissions and inclusions; as the author, I accept the responsibility for these decisions based upon my 35 years in the practice and teaching of radiology.

I. MESCHAN

CONTENTS

10

The Respiratory System

The respiratory tract can be conveniently subdivided for purposes of discussion into: (1) the upper air passages, (2) the larynx, (3) the trachea and bronchi, (4) the lung parenchyma, (5) the vascular supply, venous drainage, and lymphatics of the respiratory tract, (6) the lung hili, and (7) the thoracic cage, pleura and diaphragm.

THE UPPER AIR PASSAGES

The upper air passages are usually amenable to direct and indirect inspection to such a great extent that radiography need not often be employed. Nevertheless, because considerable useful information can be obtained by fluoroscopic and radiographic methods, a consideration of this subject is worthwhile.

Apart from the nasal air passages, which have already been described in Chapter 7, the upper air passages are referred to anatomically as the pharynx. This, in turn, consists of three fundamental areas: (1) the nasopharynx, which extends from the nasal cavity anteriorly and the base of the skull superiorly to the tip of the uvula and margin of the soft palate below; (2) the oropharynx, which extends from the soft palate above to the epiglottis and its pharyngo-epiglottic folds, opposite the hyoid bone; and (3) the laryngeal pharynx, which extends from the hyoid bone above to the upper boundary of the esophagus below, opposite the sixth cervical vertebra (posterior to the larynx). The larynx itself is considered separately.

The pharynx is approximately 12 cm. in length. It communicates with the nasal cavity, the oral cavity, the middle ear via the auditory (eustachian) tube, the esophagus, and the trachea. The vital structures on either side of the pharynx are: the carotid arteries, the jugular veins, the ninth, tenth, eleventh, and twelfth cranial nerves, the cervical sympathetic chain, important lymph nodal chains, and important fascial planes which may extend into the mediastinum.

Nasopharynx (Fig. 10–1). The anterior boundary of the nasopharynx is formed by the choanae, with the vomer of the nasal septum between them. The posterior wall lies above the level of the anterior arch or tubercle of the atlas of the cervical spine and usually contains considerable lymphatic tissue, which is continuous with a ring of lymphatic tissue around the circumference of the pharynx. The posterior wall is separated from the anterior arch of the atlas by the superior pharyngeal constrictor and longus capitis muscles (Fig. 10–1 B). The lateral nasopharyngeal walls are concave outward or sigmoidal in contour, a configuration due to the soft tissue prominence surrounding the nasopharyngeal opening of the eustachian tube, the *torus tubarius*. Posterolateral to the torus tubarius is the fossa of Rosenmüller or pharyngeal recess. The normal nasopharyngeal air shadow on basal projection does not project beyond the bony pterygoids owing to muscular structures in its lateral walls as well as its attachment to the skull base. These structures are indicated radiographically in Figure 10–1 C and D. The shadows of the oropharynx and pyriform sinuses may be superimposed upon the nasopharyngeal air column (Fig. 10–1 E and F); they may project behind the anterior arch of C1 or extend beyond the bony pterygoids, usually presenting a convex border laterally. The uvula is often identified as a nodular structure surrounded by oropharyngeal air (Fig. 10–1 E).

The adenoids of children are composed of the lymphatic tissue on the posterior wall of the nasopharynx, which tends to become atrophic in adults. As a result, the soft tissue width of the nasopharyngeal posterior wall is considerably greater in children than in adults, and tends to swell forward and downward toward the soft palate in the very young. The extent of this swelling is readily visualized on the lateral radiograph of the child's neck (Fig. 10–2) and furnishes an accurate means of evaluating the extent of adenoid hypertrophy.

Below and in front of the fossa of Rosenmüller are found the orifices of the auditive (eustachian) or auditory tubes. The elevated boundaries of the latter structures can usually be identified on the lateral radiograph of the neck.

Oropharynx. The oropharynx is the common passageway of both the digestive tract (mouth to esophagus) and the respiratory tract (nasopharynx to larynx). It is bounded anteriorly by the posterior third of the tongue, which contains lymphoid follicles, and posteriorly by the soft tissue covering of the upper three cervical spine segments.

581

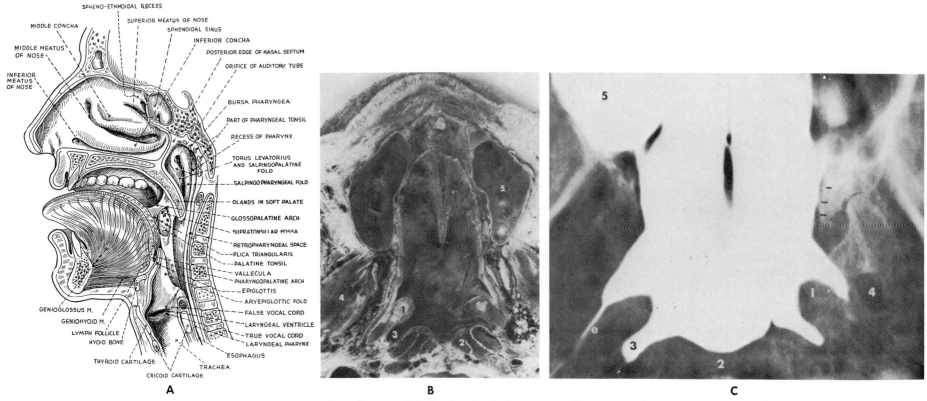

Figure 10–1. *A.* Sagittal section of the head and neck demonstrating the structure of the nasopharynx and larynx. *B,* Horizontal cross section in a postmortem specimen at the level of the nasopharynx. (1) Torus tubarius; (2) prevertebral musculature; (3) fossa of Rosenmüller; (4) internal pterygoid muscle; (5) maxillary atrium.

    C. Postmortem positive contrast radiographic examination in the base view, outlining the soft tissue structures of the lateral and posterior nasopharyngeal walls. Barium enters the eustachian tube (e). The right maxillary antrum is also opacified. Note the relationship of the barium-filled nasopharynx to the designated bony structures. (1) Torus tubarius; (2) prevertebral soft tissues; (3) fossa of Rosenmüller; (4) foramen ovale; (5) right maxillary antrum; black lines, medial pterygoid plate.

Figure 10–1 continued on the opposite page.

On each lateral wall of the oropharynx is the tonsillar fossa with its anterior and posterior pillars. Embedded between these pillars is the palatine or faucial tonsil.

Laryngeal Pharynx (Fig. 10–3). The laryngeal pharynx connects with the oropharynx above and the esophagus below. It is bounded posteriorly by the soft tissues overlying the fourth, fifth, and sixth cervical vertebrae, and anteriorly by the posterior wall of the larynx. The posterior wall of the larynx contains the arytenoid cartilages and the lamina of the cricoid cartilage. The lateral walls of this area are attached to the thyroid cartilage and to the hyoid bone. The epiglottis is situated anteriorly and superiorly, in the median plane, with the aryepiglottic folds extending posteriorly and inferiorly from the epiglottis to the arytenoids. Beneath the level of these folds on each side are the pyriform sinuses. The valleculae are hollow pockets situated between the epiglottis and the dorsal aspect of the tongue just lateral to the median plane.

THE LARYNX

The cartilaginous framework is illustrated in Figure 10–4. This consists of three large single cartilages: the thyroid, cricoid, and epiglottis; and three paired cartilages: the corniculate, cuneiform, and arytenoids.

The thyroid cartilage is composed of two wings or laminae, and two superior and two inferior horns or cornua. The superior margins of the two wings are convex and meet at the superior thyroid notch at an angle of 90 degrees in the male and 120

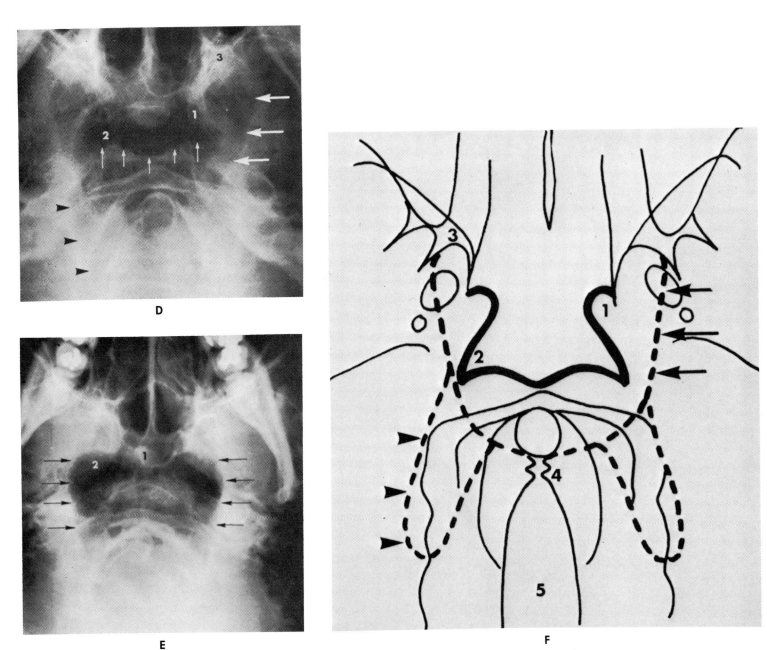

Figure 10–1 *Continued.* D. Clinical examination of the skull in the base view clearly demonstrating the outline of the nasopharynx. (1) Torus tubarius; (2) fossa of Rosenmuller; (3) pterygoid process; vertical arrows, posterior wall. The oropharynx is convex outward and laterally situated (horizontal arrows). Arrowheads define piriform sinus.

E. Clinical radiograph in the base view. The oropharyngeal air shadow (horizontal arrows) is seen with its convex lateral margins projecting beyond the lateral pterygoid processes. The uvula (1) is surrounded by oropharyngeal air. The lateral concavity formed by the torus tubarius (2) is outlined by nasopharyngeal air and is seen apart from the more inferiorly related oropharynx.

F. Composite schematic drawing of B to E. (1) Torus tubarius; (2) fossa of Rosenmüller; (3) pterygoid process; (4) vocal cords; (5) trachea; bold line, nasopharynx; arrows, oropharynx; arrowheads, piriform sinus. (B to F from Rizzuti, R. J., and Whalen, J. P.: Radiology, *104*:537–540, 1972.)

degrees in the female, which explains the greater laryngeal prominence in the male.

The cricoid cartilage attaches to and rests upon the first cartilaginous ring of the trachea, below the thyroid cartilage. It has the shape of a signet ring, being expanded posteriorly. This broad posterior aspect, or lamina, has a ridge centrally for attachment to the esophagus, an upper elliptical surface for attachment to the arytenoid cartilages, and inner impressions for attachment of the crico-arytenoid muscles. The inferior horns of the thyroid cartilage articulate with the lateral aspect of the cricoid ring.

The arytenoid cartilages are paired pyramidal cartilages surmounting the laminae of the cricoid posteriorly, while the corniculate cartilages are mounted superiorly on the arytenoids. The cuneiform cartilages are embedded in the aryepiglottic folds.

The epiglottic cartilage is situated behind the root of the tongue above the thyroid cartilage and behind the body of the hyoid bone. It lies in front of and above the superior opening of the larynx and acts to deflect the swallowed bolus of food to either side into the pyriform fossae. The aryepiglottic folds act as a sphincter, preventing the food bolus from entering the larynx and trachea.

The thyroid, cricoid, and the greater part of the arytenoid cartilages are composed of hyaline cartilage that tends to calcify late in life and may be transformed into bone. The rest of the cartilages are composed for the most part of fibrocartilage, and do not calcify. The calcification may be irregular, and these open spaces must not be misinterpreted as erosion of the cartilage. Also, these areas of calcification must not be misinterpreted as foreign bodies in the esophagus or larynx. This distinction is

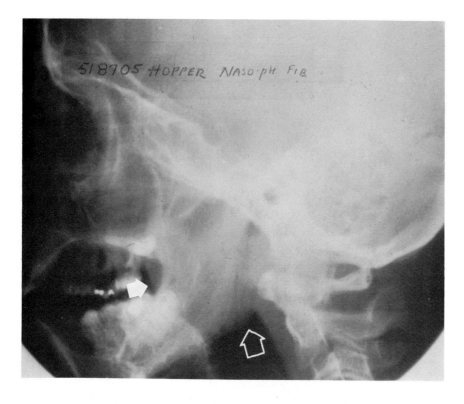

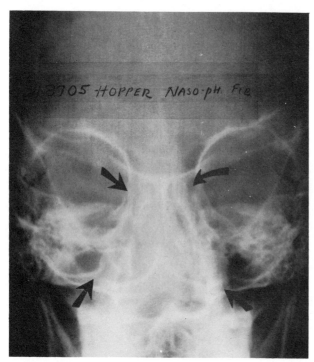

Figure 10-2   Nasopharyngeal tumor (an angiofibroma) in a child, producing a notable swelling of the posterior wall of the oropharynx and nasopharynx. A deformity (bowing) of the pterygopalatine processes is also visible.

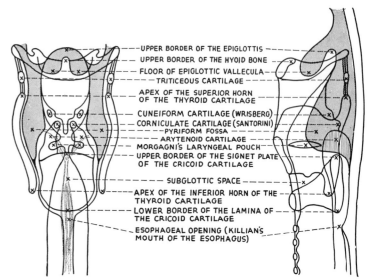

Figure 10-3.   General schematic representation of the roentgen anatomy of the larynx and pharynx.

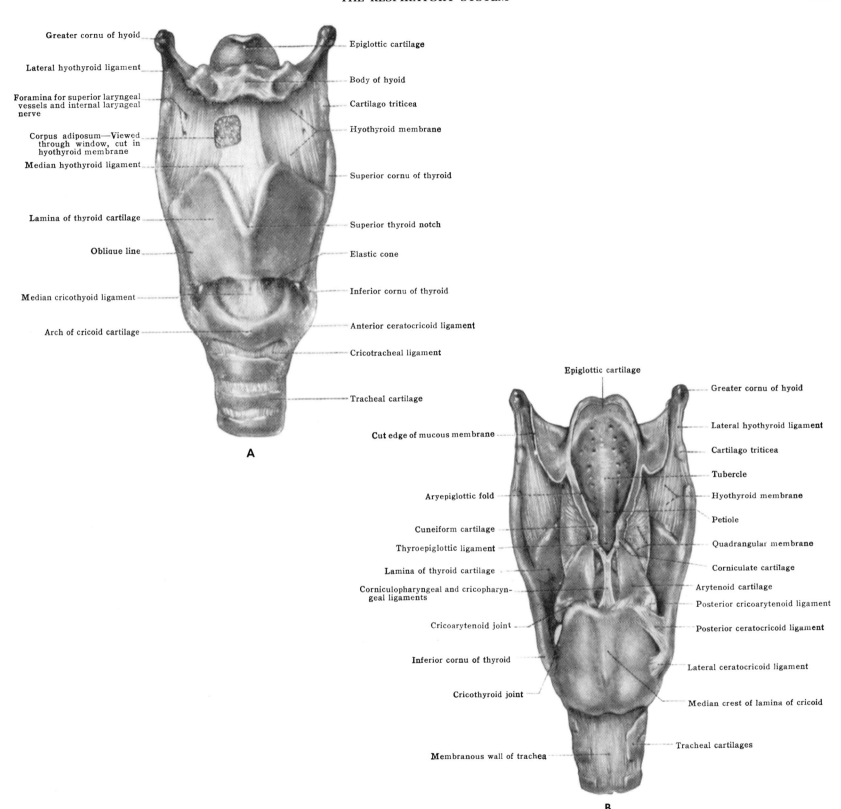

Greater cornu of hyoid

Lateral hyothyroid ligament

Foramina for superior laryngeal vessels and internal laryngeal nerve

Corpus adiposum—Viewed through window, cut in hyothyroid membrane

Median hyothyroid ligament

Lamina of thyroid cartilage

Oblique line

Median cricothyroid ligament

Arch of cricoid cartilage

Epiglottic cartilage

Body of hyoid

Cartilago triticea

Hyothyroid membrane

Superior cornu of thyroid

Superior thyroid notch

Elastic cone

Inferior cornu of thyroid

Anterior ceratocricoid ligament

Cricotracheal ligament

Tracheal cartilage

A

Epiglottic cartilage

Cut edge of mucous membrane

Aryepiglottic fold

Cuneiform cartilage

Thyroepiglottic ligament

Lamina of thyroid cartilage

Corniculopharyngeal and cricopharyngeal ligaments

Cricoarytenoid joint

Inferior cornu of thyroid

Cricothyroid joint

Membranous wall of trachea

Greater cornu of hyoid

Lateral hyothyroid ligament

Cartilago triticea

Tubercle

Hyothyroid membrane

Petiole

Quadrangular membrane

Corniculate cartilage

Arytenoid cartilage

Posterior cricoarytenoid ligament

Posterior ceratocricoid ligament

Lateral ceratocricoid ligament

Median crest of lamina of cricoid

Tracheal cartilages

B

Figure 10–4. Laryngeal skeleton. *A.* Ventral view. *B.* Dorsal view. (From Anson, B. J. (ed.): Morris' Human Anatomy, 12th ed. Copyright © 1966, by McGraw-Hill, Inc. Used by permission of McGraw-Hill Book Company.)

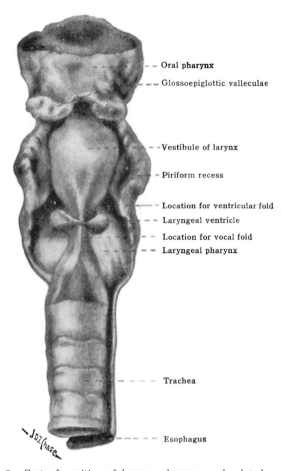

Oral **pharynx**

Glossoepiglottic valleculae

Vestibule of larynx

Piriform recess

Location for ventricular fold
Laryngeal ventricle
Location for vocal fold
Laryngeal pharynx

Trachea

Esophagus

Figure 10–5. Cast of cavities of larynx, pharynx, and related parts (ventral aspect). (From a cast by J. P. Schaeffer in The Daniel Baugh Institute of Anatomy of The Jefferson Medical College.) (From Anson, B. J. (ed.): Morris' Human Anatomy, 12th ed. Copyright © 1966 by McGraw-Hill, Inc. Used by permission of McGraw-Hill Book Company.)

with the base of the triangle formed by the ventricular folds and arytenoid cartilages posteriorly. The anterior margin of this triangle is formed by the aryepiglottic folds, and the posterior by the epiglottis.

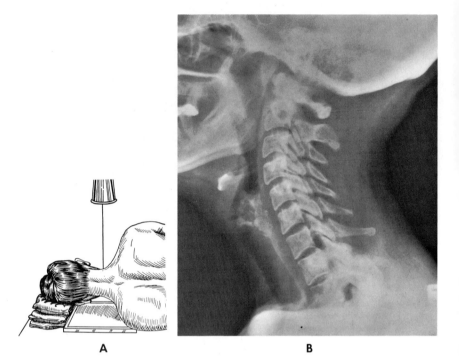

A

B

readily made if barium is administered to the patient and the barium column is then seen to go behind the larynx.

Cavity of the Larynx. The laryngeal aditus or superior laryngeal aperture or inlet is readily identified on the soft tissue films of the larynx (Fig. 10–5) as an opening bounded by the epiglottis in front and the aryepiglottic folds on each side. The pyriform recess or sinus is identified just outside the aditus on either side, between the aryepiglottic fold and the inner wall of the thyroid cartilage.

The vestibule or upper laryngeal compartment of the larynx extends from the laryngeal aditus to the ventricular folds (false vocal cords). The narrow opening between the ventricular folds is the vestibular slit. As seen on the lateral radiograph of the neck (Fig. 10–6), the vestibule of the larynx is triangular in shape,

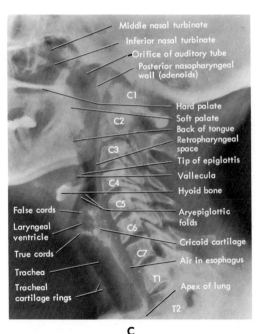

Middle nasal turbinate
Inferior nasal turbinate
Orifice of auditory tube
Posterior nasopharyngeal wall (adenoids)

C1

Hard palate
C2   Soft palate
Back of tongue
Retropharyngeal space
C3   Tip of epiglottis

C4   Vallecula
C5   Hyoid bone

False cords   Aryepiglottic folds
C6
Laryngeal ventricle
Cricoid cartilage
True cords   C7   Air in esophagus

Trachea
T1
Tracheal cartilage rings   Apex of lung
T2

C

Figure 10–6. Lateral soft tissue film of the neck. A. Position of patient. B. Radiograph. C. Labeled film of B.

The middle laryngeal compartment is situated between the ventricular folds above and the vocal folds (true vocal cords) below. The ventricular folds are undermined on each side by a small lateral outpouching forming the laryngeal ventricle.

The "rima glottidis" is an elongated slitlike opening between the true vocal folds. This is the narrowest part of the laryngeal cavity.

The portion of the laryngeal cavity below the level of the vocal folds is the lower laryngeal compartment and is the inferior entrance to the glottis. It changes from a slit to a rounded cavity surrounded by the cricoid cartilage below, and is continuous with the trachea. This portion is a favorable site for the development of edema because of its loose connective tissue.

The sensory nerve supply of the larynx above the true vocal folds is carried by the superior laryngeal nerve and below the vocal folds by the recurrent laryngeal; the motor nerve supply (with the exception of the cricothyroid muscle) is carried by the recurrent laryngeal. The cricothyroid muscle is supplied by the superior laryngeal nerve.

Articulations of the Laryngeal Cartilages. The cricothyroid articulation is lined with synovial membrane and is a typical arthrodial joint. As such it is subject to all of the diseases of the synovial joints and is of particular importance in rheumatoid arthritis or collagen diseases in which cricothyroid articular disease may occur, with esophageal cricothyroid pseudobulbar palsy and adjoining esophageal spasm. The cricoarytenoid articulation is also a typical arthrodial joint.

Position of the Larynx in the Neck. In fetal and infantile life the larynx is situated high in the neck, descending in later life. In a fetus of 6 months, the organ is in a position two vertebrae higher than in the adult. The larynx in general follows the thoracic viscera in their subsidence, which continues until old age.

At birth the space between the hyoid bone and the thyroid cartilage is relatively small and increases but little during early life.

The Normal Swallowing Function. The process of deglutition has been thoroughly studied by cineradiography in recent times. Briefly, the sequence of events is as follows:

1. There is a forward and upward movement of the tongue, which displaces the contents of the mouth backward.

2. The larynx rises and the pharyngeal space is obliterated for a fraction of a second.

3. With a backward thrust, the base of the tongue forces the bolus downward.

4. Once the bolus has passed the epiglottis, filled the pyriform recesses, and entered the esophagus, air begins to enter the nasopharynx, the soft palate relaxes, and the epiglottis and larynx begin to return to their resting position.

5. In frontal projection, the epiglottis produces the appearance of a central ovoid filling defect during the act of swallowing.

6. According to Barclay, the chief function of the epiglottis is to form, along with the vallecula, a trap for saliva running down over the back of the tongue between the acts of deglutition. When food is trapped by the epiglottis, it is forced into the vallecula, thereafter to be swallowed.

7. Below the level of the upper third of the esophagus, peristaltic action carries the food bolus down into the stomach. Peristalsis begins in the posterior pharynx and is shallow in nature, not occlusive.

8. The function of the gastroesophageal segment is complex, and will be described later in relation to the esophagus and stomach.

The laryngeal structures return to their resting position after the bolus has passed into the esophagus.

Comparison of Width of the Retro-epilaryngeal Space with the Retrotracheal Space. Figure 10–7 *A* shows the relationship of the soft tissues of the child and the adult in the specified regions at the levels of the fifth and sixth cervical vertebrae respectively. Roughly, up to the age of 1 year, the widths of these tissues equal one another and are approximately $1\frac{1}{2}$ to 2 times the anteroposterior dimension of the fourth cervical vertebral body (C); however, in the adult this ratio changes so that the retropharyngeal space measured at C5 level is about one-third the width of the retrolaryngeal space measured at C6 level. Immediately below the middle compartment of the larynx, the retrolaryngeal space is considerably wider than the retrotracheal space, and this measurement is related to the junction with the esophagus. More recent measurements as proposed by Oon are shown in Figure 10–7 *B*. Here, the posterior wall of the nasopharynx, roof of the nasopharynx, postpharyngeal space, posttracheal space, as well as diameter measurements for the trachea, are given in terms of range, mean, and standard deviation as shown.

Eller et al., on the other hand, carried out a careful statistical study of the nasopharyngeal soft tissues in males and females and plotted these against age with upper and lower tolerance limits. It was clear from this study that the amount of nasopharyngeal soft tissue in adults decreased with age and varied slightly between the sexes. However, the range of variation was so great that these investigators found this knowledge of little practical significance. It was also suggested that the involution of nasopharyngeal tissue was not complete by age 25 but continued throughout life. They recommended that other features of the nasopharynx should be regarded as more important than the measurements of the nasopharyngeal soft tissues. For example, there were two consistent features: (1) the roof thickness of the nasopharynx was always less than the thickness of the posterior wall (with one exception in which they were equal); and (2) there was a smooth concave contour of the soft tissue outline of the nasopharynx. Changes in these relationships should be regarded as significant.

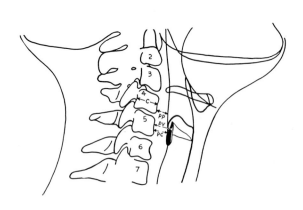

UPPER NORMAL LIMITS OF SOFT TISSUE SPACES OF NECK			
AGE	POSTPHARYNGEAL SOFT TISSUE	POSTLARYNGEAL SOFT TISSUE	
0-1	1.5c	2.c	POSTVENTRICULAR
1-2	.5c	1.5c	
2-3	.5c	1.2c	
3-6	.4c	1.2c	
6-14	.3c	1.2c	
ADULT	MALE .3c / FEMALE .3c	MALE .7c / FEMALE .6c	POSTCRICOID

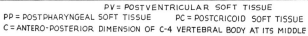

PV = POSTVENTRICULAR SOFT TISSUE
PP = POSTPHARYNGEAL SOFT TISSUE   PC = POSTCRICOID SOFT TISSUE
C = ANTERO-POSTERIOR DIMENSION OF C-4 VERTEBRAL BODY AT ITS MIDDLE

A

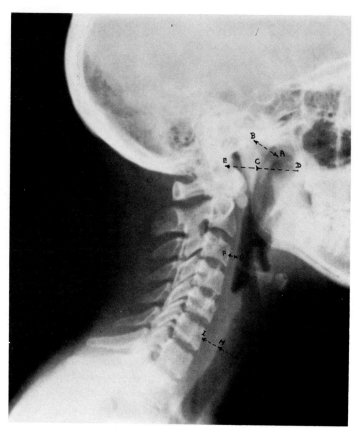

B

MEASUREMENTS SHOWN IN FIGURE 10–7B

		Range (in mm.)	Mean (in mm.)	Standard Deviation (in mm.)
A-B	Posterior wall of nasopharynx	12–24	18.4	2.5
C-D	Roof of nasopharynx	2–10.5	5.9	2.2
F-G	Postpharyngeal space	1.5–4.5	3.1	0.7
H-I	Post-tracheal space	8–17	12.4	1.9
J-H	Anteroposterior diameter of trachea (male)	15–23.5	19.2	1.8
	Anteroposterior diameter of trachea (female)	11.5–18	14.5	1.3

Figure 10–7. A. Relative width of the posterior oropharynx to the soft tissues of the neck posterior to the larynx. (After Hay.) B. Posterior wall of nasopharynx (A–B): (A) Posterior edge of the bony plate forming the nasopharynx. (B) Anterior lip of foramen magnum (basion). Soft tissue measurement is basion to posterior limit of nasopharyngeal air space.
Roof of nasopharynx (method of Ho).
    Measure along line of posterior border of lateral pterygoid plates from the skull base to the uppermost limit of the nasopharynx (E–C).
Postpharyngeal space. Midpoint of anterior border of C3 to posterior pharyngeal wall (F–G).
Post-tracheal space. From a point immediately below the inferior horns of the thyroid cartilage to the anterior border of the body of the adjacent cervical vertebra (usually C6) (I–H).
Trachea. Anteroposterior diameter in the same transverse plane as the post-tracheal space (H–J).
(Print without line overlay courtesy of Thomas Thompson, M.D., modified from Oon, C. L.: Brit. J. Radiol., *37:* 674–677, 1964.)

Radiographic Methods of Study

The air passages are moderately well demonstrated by the fluoroscope and radiograph.

In addition to identifying the anatomic structures already described, the *fluoroscopic adjunct permits visualization of the movement of the vocal cords* in the anteroposterior projection, with phonation.

1. **Soft Tissue Lateral Film of the Neck (with and without Barium)** (Fig. 10–6). Visualization of the larynx is enhanced if the hypopharynx is distended with air by an effort at expiration with the mouth and nostrils closed. It is also helpful to extend the tongue. The technique is very similar to that employed for demonstration of the cervical spine, except that a "soft exposure" technique is employed. Barium may or may not be employed in the pharynx as desired.

The structures best visualized on the lateral film of the neck are: (1) the epiglottis, (2) the aryepiglottic folds, (3) the superior laryngeal compartment, (4) the ventricular and vocal folds, with the laryngeal ventricle between, (5) the thyroid, cricoid, and arytenoid cartilages, (6) the retropharyngeal and laryngeal soft tissue spaces, and (7) the trachea, thyroid, and surrounding soft tissue structures.

At the posterior margin of the laryngeal ventricle is a spherical soft tissue mass produced by the arytenoids.

The pyriform sinuses and vallecula are best studied with the aid of barium in the pharynx.

Xeroradiography has proved to be particularly helpful in the study of the soft tissues of the neck. The vocal cords, cartilage, soft tissues, bone, and tumors, if present, have a slightly different appearance of density in this method of representation (Fig. 10–8).

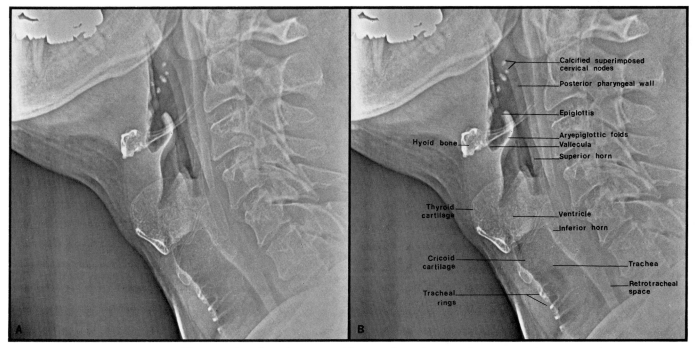

Figure 10–8. Normal larynx and trachea of a 55-year-old man is shown by (A) with structures of same xeroradiogram identified by (B). (From Xeroradiography, published by Xerox Corporation, Pasadena, California 91107. Courtesy of Dr. P. Holinger.)

2. **Soft Palate Movement Studies with Phonation** (Fig. 10–9). Soft palate movements with phonation can be studied in considerable detail to assist in analysis of speech defects. In its simplest form, these studies consist of four views, all in the lateral projection centering over the soft palate: (1) the resting state with normal breathing and no phonation; (2) the patient making the sound "ssss"; (3) the patient speaking the long vowel "eeeeee"; and (4) the patient speaking the long vowel "aaaaaa." These views can, of course, be supplemented by cineradiographic studies and special film examinations of the swallowing function, although this extra radiation exposure is a disadvantage.

3. **Anteroposterior Body Section Radiograph of the Larynx** (Fig. 10–10). If a section through the middle of the larynx in the coronal plane is obtained, the vestibule and the "zeppelin-shaped" laryngeal ventricle are clearly demonstrated, along with the true and false vocal cords. Ordinarily, such radiographs are obtained with the larynx at rest (Fig. 10–10 *A, B*); and during phonation (Fig. 10–10 *C, D*).

The laryngogram (Fig. 10–10 *F* and *G*) contributes significantly to the management of malignant laryngeal tumors by permitting an accurate classification of the lesion (Fig. 10–10 *E* [Lehman and Fletcher]).

4. **Laryngograms.** Laryngograms may also be obtained using opaque media with and without phonation. In this procedure, a topical anesthetic such as 0.5 per cent Dyclone is sprayed onto and into the pharynx and larynx, and 10 to 20 ml. of Dionosil oily is dropped slowly over the tongue during quiet inspiration. Frontal and lateral spot film radiographs are made while the patient performs nasal inspiration and phonation, strains down against a closed glottis, and breathes in against a closed glottis (Fig. 10–11). Powdered tantalum has also been utilized as a medium for human laryngography (Zamel et al.).

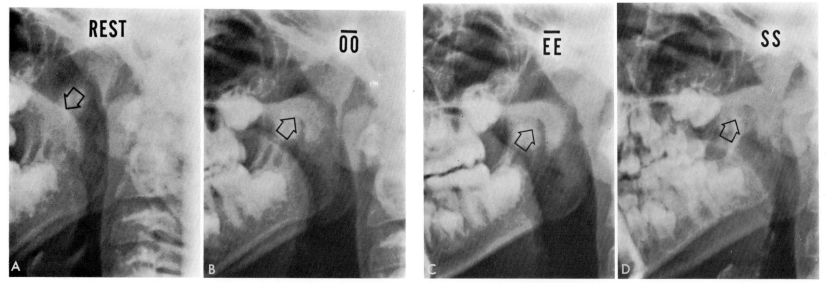

Figure 10–9. Phonation studies showing good mobility of the soft palate. *A.* Resting state. *B.* $\overline{\text{Oo}}$. *C.* $\overline{\text{Ee}}$. *D.* Ss. Note the complete approximation of the soft palate with the posterior nasopharyngeal wall in *D*.

These studies may be supplemented by cineradiographic examination and by an associated study of the swallowing function.

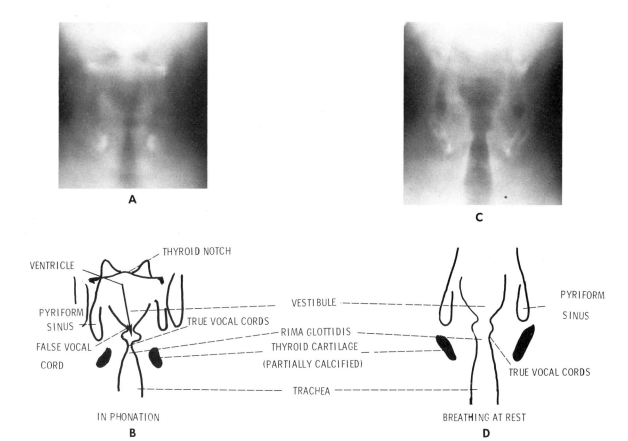

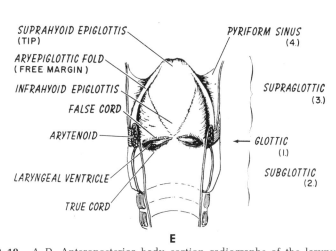

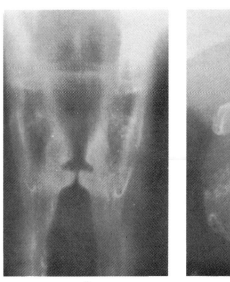 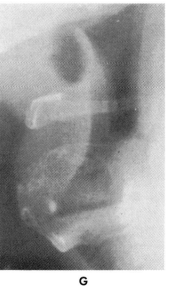

Figure 10–10. *A–D.* Anteroposterior body section radiographs of the larynx. *A.* During rest. *B.* Labeled tracing of *A. C.* During phonation. *D.* Labeled tracing of *C.*

E. Classification of laryngeal carcinoma. (1) *Glottic:* Tumors arising on any surface of the true vocal cord; (2) *True Subglottic:* Excluding subglottic extension from tumors of vocal cord origin; (3) *Supraglottic:* Tumors arising above the ventricles — on the epiglottis, false cords, or aryepiglottic folds: (4) *Laryngopharyngeal:* Tumors arising from the walls of the pyriform sinuses, adjacent pharyngeal wall, or posterior surface of the arytenoid and cricoid cartilages. *F* and *G.* Larynx tumor survey. *F. Tomogram:* The laryngopharyngeal walls, formed by the thin aryepiglottic fold above and the thicker false cord below, separate the vestibule from the pyriform sinuses. The vocal cords, approximating in the midline, delineate the ventricles above from the subglottic space below. The air-filled valleculae and midline glosso-epiglottic fold can be seen above the hyoid bone.

G. Lateral Soft-Tissue View: The hyoid bone divides the epiglottis into supra- and infrahyoid portions. The vertical position of the epiglottis during phonation may cause bulging of its lower portion, which should not be mistaken for a tumor. Air contrast outlines the valleculae, the free margin of the aryepiglottic folds, the laryngeal ventricle, and the subglottic space. Thyroid cartilage calcification and pre-epiglottic soft tissues are readily studied. (*E, F* and *G* from Lehmann, Q. H., and Fletcher, G. H.: Radiology, *83*:486–500, 1964.)

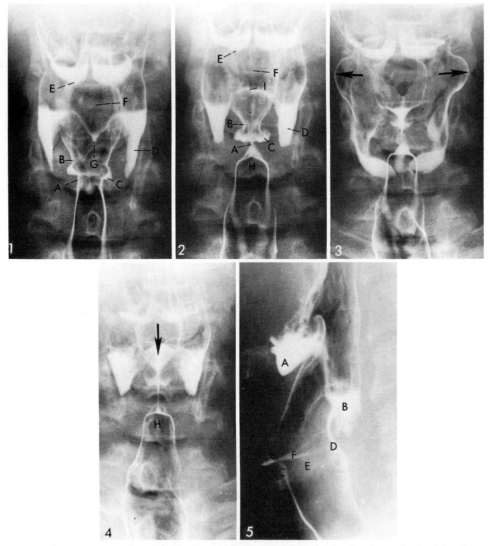

Figure 10–11. Laryngograms of a normal larynx employing Dionosil oily after local anesthesia of the pharynx and larynx: 1, Inspiration. 2, Phonation. 3, Modified Valsalva maneuver (forceful blowing against the cheek with lips closed as for blowing a horn). 4, True Valsalva maneuver (straining down against the closed glottis). 5, Lateral view in inspiration.

In parts 1, 2, 3, and 4: (A) true cords; (B) false cords; (C) collapsed ventricles; (D) pyriform sinuses; (E) valleculae; (F) laryngeal vestibules; (G) arytenoid groove; (H) subglottic angle; (I) postcricoid line. In 3, arrows point to lateral pharyngeal walls that balloon outward. In 4, arrow points to contrast material pooling above the contracted vestibule and pyriform sinuses.

In part 5, lateral view: (A) valleculae; (B) pyriform sinuses; (C) anterior commissure; (D) posterior commissure; (E) vocal cords; (F) collapsed ventricle; (G) hyoid bone; (H) epiglottis; (I) aryepiglottic folds. (From Fletcher, G. H., and Jing, B-S.: The Head and Neck. Chicago, Year Book Medical Publishers, 1968. Courtesy of Dr. Bao-Shen Jing, Department of Diagnostic Radiology, University of Texas; M. D. Anderson Hospital and Tumor Institute, Houston, Texas.)

THE TRACHEA AND BRONCHI

The Trachea. The trachea consists of a framework of cartilaginous C-shaped rings that are connected posteriorly by a dense layer of connective tissue and muscle. The cartilages present marked irregularities, and they may be partially fused with adjoining cartilage rings. The carinal cartilage is formed by the fusion of tracheal and left bronchial cartilages, and the carina tracheae is a prominent ridge running anteroposteriorly across the bottom of the trachea between the origin of the bronchi. There is very little distinction between the epithelium lining the trachea and that lining the bronchi, and four types of epithelial cells are identified: (1) basal cells, (2) intermediate cells, (3) ciliated cells, and (4) goblet cells. The latter two types predominate.

The trachea begins at the level of the cricoid cartilage (sixth or seventh cervical vertebra). It extends downward through the neck, into the superior mediastinum, and ends at the upper border of the fifth to the eighth thoracic vertebra by bifurcating into the right and left bronchi. Bifurcation is lower in the adult than in the child (Fig. 10–12), in which it usually occurs at the level of the fourth costal cartilage. The trachea moves upward upon swallowing, and downward in deep inspiration.

The trachea adheres to the midline, except toward its termination where it deviates slightly to the right. As it passes downward, it recedes from the surface, following the curvature of the vertebral column from which it is separated by the esophagus.

In the infant, the trachea may normally deviate to the right (Fig. 10–13), and tracheal shift in the infant must be interpreted with great caution. This is related to a relative redundancy of the trachea at this stage, and also to some irregularity in the position of the thymus. Lateral deviation of the trachea at the thoracic inlet occurs normally in infants and children up to 5 years of age. Since the deviation to the right is opposite the aortic arch, it is thought that the aortic arch, too, may be a major cause of this occurrence (Chang et al.). The trachea in the infant is roughly one-third the length of the adult's, growing from approximately 4 cm. in the infant to 12 cm. in the adult.

The isthmus of the thyroid gland is closely connected ventrally with the trachea, usually covering the second, third, and fourth cartilages of the trachea. More caudally, the trachea is close to the peritracheal lymph nodule and, especially in children, to the thymus gland. The innominate artery occasionally crosses the trachea obliquely in the root of the neck.

On the dorsal aspect of the trachea is the esophagus. The great vessels of the neck lie on each side of the trachea, and the inferior laryngeal nerve lies between the esophagus and the trachea.

Within the thorax, the trachea is located in the mediastinum and fixed with strong fibrous connections to the central tendon of the diaphragm. The innominate and left common carotid arteries are in close proximity to the trachea, at first ventral and then lateral to it. The left innominate vein and the thymus are situated

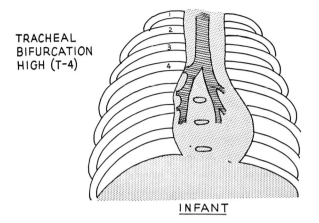

TRACHEAL
BIFURCATION
HIGH (T-4)

INFANT

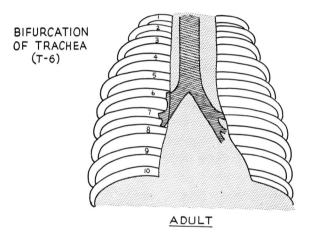

BIFURCATION
OF TRACHEA
(T-6)

ADULT

Figure 10–12. Comparison of level of bifurcation of trachea in adult and child. (After Pediatric X-ray Diagnosis, 6th ed., by Caffey, J. Copyright © 1972 by Year Book Medical Publishers, Inc., Chicago. Used by permission.)

farther away ventrally. The aortic arch is in contact with the ventral surface of the trachea near the bifurcation. On the right is the vagus nerve, the arch of the azygos vein, the superior vena cava, and the mediastinal pleura. On the left, the arch of the aorta continues, followed by the origin of the left subclavian artery and the inferior laryngeal nerve. Bronchial and peribronchial lymph nodes lie caudal to the angle of the bifurcation. As it descends, the esophagus extends toward the left and dorsal aspect of the trachea.

Calcification of the tracheal rings may occur normally in the adult.

The Bronchi. The angle which the two bronchi form with the trachea varies according to the age of the individual (Kobler and Hovorka, quoted in Miller) as follows:

Age	Right Bronchus	Left Bronchus
Newborn	10–35 degrees	30–65 degrees
Adult male	20 degrees	40 degrees
Adult female	19 degrees	51 degrees

Thus, the angle of divergence of the two bronchi from each other ranges around 60 degrees in the adult male and 70 degrees in the adult female in autopsy investigations.

Measurements made from living patients on teleoentgenograms of the chest (using a 40 inch distance for patients under 1 year of age), showed that the angle decreased uniformly up to 16 years of age and leveled off after that age. There was considerable difference in the measurements obtained from the supine and upright posteroanterior or anteroposterior positions. The 95 per cent confidence band for people under 16 years of age is shown in Figure 10–14.

In a summary of patients over 16 years of age, the mean value of the angle between the two bronchi for males was 56.40 degrees ± 5.664 degrees. The range for 95 per cent of all values was 45.298 degrees to 67.502 degrees. The mean value of this angle for females was 57.73 degrees ± 6.375 degrees; with the 95 per cent confidence limits ranging between 45.24 degrees and 70.23 degrees. Males and females, when calculated together, had a mean value of the angle of 57.16 degrees ± 6.06 degrees. The 90 per cent confidence limits for both males and females ranged between 45.28 degrees and 69.04 degrees (Alavi, Keats, O'Brien).

From each main bronchus, lateral branches are given off. The dorsal branches are usually more slender than the ventral branches.

The right main bronchus is more nearly continuous with the trachea than the left but is shorter and soon divides into two main branches—one above, and the other below the right pulmonary artery (Fig. 10–15): (1) the upper lobe bronchus (eparterial), and (2) the continuation of the main stem (hyparterial).

The right upper lobe bronchus (Fig. 10–16) has three main branches: (1) the *apical*, which in turn divides into an anterior and a posterior component; (2) the *posterior*, which supplies a pyramidal region along the axillary and posterior surface of the upper lobe; and (3) an *anterior*, which supplies the anterior segment of the upper lobe.

The right lower main stem ("intermediate bronchus") thereafter subdivides into the *middle lobe bronchus* and the *lower lobe bronchus.*

The right middle lobe bronchus has two main branches: (1) a *medial* branch that supplies the sternocardiac region of the middle lobe, and (2) a *lateral* branch that supplies the outer portion.

The *right lower lobe bronchus* has five main branches ordinarily: (1) the *superior basal branch*, which supplies the upper posterior and outer part of the apex of the lower lobe (this is sometimes an accessory lobe); (2) the *medial basal branch*, which arises directly from the inner side of the main stem and supplies the inner side of the right lower lobe. This branch arises just below the superior basal branch and above the level of the three other basal branches; (3) the *anterior basal branch*, which subdivides and supplies the anterior basal portion of the lower lobe; (4) the *posterior basal branch*, which supplies the posterior basal part of the right lower lobe; and (5) the *lateral basal branch*,

which supplies the axillary portion of the basal part of the right lower lobe. After the superior and medial basal branches have been identified the other three can be readily identified in every projection, using as a guide to orientation the first letters of the words anterior, lateral, and posterior, which spell the word "ALP."

The absence of the middle lobe modifies the pattern of the bronchi in the left side. The left main bronchus is larger than the right but leaves the trachea at a more acute angle. Opposite the inner end of the third anterior interspace, it divides into an *upper lobe branch* and a *lower lobe branch,* which continues the line of the main stem. Above the curve of the bronchus, a shadow can be seen with a free crescentic upper margin—this is the left pulmonary artery.

The *upper lobe bronchus* divides into upper and lower divisions, which almost immediately subdivide. The *upper division* has two main branches: (1) the *apical-posterior branch*, which supplies the apical and posterior portions of the left upper lobe; and (2) an *anterior branch*, which supplies the anterior portion of

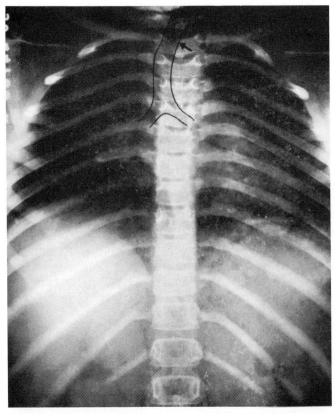

Figure 10–13. Radiograph (posteroanterior) of chest of infant to demonstrate slight normal deviation of trachea to the right, which occasionally occurs. This may result from a slight rotation of the infant's head, which may be very difficult to control, redundancy of the trachea, or slight thymic enlargement.

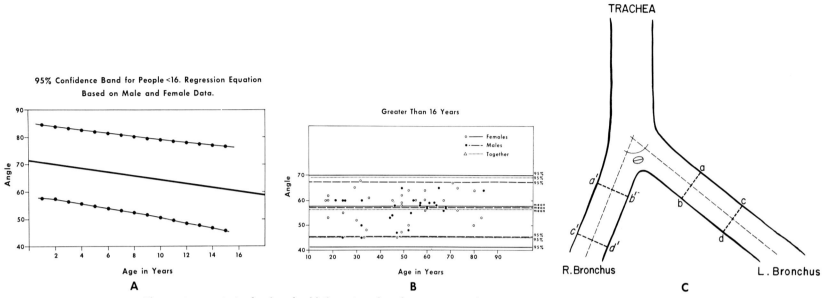

Figure 10–14.   *A.* Angle of tracheal bifurcation plotted against age with 95 per cent confidence band for people 16 years old or younger. *B.* Angle of tracheal bifurcation plotted against age demonstrates a plateau plus the 95 per cent confidence band. *C.* Diagram demonstrating the method for obtaining the most consistent angle of bifurcation. (From Alavi, S. M., Keats, T. E., and O'Brien, W. M.: Amer. J. Roentgenol., *108*:546–549, 1970.)

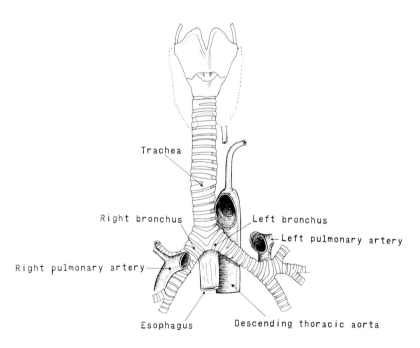

Figure 10–15.   Relationships of tracheobronchial tree to the main ramifications of the pulmonary artery.

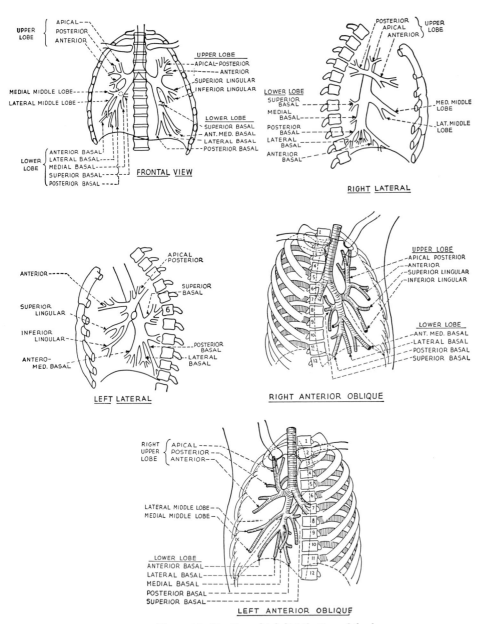

Figure 10–16.   Bronchial distribution of the lung.

the apical area. The *lower division* divides into two branches, similar to those of the right middle lobe but slightly different in direction: (1) a *superior branch* and (2) an *inferior branch,* which supply the corresponding parts of the lingula portion of the left upper lobe.

The *left lower lobe bronchus* is almost identical to its counterpart on the right side except that the medial basal branch arises from the anterior basal branch rather than as a direct off-shoot from the left lower lobe bronchus. Otherwise, the superior, an-

terior basal, posterior basal, and lateral basal branches are the same.

Bronchial Segments (Fig. 10–17).   The regions supplied by individual bronchi represent definite and separate bronchopulmonary segments of the lung that are combined according to a rather definite scheme into lobes. These are important to identify and are fully illustrated in Figure 10–17. Orientation of the lobes and fissures of the lung can be seen in Figure 10–18.

BRONCHOGRAPHY

Methods and Materials.   There are various methods and contrast media useful in visualizing the bronchi. Most methods require that the pharynx and larynx be anesthetized locally. Once that is accomplished, the simplest technique is to allow the contrast media to flow down over the back of the tongue with the tongue drawn forward and the patient leaning forward. The patient is then rotated in various positions to distribute the contrast media in the various bronchial branches. It is usually difficult to obtain a satisfactory visualization of the upper lobe in this manner, but ordinarily the lower lobe bronchi are well delineated. It is our preference to visualize the entire bronchial tree if possible—hence the catheter technique illustrated in Figure 10–19 is recommended.

Another method involves puncturing the trachea with a suitable needle and injecting the contrast media directly. Occasionally this allows considerable leakage of air into the surrounding subcutaneous tissues, causing respiratory embarrassment to the patient; this is the main disadvantage of this method.

The most suitable technique we have found for visualization of the entire bronchial tree requires the introduction of a catheter into the trachea after completely anesthetizing the throat, larynx, and upper trachea (Fig. 10–19). Small quantities of contrast media are then introduced into each major lung sector by positioning the patient as shown during the introduction of the media (Churchill's maneuvers) (see Fig. 10–19).

A variant of this technique that usually gives satisfactory results requires the injection of 20 cc. of the media while the patient is in position *B* (Fig. 10–19), instructing the patient to inspire deeply immediately thereafter; then another 20 cc. is injected in position *G*, and the patient is similarly instructed to inspire deeply once again. Thereafter posteroanterior stereoscopic erect films, both oblique projections, and a recumbent anteroposterior film are obtained in rapid sequence.

Lateral Decubitus Bronchography.   Lateral decubitus bronchography with a single bolus is illustrated in Figure 10–20 and is described as follows: The catheter is placed in either the right or the left main stem bronchus with a small amount of topical anesthetic in the usual fashion. A scout film is obtained to assure proper radiographic exposure. The patient is placed in the lateral decubitus position (Fig. 10–20) with the side to be examined dependent. He is instructed to exhale, and an additional small amount of local anesthetic is injected; he is then instructed to inhale. There should no longer be any coughing. The syringe containing the contrast medium is connected to the catheter, and once again the patient is instructed to exhale forcefully. The contrast medium is then injected rapidly under fluoroscopic control until the entire bronchial tree is outlined as a solid cast. Seven to 15 ml. should be adequate. A spot film is obtained. The patient is then instructed to breathe normally. This results in further peripheral aspiration of the contrast medium and a double contrast visualization of the bronchi. Additional spot films are obtained as required in the lateral and oblique positions. The overhead films are taken in the following sequence: lateral decubitus, posterior oblique, and anteroposterior. Generally, the films are uniformly excellent, since the opaque medium runs into various major divisions of the bronchi, which are all dependent. The patient's breathing forces the contrast bolus farther into the periphery and results in a double contrast visualization of the entire bronchial tree (Amplatz and Haut).

The ideal contrast agent has not as yet been developed for this purpose. Ideally, the agent should be nonirritating and nonsensitizing; it should be readily absorbed or expectorated so that it does not remain in the lungs for any significant period of time after the examination; if absorbed, it should not be toxic; and if any of it remains even in microscopic quantities in the lung, it should not produce any irritant or granulomatous reactions within the lung. For many years the nonabsorbable iodized oils such as Lipiodol or Iodochlorol were used, even though they clouded the lung fields for years afterward, and occasionally produced granulomas or iodine sensitivity. In more recent times, Dionosil, either aqueous or in oil suspension, has been favored by us, although this, too, is not ideal. The aqueous Dionosil is very irritating and requires a general anesthetic, which in turn makes film-making more difficult, and the procedure more time-consuming, expensive, and hazardous. Dionosil in oil suspension leaves the lungs in about 4 days, but mild pneumonitis, granulomas, and other manifestations of irritation can result.

Delayed irritative effects of contrast medium persisting in the lungs following bronchography have been well documented. Oil retention for more than 90 days in humans was regularly followed by granuloma formation in the lungs (Fischer). Granuloma formation was noted by other researchers in rats and humans and attributed to the presence of carboxy-methylcellulose following the introduction of water soluble contrast media (Werthemann and Vischer). Dionosil oily in rabbits produced foreign body granulomas in the lungs after bronchography, and this was attributed to the arachis oil in this medium (Dionosil oily is a suspension of propyliodone in arachis oil) (Bjork and Lodin). In a long-term study, Holden and Cowdell recorded the results of bronchography after 5 years of continuous use of Dionosil oily; they found: (1) no clinical evidence of long-term ill

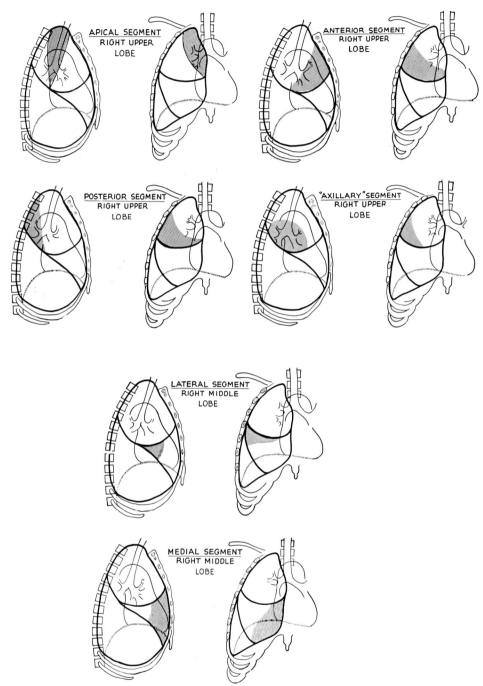

Figure 10–17. Bronchial segments of the lung.

Figure 10–17 continued on the following page.

effects; (2) immediate clinical reactions were most unusual; (3) in the survey of all resected lung tissue, no unusual reactions directly attributable to the examination were noted; (4) in only five cases was there much acute inflammatory change, in the form of either ulcerative bronchitis or small areas of bronchopneumonia.

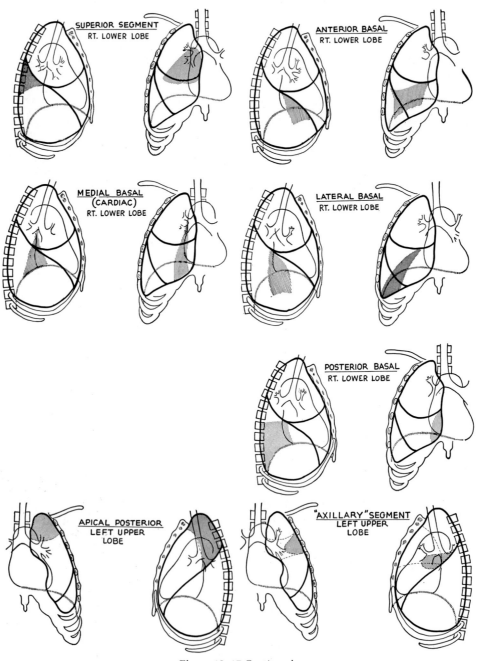

Figure 10–17 Continued.

Figure 10–17 continued on the opposite page.

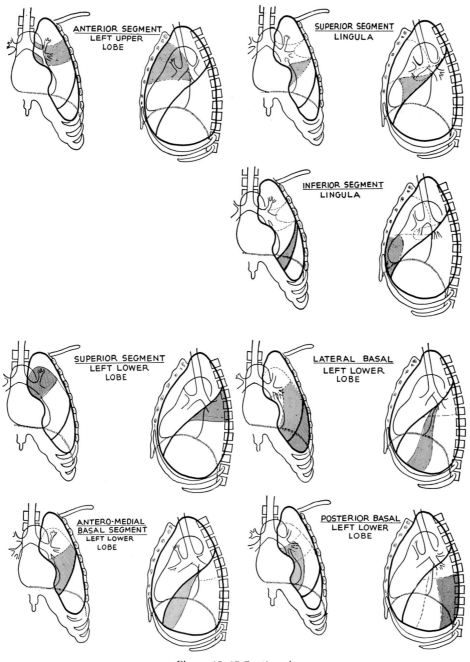

Figure 10–17 *Continued.*

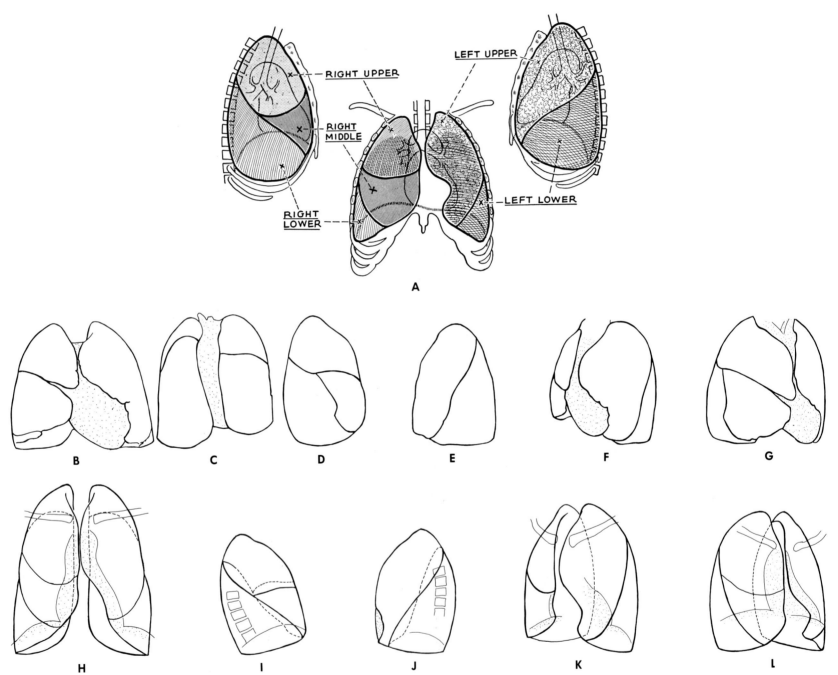

Figure 10–18. *A.* Lobes and fissures of the lung. *B* to *L.* Line diagrams illustrating the pleural demarcation zones anteriorly and posteriorly. (Also see the fissures and lobes of the lungs.) *B* through *G*: Frontal, posterior, lateral and oblique views of lungs. *H* through *L*: Similar "transparent views" with "out of view" zones projected over one another.

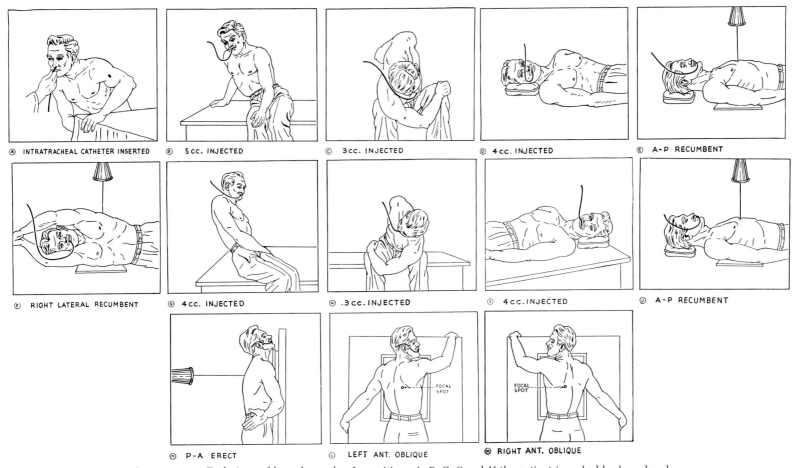

Ⓐ INTRATRACHEAL CATHETER INSERTED   Ⓑ 5 cc. INJECTED   Ⓒ 3 cc. INJECTED   Ⓓ 4 cc. INJECTED   Ⓔ A-P RECUMBENT

Ⓕ RIGHT LATERAL RECUMBENT   Ⓖ 4 cc. INJECTED   Ⓗ .3 cc. INJECTED   Ⓘ 4 cc. INJECTED   Ⓙ A-P RECUMBENT

Ⓚ P-A ERECT   Ⓛ LEFT ANT. OBLIQUE   Ⓜ RIGHT ANT. OBLIQUE

Figure 10–19. Technique of bronchography. In positions *A, B, C, G* and *H* the patient is rocked backward and forward, still maintaining the general position as indicated in the diagram. In positions *D* and *I*, the patient is rolled slightly from side to side, likewise still maintaining the general position as indicated in the diagram. This rocking or rolling motion is efficacious in obtaining a better distribution of the iodized oil medium in the bronchi.

In these five cases no evidence of granulomatous reaction to foreign material was noted more than 1 month after study. It was the belief of these investigators that these acute inflammatory changes could not be attributed to the contrast medium; (5) in no case was fatty material demonstrated in a granuloma.

The rate of elimination of the contrast material varied. In most cases, the lungs were radiologically clear within 2 days, although occasionally some remained for longer periods in cases of bronchial abnormalities. This study, however, consisted of human material already in part diseased so that interpretations were at times difficult.

Some experiments with 50 per cent colloidal barium in saline plus a 2 per cent methylcarboxycellulose mixture would appear to offer some promise but experience with this latter medium is still too limited.

Our own preference at this time is Dionosil in oil suspension, although admittedly this is not ideal in either contrast or benignity of reaction.

The following film studies are obtained after the injection of the contrast media:

1. Anteroposterior recumbent and lateral views of the side first injected, immediately after injection and before the second side is injected (Fig. 10–21 *A*, and *B* or *E*).

2. An anteroposterior view of the chest after both sides are injected.

3. An erect posteroanterior view of the chest after both sides are injected (Fig. 10–21 *D*).

4. Both oblique views after both sides are injected (stereoscopic views may be obtained if desired) (Fig. 10–21 *C* and *F*).

The above study may be combined with fluoroscopy, if a good

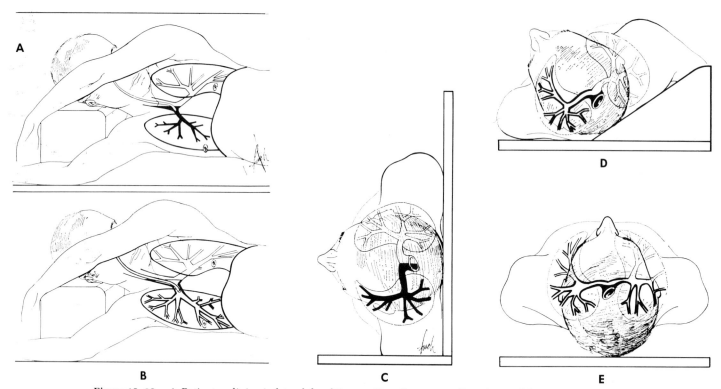

Figure 10–20. *A.* Patient reclining in lateral decubitus position. Contrast medium injected during forceful expiration allows filling of all proximal radicles with a single bolus injection. Orifices of all major bronchi are occluded by contrast medium, but distal radicles are not filled.

B. Following inhalation, the air pushes the contrast medium into peripheral radicles, resulting in double contrast visualization.

Spot-films and first overhead films made in lateral decubitus position (*C*) to be followed by posterior oblique (*D*). Last film made in supine position may result in spillage of contrast medium into contralateral lung, which is not objectionable in this view (*E*). (From Amplatz, K., and Haut, G.: Radiology, 95:439–440, 1970.)

spot-film apparatus is available that will give detail as good as the conventional studies. One advantage of the fluoroscopic examination is that it permits visualization of the filling as it occurs, so that the examiner knows immediately whether or not further filling is required. Moreover, a concept of the physiologic function of the bronchial tree is also thereby acquired. Balanced against this great advantage, however, is the fact that spot films are seldom as satisfactory in minute detail as are conventional long distance and small focal spot-film studies. The examiner must therefore adapt the technique to his requirements.

Ordinarily, both sides of the lung are injected at the same examination if the patient's respiratory capacity will permit it. In many patients, injection of only one side at a single sitting is possible.

The radiographic anatomy of the bronchi and their distribution have been illustrated in previous diagrams (see Fig. 10–16).

Bronchial Brush Biopsy and Selective Bronchography. A bronchial abrasion technique for cytologic study of peripheral

bronchial lesions was described some years ago (MacLean, 1958a). In more recent times controllable brushes, telescoping catheters, and fibroscopes have provided a means not only for obtaining microbiopsies or cytologic study of peripheral lesions, but also for segmental bronchography of these regions (Fennessy, 1967; Sovak; Bean et al., 1968; Willson and Eskridge). The most recent technique, advocated by Willson and Eskridge, is carried out as follows: The patient is given a topical anesthetic as for bronchography. The outside larger catheter of a telescoping catheter (a 45 cm. No. 16 French radiopaque polyvinyl tube) is positioned with the tip in the trachea just above the carina. Through it is inserted a specially molded telescoping bronchial catheter of radiopaque polyethylene with a precurved tip to fit the desired lobar bronchus. A controllable guidewire is used to guide this catheter into the correct position under fluoroscopic control (Fig. 10–22). Once the inner catheter is in position a special brush is passed through it to the desired location under fluoroscopic control and moved in a clockwise direction so that a scraping of the bronchial mucosa or a specimen of the lesion in question is obtained. This brush is then withdrawn back into the telescoping catheter and removed. Various specimens may be obtained by this method, including: (1) a smear of the tissue on a slide, (2) a microbiopsy specimen, or (3) cultures.

Following the procurement of satisfactory specimens, selective bronchography is carried out by injection through the catheter into the desired areas of lung, and spot films are taken of the areas in question.

Fiberoptic Bronchoscopy (Schoenbaum et al.; Kahn). A flexible bronchofiberscope was introduced by Ikeda in 1968. This instrument was inserted originally through a bronchoscope or an endotracheal tube under general anesthesia, but since that time commercial flexible fiberoptic bronchoscopes have become available.*

---

*Olympus Bronchofiberscope, Type 5 B; Olympus Bronchofiberscope, Type 5 B2, Olympus Corporation of America, 2 Nevada Drive, New Hyde Park, New York, 11040; Fiber-Bronchoscope FBS-6T with associated instruments, American Optical Machida Company, Southbridge, Mass.

These instruments vary somewhat but generally consist of a flexible tube which contains numerous bundles of thread-size glass fibers as image and light guides (Fig. 10–22 *B*). The hard tip at the end of this scope has an outer diameter of 5.2 mm. and its bending section is flexible through an angle of 160 degrees. The angle is controlled by a lever in the handle or control unit. The outer diameter of the bending section is 5.4 mm., and the flexible tube has an outer diameter of 5.7 mm. and a working length of 600 mm. A biopsy forceps or a cytology brush can be inserted through the hollow suction channel from the control unit on the handle. Photographs may be taken with the attachable Olympus camera. Various other attachments are available for teaching and evaluation by groups of two or more physicians.

Patients are given premedication with a suitable sedative, atropine, and topical anesthesia. A No. 36 French nasopharyngeal airway is passed through the nose into the oropharynx and, in most instances, the fiberoptic bronchoscope is then passed through the airway into the trachea under direct visualization.

Biopsies may be made of centrally located lesions, which may be brushed under direct visualization through the scope.

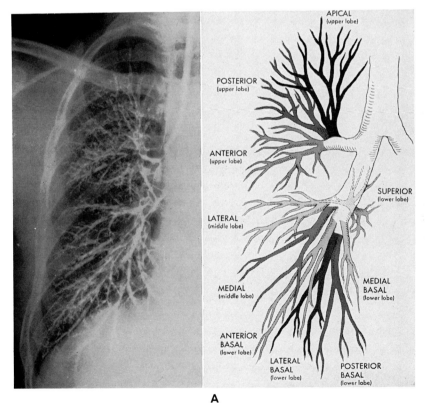
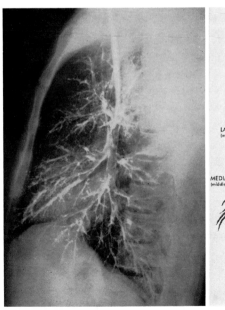
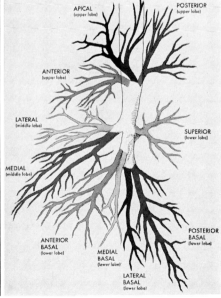

A **B**

Figure 10–21. The normal human bronchial tree. *A.* Right posteroanterior projection. *B.* Right lateral projection. (From Lehman, J. S., and Crellin, J. A.: Medical Radiology and Photography, *31*, 1955.)

Figure 10–21 continued on the following page.

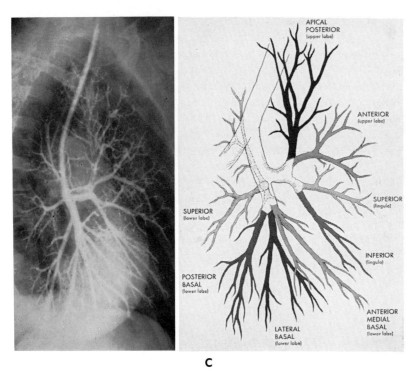

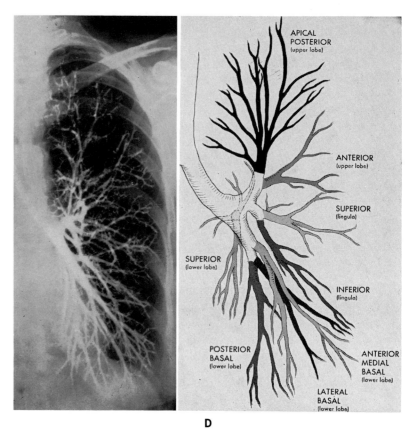

C   D

Figure 10–21 *Continued.*   *C.* Right anterior oblique projection. *D.* Left posteroanterior projection.

Figure 10–21 continued on the opposite page.

The specimen obtained is smeared on a slide coated with egg albumin and immersed immediately in 70 per cent alcohol, and is then sent for cytologic examination together with washings from the appropriate area. Biopsy specimens may be immersed in formalin and sent for histologic examination.

The fiberoptic bronchoscope may be guided to a lesion under suspicion by image-amplified fluoroscopy; bronchial brush biopsy, smears, and cultures may thereby be obtained. If a bronchogram is indicated, the fiberoptic bronchoscope is exchanged under fluoroscopic control over an appropriate angiographic guidewire for a polyethylene tube, the bronchogram then being obtained through the polyethylene catheter.

Generally, patients with heart failure, chronic obstructive pulmonary disease, asthma, pneumonia or other pulmonary problems may be studied only after careful arterial blood gas samples have been analyzed. Even the premedication should not be given to patients with borderline pulmonary functions, hypoxemia requiring oxygen, or respiratory failure.

The control handle of the instrument cannot be immersed in any liquid sterilization substance since damage may result, but the flexible section of the scope may be sterilized by soaking it in Betadine and then rinsing in isopropyl alcohol 70 per cent followed by sterile water. Cold gas sterilization may also be used, but unfortunately this procedure takes 17 to 24 hours and is not practical when more than one patient must be examined in a day.

Many investigators have used modifications of the above procedure (Smiddy et al.).

Faber et al. reported the use of the flexible fiberoptic bronchoscope in 205 cases of suspected malignancy. A positive diagnosis was obtained by brush biopsy in 76 per cent of 170 patients with proven pulmonary carcinoma. This represented an increase of 28 per cent as compared with their fixed catheter technique of obtaining such specimens.

Tracheobronchial secretion management, selective bronchography, bacteriology, and many other applications have been described for this technique. With approximately 1200 cases reported in the literature to date, there have been no reported complications (Kahn).

Schoenbaum et al. have reported the use of this technique

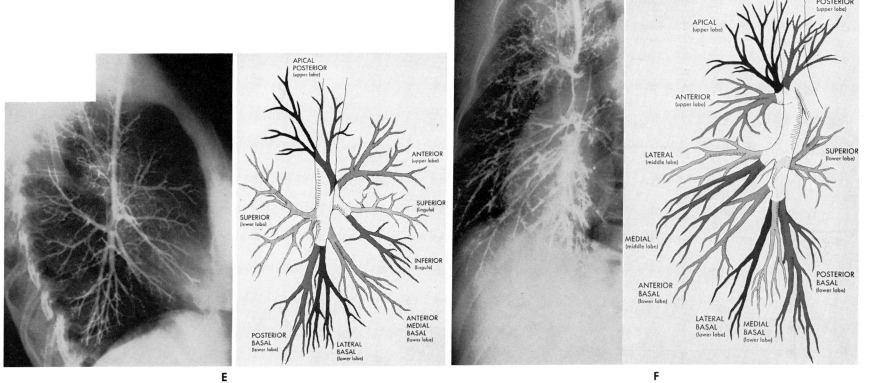

Figure 10–21 *Continued.* *E.* Left lateral projection. *F.* Left anterior oblique projection. (*C* to *F* from Lehman, J. S., and Crellin, J. A.: Medical Radiography and Photography, *31*, 1955.)

in patients with primary bronchial carcinoma and many other diseases such as bronchiectasis, tuberculosis, pneumonia, and other infections.

Selective Wedge Bronchography (Sargent and Sherwin).   In this technique a radiopaque thin-walled polyethylene tube with a distal tip slightly tapered to an external diameter of approximately 0.5 mm. is used to enter airways with the smallest diameters. This small catheter is inserted through the lumen of a larger one, thus facilitating entry into a distal selective small airway. The opaque medium is then instilled through the smaller inner catheter, and the material is allowed to enter the airway by gravity and respiratory motion.

When this study was performed on experimental animals a wide variety of opaque materials were evaluated, including: powders such as tantalum, Dionosil, micropaque (barium sulfate in an emulsion mixture), calcium tungstate, and Renografin. Oil base suspensions, such as Dionosil oily and Lipiodol, were also used. Aqueous suspensions, including aqueous Dionosil, Dionosil suspended in buffered and dextrose solutions, tantalum sus-

pended in human serum albumin, calcium tungstate suspended in reconstituted human serum albumin, stereopaque barium, Renografin-60, and Urografin in an adhesive mixture, were evaluated also.

The aqueous preparations, except for the very viscous Urografin adhesive mixtures, were the most satisfactory for ease of instillation. The powdered materials clogged the internal lumen of the small catheters used. Likewise, the oily media with their greater viscosity were not satisfactory. The tantalum and calcium tungstate suspensions in human serum albumin were the only two media extending into the periphery of the lobule that usefully filled alveolar ducts and alveoli. The commercial aqueous Dionosil preparations extended into the terminal bronchioles but rarely beyond. Oily Dionosil and Lipiodol failed to extend beyond the terminal bronchioles and a few kinds of respiratory bronchioles, and did not enter the alveoli at all. When higher pressures were used, however, bronchiolar and alveolar wall disruption occurred, resulting in loss of recognizable histologic anatomy. Thus, the best agent for demonstration of the smallest airways was found to

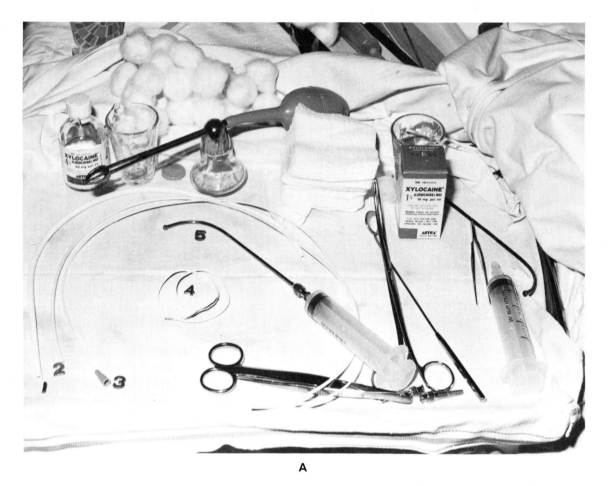

A

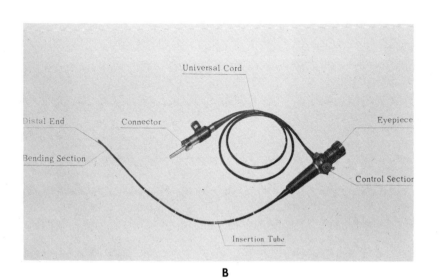

B

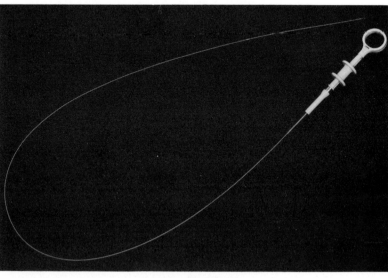

C

Figure 10–22.   A. Tray usually employed for bronchial brush biopsy when the bronchofiberscope is not available. This tray consists of three different sizes of plastic tubes and local anesthetic devices. The largest tube is passed through the nares to the larynx. A smaller tube goes through the larger one into the trachea and bronchus, and a spiral wire with a cutting helix on its end passes through the smallest tube to be used for cytologic or biopsy specimens. A very small caliber tube may also be passed for segmental or wedge bronchoscopy at this time. B. Olympic bronchofiberscope. C. Biopsy wire of bronchofiberscope which can be inserted to protrude through the distal end.

Figure 10–22 continued on the opposite page.

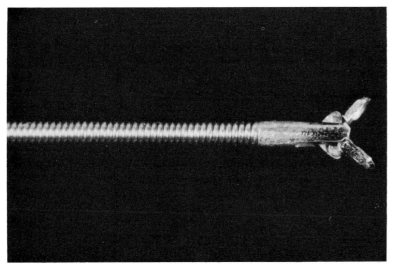

Figure 10–22 *Continued.* *D.* Close-up of claw mechanism of bronchofiberscope used for biopsy.

be tantalum suspended in human serum albumin. The technique of selective wedge bronchography is designed to limit the filling of selective portions of the lung so that only one or a few secondary lobules are filled, and superimposition of filling in adjacent areas is avoided.

From this study it was concluded that, in the normal lung, oily suspensions immediately fill airways beyond the first order respiratory bronchioles up to the alveolar region without using excessive tissue disruptive pressures. However, with the more viscous oily substances, no filling beyond the terminal bronchioles occurred unless excessive pressures were applied. The longer the media were permitted to remain in the distal airways, the greater the chance of alveolar filling.

The "alveolar image" seen on the usual bronchogram in clinical practice is actually a conglomeration of shadows with superimposition of secondary lobules which probably cannot be accurately correlated morphologically.

Unfortunately, tantalum has been demonstrated in experiments to remain in the lung as long as 12 months after bronchography (Nadel et al.). The long-term retention of tantalum in experimental bronchography is about 20 per cent of the administered tantalum dose (Upham et al.). Unfortunately also, the diatrizoates can produce pulmonary edema, and barium sulfate suspensions can obstruct airways by a mechanical inspissation (Reich).

Dionosil has the advantage of being only slightly soluble in saline and serum. It is hydrolized enzymatically in the body, and the resulting organic iodopyracet is not further metabolized or degraded but is secreted rapidly by the kidneys (Fischer and Balug). Oily Dionosil, which contains peanut oil, can cause changes resembling those produced by Lipiodol, such as late pulmonary granuloma and fibrotic alterations. Aqueous Dionosil

contains carboxymethylcellulose, which is said to be the source of granuloma formation, particularly in emphysematous lungs. Although emulsified Ethiodol has been suggested as a bronchographic medium, toxicity studies are not available at this time (L'Heureux and Baltaxe). Thus, it was concluded in this study that of all the media tried, aqueous Dionosil might fulfill the ideal requirement for human use. However, aqueous tantalum suspended in human serum albumin was superior for roentgenographic opacification of the smallest airways (Sargent and Sherwin).

THE LUNG PARENCHYMA; THE AIR SPACES

The Primary Lobule (Fig. 10–23). The bronchi continue to ramify until a point is reached when the walls no longer contain cartilage. forming the tubular bronchioli. Eventually the tubular character changes, and small projections appear on all sides of the bronchiolus known as alveolar ducts (Fig. 10–23). At the distal end of each alveolar duct, there are three to six spherical cavities called atria. These atria, in turn, communicate with a variable number of larger and more irregularly shaped cavities called air sacs. Projecting from the wall of each air sac and atrium there are a number of smaller spaces called pulmonary alveoli This entire

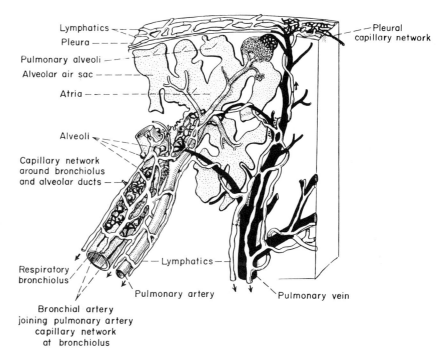

Figure 10–23. Primary lobule of the lung. (Modified from Miller, The Lung. Courtesy of Charles C Thomas, Publishers, Springfield, Illinois.)

group of structures together with the accompanying blood vessels, lymph vessels, and nerves forms a primary lobule. The primary lobules are grouped into bronchial segments, in accordance with the pattern previously described.

The epithelium of the alveoli, like that of the bronchi and bronchioli rests upon a network of reticulum, which is of some importance in connection with interstitial disease processes of the lungs.

The interchange of gases takes place in the alveoli, and the entire structure of the lungs is subservient to this end.

Secondary Lobule. When a bronchial pathway is followed to its end, a point is reached where branching of parallel walls of the pathway occurs about every 0.5 to 1.0 cm. After three or four such branchings an abrupt transition takes place after which the branching patterns occur much more frequently—at 2 to 3 mm. intervals. Reid and Simon have called these the centimeter and

millimeter patterns respectively. The centimeter pattern represents small bronchi and bronchioles; the millimeter pattern represents terminal bronchioles. A cluster of 3 to 5 terminal bronchioles in this millimeter pattern, together with the respiratory tissue that they supply, constitutes one *secondary lobule*. Generally, a secondary lobule is a unit with a diameter of about 1.0 to 1.5 cm., allowing 2 mm. as the distance between terminal bronchiolar branches and 5 mm. as the depth of respiratory tissue beyond the terminal bronchiole.

This concept of the secondary lobule is different from that of a lung unit demarcated by septal connective tissue passing into the lung from the pleura (Miller; VonHayek).

The secondary lobule as defined by Reid and Simon is morphologically recognizable on films, particularly following bronchographic study, or when this sector of the lung contains a water density material. A "mulberry-like" shadow is produced (Fig. 10–24 and 10–26 *B, C*).

The *acinus* represents that portion of the lung parenchyma encompassing all the tissues distal to one terminal bronchiole, i.e., all of the respiratory bronchioles, alveolar ducts, and alveoli (Fig. 10–25). Thus, a secondary lobule contains a cluster of three to five terminal bronchioles supplying three to five acini. Very likely, then, an acinus measures 5 to 7 mm. in diameter, in contrast to a secondary lobule which is approximately 1.0 to 1.5 cm. in diameter.

Each alveolar duct, in contrast, supplies a family of approximately 20 to 25 alveoli. The primary lobule of Miller comprises only the air spaces supplied by one alveolar duct and is probably 1.0 to 1.5 mm. in diameter; it is not to be confused with the much larger secondary lobule recognizable macroscopically. Distal to one terminal bronchiole are some 400 alveolar duct units and 8000 alveoli, all contained in an area of about 5 mm. on the roentgenogram (Sargent and Sherwin).

Various histologic measurements of airway passages and alveoli are given for reference (Davies; Weibel; Pump).

The secondary pulmonary lobule furnishes a practical concept for interpretation of both normal and abnormal chest radiographs (Heitzman et al.).

Canals of Lambert. In the distal portions of the bronchiolar tree there are a number of epithelium-lined tubular communications that apparently provide an accessory route for the passage of air directly from the bronchioles into the alveoli. These are known as the *canals of Lambert* (Lambert).

Alveolar Pores (the Pores of Kohn). These pores in the alveoli are openings or discontinuities of the alveolar wall that measure about 10 to 15 microns in diameter. These apparently permit the transfer of gases, fluids, or particulate matter between lobules. They exist only between segments of a lobe; the total lobe remains an isolated unit with no collateral channel communications with adjacent lobes. However, if segmental or sub-

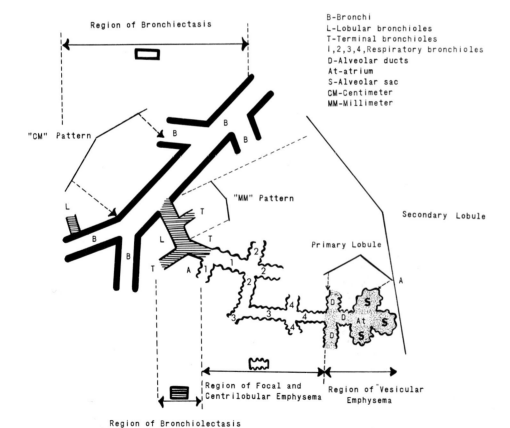

Figure 10–24. The "secondary lobule" (diagram).

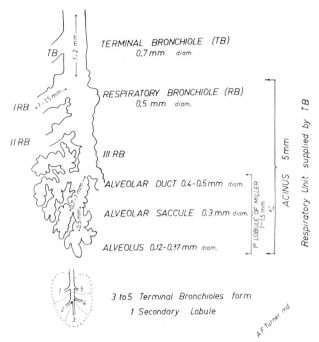

Figure 10–25. Anatomic drawing of terminal bronchiole and components of one acinus. (From Sargent, E. N., and Sherwin, R.: Amer. J. Roentgenol., *113*:660–679, 1971.)

segmental bronchial occlusion exists, ventilation of the occluded segment may be brought about through these collateral channels. Hence, this is known as "collateral air drift." McLean has suggested that the positive pressure of expiration produces a collapse of the pores of Kohn and that this causes a check-valve mechanism to operate at each of these collateral pathways. Reich and co-workers have referred to this as "an interalveolar air drift," and represent this as an integral part of the mechanism of coughing. They have discussed these anatomic structures in relation to various pathologic entities (Fig. 10–26 *A, B, C*) (Macklin).

Fissures and Lobes of the Lungs (Fig. 10–18 *A*). The right lung is subdivided into three lobes, an upper, middle, and lower, by two interlobar fissures. The major fissure separates the lower lobe from the middle and upper lobes. With minor differences to be described soon, this fissure corresponds to the major fissure on the left side. The other fissure, or minor fissure, separates the upper from the middle lobe.

The left lung contains only a major fissure, and is subdivided into two lobes, an upper and a lower.

Each lobe of the lung is almost completely covered by visceral pleura, and each interlobar fissure is composed, therefore, of the visceral pleura of the two adjoining lobes that have extended down the fissure.

There is a considerable variation in the normal configuration and exact position of each fissure. From the radiologic point of view, the configuration of the entire surface of the interlobar fissure is of great importance. Each fissure must be visualized not as it is projected onto the surface of the thorax, but rather as a three-dimensional structure (Figs. 10–18, and 10–27).

Shape of the Interlobar Surfaces (Figs. 10–18, 10–27). The major fissure on the right side has the shape of an elongated and concave semi-ellipse. On the left side, it is rather crescentic. The major fissures reach to a variable distance from the hilus, and the minor (middle lobe) fissure is closed on the hilar surface.

Pleural bridges unite the various surfaces. There are also parenchymatous bridges uniting the various lobes with one another, particularly on the hilar and posterior aspects.

The right minor or middle lobe fissure is triangular, with the apex directed anteriorly. The base of the triangle is formed by the junction of the middle lobe fissure and the major fissure.

The upper part of the interlobar surface of the lower lobe faces anteriorly and somewhat laterally, while the lower part of this surface faces anteriorly and inward. This gives this surface a somewhat spiral appearance (resembling a propeller).

The minor (middle lobe) fissure on the right side is horizontal, at the level of the fourth costal cartilage.

The upper limit of the lower lobe posteriorly is at the vertebral end of the third rib or medial end of the spine of the scapula. The lower end is opposite the lateral part of the sixth costal cartilage.

The left upper lobe forms about one-eighth of the diaphragmatic surface of the left lung in its anteromedian portion. On the right side, a rather large part of the middle lobe is in contact with the diaphragm (as much as one-half).

The major fissure is steeper on the left side than on the right, forming an angle of about 60 degrees with the horizontal as against 50 degrees on the right side.

In addition to the spiral curvature of the major fissure, there is an upward convexity of the surface as well.

Radiographic Visualization of the Fissures. The interlobar fissures are areas in which the visceral pleura can be visualized on roentgenograms owing to the double thickness of the investing pleura of adjacent lobes and the contrasting air on either side of the fissure line (Felson; Fleischner et al.; Robbins and Hale, 1945a). Fairly large planes of the fissures must be parallel with the roentgen ray beam in order to permit visualization. Thus the interlobar fissure between the upper and middle lobes on the right is seen often, since much of its surface is thrown into tangential projection in the posteroanterior projection. In the straight lateral projection, the major fissure may likewise be seen at least in part for the same reason. It is conceivable that if one were to try carefully to obtain a good surface tangential view of the various portions of the surface of any of the fissures, it would

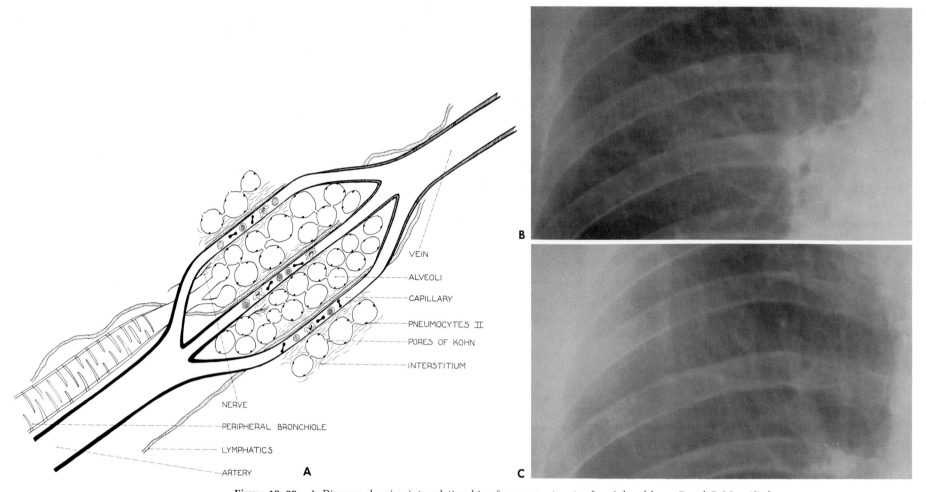

Figure 10–26. *A.* Diagram showing interrelationship of component parts of peripheral lung. *B* and *C.* Magnified view of air space consolidation in acute pulmonary edema before and after diuresis. Some discrete acinar shadows are shown before diuresis.

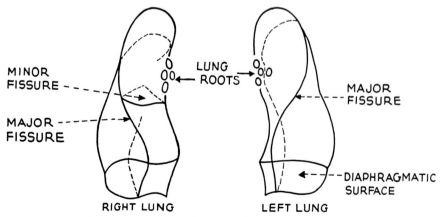

Figure 10–27. Three-dimensional concept of interlobar fissures.

be possible to demonstrate successively the various portions of the fissures.

Visualization of the fissures is helpful in detecting and localizing disease, and in determining its nature. Bean et al. found that approximately 70 per cent of normal chest roentgenograms in the newborn demonstrate fissure lines. This percentage decreases to about 50 per cent at 1 month, and then progressively increases with age, reaching 70 per cent at about 9 years, and about 100 per cent beyond 20 years of age. In the presence of acute inflammatory diseases of the chest the fissures are accentuated, either by fluid in the pleural space or in the lung adjacent to the pleura. After the acute phase, this accentuated appearance disappears and the per cent of visualization returns to the expected normal. This return to normal, however, does not occur in children with tuberculosis or cystic fibrosis.

In the adult, fissure lines are accentuated when a tumor adjoins an interlobar fissure.

The Pleura. The pleura is a thin continuous layer of endothelial cells resting on a thin membrane of connective tissue, which in turn contains blood vessels, lymphatics, and nerves. This lining membrane covers the entire inner aspect of the thoracic cavity as a closed space and also invests the lungs as well. That portion lining the thoracic cavity is called the *parietal* pleura, and that investing the lungs is called the *visceral* pleura. The interlobar fissures are formed by invagination into the lungs of two closely approximated layers of visceral pleura.

Ordinarily the pleura is not visualized unless it contains excessive fluid or foreign tissue as with inflammation or neoplasm. When the pleural shadow can be identified it is usually indicative of an active or previous abnormality.

The costophrenic and cardiophrenic angles are ordinarily rather sharply delineated also. Since the costophrenic angles represent the most dependent portions of the chest when the patient is in the erect position, it is in this location that excessive fluid accumulates first. The cardiophrenic angles vary considerably in appearance, depending on the variable appearance of the pericardial fat pad (to be described later with the heart).

Segments of the Lungs (Fig. 10–17). Although the segments of the lung do not have definite visceral pleural subdivisions as do the various lobes of the lungs, there is a certain amount of separability of these segments within the lung parenchyma. Each segment is supplied by a separate bronchial and arterial subdivision (see Fig. 10–34), and thus is a separate entity surgically.

Accessory Lobes of the Lungs

Inferior Accessory Lobe (Fig. 10–28). The segment of lung supplied by the medial basilar branch of the lower lobe bronchus on the right or the corresponding medial basilar branch of the anterior basilar branch of the left lower lobe bronchus may exist wholly or partially as a separate lobe. Schaffner found it in 45 per cent of 210 postmortem examinations, and radiologically it may be found in about 8 per cent of chest films (Twining). Fleischner has noted the variation in direction of the fissure of this lobe, and hence its variable appearance must be constantly borne in mind. It resembles closely at times an abnormally large pericardial fat pad in the right cardiophrenic angle, or any other abnormality that may be projected in this location.

Posterior Accessory Lobe. The segment supplied by the superior branch of the lower lobe bronchus may not infrequently be an accessory lobe. It is probable, however, that it need not necessarily be a separate lobe even if it is shown sharply demarcated from the surrounding lung in disease, since the segmental distribution of the bronchi is discrete in any event.

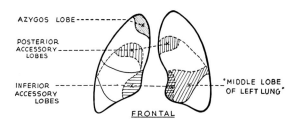

OCCASIONAL ACCESSORY LOBES OF LUNGS

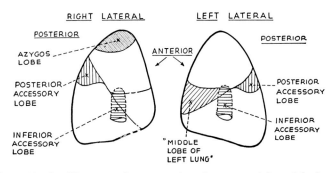

Figure 10–28. Diagrammatic presentation of accessory lobes of the lungs.

Middle Lobe of Left Lung. Although the lingular portion of the left upper lobe is separated from the rest of the upper lobe by a relatively avascular portion and occasionally by an incomplete fissure, it is practically never a completely separate accessory lobe as in the case of the other lobes.

Accessory Azygos Lobe (Figs. 10–28 *B*, and 10–29). Embryologically the azygos vein runs just lateral to the apex of the right upper lobe. As the apex grows upward, the azygos vein ordinarily glides medially so that it lies medial to the right lung apex.

If this gliding movement is interrupted as the apex of the right upper lobe grows upward, the azygos vein produces an indentation into the right upper lobe medially, carrying with it a fold of both visceral and parietal pleura. Thus, unlike the true fissures between lobes that consist of two layers of visceral pleura, this artificial fissure consists of four layers, two visceral and two parietal.

This false fissure appears radiologically as a thin, outwardly convex line, always in the right upper lobe medially. It is usually thicker at its lower end, a characteristic probably related to the fact that the azygos vein is situated in this location, or possibly this is to be associated with a fold of pleura. This thicker area must be carefully differentiated from any abnormality in the lung.

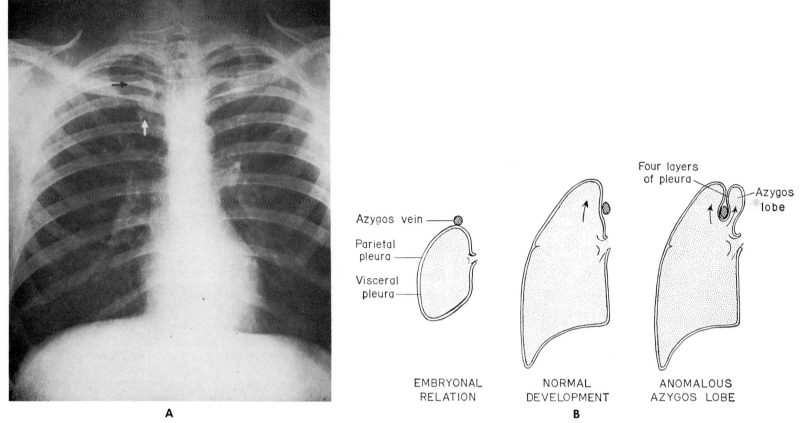

A

Azygos vein
Parietal pleura
Visceral pleura
EMBRYONAL RELATION

NORMAL DEVELOPMENT

Four layers of pleura
Azygos lobe
ANOMALOUS AZYGOS LOBE

B

Figure 10–29. *A.* Radiograph of chest showing position and appearance of the azygos lobe. *B.* Anatomic concept of "azygos" lobe. Normally the azygos vein migrates into its normal suprahilar position by moving "around" the apex of the right upper lobe. In some cases it takes a shorter route, and indents both the parietal and the visceral pleura, producing the anomalous "fissure." Unlike a true interlobar fissure, this one consists of four mesothelial layers—two from the parietal and two from the visceral pleura. The true interlobar fissure consists of only two layers of visceral pleura.

VASCULAR SUPPLY, VENOUS DRAINAGE, AND LYMPHATICS OF THE RESPIRATORY TRACT

Blood Vessels of the Lungs. *Pulmonary Artery.* The pulmonary artery (Figs. 10–15, 10–30) follows closely the subdivisions of the bronchial tree. It arches over the right main-stem bronchus and lies dorsal and slightly lateral to the bronchus. The artery diminishes more rapidly in size than the bronchus it accompanies, and by the time it reaches the primary lobule, it is about one-fourth or one-fifth the size of the ductulus alveolaris. It finally ends in a capillary network surrounding the alveolus. The pulmonary vein takes origin from the latter capillary network.

The common pulmonary artery divides into right and left pulmonary arteries (Fig. 10–31). The right pulmonary artery

passes under the aortic arch below the tracheal bifurcation and crosses in front of the right bronchus between its upper lobe and lower division branches. It divides into three branches, two going to the upper lobe, and one supplying the middle and lower lobes. Each of the branches of these subdivisions follows the corresponding branches of the bronchial tree rather closely, with the artery lying along the upper side of the bronchus most of the way. The left pulmonary artery is seen just below the aortic knob as it arches posteriorly into the left lung, forming the crescentic shadow of the left hilus above the downward curving left bronchus. It enters the hilus as three branches and then subdivides into nine principal branches, five of which go to the upper lobe and four to the lower lobe following corresponding bronchial branches. (The relationships of the heart, major vessels, and other structures of the mediastinum will be discussed in greater detail in Chapters 11 and 12.)

Capillaries. The network of capillaries is situated in the walls of the alveoli, and each capillary is common to two alveoli.

The mesh of capillaries in the walls of the alveoli situated beneath the pleura is much coarser than that within the lung. The same holds true for the capillaries situated near the fibrous septa and larger blood vessels.

Pulmonary Veins. Unlike the pulmonary artery, which is virtually in the same sheath as the bronchus, the more peripheral pulmonary veins are situated far removed from the corresponding bronchus in the septa that unite several lobules. The pulmonary veins have four sources of origin: (1) the capillary network of the pleura, which is derived from the bronchial artery; (2) the capillary network of the alveoli; (3) the bronchopulmonary veins, which are situated on either side of the junction of two bronchi or

bronchioli; and (4) the capillary network in the alveolar ducts, which gives origin to two venous radicles, one on either side of the duct.

The veins and arteries come closer together at about the fourth bronchial bifurcation, the veins lying anterior to and below the arteries. As they approach the hilum, they again become dissociated, the veins lying below and anterior to the arteries and diverging from them to enter the left atrium.

THE ESTIMATION OF PULMONARY VENOUS AND ARTERIAL PRESSURES FROM ROUTINE CHEST ROENTGENOGRAMS. There have been many attempts to estimate pulmonary vascular pressures from routine chest radiographs (Davies et al.; Jacobson et al.; Milne;

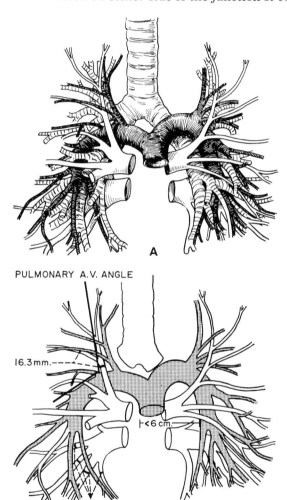

PULMONARY A.V. ANGLE

16.3 mm.

⊢<6 cm.⊣

18.1 mm.

A

B

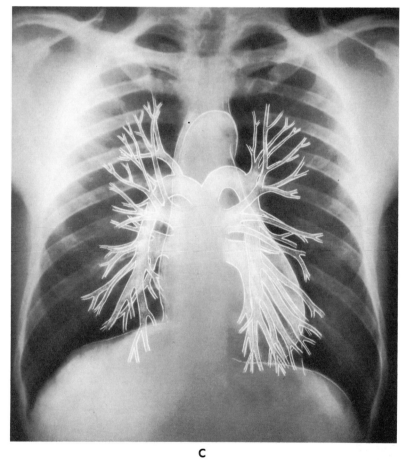

C

Figure 10–30. *A.* Relationship of major ramifications of pulmonary artery and tracheobronchial tree to one another, also showing the relationship to major pulmonary veins. Note that left pulmonary artery is slightly more cephalad than right. *B.* The pulmonary arteriovenous angle, which becomes more obtuse with passive hyperemia of the lungs. Also shown are several measurements which are occasionally quoted in the literature (after Logue et al.). The measurement 16.3 mm. indicates the sum of the diameters of the apical vein of the right upper lobe at the level of the right upper lobe bronchus, and the posterior segmental vein of the right upper lobe at the point at which it is crossed by the anterior segmental artery. The 18.1 mm. is the sum of the diameters of the superior and inferior basal veins of the right lower lobe measured 1 cm. from their junction. (From Lavendar et al.: Brit. J. Radiol., 35:413, 1962.) *C.* Diagrammatic intensification of pulmonary arteries and veins on a routine posteroanterior radiograph.

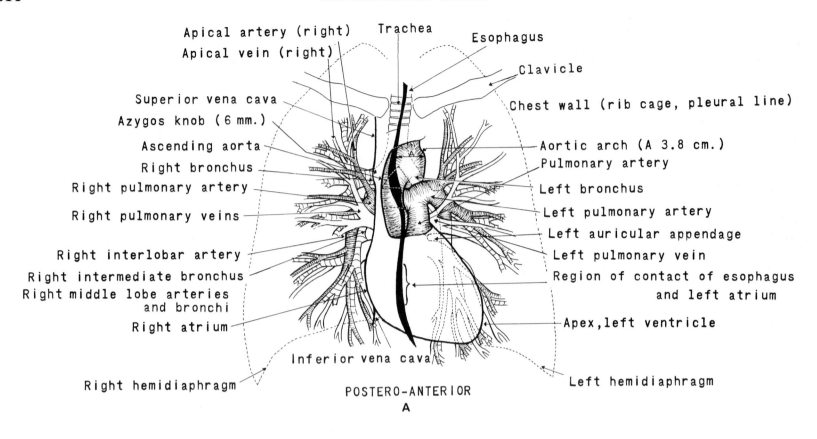

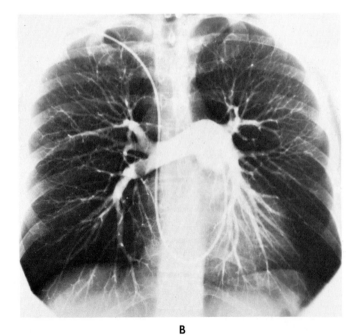

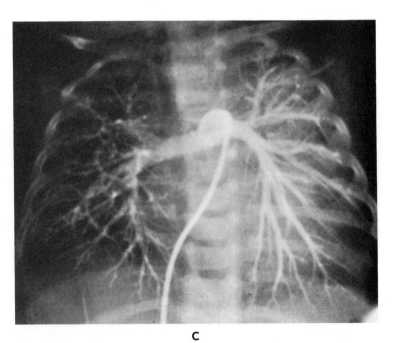

Figure 10–31. *A.* Diagram of chest film showing arteries, veins, and relationships to bronchi. *B.* Pulmonary arteriogram, arterial phase. *C.* Pulmonary arteriogram in an infant, arterial phase.

Simon, 1963; Steiner; Turner et al.). Since the pulmonary vascular bed is a low resistance bed, it can be readily surmised that in pulmonary circulation the blood flows forward across the capillary bed for oxygenation, and returns to the left atrium by means of a postcapillary or pulmonary venous pressure component. The precapillary pressure requirements are assessed by changes in the main pulmonary artery and its visualized major branches. The pulmonary venous pressure or postcapillary component is evaluated by studying the regional distribution of pulmonary blood flow.

Considerable change in blood-flow through the lungs occurs as body position changes, since, normally, blood-flow is directed into the lower lung zones largely by gravity. Normally, the size and number of vessels per unit area in the lower lung are greater than they are in the upper zones in the upright position. Normally, the pulmonary vessels show an orderly tapering and branching toward the periphery, so that for perhaps 2 or 3 cm. in the immediate subpleural area the vessels become virtually invisible. Moreover, the distribution of vessels is considerably greater in the lower lung in the erect position by at least a factor of 3. Various methods of studying redistribution of the numbers of vessels in the lower and upper lung have been devised (Turner et al.). Redistribution is then interpreted in terms of postcapillary pressure.

ASSESSMENT OF PRECAPILLARY OR ARTERIAL PRESSURE. Precapillary or arterial pressure is assessed by: (1) studying the *size of the main pulmonary artery* and its major branches, and (2) studying the *degree of tapering* of the vessels as they branch in the midzone of the lungs. Experience and correlation with cardiac catheterization values is remarkably good. Unfortunately, pulmonary parenchymal disease and increased total pulmonary blood-flow are the major sources of inaccurate estimations.

The upper lobe pulmonary veins are most consistently visualized at the main pulmonary artery level. Superimposition of artery and vein occurs in about 40 to 50 per cent of examinations, but otherwise the vein is almost invariably lateral to the artery. The pulmonary vessels are usually vertical in the left upper lobe and either vertical or oblique in the right upper lobe. Considerable significance can be ascribed to the detection of a change in diameter of upper lobe pulmonary veins in serial chest roentgenograms (Burko et al.).

Doppman and Lavender proposed a careful study of the hilum on the right as an indicator of left atrial pressure (Fig. 10–32). In the normal individual an angle of approximately 120 degrees is formed by the intersection of the superior pulmonary vein and the descending pulmonary artery (Figs. 10–30, 10–32 A). This concave hilar angle is obliterated early with rising left atrial pressure (Fig. 10–32 B).

Bronchial Artery. The bronchial arteries vary in number and origin. They may arise from the aorta (in over 90 per cent of cases), or from any of the first three intercostal subclavian or internal mammary arteries. In about 80 per cent of cases, their level of origin is opposite the fifth and sixth dorsal vertebrae. They supply the bronchi, visceral pleura, walls of pulmonary vessels, and interstitial supporting structures of alveoli. No precapillary anastomoses are present between pulmonary and bronchial arteries in normal lungs. The middle third of the esophagus, the hilar lymph nodes, vagus nerve, and mediastinal fascia are also nourished by bronchial arterial circulation. Anastomoses with other systemic arteries may occur.

The variations in origin of the bronchial arteries have been carefully cataloged by Cauldwell et al. In 74 per cent of their dissections, the right and left bronchial arteries arose independently, while in the remainder, a common trunk divided into right and left bronchial arteries. Rarely, the bronchial artery originated from the subclavian. The bronchial arteries are embedded in the connective tissue surrounding the bronchi and usually form an acute angle with the aorta at their origin, coursing upward and anteriorly initially, and following the course of the bronchi closely. The vessels end in an arterial plexus that anastomoses with the pulmonary capillary plexus (Newton and Preger; Viamonte et al.; Cudkowicz and Armstrong) (Fig. 10–33). The capillaries in the alveolar walls are derived from the pulmonary artery and not from the bronchial artery. (It is interesting to note that this point of transition from the bronchial to the pulmonary circulation is a favorite site for tubercle formation.)

Bronchial Veins. True bronchial veins are found only at the hilus of the lung. These arise from the first or first two dividing points of the bronchial tree, and receive branches from part of the pleura close to the hilus. These bronchial veins empty into the azygos, the hemiazygos, or one of the intercostal veins. Communications exist between the bronchial arteries and pulmonary veins via the capillaries, but Guillor (Miller) could not demonstrate such communication with the pulmonary artery directly. These vascular phenomena are of considerable importance from the standpoint of much of the circulatory pathology of the lungs.

Lymphatics of the Lungs (Figs. 10–34, 10–35). The lung is provided with a great abundance of lymphatics, more than the liver, spleen, or kidney (Miller). They may be divided grossly into a superficial set and a deep set. The superficial lymphatics are situated in the pleura; the deep group are situated along the pulmonary artery, veins, and bronchi, and form a dense network between the secondary lobules in the connective tissue septa. These two sets of lymphatics communicate with one another at the pleura and in the hilus. The pleural lymphatics have unusually large diameters and are arranged in the form of irregular polyhedral rings. Numerous valves, 1 to 2 mm. apart, direct the flow of lymph in both pleural and intrapulmonary lymphatics.

Normal lymph nodes may be found in the substance of the lung far from the hilum (Trapnell, 1964).

Lymphatics of the Bronchi. The larger bronchi have two sets of lymphatics which intercommunicate with one another, but

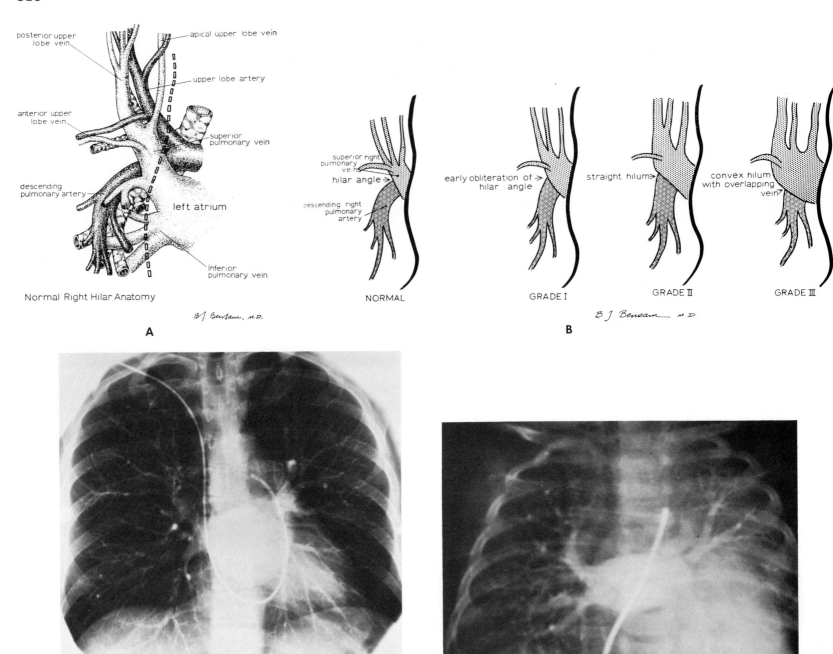

Figure 10–32. *A.* Diagrammatic representation of vasculature of right lung. Note the concave hilar angle formed by the intersection of the superior pulmonary vein and the descending pulmonary artery. *B.* Progressive changes in hilar contour with rising left atrial pressure. Grade I shows partial obliteration of the hilar angle by the enlarging upper lobe vein. Grade II shows complete effacement of the hilar angle with a straight lateral border to the hilum. The clear space between descending pulmonary artery and right atrium is encroached upon. Grade III shows a convex hilum with the horizontal inferior margin of the upper lobe vein crossing the artery. (From Doppman, J. L., and Lavender, J. P.: Radiology, *80*:931–936, 1963.) *C.* Pulmonary arteriogram, venous phase. Note that the major veins which return blood to the left atrium are situated partially over the spine and are concealed by the cardiac silhouette. *D.* Venogram phase of a pulmonary arteriogram in a normal infant.

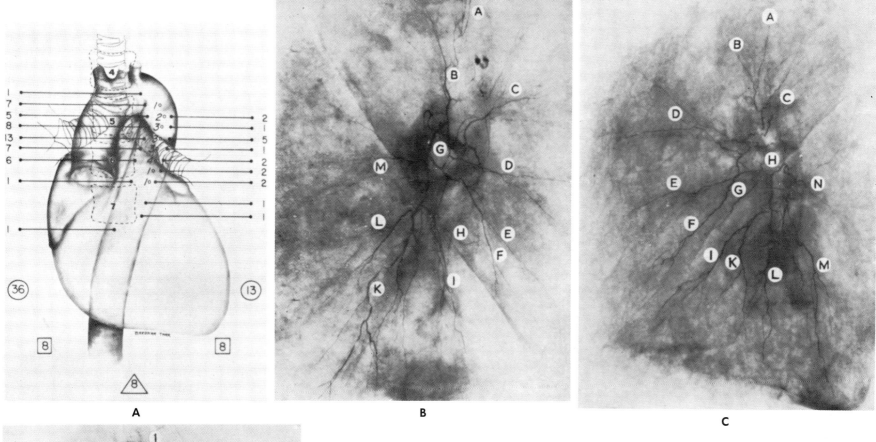

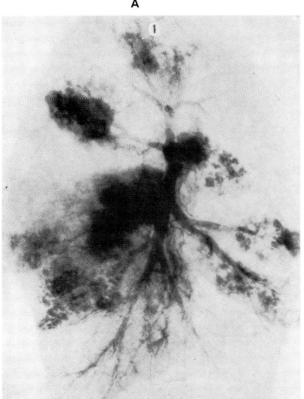

Figure 10–33. *A.* Diagram showing levels of origin of the right and left bronchial arteries and of common trunks (central circles) that were studied. Lateral circles indicate the number of lesions studied on each side. In the squares are the number of bilateral lesions. In the triangle, the number of midline lesions is indicated.

Note: First 71 studies. (From Viamonte, M., Parks, R. E., and Smoak, W. M. III: Radiology, *85*:205–230, 1965.)

B. Standard pattern of left bronchial arteries seen in a lateral view of a left lung (Case 6). (Hilum faces x-ray tube.)

Upper lobe: (A) apical pleural branch, (B) posterior branch, (C) apical branch, (D) anterior branch, (E) superior lingual branch, (F) inferior lingular branch, (G) annulus. *Lower lobe:* (H) interlobar pleural branch, (J) anterior branch, (K) lateral branch, (L) posterior branch, (M) apical branch.

C. Standard pattern of right bronchial arteries seen in a lateral view of a right lung (Case 7). (Hilum faces x-ray tube.)

Upper lobe: (A) apical pleural branch, (B) apical branch, (C) posterior branch, (D) anterior branch. *Middle lobe:* (E) lateral branch, (F) medial branch, (G) interlobar pleural branch, (H) annulus. *Lower lobe:* (I) anterior branch, (K) cardiac (medial) branch, (L) lateral branch, (M) posterior branch, (N) apical branch.

D. Lateral view (Case 3) of right bronchial tree superimposed on right bronchial arterial pattern. (1) Apical pleural branch. Some alveolar fogging has occurred. The hilum faces away from x-ray tube. About one-third of normal size. (*B, C,* and *D* from Cudkowicz, L., and Armstrong, J. B.: Thorax, 6:342–358, 1951.)

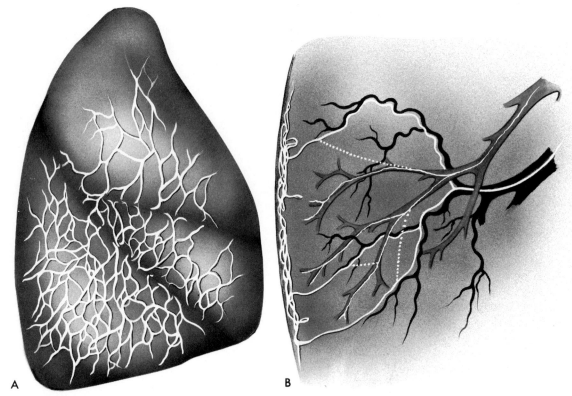

Figure 10–34. The lymphatic drainage of the pleura and lungs. *A.* A drawing of the lateral aspect of the right lung shows the pleural lymphatics to be much more numerous over the lower half of the lung than over the upper. *B.* In a coronal section through the midportion of the lung, lymphatic channels from the pleura enter the lung at the interlobular septa and extend medially to the hilum along venous radicals (dark shaded vessels); lymphatic channels originating in the peripheral parenchyma extend medially in the bronchovascular bundles (light shaded vessels). Communicating lymphatics (dotted lines) extend between the peribronchial and perivenous lymphatics. (From Fraser, R. G., and Paré, J. A. P.: Diagnosis of Diseases of the Chest. Philadelphia, W. B. Saunders Co., 1970.)

the smaller bronchi have only a single plexus of lymphatics which terminates at the alveolar ductules. Here they join the lymphatics accompanying the pulmonary veins that form at this point.

There are no lymphatics in the walls of the air spaces distal to the alveolar ductules.

Lymphatics of the Pulmonary Artery. The larger branches of the pulmonary artery are accompanied by two lymph channels, one of which is situated between the artery and its accompanying bronchus. These intercommunicate freely by means of a rich plexus. The smaller arterial branches are accompanied by only single lymph channels. Communications between the periarterial and peribronchial lymphatics occur in many places but predominantly in the region of bifurcations and at the distal end of the alveolar ductules.

Lymphatics of the Pulmonary Veins. As in the case of the arteries and bronchi, lymph channels accompany all of the veins, except in the region of the alveolar sacs.

Lymphatics of the Pleura. There is only a single plexus of lymphatics in the pleura, arranged in polyhedral rings. There are smaller rings within these larger ones, with smaller lymph channels.

Direction of Lymph Flow. The valves situated in the hilus, pleura, and at the junction of the deep and superficial systems permit flow in one direction only. *The flow in the peribronchial, periarterial, and perivenous lymphatics is toward the interior of the lung* or hilus.

The *valves situated just beneath the pleura permit flow of lymph toward the pleura.* In the subpleural region, the pleural lymphatics occasionally dip into the lung and then return to the surface to become pleural again (Trapnell, 1963).

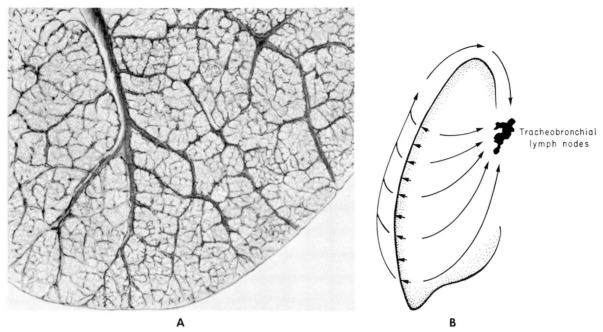

Figure 10–35. *A.* Drawing of lower surface of middle lobe showing lymphatic vessels outlining the lobules and acini of the lung parenchyma. (From Twining, E. W.: A Textbook of X-Ray Diagnosis. H. K. Lewis & Co., Publishers, *B.* Diagrammatic illustration of the drainage of the lymphatics of the lungs. The superficial lymphatics are situated in the pleura and drain into the pleural space and around to the hili thereby. The deep lymphatics follow along the pulmonary arterial branches, veins, and bronchi and drain toward the hilus. The two sets of lymphatics communicate with one another immediately adjoining the pleura and in the region of the hilus, but are otherwise separate.

The valves situated in the pleura allow free circulation of the lymph within this space. The pleural lymphatics together with the lymphatics from the interior of the lung all enter the tracheobronchial lymph nodes.

In the presence of an obstructed lymph channel, a reversal of lymph flow can occur. These obstructed and distended lymphatics appear linear and stellate in relation to hilar lymph nodes.

Lymphoid Tissue. Lymphoid tissue may occur in the form of lymph nodes, lymph follicles, or small masses of lymphoid tissue. Lymph nodes in the normal lung are associated with the larger divisions of the bronchi, and are situated at the places where branching takes place (Fig. 10–36). There is in old age a definite increase in the lymphoid tissue independent of that produced by disease, but dependent to a great extent on the amount of irritating particles inhaled (such as carbon). In the normal lung, lymph nodes are not present in the pleura.

The following groups of lymph nodes occur (Fig. 10–36): (1) the paratracheal group; (2) the tracheobronchial group, the right being more constant than the left, but those on the left are in close proximity to the recurrent nerve (they are connected with the anterior and posterior mediastinal nodes, and also with the inferior deep cervical nodes); (3) the bifurcation group, which are likewise in communication with the posterior mediastinal nodes; (4) the bronchopulmonary group, lying in the hilus of the corresponding lung, in the angles between the branches of the bronchi;

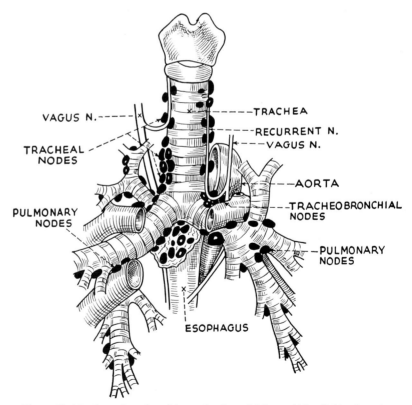

Figure 10–36. Lymph nodes of the tracheobronchial tree. (After Sukienikow.)

(5) the pulmonary groups, lying in the lung substance, usually in the angles of the branching bronchi up to the third branching. The nodes in the left upper lobe may lie in the anterior mediastinum in close proximity with the aorta and ductus arteriosus.

The hilar nodes receive lymph not only from the more peripheral lymphatics of the lung but also from the pleura, by lymph channels which drain along the interlobar fissures and over the anterior and posterior lung surfaces toward the hilus. This accounts for the great frequency with which these fissures are visible in both pleural and pulmonary disease.

Lymphatic Pathways of the Mediastinum. Fraser and Paré have divided the lymphatic pathways of the mediastinum according to the three conventional compartments of the mediastinum (see Chapter 11), although usually the intrathoracic lymph nodes are considered to be divided into a parietal group and a visceral group. The parietal lymph nodes drain the thoracic wall and certain extrathoracic tissues, whereas the visceral group are involved mostly with intrathoracic structures.

Group 1: Lymph Nodes of the Anterior Mediastinal Compartment

(1) *The sternal, anterior parietal, or internal mammary group.* This group of nodes is distributed along the internal mammary arteries behind the anterior costochondral cartilages bilaterally. They drain the upper anterior abdominal wall, the anterior thoracic wall, the anterior portion of the diaphragm, and the medial portions of the breast. They communicate with a visceral group of anterior mediastinal lymph nodes and cervical nodes.

(2) *The anterior mediastinal lymph node group.* These are visceral nodes, lying posterior to the sternum in the lower thorax, along the superior vena cava and innominate vein on the right and in front of the aorta and carotid artery on the left. Some of these nodes are situated anterior to the thymus.

Group 2: The Posterior Mediastinal Lymph Nodes (Fig. 10–38)

This group of lymph nodes lies posteriorly in the intercostal spaces and in paravertebral areas. They drain the parietal pleura and vertebral column. This group consists of parietal nodes and mediastinal visceral nodes, which communicate with each other. The posterior mediastinal group of visceral nodes lie along the lower esophagus and descending aorta, and drain the posterior portion of the diaphragm, the pericardium, the esophagus, and the lower lobes of the lungs.

Group 3: The Middle Mediastinal Lymph Nodes (Fig. 10–39)

The parietal group of lymph nodes in this chain are located mainly around the pericardial attachment to the diaphragm, whereas the visceral group consists mainly of the tracheobronchial and bifurcation nodes and bronchopulmonary nodes (see also Figure 10–36).

The lymph from the anterior mediastinal nodes flows into the right lymphatic duct or bronchomediastinal duct, and the thoracic duct on the left. The posterior mediastinal lymph nodes drain into the thoracic duct and the cisterna chyli from the lower thoracic region. They also communicate with the visceral mediastinal lymph nodes draining mainly via the thoracic duct.

The middle mediastinal lymph nodes communicate with anterior mediastinal and posterior nodes, and also drain into the bronchomediastinal trunk on the right and the thoracic duct on the left (Rouviere). The bronchomediastinal trunk receives the lymph from the right lung and empties via the right lymphatic duct into the beginning of the innominate vein. Near their terminations, both thoracic ducts lie close to the lower deep cervical lymph nodes.

THE LUNG HILI

The hilus of the lung (Fig. 10–40) is a wedge-shaped depressed area on the mediastinal surface of the lung above and behind the pericardial impression on the lung, within which the blood vessels, lymph vessels, nerves, and bronchi enter and leave the lung. Bronchial lymph nodes are located among those structures. The hilus is surrounded by the reflection of the pleura from the surface of the lung on to the pulmonary root. The mediastinal surface of the lung presents the pericardial impression produced by structures in the posterior mediastinum and the superior mediastinum in addition to the hili.

The term "root of the lung" is, strictly speaking, applied to a number of structures that enter and leave the lung on its mediastinal surface. It constitutes a pedicle that attaches the lung to the mediastinal wall of the pleural cavity. The large structures forming the pulmonary root are: (1) the two pulmonary veins, (2) the pulmonary artery, (3) the bronchus, (4) bronchial arteries and veins, (5) pulmonary nerves, and (6) lymph vessels and some lymph nodes (bronchial).

In the case of the left lung, the major arteries and veins and their branches are arranged in the form of a triangle, with the pulmonary veins forming the anterior and inferior apices of the triangle and the left pulmonary artery forming the superior apex; the bronchus is in the center of the triangle. The pulmonary artery lies higher in the left root than in the right, and crosses the bronchus on the left before it divides into its branches.

These root structures can be moderately well distinguished on radiographs in the posteroanterior and oblique projections. By common usage, the terms "hilus" and "root" are used interchangeably.

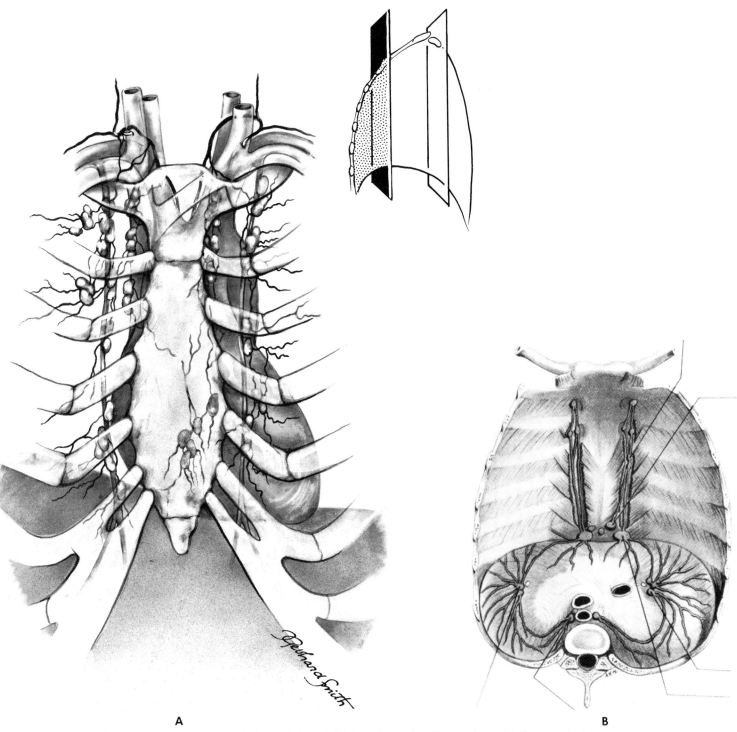

Figure 10–37. A. Anterior Mediastinal Lymph Nodes. The nodes illustrated are chiefly those of the anterior parietal group scattered along the internal mammary arteries and behind the anterior intercostal spaces and costal cartilages bilaterally. The prevascular (visceral) group relate to the superior vena cava and innominate vein on the right and to the aorta and carotid artery on the left. (From Fraser, R. G., and Paré, J. A. P.: Diagnosis of Diseases of the Chest. Philadelphia, W. B. Saunders Co., 1970.) B. The anatomy of the internal mammary lymph nodes. From Cunningham's Textbook of Anatomy, 10th ed. London, Oxford University Press, 1964.)

Figure 10–37 continued on the following page.

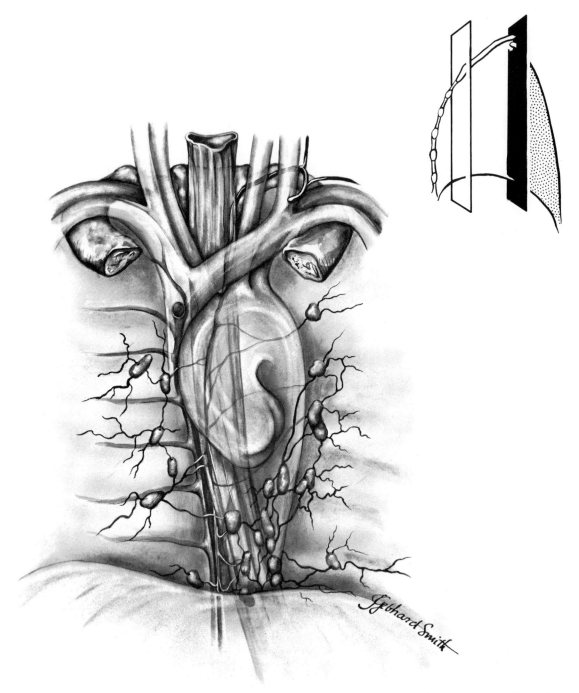

Figure 10–38.   Posterior Mediastinal Lymph Nodes. The intercostal (posterior parietal) group lies laterally, in the intercostal spaces, and medially, in the paravertebral areas adjacent to the heads of the ribs. The visceral group of posterior mediastinal nodes is situated along the lower esophagus and descending aorta. (From Fraser, R. G., and Paré, J. A. P.: Diagnosis of Diseases of the Chest. Philadelphia, W. B. Saunders Co., 1970.)

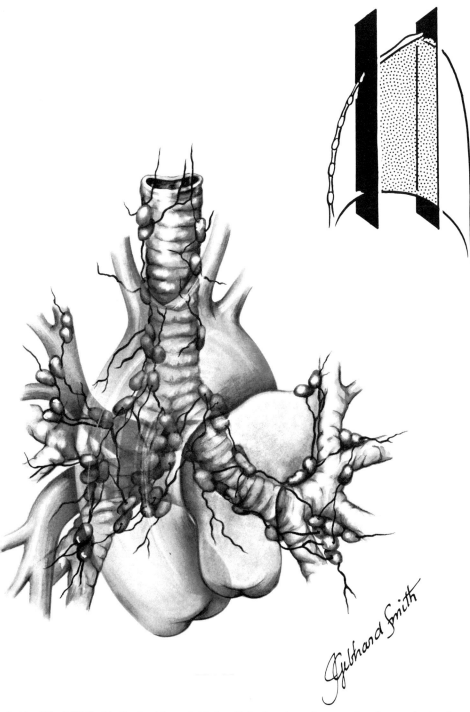

Figure 10–39.   The Middle Mediastinal Lymph Nodes. Only the visceral group of nodes are depicted, consisting of the tracheobronchial, carinal, and bronchopulmonary nodes. See text for description. (From Fraser, R. G., and Paré, J. A. P.: Diagnosis of Diseases of the Chest. Philadelphia, W. B. Saunders Co., 1970.)

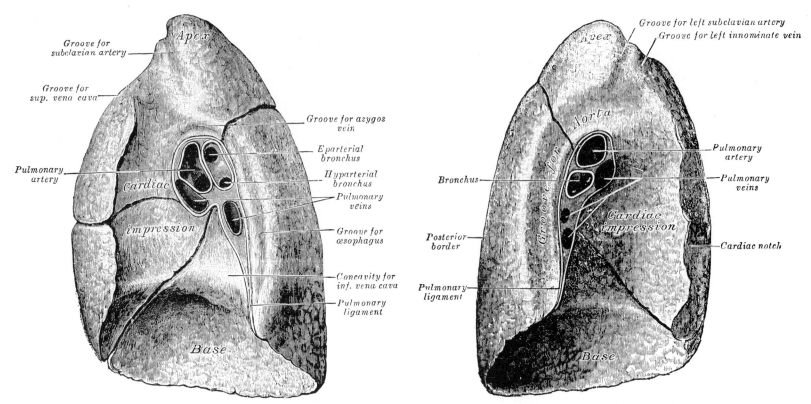

Figure 10-40. Structures in the lung hili. (From Gray's Anatomy of the Human Body, 29th edition. Goss, C. M. (ed.) Philadelphia, Lea & Febiger, 1973.)

THE THORACIC CAGE, PLEURA, AND DIAPHRAGM

There are several important component parts of the thoracic cage, all of which may be visualized to some extent radiographically. These are: (1) the soft tissue structures of the thoracic wall, such as the skin, breasts, and muscular tissues; (2) the bony structures of the thoracic cage, consisting chiefly of ribs, costal cartilage, sternum, and thoracic spine; (3) the pleura, both visceral and parietal; and (4) the diaphragm.

Soft Tissue Structures of the Thoracic Wall

Skin and Subcutaneous Tissues. The skin and subcutaneous tissues of the thoracic cage cannot be entirely ignored in the consideration of the radiographic anatomy of the chest. Normally, these tegmental layers are seen only over the clavicle (Fig. 10-41), and as outlining shadows of the thoracic cage; abnormally,

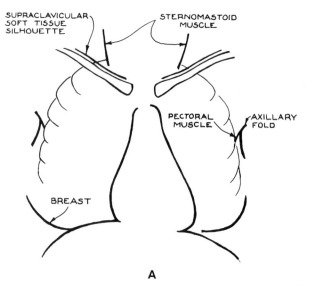

Figure 10-41. A. Soft tissues of the thoracic cage as seen radiographically.

Figure 10-41 continued on the opposite page.

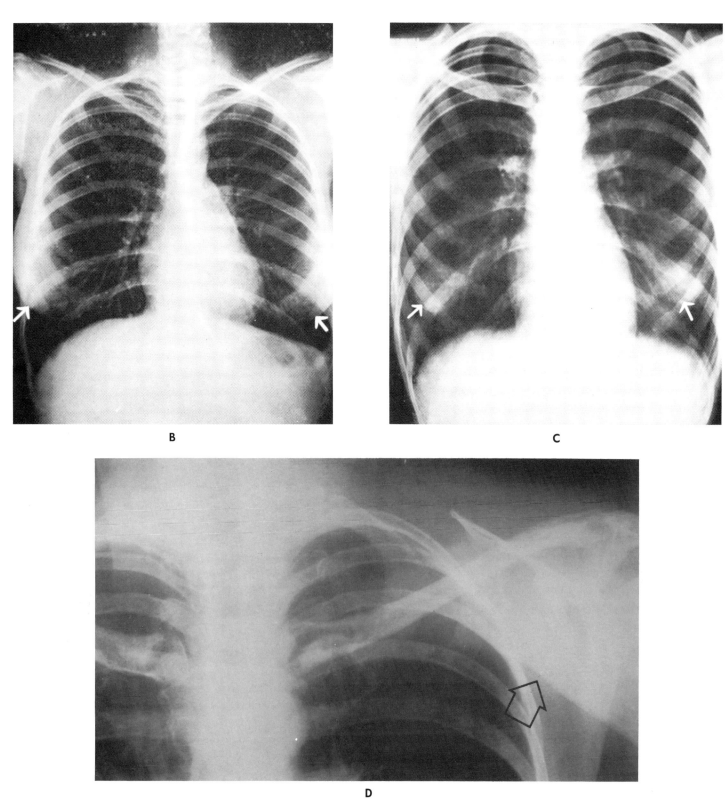

Figure 10–41 *Continued.* *B.* Projection of female breast shadows over the lung substance. *C.* Radiograph showing areola and nipple shadows. *D.* Close-up view of the axilla in a patient following radical mastectomy. There is complete absence of the pectoral muscles.

shadows contained within the skin and subcutaneous tissues can produce very dense shadows that must be differentiated from pulmonary constituents. Free air in the skin and subcutaneous tissues also produces its individual appearance. The fact that structures contained within the skin have radiographic significance must not be overlooked.

The Breasts. The breasts are situated in the superficial fascia covering the anterior aspect of the thoracic cage, and in the female usually extend from the level of the second or third rib to the level of the sixth. The hemispherical shadow of the female breast is cast over that of the pectoralis major muscle (Fig. 10–41 *B*), and together they form a notable haziness that may obscure to a great extent the lung substance proper. At the level of the fourth or fifth rib, the nipple, in turn, may cast an even denser shadow than that of the breast (Fig. 10–41 *C*), and has the ap-

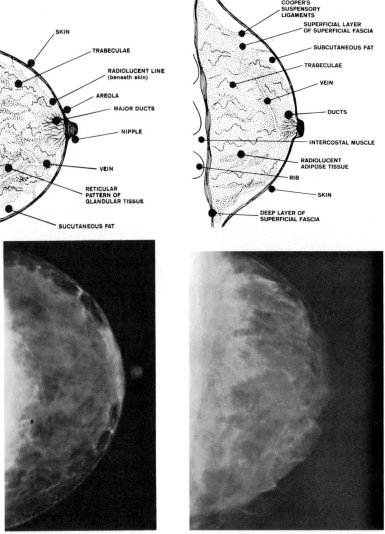

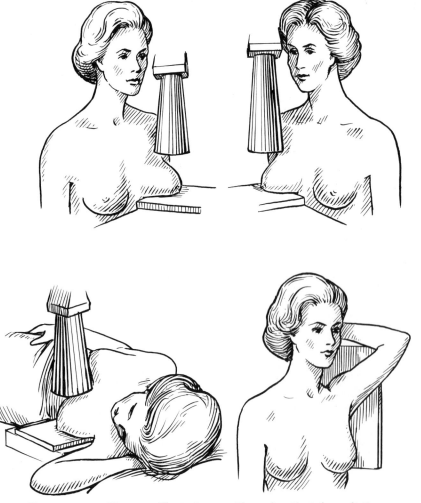

Figure 10–42. Diagrams illustrating position of patient for soft tissue mammography.

Figure 10–43. Representative mammograms in the craniocaudad (*left*) and mediolateral (*right*) projections and labeled line drawings of each. (From Egan, R. L.: Mammography, 1964. Courtesy of Charles C Thomas, Publisher, Springfield, Illinois.)

Figure 10–43 continued on the opposite page.

pearance of a rather dense nodule. Occasionally the areola around the nipple may also be distinguished. Of course, the size and shape of the breasts vary considerably among both women and men, and will vary in the same woman according to the physiologic state of the breast.

The breast may be investigated radiographically in several ways: (1) soft tissue study tangential to the breast (Figs. 10–42 and 10–43); (2) study of the breast following injection of CO_2 into tissues around the breast (Fig. 10–44); and (3) injection of opaque media into the lactiferous ducts (Fig. 10–45).

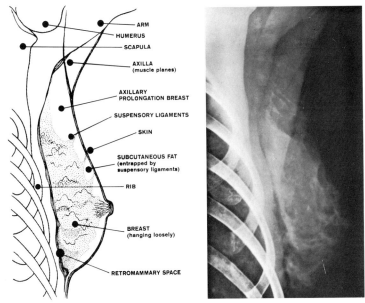

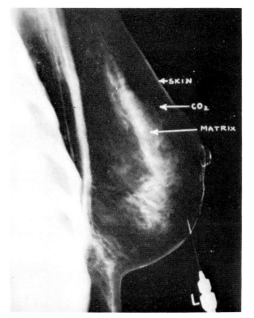

Figure 10–43 *Continued.* Representative mammogram in the axillary projection with labeled line drawing. (From Egan, R. L.: Mammography. 1964. Courtesy of Charles C Thomas, Publisher, Springfield, Illinois.)

Figure 10–44. Study of breast following injection of soft tissues with air. (From N. F. Hicken et al., Amer. J. Roentgenol., *39*, 1938.)

The main purpose of these studies is to demonstrate abnormal mass lesions within the breast.

Muscular Tissues. The following muscles of the thoracic cage may produce a shadow upon the radiograph: (1) the pectoralis major and minor; (2) the sternocleidomastoid; (3) the serratus anterior; and (4) the intercostal muscles (may be seen on oblique views of the ribs and chest). Their importance lies chiefly in the fact that they must be differentiated from abnormal shadows in the chest. By the injection of air, these muscle shadows can be delineated more clearly.

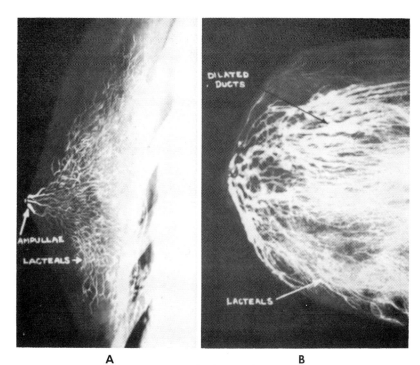

Figure 10–45. Radiographs of breast after injection of the ducts with lipiodol. *A.* Virginal breast. *B.* Multiparous breast.

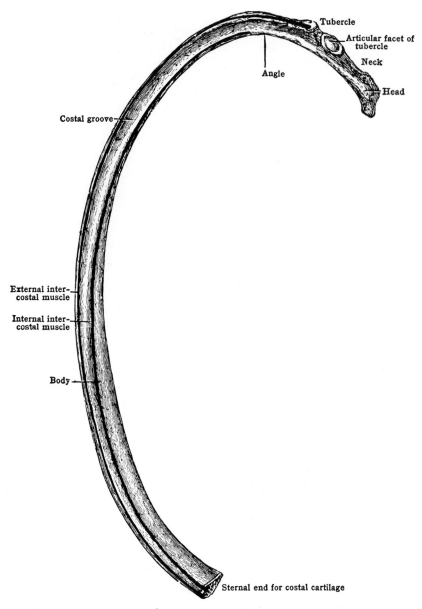

Figure 10-46.   Anatomic drawing of a typical rib. (From Anson, B. J. (ed.): Morris' Human Anatomy, 12th ed. Copyright © 1966 by McGraw-Hill, Inc. Used by permission of McGraw-Hill Book Company.)

The Ribs

Gross Anatomy Related to Radiographic Anatomy.   The typical rib (Fig. 10–46) consists of a head, neck, tubercle, body or shaft, and costal cartilage. The body has an angle and a costal groove. The heads of the upper nine ribs articulate with two thoracic vertebrae—the one with which each rib is in numerical correspondence, and the one above. Each rib has two articular facets for this purpose. The tenth, eleventh, and twelfth ribs have only one articulation, and articulate with only one vertebral body.

Anatomic Features of Radiographic Significance.   The inferior aspect of the neck may have a notched appearance (Fig. 10–47), and this notching must not be confused with the abnormal notching and undulation that occur more peripherally in association with dilated intercostal arteries (as in coarctation of the aorta) (Fig. 10–48 *A, B, C, D*).

The inferior margin of the rib where the costal groove is identified may have a somewhat irregular appearance, particularly at the angle of the rib. This irregularity at the angle is due to the fact that the bone is slightly thickened in this location (Fig. 10–49).

There is usually a slight widening of the rib as it joins the costal cartilage, and a ring-like shadow may be seen in this location (see Fig. 10–50 *A* and *B*). This slight flare of the ribs must not be confused with the abnormal rosary which occurs in vitamin D deficiency in children (Fig. 10–50 *C*).

When it is desired to differentiate any of these soft tissue structures, it is well to mark or delineate the structures with wire, and compare a radiograph so obtained with one obtained without the delineation. This permits the radiologist to distinguish at a glance the cause of the shadow.

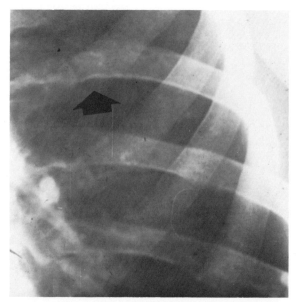

Figure 10-47.   Magnified view of neck of rib to show normal concavity.

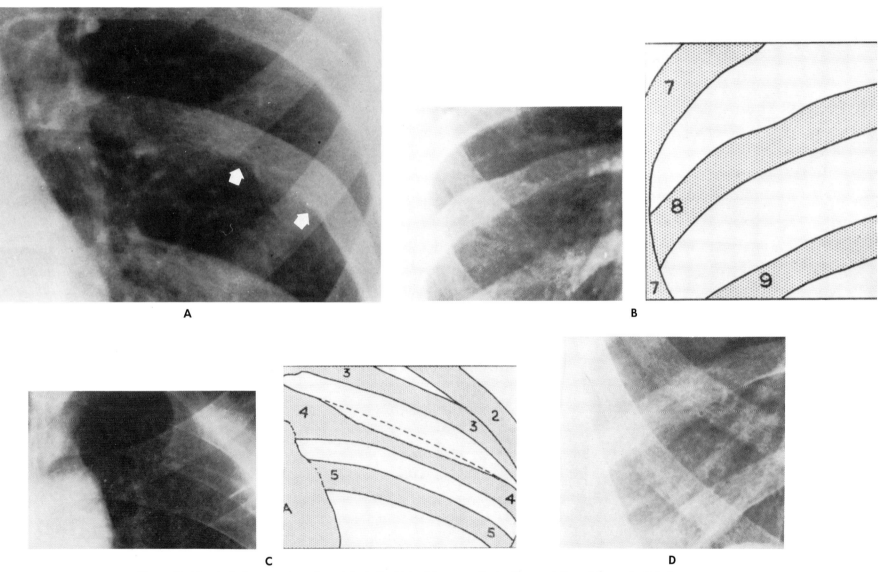

Figure 10–48. *A.* A close-up view of a notched rib obtained from a patient with coarctation of the aorta. *B. Left,* Shallow indentation of posterior aspect of eighth rib as often seen in healthy individuals. Note sharp cortical margin. *Right,* Diagram of left radiograph. *C.* Varying extent of erosion of the upper cortical rib margin. Note fuzzy outline of lesions. *Left,* Shallow, long erosion of left fourth rib. *Right,* Diagram of radiograph. *D.* Short, shallow erosions of right ninth rib. (*B, C,* and *D* from Noetzl, M., and Steinbach, H. L.: Amer. J. Roentgenol., *87:* 1058, 1962.)

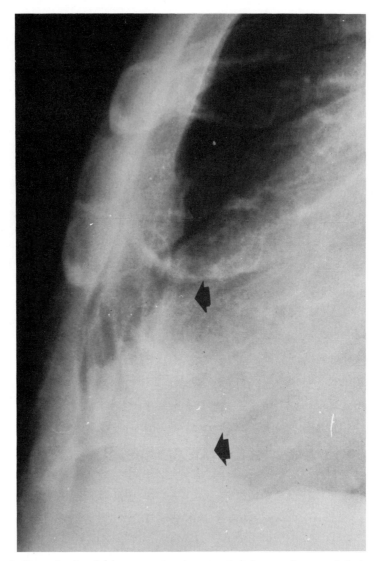

Figure 10–49. Radiograph of a rib, demonstrating the normal slight irregularity and thickening at its angle.

The gas shadows over ribs are very disturbing at times, and make a study of bony detail extremely difficult. These gas shadows must not be confused with areas of true bone absorption or replacement.

The last rib may simulate a transverse process of the lumbar spine, but can be identified frequently by its articulation with the twelfth thoracic vertebra. This transition between the ribs and the transverse processes of the lumbar vertebrae is usually a gradual one, and is exemplified in the anatomic changes visible in the last three thoracic ribs.

Mode of Radiographic Examination of the Ribs.   Ribs may be studied in any of the routine radiographs of the chest. Ordinarily, however, for greatest accuracy, special studies of the ribs are desirable. These are obtained by placing the ribs in question in various degrees of obliquity (essentially the same as that shown in Fig. 10–53), centering over the area of maximum suspicion and obtaining movable grid films. Usually at least three such views are obtained. *It is not unusual to find that routine radiographs of the chest are inadequate for rib detail, and that the study is considerably better when done as a special or separate procedure*

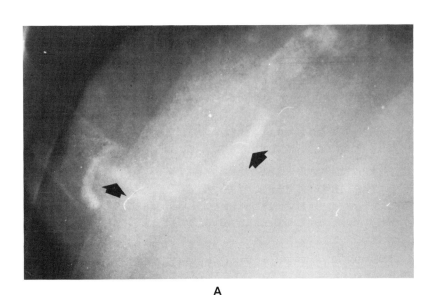

A

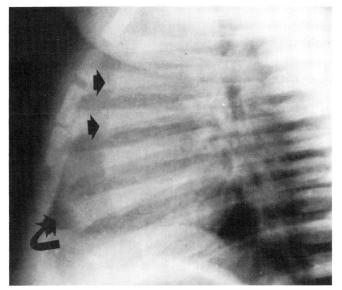

B

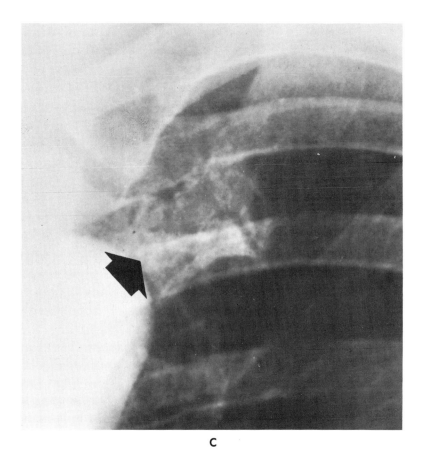

C

Figure 10–50. *A.* Calcified costal cartilage, lower chest. *B.* Costochondral junctions in a newborn infant as seen in lateral view. The curvilinear area is the costochondral junction farthest from the film, whereas the straight areas are those closest to the film. *C.* Calcified costochondral cartilage in the upper chest adjoining the manubrium.

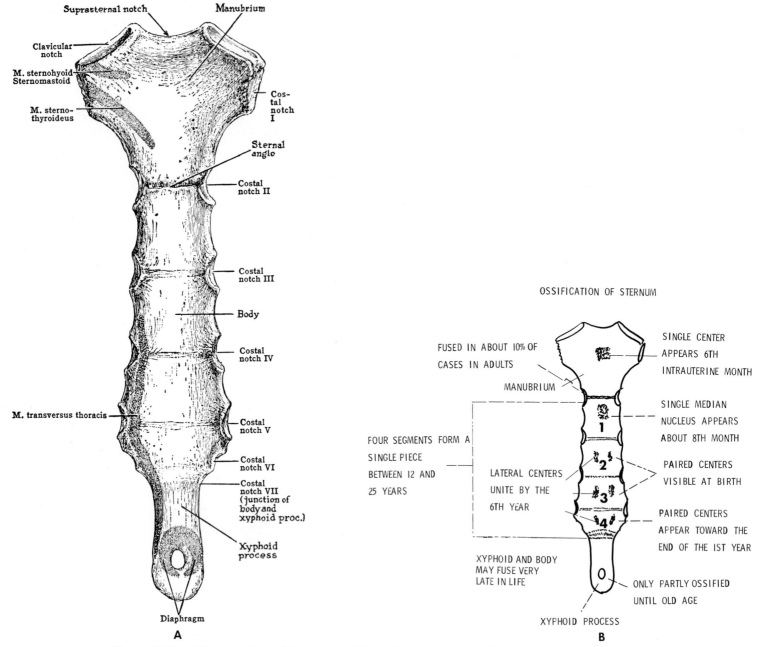

OSSIFICATION OF STERNUM

Figure 10–51.   *A.* Gross anatomy of the sternum. (Adapted from Anson, B. J. (ed.): Morris' Human Anatomy, 12th ed. Copyright © 1966 by McGraw-Hill, Inc. Used by permission of McGraw-Hill Book Company.) *B.* Ossification of sternum.

The Sternum

Gross Anatomy and Correlated Radiographic Anatomy. The sternum consists of the manubrium, body, and xiphoid process. The body in youth consists of four segments. The manubrium ordinarily is united with the sternal body by a cartilaginous union only, until old age. The manubrium has a suprasternal notch (Fig. 10–51), a clavicular articular surface on either side for articulation with the clavicle, and a rough portion just below the clavicular articulation where the cartilage of the first rib is implanted.

The angle between the body of the sternum and the manubrium is called the sternal angle, and the cartilage of the second rib joins the sternum at this point.

The body of the sternum is composed of four segments that fuse in adolescence, leaving a transverse ridge at each site of fusion. There are small protuberances on either side of the sternum at these junction lines, and the rib cartilages for the third, fourth, and fifth ribs join the sternum at these protuberances.

The seventh rib cartilages join the sternum at the junction of the body and xiphoid process, and the sixth rib cartilages join the sternum slightly above this level.

The upper margin of the manubrium is at the level of the lower border of the body of the second thoracic vertebra; the sternal angle, with the upper border of the body of the fifth thoracic vertebra; and the xiphoid process, with the eighth or ninth thoracic vertebra (Fig. 10–52).

With the exception of the manubrium, the sternum will ordinarily not be visible on straight posteroanterior views of the chest, and requires special projections for the demonstration of its radiographic anatomy (Fig. 10–53).

Variations with Growth and Development (Figs. 10–51 *B*, 10–54). Ordinarily, there are one or two centers of ossification already present and ossified at birth for four of the segments of the sternum. The paired centers of the fourth segment of the body of the sternum appear toward the end of the first year of life, but the center of ossification for the xiphoid process usually does not appear until about 3 years of age.

The segments of the body of the sternum unite from below upward. First the paired lateral centers unite with one another by the sixth year. Then the four segments of the body form a single bony piece between 12 and 25 years. The manubrium and body fuse in about 10 per cent of adults, and the body and xiphoid process fuse late in life in about 30 per cent of adults. The xiphoid process may remain only partly ossified until old age (Anson; Gabrielsen and Ladyman).

Generally, the enchondral ossification of the sternum is very slow and irregular.

These normal lines of fusion of the various segments must not be confused with fractures.

Modes of Radiographic Examination. *1. Oblique View of the Sternum* (Fig. 10–53). Since the sternum overlies the heart and mediastinal structures, it must be projected away from these structures to be visualized radiographically. Either oblique projection may be employed as illustrated. In either case, the lung structures are projected over the sternum, so that bony texture is very difficult to evaluate accurately. Gross abnormalities are readily manifest, but minute changes in the sternum can escape detection.

The manner in which the film is obtained, and the associated anatomy are shown in Figure 10–53.

2. Lateral View of the Sternum (Fig. 10–55). This view is particularly helpful since it shows the structure of the sternum

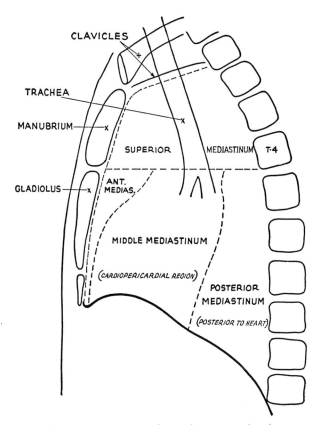

Figure 10–52. The compartments of the mediastinum, also demonstrating the usual topographic relationship of the sternum to the spine.

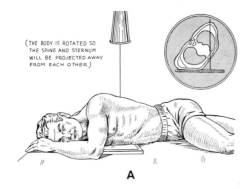

(THE BODY IS ROTATED SO THE SPINE AND STERNUM WILL BE PROJECTED AWAY FROM EACH OTHER.)

A

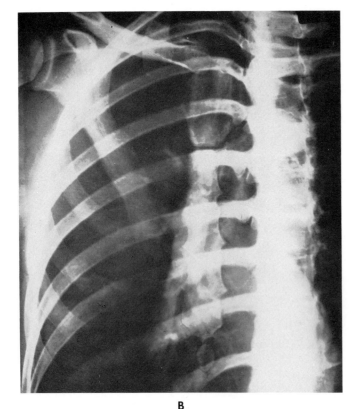

B

Figure 10–53. Oblique view of sternum and sternoclavicular joints (also ribs). *A*. Position of patient similar in both. *B*. Radiograph of sternum. *C*. Labeled tracing of *B*.

Figure 10–53 continued on the opposite page.

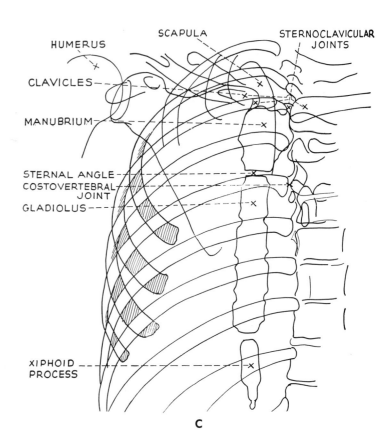

C

Points of Practical Interest With Reference to Figure 10–53, and Comments Relating to Body Section Radiography of the Sternum

1. Sometimes the sternum is difficult to visualize with sufficient clarity in this view. Under these circumstances, body section radiography is recommended. The best technique for this is as follows:
   (a) A mobile cart is placed at right angles to the x-ray table, and the patient lies prone on the cart, with his chest overlapping the table, so that he is as nearly as possible *perpendicular to the x-ray table.*
   (b) *The long axis of the sternum is therefore in contact with the surface of the x-ray table but at right angles to the long axis of this table.*
   (c) The cassette is placed in the tray so that its long axis corresponds to that of the sternum.
   (d) The body section study is thereafter made in the usual manner, and two or three "cuts" may be made.

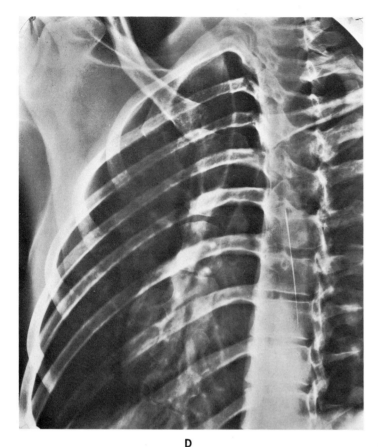

D

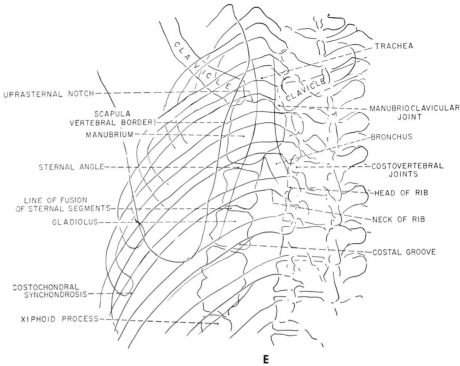

E

Figure **10–53** *Continued.* D. Radiograph of sternoclavicular joints. E. Labeled tracing of D.

without the interference of overlying structures. This is only one perspective, however, and one cannot ordinarily obtain a clear anatomic concept from one projection alone. Moreover, in certain people, the sternum is somewhat depressed and the ribs overlie the sternum in considerable part. It is most difficult to obtain a clear idea of the structure of the sternum in such people.

This view is also valuable since it shows the relationship of the sternum to the underlying structures.

The method by which this view is obtained, along with film and tracing, are illustrated in Figure 10–55.

3. Body Section Radiographs of the Sternum (Fig. 10–56). Body section radiographs must frequently be employed to obtain an unobstructed view of the sternum. A much more detailed visualization of the bony texture and structure can thus be obtained. Several sections are necessary, and caution must be used in interpretation since the entire sternum is not visualized at one level.

A study of the bony texture of the sternum is of particular interest and importance since the sternal marrow is one of the important hematopoietic organs, and as such can be readily affected by diseases of the blood-forming apparatus, lymphoid structures, or any of the cellular components of the marrow.

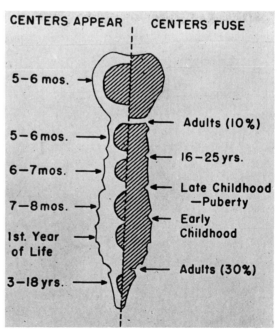

Figure **10–54.** Ossification and fusion of the various sternebrae (infant and adult sternum) (Also see Fig. 10–51 A). (From Currarino, G., and Silverman, F. N.: Radiology, *70:*532–540, 1958.)

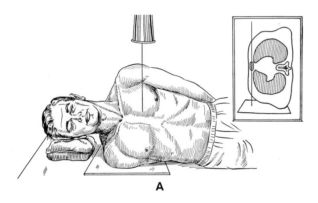

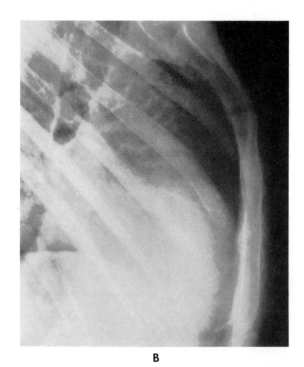

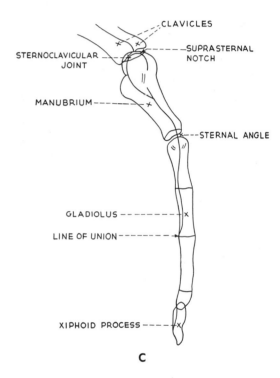

Figure 10–55. Lateral view of sternum. *A.* Position of patient. *B.* Radiograph. *C.* Labeled tracing of *B.*

Points of Practical Interest With Reference to Figure 10–55

1. This view of the sternum gives us maximum clarity of the sternum, but unfortunately has the following disadvantages:
   (a) When the sternum is depressed at all, it is concealed behind the costal cartilages and some lung in this projection. This is especially true of the condition called "pectus excavatum."
   (b) Abnormalities which do not affect the entire width of the sternum may be obscured by the unaffected portion. Body section radiographs are helpful when this is suspected.
   (c) The various segments of the sternum must be recognized and differentiated from other abnormalities which may be stimulated at the costosternal junctions.
2. The retrosternal mediastinal and pleural shadows should always be examined very carefully. This is also true of the shadows which are superficial to the sternum. The clue to abnormality is often found here where it may escape detection by inspection of the sternal shadow only.

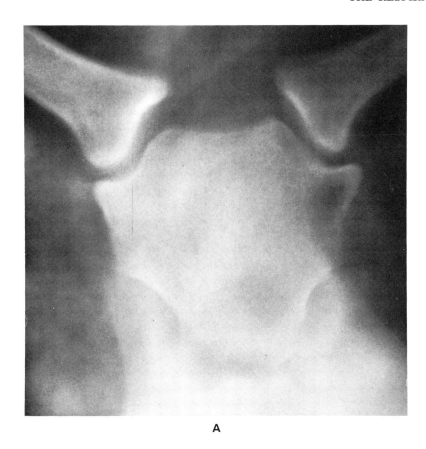

A

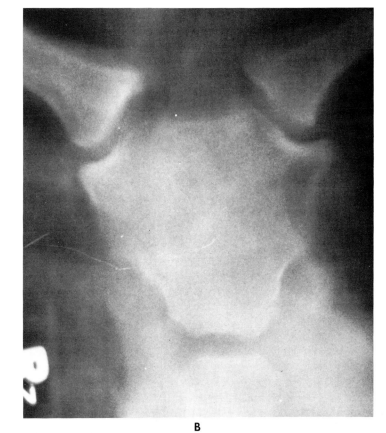

B

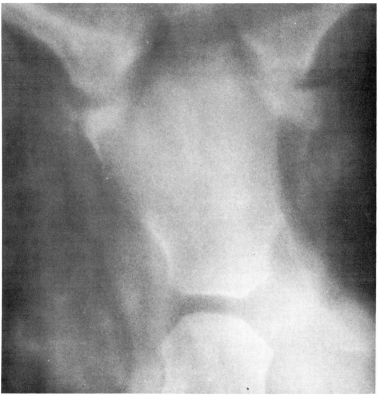

C

Figure 10–56. *A* and *B*. Tomographs of manubrium. *C*. Tomograph of sterno-manubrial junction.

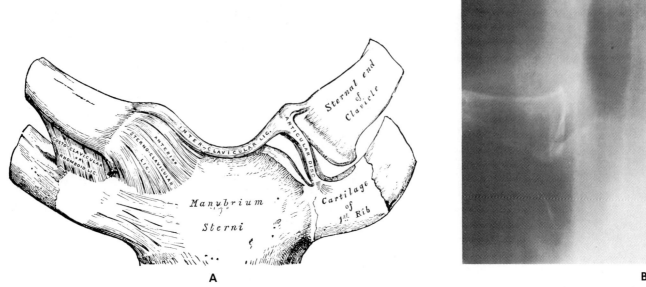

Figure 10–57.   A. Gross anatomy of sternoclavicular joint. (From Gray's Anatomy of the Human Body, 29th ed. Goss, C. M. (ed.) Philadelphia, Lea & Febiger, 1973.) B. Body section radiograph of the sternoclavicular joints. This is obtained in the prone position, centering over the sternoclavicular joints.

Sternoclavicular Joints (Fig. 10–57).   The sternoclavicular joint is a two-chambered synovial or diarthrodial joint with an articular disk between the two chambers. Each chamber is usually distinct and separate from the others, unless the articular disk happens to be unusually thin (as in the case of the temporomandibular joint).

These joints are usually demonstrated on oblique projections such as those employed for the sternum proper (Fig. 10–53), except that the tube is centered over the joint. *A comparison film of the opposite side is always obtained so that the two sternoclavicular joints can be compared in the same patient.*

The Pleura

Gross Anatomic Features as Applied to Radiographic Anatomy.   The pleura lines the entire thoracic cavity and invests the entire lung, and invaginations of the pleura form the interlobar fissures. That portion lining the thoracic cavity is called the *parietal pleura,* and that investing the lung is called the *visceral pleura.* The interlobar fissures are formed by invagination into the lung of two closely approximated layers of visceral pleura.

The lines of pleural reflection do not accurately correspond on the two sides of the thorax. These lines of reflection also vary in different subjects, depending upon body habitus.

The pleura is composed of a layer of endothelial cells resting on a membrane of connective tissue, within which are situated blood vessels, lymphatics, and nerves.

There is a thin layer of serous fluid between the two opposing layers of pleura ordinarily, with a slow and steady filtration and absorption occurring normally. The visceral pleural blood supply is obtained from the bronchial arteries as previously indicated, whereas the parietal pleura is supplied by systemic arteries that are branches of the subclavian artery and thoracic aorta. Also, the reader is referred to the previous discussion of the lymphatics in connection with the lung. The superficial lymphatics drain the visceral pleura outward, and communicate by means of short tributaries with the deep lymphatics that drain in the opposite direction toward the lung hilus. The parietal lymphatics do not drain directly into the hilar lymph nodes but rather into the lymph trunks at the junction of the internal jugular and subclavian veins.

Ordinarily, the pleura does not cast a significant radiographic shadow, except perhaps minimally in the costophrenic angles. When the pleural shadow can be identified, it is usually indicative of an abnormality.

There are usually small blebs or ruptured alveoli at the lung apices (Cunningham) which cast a shadow on the chest radiograph (Fig. 10–58). This may simulate pleural disease and must not be confused with an abnormal appearance of the pleura or lungs in this location.

Ordinarily, the costophrenic angles are sharply delineated, and any significant degree of blunting is indicative of previous

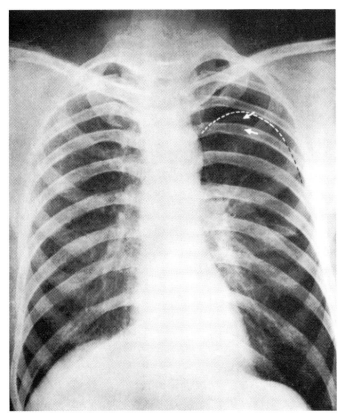

Figure 10–58. Chest film to demonstrate small blebs or ruptured alveoli at lung apices: chest film of patient with spontaneous rupture into the pleural space of one of these blebs on the left. There are similar blebs in the right apex.

pleural disease; since these areas represent the most dependent portions of the pleura, disease is readily seen in these locations.

The cardiophrenic angles, however, vary considerably in appearance, and although the reflection of the pleura is normally sharp in this location also, a greater variability exists in the appearance of the pleural shadow here. An increased acuity of the appearance of this angle is of significance in detecting excessive fluid within the pericardial space, and thus an accurate conception of these angles must be constantly borne in mind.

The Diaphragm

Composition and Normal Attachments of the Diaphragm. The diaphragm consists of a peripheral muscular portion that completely surrounds an aponeurotic membrane and arches over the abdominal contents, separating the abdomen from the chest. There is extensive peripheral attachment to the xiphoid process, the lower six costal cartilages, the ribs, the first three lumbar vertebrae on the right side, and the first two on the left side. With varying degrees of curvature, the fibers arch centrally

and end in the central tendon. This latter tendon is more anterior than posterior and thus is not truly central. It is incompletely divided into three lobes or leaflets. The middle one is anterior and intermediate in size, whereas the right lateral one is the largest and the left lateral the smallest. The crura of the diaphragm are two elongated musculotendinous bundles that arise on each side of the aorta and are partly separated from the lumbar vertebrae by the upper lumbar arteries, but are firmly attached to the upper three vertebrae on the right and the upper two on the left. There is a tendency for the cupola of the diaphragm to descend with age (Fig. 10–59).

Normal Openings in the Diaphragm (Fig. 10–60). The diaphragm is pierced by numerous structures: the superior epigastric artery, the musculophrenic artery, the splanchnic nerves, and the sympathetic trunks behind; the aorta, azygos vein, and thoracic duct passing between the crura; the inferior vena cava,

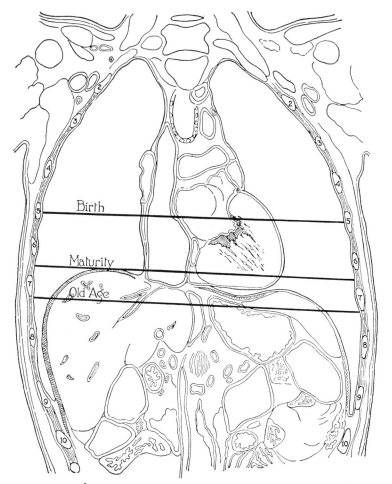

Figure 10–59. Diaphragm at various ages. (From Scamon, in Meyers and McKinlay, The Chest and the Heart, Charles C Thomas, Publishers.)

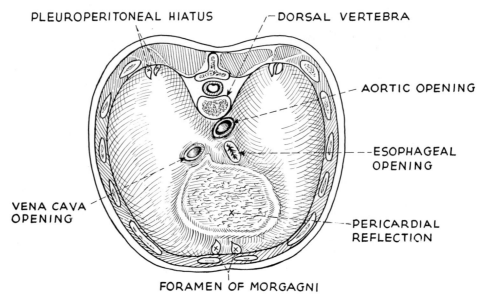

PLEUROPERITONEAL HIATUS   DORSAL VERTEBRA

AORTIC OPENING

ESOPHAGEAL
OPENING

VENA CAVA
OPENING

PERICARDIAL
REFLECTION

FORAMEN OF MORGAGNI

Figure 10-60.   Normal openings of the diaphragm.

and small branches of the right phrenic nerve passing through the foramen venae cavae; and the esophageal opening, transmitting the esophagus and two vagus nerves.

Three-Dimensional Concept of the Diaphragm (Fig. 10–61). The posterior attachment of the diaphragm is considerably lower than the anterior, and there is much lung substance and diaphragm which cannot be seen from the posteroanterior projection.

Moreover, much of the pleural space is likewise obscured from view by virtue of the attachments of the diaphragm. For that reason, it is important to attempt to visualize the structures behind it and frequently to obtain lateral and oblique projections.

Occasionally, the diaphragm may have a slightly irregular appearance, and by projection, a structure which actually lies beneath the diaphragm will be projected above a portion of it. Every effort must be made to obviate such projection phenomena and understand them when they occur.

Tenting and Scalloping of the Diaphragm.   Occasionally, the contour of the diaphragm is broken into two or more arches, the outlines appearing as a scalloped margin (Fig. 10–62). This is usually caused by an irregular contraction of the diaphragmatic musculature, and usually these irregularities become less evident in expiration.

Occasionally, several peaks are present on the diaphragmatic surface that are likewise due to the rib attachments of the diaphragm. Occasionally, these are due to abnormal pleurodiaphragmatic adhesions, and the two processes must not be confused. This is spoken of as "tenting" of the diaphragm.

Overlapping Shadows Due to Diaphragm, Liver, and Heart Anteriorly (Fig. 10–63).   The anteromedian part of the diaphragmatic dome, the heart shadow, and the anterior margin of the

liver overlap one another in the lateral projection, producing a triangular shadow that may be confused with an interlobar effusion or consolidation of the inferior portion of the right middle lobe. Care must be exercised not to make this error of interpretation.

Roentgen Significance of the Transverse Thoracis Muscle (Shopfner et al.).   The transverse thoracis muscle is the plane of muscular and tendinous fibers and muscle situated on the front wall of the thoracic cage (Fig. 10–63 B). It originates on either side from the lower third of the posterior surface of the sternal body xiphoid process and medial ends of the costal cartilages of the lower three or four true ribs. It is inserted by slips into the lower borders and inner surface of the costal cartilages of the second, third, fourth, fifth, and sixth ribs. Usually, it is directed obliquely downward, producing a density of varying size and contour in the lateral chest roentgenogram that may cause difficulty in differential diagnosis since it may resemble a retrosternal mass (Fig. 10–63 C and D).

The thickness of the muscle varies, depending upon the size of the patient, between 2 and 4 mm. Its appearance varies somewhat, depending upon the degree of rotation of the patient from the true lateral. It is ordinarily not visualized in oblique projections of 45 to 60 degrees. Actually, perfectly positioned lateral roentgenograms likewise do not show this shadow, which is apparent only when there is a slight rotation from the true lateral position which throws this muscle into relief. It is not important except that it should be recognized as a normal anatomic structure not to be confused with possible pathologic entities. Generally, a true lateral view with expiration can prevent its visualization since it blends imperceptibly with the

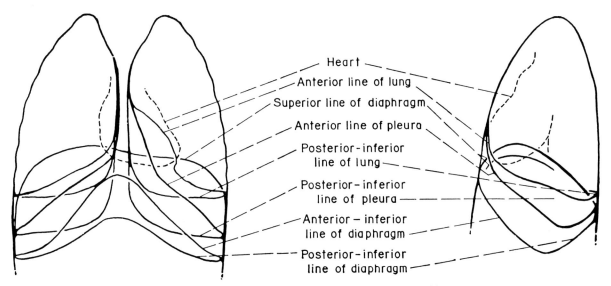

Figure 10–61. Isometric concept of the diaphragm on frontal and lateral views.

shadow of the sternum. Slight obliquity and deep inspiration allow the lower portion of the muscle to appear on one side as a linear density. Differentiation can thereby be achieved with reasonable accuracy.

Diaphragmatic Movements. On quiet breathing, the range of motion of the diaphragm is about 1 to 2 cm. On deep breathing it will increase to 3 to 5 cm., or even somewhat more. There is usually an accompanying flare of the ribs upward and outward (Fig 10–64). Occasionally, half of the diaphragm will move somewhat more than the other, or in slightly different sequence, but marked differences in any area of the diaphragm or inequalities between the two sides are of definite pathologic significance.

The diaphragmatic position at rest is also of considerable im-

portance, whether it be elevated or depressed, and localized elevations are likewise noteworthy, since they may be related to masses underlying the diaphragm.

ROUTINE POSITIONS IN THE RADIOGRAPHY OF THE CHEST

Chest Fluoroscopy. Fluoroscopy offers the first mode of examination of the chest. However, for consistent demonstration of fine detail, for avoidance of considerable magnification, and for the sake of permanent record and future comparison, radiography has no substitute.

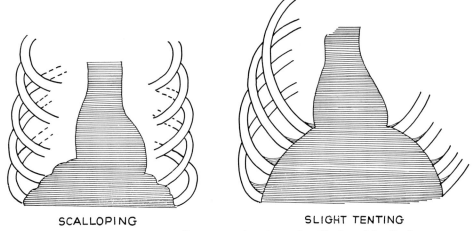

SCALLOPING   SLIGHT TENTING

Figure 10–62. Diagrammatic illustration of tenting and scalloping of the diaphragm.

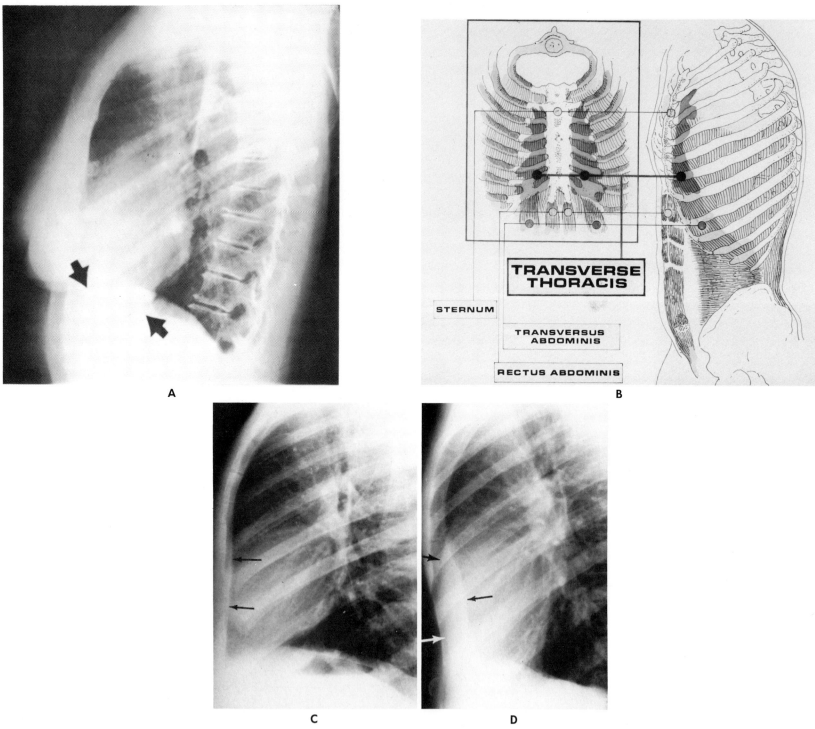

Figure 10–63. *A.* Lateral view of the chest, demonstrating a rather dense ovoid area produced by overlapping shadows of the heart, liver, and diaphragm anteroinferiorly. This must not be confused with an interlobar effusion. *B.* Artist's sketch of transverse thoracis muscle showing its relationship to other anatomic structures in the anteroposterior and lateral views. *C.* True lateral chest roentgenogram of 7-year-old female. The transverse thoracis muscle shows a thin strip of density (arrows) contiguous to the sternum. *D.* Same patient as in *C.* Slight rotation from the true lateral position causes the origin and lowest inserting fibers of the muscle to cast a triangular density (arrows). Only slight rotation from the true lateral is necessary to produce the density because of the sternal width being interposed between the muscle of the two sides. (*B, C,* and *D* from Shopfner, C. E., Jansen, C., and O'Kell, R. J.: Amer. J. Roentgenol., *103*:140–148, 1968.)

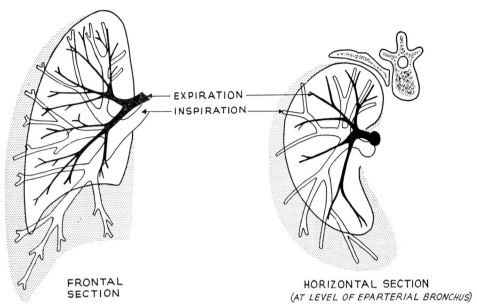

EXPIRATION
INSPIRATION

FRONTAL
SECTION

HORIZONTAL SECTION
(*AT LEVEL OF EPARTERIAL BRONCHUS*)

Figure 10–64. Longitudinal and transverse sections through thorax, showing mode of expansion of lungs with respiration. (After Caffey, J.: Pediatric X-ray Diagnosis, 6th ed. Springfield, Illinois, Charles C Thomas, 1972.)

A very useful routine to follow in fluoroscopy of the chest is as follows:

1. Notation of the position and contour of the trachea and larynx, in phonation and at rest.
2. Detection of the movement and symmetry of the two halves of the diaphragm.
3. Notation of the clarity of the costophrenic and cardiophrenic angles.
4. Examination of the lung fields, bilaterally, for notation of any differences in clarity of the two sides.
5. Examination of the lung apices, requesting the patient to move his scapula forward so as to improve the visibility of the lung apices.
6. Notation of the type of rib movement and flare with respiration.
7. Simultaneously, the heart and mediastinum must also be studied, as well as the esophagus in its entirety. (These structures will be described subsequently.)

Fluoroscopy has the great advantage of offering the immediate opportunity of turning the patient in any degree of obliquity, or into the erect or recumbent positions. Spatial relationships as well as physiologic function are thus elucidated.

It has the disadvantage of requiring the exposure of the radiologist as well as the patient to considerably greater x-ray exposure than would be necessary by the film studies alone. Even though we may be well below presently considered tolerance levels for exposure to x-ray irradiation, any exposure must be regarded as potentially dangerous.

Posteroanterior View of the Chest (Fig. 10–65). This view is ordinarily obtained with a 6-foot film-target distance so that it can be utilized for study of cardiac size and contour as well. The patient's shoulders are rotated forward so that the scapulas are projected away from the lung fields, and the patient is asked to stop respiration after full inspiration and hold his breath for the film in inspiration, and similarly to stop respiration after forced exhalation for the film in expiration. Both of these studies have definite characteristics. The film in inspiration will show the aerated lung to best advantage, and if there are any unaerated portions, they can be demonstrated by contrast. The film in expiration, on the other hand, will demonstrate any areas that are unusually well aerated. In either case, the mediastinum will normally remain stationary, but abnormally it will shift to one side or the other if unfixed by disease. The excursion of the diaphragm in the two phases of respiration may also be studied in this manner.

Films in both inspiration and expiration (exhalation) are particularly valuable in children. Needless to say, it is not always possible to time the exposure in a child or infant exactly as one would desire it. The value of these views in children is as follows: (1) the history in relation to a child's chest abnormality is notoriously poor, since often it is obtained from the parent who may be unaware of the fact that the child may have inhaled a foreign body; (2) the two frontal views of the chest, even though they may not be perfectly timed in relation to inspiration or expiration, usually supplement one another in any case in an area of difficult diagnosis. Sometimes one of the films is

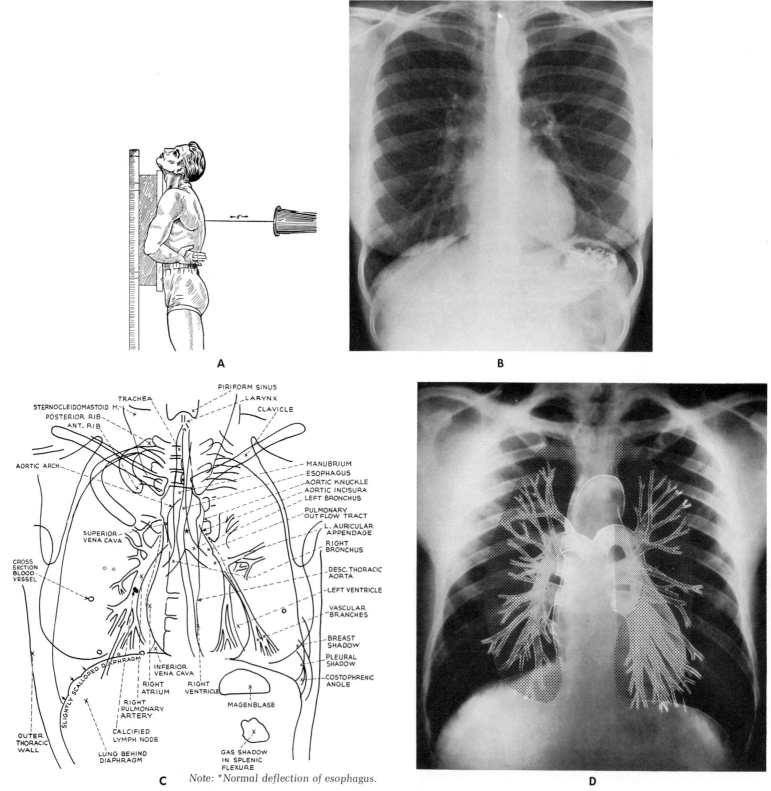

Figure 10–65.   Posteroanterior view of chest. *A*. Position of patient. *B*. Radiograph (female). *C*. Labeled tracing of *B*. *D*. Normal radiograph of chest showing three zones of study in the parenchyma.

faulty because of motion on the film or some other feature in the roentgen technique difficult to control in an infant or child. We are then particularly happy to have the two films for comparison. Actually, in infants at least eight ribs should appear above the level of the diaphragm when counted posteriorly in inspiration (White). On the other hand, when nine or more ribs are visible, overinflation, such as may occur with air trapping in bronchiolitis, is to be suspected.

Gross Subdivisions of the Lung Fields (Fig. 10–65). Arbitrarily one can subdivide the lung fields into three zones, depending on the size of the vascular radicles. The vascular branches gradually assume a smaller caliber proceeding from the hilus to the lung periphery. The inner one-third zone contains the largest channels; the middle one-third zone contains vessels of intermediate size; and the peripheral one-third zone usually has vessels that are 1 mm. or less in diameter. This arbitrary subdivision permits the radiologist to attribute definite significance to shadows that are inordinately large in diameter or size, particularly in the middle and outer zones. (See final section in this chapter: Methods of Studying Radiographs of the Chest.)

Lateral Views of the Chest (Fig. 10–66). When a lateral view of one lung is desired, that side of the patient is placed closest to the film, and the arms are raised out of the projection as much as possible. A relatively close film-to-target distance (36 to 48 inches) is desired in this instance to "blur out" the lung that is farthest from the film.

The anatomic parts are illustrated in Figure 10–67. A detailed discussion of the anatomy will be deferred until after the entire thorax and its contents have been reviewed from the correlated gross anatomic standpoint.

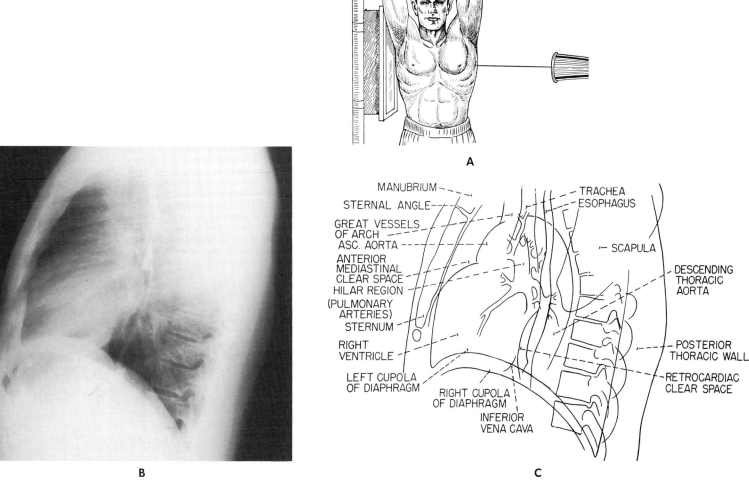

Figure 10–66.   Lateral view of chest. *A.* Position of patient. *B.* Radiograph. *C.* Labeled tracing of *B.*

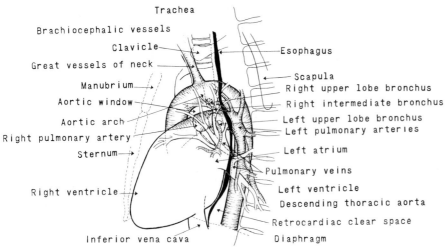

Trachea
Brachiocephalic vessels
Clavicle
Great vessels of neck
Manubrium
Aortic window
Aortic arch
Right pulmonary artery
Sternum
Right ventricle
Inferior vena cava

Esophagus
Scapula
Right upper lobe bronchus
Right intermediate bronchus
Left upper lobe bronchus
Left pulmonary arteries
Left atrium
Pulmonary veins
Left ventricle
Descending thoracic aorta
Retrocardiac clear space
Diaphragm

Figure 10–67.   Lateral view of the chest showing anatomic relationships.

Oblique Views of the Chest (Figs. 10–68 to 10–71).   These projections are obtained by rotating the thorax 45 degrees, with the side in question closest to the film. In posteroanterior oblique views the anterior aspect of the patient is closest to the film. On the other hand, in anteroposterior oblique views the posterior aspect of the patient is closest to the film.

The left posteroanterior oblique view (Fig. 10–69) (or right anteroposterior oblique) is ordinarily best for visualization of the trachea and its bifurcation. A portion of the left lung is obscured by the spine, but other portions of the left lung are seen in better detail. The right posteroanterior (or left anteroposterior) oblique (Figs. 10–70 and 10–71), on the other hand, gives the clearest visualization of the right retrocardiac space and right lung.

Anteroposterior View of the Chest (Fig. 10–72).   This projection has the disadvantage of not permitting the scapulas to be projected out of the lung fields as readily as in the posteroanterior

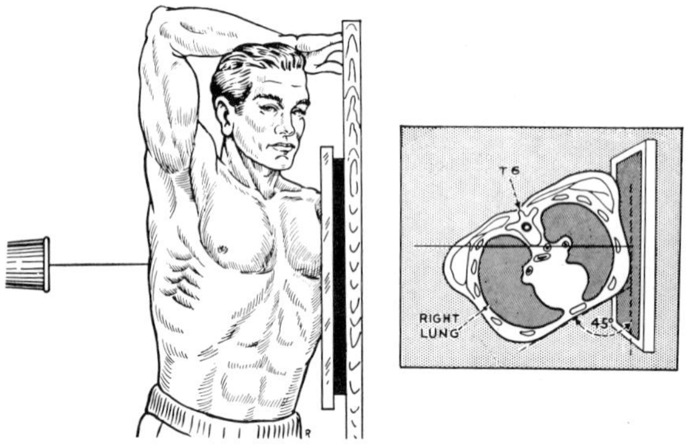

A

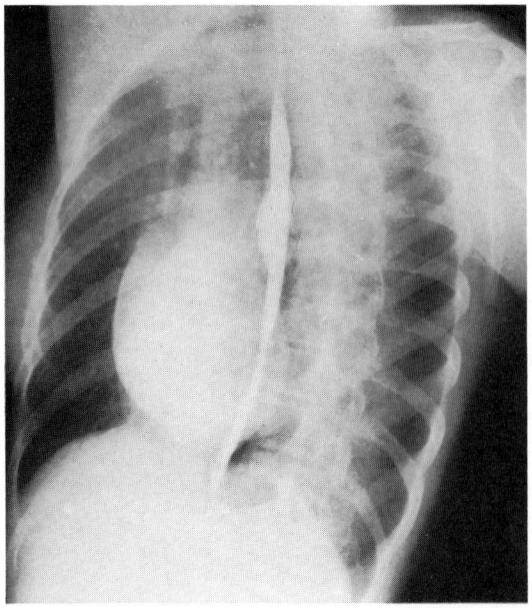

B

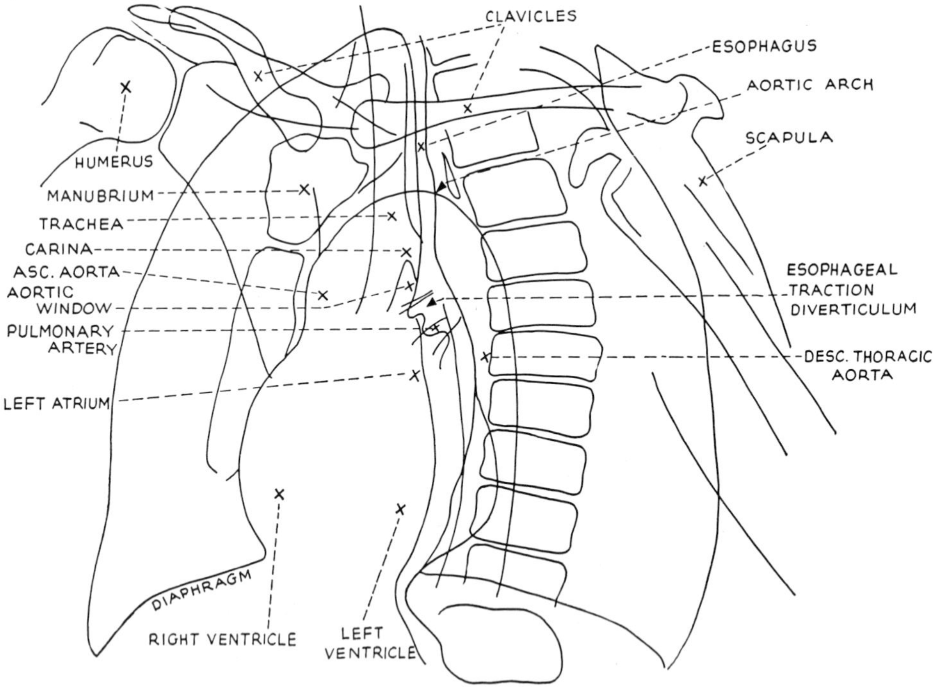

CLAVICLES
ESOPHAGUS
AORTIC ARCH
SCAPULA
HUMERUS
MANUBRIUM
TRACHEA
CARINA
ASC. AORTA
AORTIC WINDOW
PULMONARY ARTERY
ESOPHAGEAL TRACTION DIVERTICULUM
LEFT ATRIUM
DESC. THORACIC AORTA
DIAPHRAGM
RIGHT VENTRICLE
LEFT VENTRICLE

C

Figure 10–68.   Left posteroanterior oblique view of chest. *A.* Position of patient. *B.* Radiograph. *C.* Labeled tracing of *B*.

Points of Practical Interest With Reference to Figure 10–68

1. The 45-degree obliquity may be increased to 50 or 55 degrees on occasion, to obtain maximum clearance of the spine.
2. Ordinarily the left ventricle clears the spine, and the right ventricle forms a smooth uninterrupted convexity with the ascending portion of the arch of the aorta.
3. This view gives maximum clarity of the bifurcation of the trachea, the arch of the aorta, and the posterior basilar portion of the left ventricle. Pulsations are ordinarily of maximum amplitude in this portion of the cardiac silhouette.
4. Although the right ventricle is seen very adequately in most instances in this view, the straight lateral is preferable, since the relationship of the right ventricle to the retrosternal space is more informative. Likewise, the left ventricle is more accurately evaluated in the straight lateral view by noting its relationship to the shadow of the inferior vena cava. It should not normally project more than 5 or 6 mm. beyond this shadow in the lateral projection.

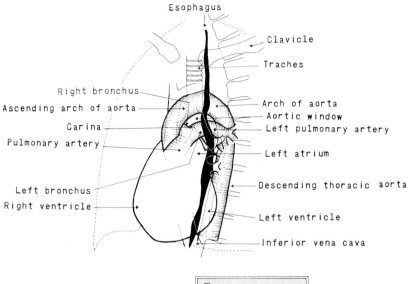

CHEST, LEFT ANTERIOR OBLIQUE
VIEW

Esophagus

Clavicle

Traches

Right bronchus

Ascending arch of aorta

Carina

Pulmonary artery

Left bronchus

Right ventricle

Arch of aorta

Aortic window

Left pulmonary artery

Left atrium

Descending thoracic aorta

Left ventricle

Inferior vena cava

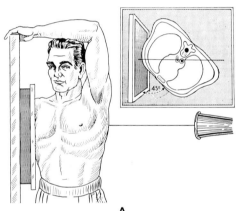

A

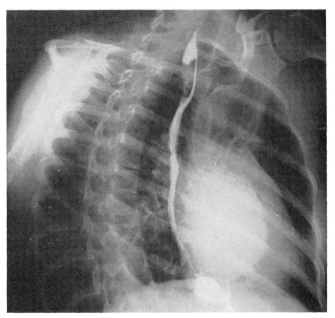

B

Figure 10–69. Left anterior oblique view of the chest showing anatomic relationships.

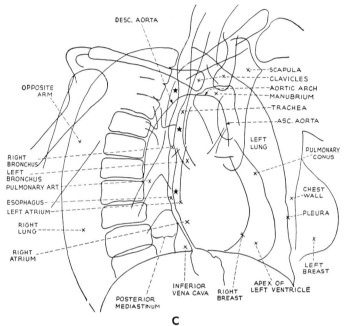

DESC. AORTA

OPPOSITE ARM

RIGHT BRONCHUS
LEFT BRONCHUS
PULMONARY ART.

ESOPHAGUS
LEFT ATRIUM

RIGHT LUNG

RIGHT ATRIUM

SCAPULA
CLAVICLES
AORTIC ARCH
MANUBRIUM
TRACHEA
ASC. AORTA

LEFT LUNG

PULMONARY CONUS

CHEST WALL

PLEURA

LEFT BREAST

POSTERIOR MEDIASTINUM

INFERIOR VENA CAVA

RIGHT BREAST

APEX OF LEFT VENTRICLE

C

Note: *Undulation of esophagus in regions of . . .
1. Above arch of aorta
2. At arch of aorta and pulmonary art.
3. Left atrium (slightly prominent in this case)

Figure 10–70. Right posteroanterior oblique view of chest. *A.* Position of patient. *B.* Radiograph. (The left atrium is enlarged slightly but is shown for demonstration of its indentation upon the esophagus.) *C.* Labeled tracing of *B.*

Points of Practical Interest with Reference to Figure 10–70

1. The patient's right shoulder is placed against the film and the body turned approximately 45 degrees from the film, with the left arm resting in a convenient position, away from the body.
2. The central ray is directed just medial to the scapula nearest the x-ray tube at approximately the level of the sixth or seventh thoracic vertebra.
3. The patient is placed in proper position and then barium paste is administered. He is instructed to swallow and then take a deep breath and hold it while the x-ray exposure is made.
4. The maximum area of the right lung field is demonstrated in this view, but it is partially obscured by the shadow of the spinal column.
5. This view is most advantageous for demonstration of the left atrium and its possible enlargement, since any slight enlargement will cause a significant impression upon the esophagus, as indicated.
6. This view is also valuable for demonstration of the anterior apical portion of the left ventricle, which is most significantly involved in anterior apical myocardial infarction, a rather common disease entity.

CHEST,RIGHT ANTERIOR OBLIQUE
VIEW

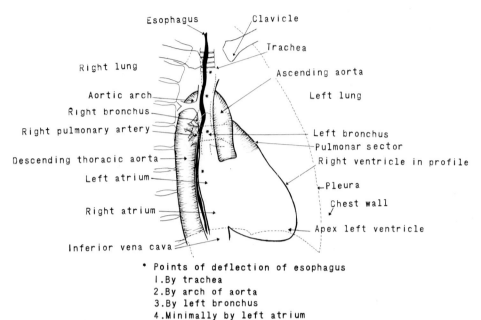

* Points of deflection of esophagus
  1. By trachea
  2. By arch of aorta
  3. By left bronchus
  4. Minimally by left atrium

Figure 10–71.   Normal right anterior oblique view of chest.

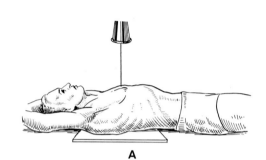

A

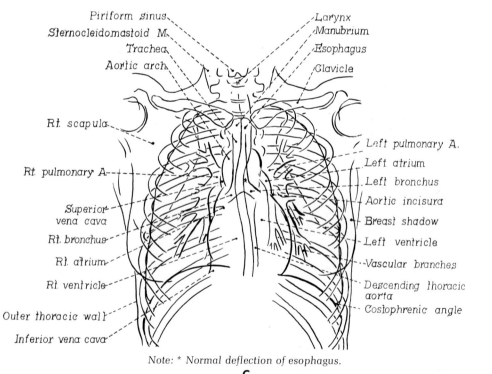

Note: * Normal deflection of esophagus.

B

C

Figure 10–72.   Anteroposterior view of chest. *A.* Position of patient. *B.* Radiograph. The main differences between Figures 10–65 and 10–72 are: (1) the projection of the clavicles; (2) the scapulas are projected over the lung fields in the anteroposterior view; (3) the superior mediastinal structures appear somewhat fuller in the anteroposterior view; (4) the obliquity of the ribs is different. *C.* Labeled tracing of *B.*

projection The clavicle, however, is projected out of the subapical portion of the lung fields, and thus this view has this slight advantage. This projection is usually the only one possible in a very sick patient who cannot sit or stand up, and who cannot be rolled over onto his abdomen readily.

It will be noted that the rib structures have a different appearance in this projection compared with that in the posteroanterior view.

Apical Lordotic View (Fig. 10–73). This projection is particularly useful for clear demonstration of the lung apices and subapical areas. It also has its application in demonstrating the anterior mediastinum tangentially. Distortion of the lower chest areas is maximum in this view.

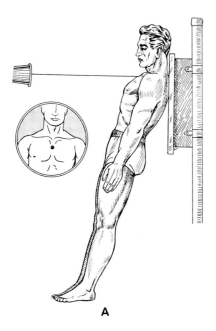

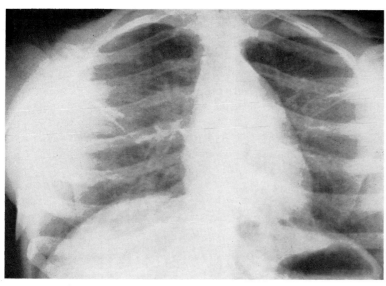

B

Figure 10–73. Apical lordotic view of chest. *A.* Position of patient. *B.* Radiograph. *C.* Labeled tracing of *B.*

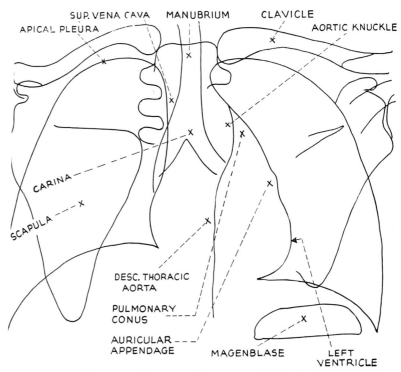

Note: *Apical portion of lung is completely clear*

C

Points of Practical Interest with Reference to Figure 10–73

1. By standing the patient approximately 1 foot in front of the vertical cassette stand and then having him lean directly backward, a proper obliquity of the chest is obtained.
2. The top of the cassette is adjusted so that the upper border of the film is about 1 inch above the shoulders.
3. The central ray passes through the region of the manubrium. Occasionally a slight angle of 5 degrees toward the head may prove to be of advantage in demonstrating the apices more clearly.
4. This view gives a very distorted picture of the lung fields and mediastinum, but is particularly valuable in showing more clearly: (1) the apices; (2) the interlobar areas of the lungs; and (3) the region of the pulmonary sector of the cardiac shadow.

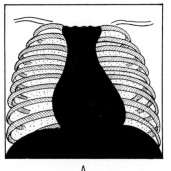 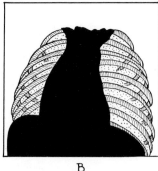 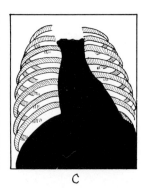

A   B   C

Figure 10–74. Diagram illustrating changes in appearance of mediastinum with position of patient. A. Upright. B. Lying on right side. C. Lying on left side.

Lateral Decubitus Film Studies. By placing the patient on one side or the other and utilizing a horizontal x-ray beam, a posteroanterior projection can be obtained. By gravity, the mediastinal structures will shift downward, and thus show the paramediastinal lung areas to better advantage (Fig. 10–74). If there is any free fluid in the chest, it will shift away from the side of the chest which is uppermost, and thus it is possible to obtain a clearer concept of a portion of lung or pleura that would otherwise be obscured. Also, this method offers an accurate means of estimating small amounts of free pleural fluid that might otherwise escape detection.

It is possible to detect amounts of fluid in excess of (but not less than) 100 cc in this manner, whereas on other conventional views of the chest one cannot ordinarily detect fluid unless it exceeds about 300 cc. in volume.

Air Gap Technique. The air gap technique provides a positioning frame that displaces the patient's chest 6 to 10 inches from the cassette (Fig. 10–75). This has two advantages: (1) The air gap of 6 to 10 inches acts as a filter for secondary radiation, making this procedure a "gridless technique." There are no grid lines to interfere with the interpretation of the film (Watson; Jackson). The air gap roentgenogram is considered by some to be of greater value than the over-penetrated grid roentgenogram on this basis. The kilovoltage is raised to 120 Kv., since lower values are found to give inadequate penetration. Also, the use of these higher voltages reduces the patient's dose (Trout et al.). (2) The air gap roentgenogram may be considered a midchest laminagram since the structures in the midchest are seen in greatest detail, whereas the anterior and posterior chest regions are perhaps diminished in sharpness. Ideally, the distance of the tube-target from the film should be 10 feet for optimum results (3.05 meters).

Most adults require an exposure of 1000 Ma., 120 Kv., and one-40th of a second. Infants and children require an exposure of at least 300 Ma., 110 Kv., and one-60th of a second.

The disadvantage of this technique is that soft pulmonary infiltrates and small densities tend to be obscured. Moreover, a patient with a wide chest is most difficult to fit on the frame, unless the cassette is placed crosswise to the beam. If the anteroposterior position is utilized, it is important to move the scapulae out of the way by special positioning of the patient.

Positive Pressure Radiography. The Valsalva maneuver may be utilized in radiologic diagnosis to increase intrathoracic pressure and lower the effective filling pressure of both cardiac ventricles. This maneuver, originally described by Valsalva in 1704 for use in patients with middle ear disease and tympanic membrane perforation, requires the patient to blow against the closed mouth and nose to aid in diagnosis and therapy. Weber in 1951 emphasized a similar pressure against a closed glottis with its associated alteration in heart sound and pulse. More recently, Whitley and Martin have utilized this procedure as a diagnostic tool in chest disease. A mercury column is positioned so that it is superimposed over the edge of the posteroanterior film of the chest (Fig 10–77), and thus an instantaneous record of the pressure at the moment the film is made is obtained. The exposure is made approximately 5 to 6 seconds after initiation of the patient's positive pressure effort. This timing is important because after 8 to 10 seconds there is a return to normal pressures and cardiac output. The miminum level of intrabronchial pressure to assume a consistent response has been estimated to be between 30 and 40 mm of mercury. A precise level in any individual is determined by his lung compliance, venous pressure, and vasomotor tone. In the overshoot or post-Valsalva maneuver phase following the release of the pressure, the visualization of the enlarged left atrial appendage is improved, as might occur in mitral stenosis. The overshoot phenomenon is best determined approximately 8 to 10 seconds after the cessation of the Valsalva maneuver. During the maneuver, there is a diminution in cardiac size and intrapulmonary vasculature, since cardiac output has been lowered temporarily and visualization of the pulmonary vascular bed and the aorta and its principal branches has been improved by increased aeration of surrounding lung and diminished size of vasculature.

The Valsalva maneuver, as utilized above, has been found useful in the following circumstances: (1) differentiation of en-

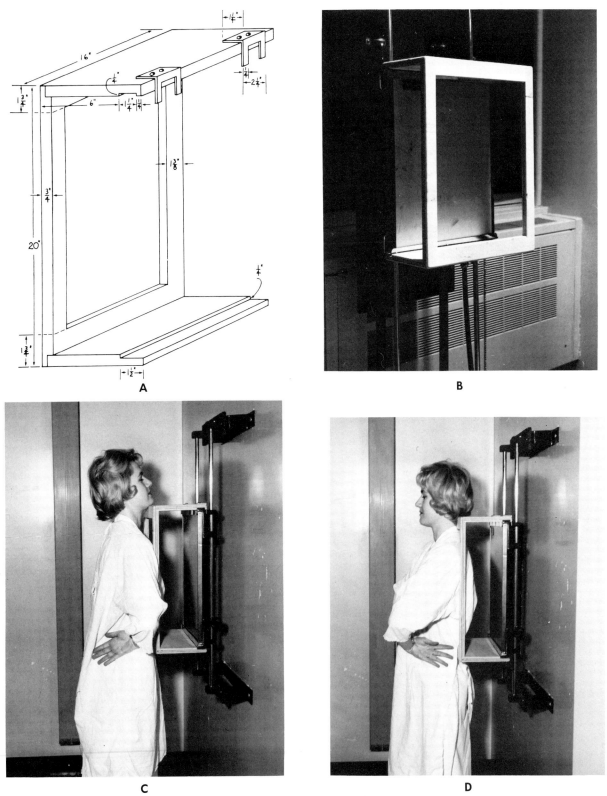

Figure 10–75. *A.* A drawing of the frame, indicating its dimensions. *B.* The frame is ready for use. *C.* The patient is positioned against the frame for a posteroanterior roentgenographic study. *D.* The patient is positioned for an anteroposterior study. (From Jackson, F. I.: Amer. J. Roentgenol., *92*:688–691, 1964.)

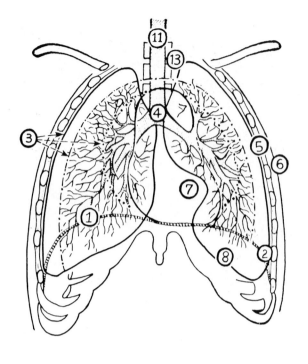
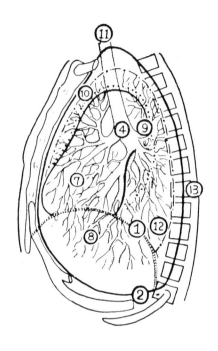

1. DIAPHRAGM	5. RIBS AND PLEURA	9. HILI ON LATERAL VIEW
2. COSTOPHRENIC SINUSES	6. THORACIC WALL	10. ANT. MEDIASTINUM
3. ZONES OF LUNG FIELDS	7. HEART	11. TRACHEA IN NECK
4. TRACHEA IN THORAX AND HILI	8. UNDER DIAPHRAGM	12. POST. MEDIASTINUM
		13. VERTEBRA

Figure 10–76. A suggested routine to be followed in examining radiographs of the chest.

larged hilar vessels from hilar lymphadenopathy; (2) differentiation of hyperemia, both isolated and associated with other abnormalities, from infiltration and fibrosis of the lung; (3) differentiation of pulmonary arteriovenous fistula from solid tumors; (4) visualization of the miliary and small nodular pulmonary densities; (5) differentiation of focal nodular areas of hyperemia and infiltration from ill-defined tumor nodules.

METHOD OF STUDYING RADIOGRAPHS OF THE CHEST (Fig. 10–76)

1. Localize the abnormal shadow with respect to the chest wall, pleura, lung parenchyma, or mediastinum. If localized in the lung, determine the exact lobe or segment involved if possible

2. Study the level of the diaphragm on each side, noting its general contour and position and any abnormalities contiguous with it.

3. Study the costophrenic and cardiophrenic sinuses in relation to their clarity and sharpness for indication of pleural disease

4. Survey the lung fields. First compare the two sides in relation to one another. Second, divide the lung fields into three zones as shown in Figure 10–65 D. The innermost zone contains hilar blood vessels of large caliber, the intermediate or middle zone contains the medium-sized blood vessels, and the outer zone contains the very small blood vessels, usually so small that only minimal detection is obtained in the usual radiographs. When any shadows that are extraordinary in any respect appear, therefore, in any of these zones, they are immediately suspicious of abnormality.

5. Note the lung apices particularly, and take care to look

tion is noted? Is there an accentuation of the interstitial pattern? Is there arterial distention?

7. Study the thoracic cage, tracing each rib carefully. The widths and symmetry of the intercostal spaces are evaluated simultaneously. The clavicle, scapulae, and visible bony structures of the neck should be noted. Although the skeletal structures of the dorsal spine are not seen adequately enough for careful diagnosis, it can be noted whether or not there is a scoliosis or other significant spine deformity which may affect the radiographic diagnosis of chest lesions. Is there a sternal depression or deformity, pectus excavatum, or pectus carinatum?

8. Study the soft tissue structures of the thoracic cage (Fig. 10–41 *A*). Identify the breasts, nipples, areoli, muscular shadows, particularly the pectoralis major and minor, and the sternocleidomastoids, which very often cast a significant soft tissue shadow across the medial aspect of the lung apices. A tegmental shadow, ordinarily seen above the superior border of the clavicle, must be identified and distinguished from the abnormal.

9. Any unusual pleural shadows are identified. The pleura does not ordinarily cast a significant visible shadow, except occasionally the posterior mediastinal (paraesophageal) stripe to a minimal degree in the costophrenic sinuses (Fig. 10–78) and

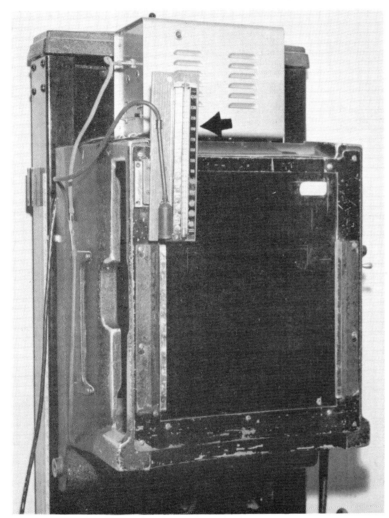

Figure 10–77. Stereoscopic 14 × 17 inch cassette changer equipped with a manometer (arrow) which will register the extent of positive pressure obtained during positive pressure film studies. The film exposure is triggered after maximum pressure is achieved by the electronic device in the box above the cassette holder. (From Whitley, J. E., and Martin, J. F.: Amer. J. Roentgenol., 91:297–306, 1964.)

"under the bones" so that no actual pulmonary markings of unusual character are overlooked.

6. Study the hilar blood vessels and mediastinum. The position of the trachea and its major ramifications should be noted. The trachea is ordinarily located near the midline. A further analysis of the mediastinum will follow in later chapters; here, it is enough to say that a study of the mediastinum cannot be separated from a study of the respiratory system.

The major hilar blood vessels should be traced so that arteries and veins are distinguished, especially in the lung apices and the lung bases. Is there a "deflection" or "cephalization-of-flow" phenomenon in the upright position so that venous disten-

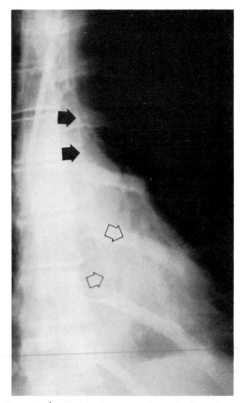

Figure 10–78. Posterior mediastinal (paraesophageal) pleural stripe. Air bronchogram (open arrows) with atelectasis of the left lower lobe and deflection of the posterior mediastinal stripe to the left (closed black arrows).

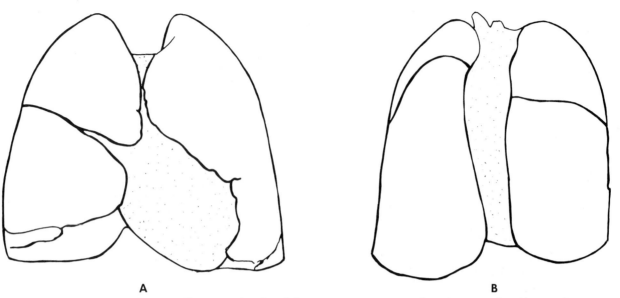

A   B

Figure 10–79. Line diagrams illustrating the pleural demarcation zones anteriorly and posteriorly. (Also see the fissures and lobes of the lungs.) *A* and *B*. Frontal and posterior views of lungs.

overlying the lung apices. In the region of the lung apices small blebs may occur normally. They are without pathologic significance and must be identified and distinguished from a pathologic process.

10. Identify structures underlying the diaphragm. A posteroanterior erect chest film offers a very good opportunity for visualizing free air under the diaphragm. Dense areas of calcification such as calcified cysts of the liver are also identified. The distance of the stomach (fundal air bubble or Magenglase) from the left hemidiaphragm should be noted. Is there a filling defect in the fundus? Is the spleen enlarged?

11. In the lateral projection of the chest it is particularly important to identify the *mediastinal shadow* and to form in the mind's eye a concept of the normal in this regard. Identify the left and right pulmonary artery, the trachea, and the bifurcations. We find the lateral projection extremely valuable in detecting abnormal lymphadenopathy or tumor masses in the central mediastinum.

12. In the lateral view identify the *anterior mediastinal clear space* which is just anterior to the cardiac silhouette and underlies the sternal shadow. On occasion the lateral view is the only projection in which the clear space is obliterated in the presence of a space-occupying lesion in the anterior superior mediastinum.

13. In the lateral projection, *the pleural reflection over the internal mammary vessels should be studied*. Metastases will at times produce detectable masses in this location.

14. In the oblique projections, further care must be exercised to identify the trachea and bronchial structures which can be seen to excellent advantage. The oblique views are also particu-

larly valuable in analysis of the cardiac silhouette, especially when barium delineates the esophagus (this will be described in Chapters 11 and 12).

15. Study the clear pneumonic space in the posterior mediastinum and identify the relationship it has with the posterior margin of the left ventricle and the reflection of the inferior vena cava especially.

16. Study the dorsal spine.

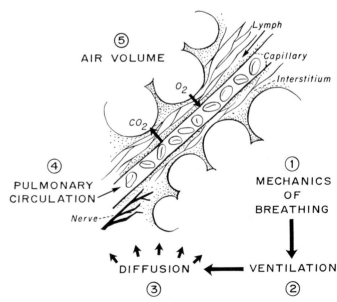

Figure 10–80. Diagrammatic basis for various pulmonary function tests.

Appendix 1

PULMONARY PHYSIOLOGY — ITS PLACE IN PULMONARY ROENTGEN DIAGNOSIS
(Tables 10–1, 10–2)

The morphology of the chest provides:

1. An adequate delivery of oxygen to the alveolus.

2. An adequate permeation of oxygen from the alveolus to a capillary and its red cell content and plasma.

3. A reverse passage of carbon dioxide from the capillary and its contents to the alveolus.

4. An efficient delivery of blood to and from the primary lobule of the lung.

5. Adequate compliance of the chest in overcoming frictional resistance and other forces resistant to exchange of gases and flow of blood (Fig. 10–80).

Thus, in evaluating the chest film we must think of the chest as a model of a gaseous volume and a blood circulatory space. Both of the compartments in this model must be analyzed.

The physiologic tests of pulmonary function indicate how the disease has altered this function. An anatomic, bacteriologic, or pathologic concept such as may be obtained radiographically is usually not rendered.

The radiologist may supplement the tests of pulmonary function that measure pressure, blood flow, vascular resistance, and the distribution of blood in the pulmonary circulation by defining the size of veins and arteries, the presence of venous arterial shunts, the presence or absence of vascular occlusion, pulmonary venous or arterial hypertension, and diminution in pulmonary capillary volume. In some instances it is possible to locate specific areas which may be so involved.

Apart from these considerations, the interstitium of the lung must also occupy the attention of the radiologist. In certain patients, a tentative diagnosis of "alveolar-capillary block" or impairment of diffusion is justified on the basis of the classical clinical picture. Physiologic tests can confirm this diagnosis. Only microscopic examination of the pulmonary tissues can actually establish the exact cause of the alteration. Such may occur in patients with Boeck's sarcoid of the lung, granulomatoses, pulmonary scleroderma, alveolar cell carcinoma, diffuse metastatic lesions in the lungs, and occasional cases of chemical poisonings of the lungs when the diffusion apparatus is disturbed.

With regard to evaluation of pulmonary disability, there may be gross roentgen changes in the lungs of patients with completely normal function, as in some cases of silicosis. Minor anatomic roentgen lesions in the lungs of patients may be associated with severe disturbances of pulmonary function, as in chronic obstructive pulmonary emphysema. In evaluation of pulmonary disability, tests of *function* of the lungs should replace tests that

TABLE 10–1 ROLES OF THE PULMONARY PHYSIOLOGIST AND RADIOLOGIST IN CHEST DISEASE EVALUATION

	Pulmonary Physiologist Evaluates	Radiologist Evaluates
Mechanical factors in ventilation	Yes	To some extent
Lung volume	Yes	To a limited extent
Distribution of air ventilating alveoli	Yes	No
O_2 and CO_2 diffusion	Yes	Qualitatively
Pulmonary capillary blood flow	Yes	To some extent
Lung compliance on resiliency	Yes	To some extent
How disease has altered function	Yes	
Anatomic, bacteriologic, or pathologic diagnosis	No	Yes, well
Differentiation of types of edema or alveolar infiltrate	No	To a considerable extent
Presence of small regional impairments	No	Yes, well
Arterial pressure	} Not by usual studies	Yes
Venous pressure		Yes
Interstitial pressure		Yes
Asymmetry of vascularity		Yes

evaluate only anatomic alterations in the lungs. In general, compensation cases should be settled by such objective tests as airway resistance, pulmonary compliance, arterial blood studies, thoracic mass volume, and diffusing capacity; these do not require the claimant's cooperation. Neither the physician nor the physiologist can ever conclude that the dyspneic patient does not in fact have dyspnea. It is possible that the patient's complaint may be caused by rather elusive factors such as chronic irritation of nerve endings somewhere in the respiratory tract, or the existence of some alveoli with decreased compliance and consequent under-inflation. Every effort should be made to determine (1) the presence or absence of functional impairment; (2) the nature of the impairment; (3) the severity of the disturbance; and (4) whether the degree of abnormality is compatible with the claim of disability.

TABLE 10–2 ROLE OF THE RADIOLOGIST IN THE STUDY OF VASCULARIZATION OF THE LUNGS

I. Distribution of vascularization: is it normal?

II. Size of pulmonary arteries and veins.

   A. Rapid tapering of pulmonary arteries, resulting in pulmonary artery hypertension greater than 25 to 35 mm. Hg.

      1. Interstitial edema with loss of compliance.

      2. Intra-alveolar edema.

   B. Pulmonary venous hypertension.

      1. Venous distention.

      2. Upper lobe veins more distended than others.

III. Septal lines of interstitium: capillary pressure 18 mm. or greater and pulmonary artery diastolic pressure of greater than 25 mm. Hg.

REFERENCES

Alavi, S. M., Keats, T. E., and O'Brien, W. M.: The angle of tracheal bifurcation: its normal mensuration. Amer. J. Roentgenol., *108*:546–549, 1970.

Amplatz, K., and Haut, G.: Lateral decubitus bronchography with a single bolus. Radiology, *95*:439–440, 1970.

Anson, B. J. (ed.): Morris' Human Anatomy. 12th edition. New York, McGraw Hill, 1966.

Bean, W. J., Graham, W. L., and Jordon, R. B.: Diagnosis of lung cancer by transbronchial brush biopsy technique. J.A.M.A., *206*:1070–1072, 1968.

Bean, W. J., Jordan, B., Gentry, H., and Nice, C. M.: Fissure lines in the pediatric roentgenogram. Amer. J. Roentgenol., *106*:109–113, 1969.

Bjork, L., and Lodin, H.: Pulmonary changes following bronchography with Dionosil oily (animal experiment). Acta Radiol., *47*:177, 1957.

Burko, H., Carwell, G., and Newman, E.: Size, location and gravitational changes of normal upper lobe pulmonary veins. Amer. J. Roentgenol., *111*:687–689, 1971.

Cauldwell, E. W., Siekert, R. G., Lininger, R. E., and Anson, B. J.: The bronchial arteries; an anatomic study of 150 human cadavers. Surg. Gyn. Obst., *86*:395–412, 1948.

Chang, L. W. M., Lee, F. A., and Gwinn, J. L.: Normal lateral deviation of the trachea in infants and children. Amer. J. Roentgenol., *109*:247–251, 1971.

Cudkowicz, L., and Armstrong, J. B.: Observations on the normal anatomy of the bronchial arteries. Thorax, *6*:342–358, 1951.

Cunningham, D. J.: Manual of Practical Anatomy. 12th edition. London, Oxford University Press, 1958.

Davies, C. N.: Inhaled particles and vapours. A formalized anatomy of the human respiratory tract. Elmsford, New York, Pergamon Press, 1961.

Davies, L. G., Goodwin, J. F., Steiner, R. E., and Van Leuven, B. D.: Clinical and radiological assessment of pulmonary arterial pressure in mitral stenosis. Brit. Heart J., *15*:393–400, 1953.

Doppman, J. L., and Lavender, J. P.: The hilum and the large left ventricle. Radiology, *80*:931–936, 1963.

Eller, J. L., Roberts, J. F., and Ziter, F. M. H., Jr.: Normal nasopharyngeal soft tissue in adults: a statistical study. Amer. J. Roentgenol., *112*:537–541, 1971.

Faber, L. P., Monson, D., Amato, J. J., and Jensik, R. J.: Flexible fiberoptic bronchoscopy (Abstract). Presented at Ninth Annual Meeting of Society of Thoracic Surgeons, Jan. 22–24, 1973.

Felson, B.: Lobes and interlobar pleura. Fundamental roentgen considerations. Amer. J. Med. Sci., *230*:572–584, 1955.

Fennessy, J. J.: Bronchial brushing in the diagnosis of peripheral lung lesions; preliminary report. Amer. J. Roentgenol., *98*:474–481, 1968.

Fennessy, J. J.: Transbronchial biopsy of peripheral lung lesions. Radiology, *88*:878–882, 1967.

Fischer, F. K.: The bronchial tree: technique of bronchography. *In* Schinz, H. C., et al.: Roentgen Diagnostics, Vol. 3. First American edition. London, Heinemann, 1953, p. 2023.

Fischer, H. W., and Balug, S. M.: Aerosol bronchography. Radiology, *92*:150–154, 1969.

Fleischner, F., Hampton, A. O., and Castleman, B.: Linear shadows in lung: interlobar pleuritis, atelectasis and healed infarction. Amer. J. Roentgenol., *46*:610–618, 1941.

Fraser, R. G., and Paré, J. A. P.: Diagnosis of Diseases of the Chest. Philadelphia, W. B. Saunders Company, 1970.

Gabrielsen, T. O., and Ladyman, G. H.: Early closure of sternal sutures. Amer. J. Roentgenol., *89*:975–983, 1963.

Heitzman, E. R., Markarian, B., Berger, I., and Dailey, E.: Secondary pulmonary lobule: A practical concept for interpretation of chest radiographs. Radiology, *93*:507–519, 1969.

Holden, W. S., and Cowdell, R. H.: Late results of bronchography using Dionosil oily. Acta Radiol., *49*:105–112, 1958.

Ikeda, S., Yanai, N., Ishikawa, S.: Flexible bronchofiberscope. Keio J. Med., *17*:1–16, 1968.

Jackson, F. I.: The air gap technique: An improvement by anteroposterior positioning for chest roentgenography. Amer. J. Roentgenol., *92*:688–691, 1964.

Jacobson, G., Schwartz, L. H., and Sussman, M. L.: Radiographic estimation of pulmonary artery pressure in mitral valvular disease. Radiology, *68*:15–24, 1957.

Johannesson, S.: Roentgenologic investigation of nasopharyngeal tonsil in children of different ages. Acta Radiol. (Diag.), *7*:299–304, 1968.

Kahn, B. S.: Bronchofiberoscopy. J. Wadsworth Hospital, Los Angeles, Calif., Aug. 1933.

Lambert, M., and Waugh, W.: Accessory bronchiole-alveolar communications. J. Path. Bact., *70*:311–314, 1955.

Lehmann, Q. H., and Fletcher, G. H.: Contribution of the laryngogram to the management of malignant laryngeal tumors. Radiology, *83*:486–500, 1964.

L'Heureux, P. R., and Baltaxe, H. A.: Emulsified Ethiodol as bronchographic contrast agent. Radiology, *95*:273–275, 1970.

MacLean, K. S.: Bronchial abrasion microbiopsy instrument. J.A.M.A., *166*:2160–2161, 1958a.

McLean, K. H.: Pathogenesis of pulmonary emphysema. Amer. J. Med., *25*:62–74, 1958b.

Macklin, C. C.: Alveolar pores and their significance in the human lung. Arch. Path., *21*:202–216, 1936.

Milne, E. N.: Physiological interpretation of plain radiographs in mitral stenosis, including review of criteria for radiological estimation of pulmonary arterial and venous pressures. Brit. J. Radiol., *36*:902–913, 1963.

Miller, W. S.: The Lung. Second edition. Springfield, Ill., Charles C Thomas, 1950.

Nadel, J. A., Wolfe, W. G., Graf, P. D., Youker, J. E., Samel, H., Austin, J. H., Hinchcliffe, W. A., Greenspan, R. H., and Wright, R. R.: Powdered tantalum. New Eng. J. Med., *283*:281–286, 1970.

Newton, T. H., and Preger, L.: Selective bronchial arteriography. Radiology, *84*:1043–1051, 1965.

Noetzl, M., and Steinbach, H. L.: Subperiosteal erosion of the ribs in hyperparathyroidism. Amer. J. Roentgenol., *87*:1058, 1962.

Owsley, W. C., Jr.: Palate and pharynx. Amer. J. Roentgenol., *87*:811–821, 1962.

Pump, K. K.: Morphology of finer branches of bronchial tree of human lung. Disease Chest, *46*:370–398, 1963.

Reid, L.: Secondary lobule in adult human lung, with special reference to its appearance in bronchograms. Thorax, *13*:110–115, 1958.

Reich, S. B., and Abouav, J.: Interalveolar air drift. Radiology, *85*:80–86, 1965.

Reich, S. B.: Production of pulmonary edema by aspiration of water soluble non-absorbable contrast media. Radiology, *92*:367–370, 1969.

Reid, L. M.: Selection of tissue for microscopic study from lung injected with radiopaque material. Thorax, *10*:197–198, 1955.

Reid, L. M., and Simon, G.: Peripheral pattern in normal bronchogram and its relation to peripheral pulmonary anatomy. Thorax, *13*:103–109, 1958.

Rizutti, R. J., and Whalen, J. P.: The nasopharynx: Roentgen anatomy and its alteration in the base view. Radiology, *104*:537–540, 1972.

Robbins, L. L., and Hale, C. H.: Roentgen appearance of lobar and segmental collapse of lung: Preliminary report. Radiology, *44*:107–114, 1945a.

Robbins, L. L., and Hale, C. H.: Roentgen appearance of lobar and segmental collapse of lung. IV. Collapse of lower lobes. Radiology, *45*:120–127, 1945b.

Rouviere, H.: Anatomy of the Human Lymphatic System. Tobias, M. J., Trans. Edwards, Ann Arbor, Michigan, 1938.

Rubin, P., Bunyagidj, S., and Poulter, C.: Internal mammary lymph node metastases in breast cancer: detection and management. Amer. J. Roentgenol., *111*:588, 1971.

Sargent, E. N., and Sherwin, R.: Selective wedge bronchography: Pilot studies in animals for development of a proper technique. Amer. J. Roentgenol., *113*:660–679, 1971 (29 ref.).

Schoenbaum, S. W., Pinsker, K. L., Rakoff, S. J., Peavey, H. H., and Koerner, S. K.: Fiberoptic bronchoscopy: complete evaluation of the tracheobronchial tree in the radiology department. Radiology, *109*:571–575, 1973. (Also several personal communications.)

Shopfner, C. E., Jansen, C., and O'Kell, R. T.: Roentgen significance of the transverse thoracis muscle. Amer. J. Roentgenol., *103*:140–148, 1968.

Simon, M.: Pulmonary veins in mitral stenosis. J. Fac. Radiol., *9*:25–32, 1958.

Simon, M.: Pulmonary vessels: their hemodynamic evaluation using routine radiographs. Radiol. Clin. N. Amer., *1*:363–376, 1963.

Smiddy, J. F., Ruth, W. E., Kerby, G. R., Renz, L. E., and Raucher, C.: Flexible fiberoptic bronchoscope [Letter]. Ann. Intern. Med., *75*:971, 1971.

Sovak, M.: Bronchography with a directable double catheter. Radiology, *90*:152, 1968.

Steiner, R. E.: Radiology of pulmonary circulation: Chamberlain lecture. Amer. J. Roentgenol., *91*:249–264, 1964.

Trapnell, D. H.: Recognition and incidence of intrapulmonary lymph nodes. Thorax, *19*:44–50, 1964.

Trapnell, D. H.: The peripheral lymphatics of the lung. Brit. J. Radiol., *36*:660–672, 1963.

Trout, E. D., Graves, D. E., and Slauson, D. B.: High kilovoltage radiography. Radiology, *52*:669–683, 1949.

Turner, A. F., Law, F. Y. K., and Jacobson, G.: A method for the estimation of pulmonary venous and arterial pressures from the routine chest roentgenogram. Amer. J. Roentgenol., *116*:97–106, 1972.

Upham, T., Graham, L. S., and Stecke, R. J.: Determination of in vivo persistence of tantalum dust following bronchography, using reactor activated tantalum and total body counting. Amer. J. Roentgenol., *111*:690–694, 1971.

Viamonte, M., Parks, R. E., and Smoak, W. N. III: Guided catheterization of the bronchial arteries. Part I. Technical considerations. Radiology, *85*:205–230, 1965.

Von Hayek, H.: The Human Lung. New York, Hafner Publishing Co., Inc., 1970.

Wanner, A., Zighelboim, A., and Sackner, M. A.: Nasopharyngeal airway: a facilitated access to the trachea. For nasotracheal suction bedside bronchofiberoscopy and selective bronchography. Ann. Intern. Med., *75*:593–595, 1971.

Watson, W.: Gridless radiography at high voltage with air gap technique. X-ray Focus (Ilford), 2:12, 1958.

Weibel, E. R.: Morphometry of the Human Lung. New York, Academic Press, 1963.

Werthemann and Vischer, quoted in Holden, W. S., and Cowdell, R. H.: Late results of bronchography using Dionosil oily. Acta Radiol., 49:105–112, 1958.

White, H.: Respiratory disease in later infancy. Sem. Roentgenol., 7:85–121, 1972.

Whitley, J. E., and Martin, J. F.: The Valsalva maneuver in roentgenologic diagnosis. Amer. J. Roentgenol., 91:287–306, 1964.

Willson, J. K. V., and Eskridge, M.: Bronchial brush biopsy with a controllable brush. Amer. J. Roentgenol., 109:471–477, 1971.

Xerox Corporation: Progress report: Xeroradiography. No. 3, September, 1972. Xerox Corp., P.O. Box 5786, Pasadena, California 91107.

Zamel, N., Austin, J. H. M., Graf, P. D., Dedo, H. H., Jones, M. D., and Nadel, J. A.: Powdered tantalum as a medium for human laryngography. Radiology, 94:547–553, 1970.

11

The Mediastinum, Excluding the Heart

BASIC ANATOMY

Mediastinal Boundaries

The mediastinum is that compartment of the thoracic cage that is bounded laterally by the parietal pleural reflections along the medial aspects of both lungs, superiorly by the thoracic inlet, inferiorly by the diaphragm, anteriorly by the sternum, and posteriorly by the anterior surfaces of the thoracic vertebral bodies.

Arbitrary Compartments of the Mediastinum

For descriptive purposes the mediastinum is divided into four compartments (Fig. 11–1): (1) the *superior mediastinum,* bounded superiorly by the thoracic inlet and inferiorly by a line drawn from the manubriosternal angle to the intervertebral disk between the T4 and T5 vertebrae. Below this imaginary line the *inferior mediastinum* has three compartments or subdivisions; (2) an *anterior mediastinum* bounded anteriorly by the sternum and other tissues beneath the sternum, and posteriorly by the pericardium covering the heart and major vessels anteriorly; (3) a *middle mediastinum,* which contains the heart, the aorta, the origin of the great vessels to the upper extremities and neck, the pulmonary arteries, superior and inferior venae cavae, and the vessels of the root of the lung; and (4) the *posterior mediastinum,* which is bounded anteriorly by the heart and posteriorly by the thoracic spine.

Major Anatomic Structures Contained in the Mediastinum

When the mediastinum is viewed from its *right side* with the mediastinal and costal parts of the pleura removed and the pericardium open (Fig. 11–2 *A*), the major structures visualized are (from top to bottom): esophagus, trachea, right vagus nerve, right phrenic nerve, azygos vein, superior vena cava, right atrium of

the heart, inferior vena cava, greater splanchnic nerve, and a number of intercostal veins, arteries, and nerves. In cross section the superior and middle right pulmonary arteries, the superior and inferior pulmonary veins, and the right bronchus may be visualized.

Similarly, when the *left side* of the mediastinal septum is viewed (Fig. 11–2 *B*) with the mediastinal and costal parts of the pleura removed, the pericardium opened, and the structures exposed and partly dissected, the following structures can be seen (from top to bottom): esophagus, major vessels arising from the

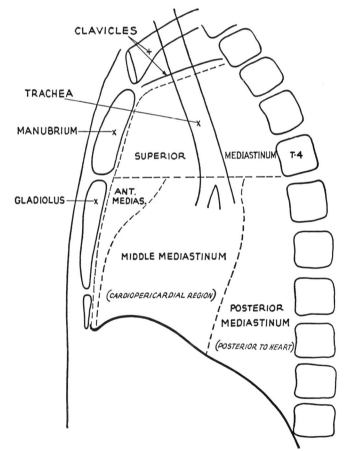

Figure 11–1. Compartments of the mediastinum.

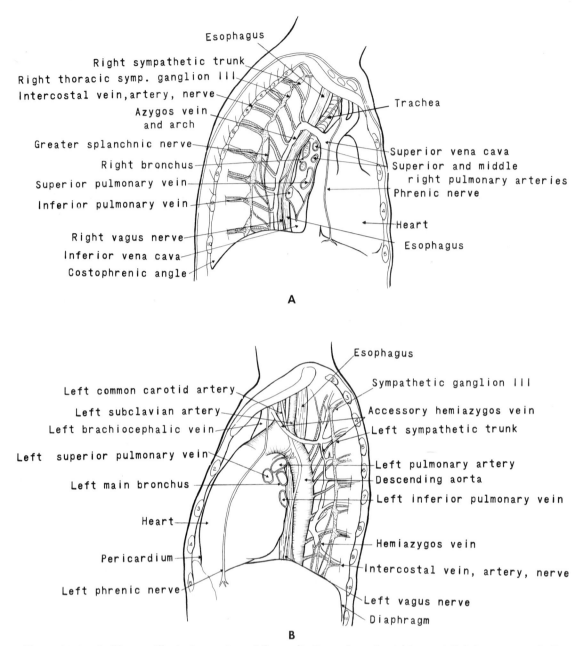

Figure 11–2. *A.* Diagram illustrating a view of the mediastinum from its right aspect (left lung removed). *B.* Diagram illustrating a view of the mediastinum from its left aspect (right lung removed). (After Pernkopf, E.: Atlas of Topographical and Applied Human Anatomy, Vol. 2. Philadelphia, W. B. Saunders Co., 1964.)

arch of the aorta (including the left common carotid artery and the left subclavian artery), left brachiocephalic vein, the entire arch and descending aorta, hemiazygos vein, left vagus nerve, left phrenic nerve, left ventricle of the heart, and, in cross section, the left pulmonary artery, left inferior pulmonary vein, left superior pulmonary vein, and left main bronchus. There are, in addition,

the segmental intercostal veins, arteries, and nerves, as well as the left sympathetic trunk, and some of the sympathetic ganglia.

In *sagittal section,* along the line of the superior and inferior venae cavae, passing through the right aspect of the cavity of the left atrium, one may visualize: the right innominate vein and the opening of the left innominate vein, a small portion of the ascending aorta, the auricle of the right atrium, the right ventricle, left atrium, superior vena cava, right pulmonary artery in cross section, and the right bronchus with the azygos vein above it (Fig. 11–3).

Figure 11–3 is also useful as a supplement to cross-sectional diagrams of the chest, which help greatly in further understanding the structures of the mediastinum.

In *frontal perspective,* a diagram of a radiograph is very helpful in revealing the structures of the mediastinum (Fig. 11–4). Thus, the following structures can be identified: the trachea with its left and right main bronchi, the pulmonary arteries and veins, the azygos knob adjoining the inferior margin of the superior vena cava and producing an ovoid shadow in the right tracheobronchial angle, the arch of the aorta and descending thoracic aorta, the thoracic spine with its paraspinal lines, and the pleural contours of the mediastinum medially. These will be identified more clearly as the radiographs of the mediastinum are shown in greater detail.

A line drawing showing the *boundaries of the anterior and posterior mediastinal pleura* as they adjoin the mediastinum is shown in Figure 11–5. Anteriorly, the lower left mediastinal

pleura diverges from the midline to accommodate the heart and pericardium. Beneath the sternum, the soft tissue space is identifiable where the costal and mediastinal pleurae meet. The pleura at the level of the manubrium passes backward over the superior mediastinum from the sternum to the vertebral column and is reflected over the apex of lung; it protrudes slightly above the first rib laterally but no higher than the first rib posteriorly. The anterior margins of the two pleurae converge behind the sternoclavicular joints and come into apposition with each other at the lower border of the manubrium, remaining in apposition to approximately the fourth costal cartilage. The left pleura at this level turns away from the median plane as much as 2 to 3 cm. and finally reconverges with the right pleura at the level of the xiphoid process.

The fat and remains of the *thymus* (in the adult) lie beneath the manubrium and anterior to the innominate veins. Somewhat laterally, beneath the costal cartilages, the internal mammary vessels descend deeply to the pectoralis muscles. The thymus in the adult cannot be identified unless it is enlarged or unless it is the site of tumor formation.

A study of the *caudal cross section* of the superior medias-

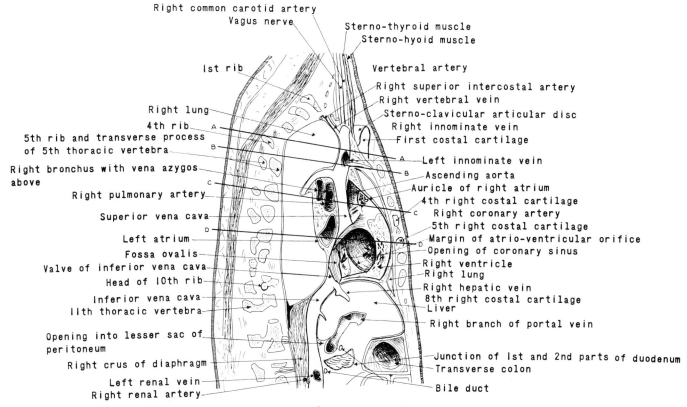

Figure 11–3. Line drawing illustrating the sagittal anatomy of the chest along the line of the superior and inferior venae cavae. (After Cunningham's Textbook of Anatomy, 6th ed. London, Oxford University Press, 1931.)

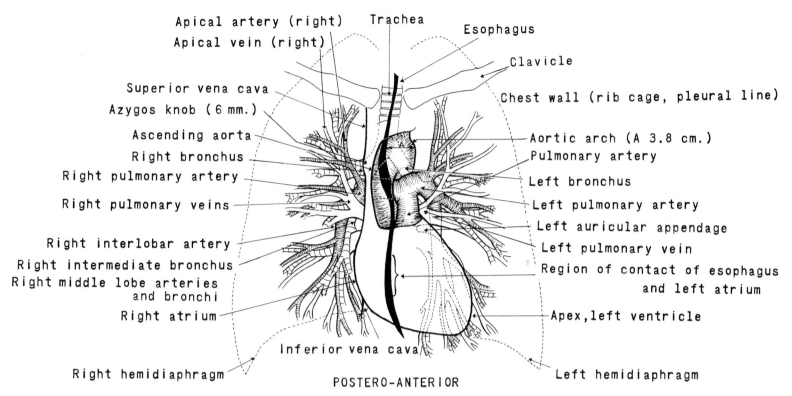

Figure 11–4.   Diagram of chest film showing arteries, veins, and relationships to bronchi.

tinum (Fig. 11–6) reveals the structures that descend from the neck into the inferior mediastinum. Thus, anteriorly the fat and remains of the thymus can be identified, as well as the left and right innominate veins, the trachea, esophagus, left subclavian and left common carotid arteries and innominate artery, and nerves such as the right and left phrenic, right and left vagus, and laryngeal (cross section at the level of the third thoracic vertebra).

The *innominate veins and innominate artery* lie anterior to the trachea. At the level of the trachea the left common carotid artery can be identified. The left subclavian artery and the esophagus lie posterior to the level of the trachea. The trachea lies just to the right of the midline, while the esophagus, more posteriorly, lies in the midline closely applied to the thoracic vertebrae.

Descending into the *inferior mediastinum,* the cross-sectional diagrams allow us to detect more accurately the contents of the anterior, middle, and posterior compartments. At the inferior margin of the superior mediastinum, fourth thoracic level, the pericardium comes into intimate contact with the substernal connective tissue and fat, separating the right and left pleural sacs (Fig. 11–7). The internal mammary vessels lie immediately anterior to the pericardium at this level, just anterior to the pleural margins. These are important anatomic landmarks, since enlargement of the internal mammary vessels (as in coarctation of the aorta), or enlargement of the lymph nodes and lymphatics that course along the internal mammary vessels, or infiltration

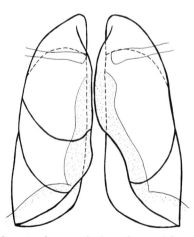

Figure 11–5.   Line diagram showing the boundaries of the anterior and posterior mediastinal pleura.

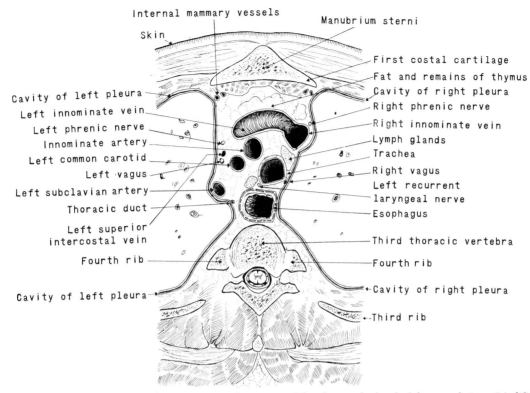

Figure 11-6. Line drawing of the cross-sectional anatomy of the chest at the level of the manubrium. (Modified from Cunningham's Textbook of Anatomy, 6th ed. London, Oxford University Press, 1931.)

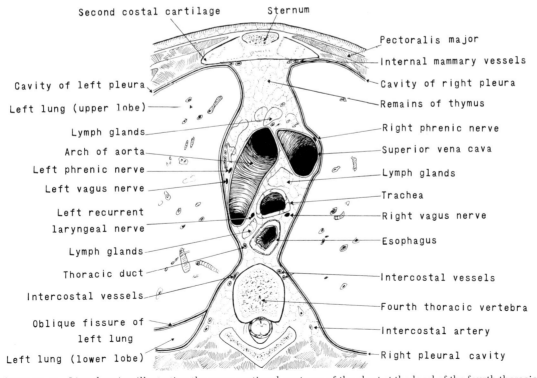

Figure 11-7. Line drawing illustrating the cross-sectional anatomy of the chest at the level of the fourth thoracic vertebra. (Modified from Cunningham's Textbook of Anatomy, 6th ed. London, Oxford University Press, 1931.)

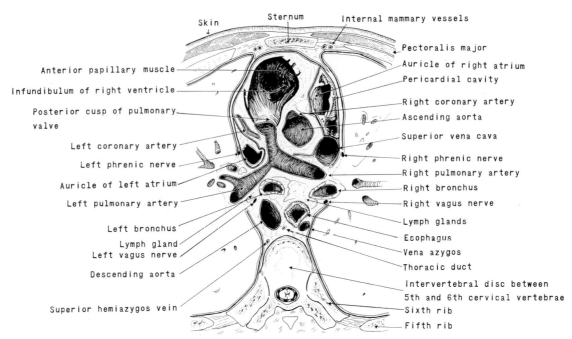

Figure 11–8. Line drawing illustrating the cross-sectional anatomy of the chest at T5 level, just below the inferior boundary of the superior mediastinum. (Modified from Cunningham's Textbook of Anatomy, 6th ed. London, Oxford University Press, 1931.)

by any neoplasia or fluid, may be recognized beneath the sternum in a lateral view of the chest at this level.

The remains of the thymus, fat, and areolar tissue, as well as lymph nodes, compose the rest of the anterior mediastinum at this level. In the midmediastinum, the major vessels such as the arch of the aorta, the superior vena cava, and adjoining lymph nodes come into view. The phrenic nerves, vagus nerves, and trachea with the left recurrent laryngeal nerve adjoining may be identified here as well. In the posterior mediastinum, the main structures are the esophagus, thoracic duct, and lymph nodes. The thoracic duct is situated to the left of the esophagus. Occasionally the esophagus can be seen on radiographs when it contains air in sufficient quantities, but otherwise it requires barium esophagrams for delineation.

In infancy and early childhood, the thymus gland extends into the anterior mediastinum, producing a distinct shadow in lateral and frontal projections. Farther down in the mediastinum the following structures can be seen (Figs. 11–8, 11–9). *At the level of the intervertebral disk between the fifth and sixth thoracic vertebrae,* the heart and pericardium are in contact with the internal aspect of the covering structures of the sternum. At this level the infundibulum of the right ventricle is shown anteriorly, and the pulmonary arteries are shown posteriorly in the cardiac cross section. The left and right bronchi are also shown in cross section,

the left being closer to the midline. In the posterior compartment, the esophagus and the azygos vein are shown to the right of the midline and the descending aorta to the left. The azygos vein lies slightly posterior and lateral to the esophagus, and very close to it. All of these structures are in close proximity with the soft tissues covering the spine. The superior hemiazygos vein and the thoracic duct also lie in this posterior compartment, with the thoracic duct lying between the descending thoracic aorta and esophagus, and the superior hemiazygos vein lying posterior to the descending thoracic aorta.

Descending the mediastinum farther still (Fig. 11–9) to the interspace between the seventh and eighth thoracic vertebrae, the heart can be seen occupying most of the mediastinum at this level. The left atrium and pulmonary veins are seen in the posterior aspect of the cardiac silhouette. The esophagus and descending thoracic aorta are closely applied against the left atrium, which explains why a slight enlargement of this cardiac chamber causes a significant displacement of the esophagus. The descending thoracic aorta lies just to the left of and almost in the same sheath as the esophagus. It can be readily understood why the esophageal displacement is a "tug of war" between the left atrium on the one hand and the descending thoracic aorta on the other. This is an important concept in understanding the radiographic pathology of this region. The azygos vein and superior hemia-

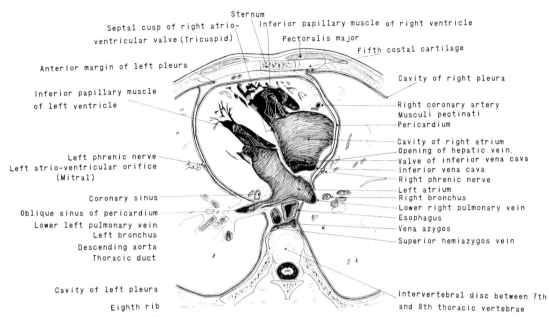

Figure 11-9. Line drawing illustrating the cross-sectional anatomy of the chest at the interspace between T7 and T8 levels. (Modified from Cunningham's Textbook of Anatomy, 6th ed. London, Oxford University Press, 1931.)

zygos vein lie to the right of the esophagus, posteriorly on the one hand (azygos vein), and directly posterior to the descending thoracic aorta (superior hemiazygos vein), on the other.

Thoracic Gutters. The posterior mediastinum is a very narrow structure at this level, narrower than the width of the spine. Note also how far the lung extends posterior to the posterior mediastinum in Figures 11-8 and 11-9. These concavities compose the so-called *thoracic gutters.* The space between the right and left pleurae is approximately 2 cm. or less in the posterior mediastinum at this level, just enough to allow easy visibility for the paraspinous ligamentous silhouette (Fig. 11-10). The vagus nerves are closely applied to the esophagus on each side. There are also numerous paravertebral lymph nodes in this region that can be particularly important when enlarged and detectable.

In a line diagram of the *left lateral roentgenogram* of the chest with barium in the esophagus, the following important indentations in the esophagus can be seen (Fig. 11-11): (1) indentation to the left and slightly posteriorly at the level of the aortic arch, (2) slight indentation anteriorly by the left main bronchus close to the bifurcation of the trachea, and (3) a minimal impression at the level of the left atrium, unless the left atrium is significantly enlarged.

The trachea, on the other hand, is slightly indented on its left side by the arch of the aorta.

In the *lateral view,* the relationship of the sternum to the thoracic vertebral column varies somewhat, depending on body build, the presence of kyphosis, the shape of the sternum, and the presence or absence of air-trapping in the anterior lung fields. In

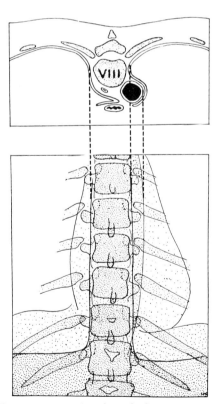

Figure 11-10. *Upper,* cross section through the posterior mediastinum at the level of the eighth thoracic vertebra. *Lower,* diagram taken from a roentgenogram depicting the posterior portions of the visceral or parietal pleura as lines along the vertebral column. Dotted lines indicate anatomic substrates of pleural lines and aortic lines in cross section. (From Lachman, E.: Anat. Rec., *83:*521, 1942.)

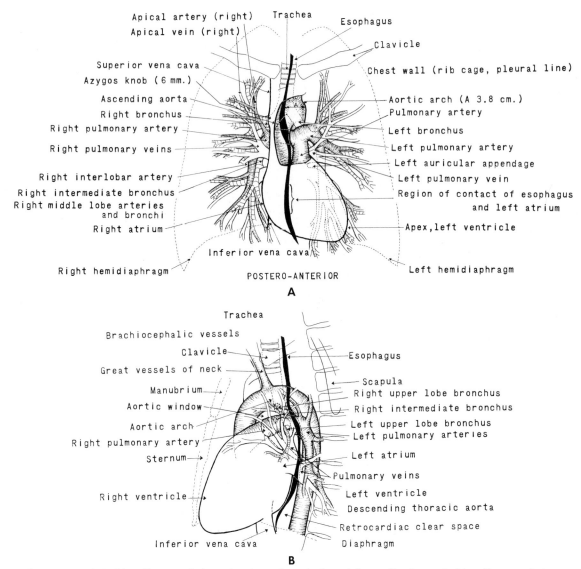

Figure 11–11. *A.* Line diagram of chest showing a frontal view of the mediastinum. *B.* Line diagram of chest showing a left lateral view.

general, however, in a young man of average build the following relationships are demonstrated:

Upper border of manubrium	Opposite interspace between T2 and T3
Sternal angle (junction of manubrium and sternum)	Lower border of T4
Xiphisternal joint	T9

Azygos and Hemiazygos Veins. Line drawings illustrating the anatomy of the azygos and hemiazygos veins and their tributaries are shown in Figure 11–12 *A* and *B*. The azygos and as-

cending lumbar veins constitute a continuous channel for venous drainage of the posterior body wall. In the abdomen the ascending lumbar veins receive the intercostal lumbar veins; in the thorax the azygos veins receive the thoracic posterior intercostal veins. In the thorax also the azygos ultimately terminates in the superior vena cava, forming a small knob at this point which can be identified on most roentgenograms of the chest (posteroanterior view) and measured. The size of the azygos knob becomes significant when interpreting distention of the azygos system such as occurs in certain decompensated states. Together with the lumbar veins, the azygos system constitutes a bypass between the superior and inferior venae cavae.

Azygos Venous System. The azygos venous system of the

thorax is composed of three primary channels: (1) the azygos vein and right superior intercostal vein on the right, (2) the hemiazygos, and (3) the accessory hemiazygos veins forming a continuous channel on the left. Other thoracic channels drain into the azygos system, including the left intercostal, esophageal, bronchial, pericardiac, mediastinal, and phrenic veins.

Thus, the azygos vein has its origin in the thorax at the level of the twelfth thoracic vertebra. It first lies ventral to the fifth to

the twelfth right intercostal arteries and to the right of the thoracic duct and thoracic aorta. Near the sternal angle it bends forward, arching cranially over the root of the right lung, and then empties into the superior vena cava just before the latter pierces the pericardium.

On its left margin the azygos receives the hemiazygos vein as a single or double communication at the eighth or ninth vertebral level. A little higher, at the sixth or seventh thoracic level, it re-

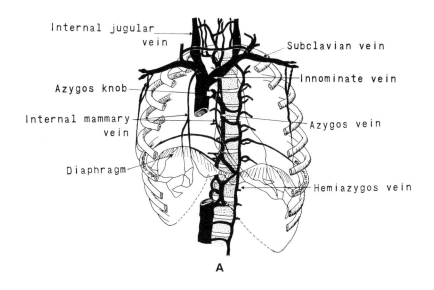

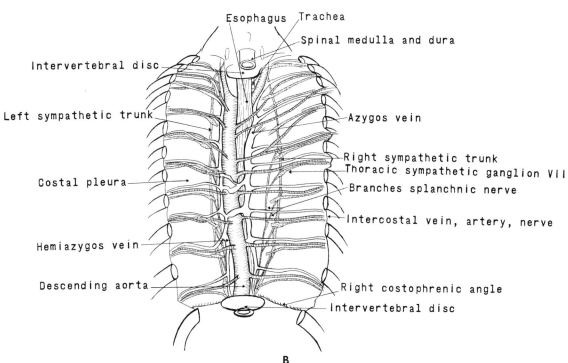

Figure 11–12. Line drawings illustrating the anatomy of azygos and hemiazygos venous systems.

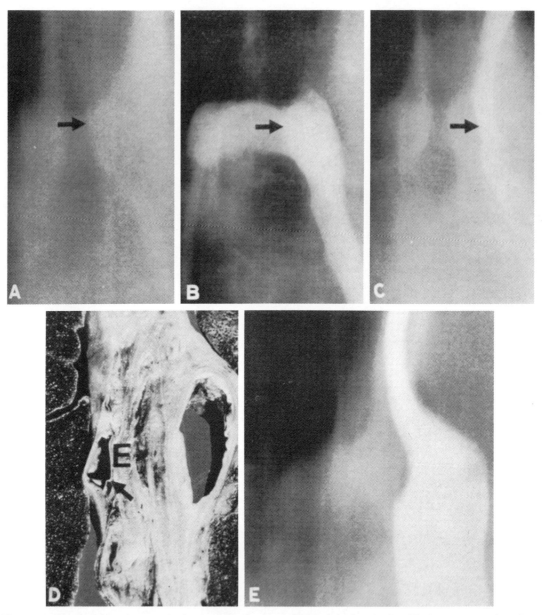

Figure 11–13. *A.* An anteroposterior laminagram shows an elliptical shadow outlined by lung on its right side at the level of T5 (arrow). *B.* An anteroposterior azygogram (same patient) shows this shadow to represent the posterior portion of the azygos arch, the "azygos knob" (arrow). *C.* An anteroposterior laminagram with barium in the esophagus demonstrates the imprint of the posterior azygos arch on the esophagus (arrow). *D.* A coronal section of the thorax through the level of the posterior azygos arch shows the intimate relationship of this structure (arrow) to the esophagus (E). *E.* Left posterior oblique esophagram shows the azygos "imprint" on the esophagus. (From Heitzman, E. R., Scrivani, J. V., Martino, J., and Moro, J.: Radiology, *101*:249–258, 1971.)

ceives the accessory azygos vein. In about 15 per cent of individuals the intercostal veins of the left side of the thorax drain directly into the azygos vein and the hemiazygos and accessory hemiazygos veins are incompletely formed.

The *hemiazygos vein,* formed from a number of venous roots, perforates the diaphragm just lateral to the left crus and courses along the left margin of the thoracic vertebral bodies, receiving intercostal veins along its left side. It lies just dorsal to the esophagus and to the left of the aorta. Throughout its entire course it lies in contact with the left mediastinal pleura. At the level of the ninth vertebra the hemiazygos vein turns to the right, passes behind the aorta and joins the azygos vein. In about 40 per cent of people, the hemiazygos vein is continuous above with the accessory hemiazygos vein (Anson).

The *accessory hemiazygos vein* is a longitudinal vein lying on the left margin of the fifth through the seventh thoracic vertebral bodies, and receiving posterior intercostal veins. It empties into the azygos veins through a trunk that crosses to the right behind the aorta, usually at the level of the seventh thoracic vertebra. There are usually valves in this venous system at the junctions of the azygos and intercostal veins, the hemiazygos and accessory hemiazygos veins with the azygos trunk, and, especially, the azygos and the superior vena cava.

The Azygos Knob. The azygos "knob" is that portion of the azygos vein that turns at a sharp angle from a prespinal location to join the superior vena cava. The knob is very close to the esophagus, which lies to the left and slightly anterior to it.

Knowledge of the normal dimension of the azygos knob has proved to be useful in the differentiation of a number of chest conditions, particularly inflammatory and neoplastic pulmonary infiltration from acute congestive pulmonary interstitial edema. In congestive pulmonary interstitial edema, the azygos knob measurement is increased, whereas in inflammatory or neoplastic pulmonary infiltrative diseases (which may resemble interstitial edema), the azygos knob is normal in size (Keats et al.). However, once the acute phase of interstitial pulmonary edema gives way to actual pleural effusion, the azygos arch dilatation may disappear. The azygos knob is also slightly dilated in pregnancy. In contrast with the normal measurement in women (3 to 7 mm.), in pregnant women the azygos knob ranges from 3 to 15 mm., with an average of 7.14 mm. Azygos measurement may be erroneous in the presence of lymph node enlargement in the area of the azygos arch. Differentiation, however, is possible, since the azygos arch enlarges in the supine position while an azygos lymph node in this immediate location will not.

The method of measurement of the azygos knob proposed by Keats et al. is shown in Figure 11–14. This measurement is obtained on *erect* teleroentgenograms of the chest, and is possible in 56 per cent of the normal patients surveyed.

Others have indicated other maximum dimensions: Felson, 10 mm.; Fleischner and Udis, 6 mm. Doyle et al. and Wishart used tomography to obtain comparable measurements. In the *supine* position on tomography, Doyle's maximum was 14.2 ± 2.6 mm. Felson's technique was apparently comparable to that of Keats et al. (Table 11–1).

The normal vein width in children was studied by Wishart in 762 chest radiographs of patients from birth to 14 years of age with the results shown in Table 11–1. The azygos vein does not increase uniformly in size with age. Respiratory activity, posture,

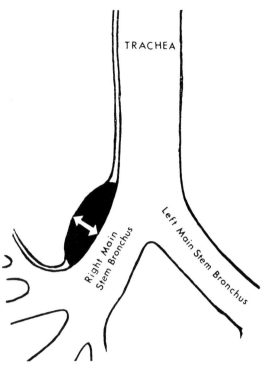

Figure 11–14. Method of measurement of azygos "knob" proposed by Keats et al. (From Keats, T. E., Lipscomb, G. E., and Betts, C. S., III: Radiology, *90*:990–994, 1968.)

and anatomic arrangement may cause changes in its width from subject to subject and from time to time in the same subject, making clinico-radiologic correlation somewhat uncertain. It was pointed out by Preger et al. that when the width of an azygos vein

TABLE 11–1 AVERAGE VALUES FOR AZYGOS VEIN SHADOW WIDTH*

Investigator	Conditions of Measurement	Normal Range
Fleischner and Udis, 1952	Upright posteroanterior teleroentgenogram	Up to 6 mm.
Doyle et al., 1961	Supine anteroposterior tomograms	14.2 ± 2.6 mm.
Felson, 1967	Upright anteroposterior teleroentgenograms	Up to 10 mm.
Keats et al., 1968	Erect teleroentgenogram	3 – 7 mm.

	Age	Mean ± 1 Standard Deviation
Wishart, 1972	Birth to 6 months	3.5 ± 1.3 mm.
	6 to 24 months	4.1 ± 1.0 mm.
	2 to 7 years	4.8 ± 1.2 mm.
	8 to 14 years	5.1 ± 1.6 mm.

*Modified from: Wishart, D. L.: Normal azygos vein width in children. Radiology, *104*:115–118, 1972.

is greater than 15 mm. as measured on a *supine* adult chest roentgenogram, it is associated with a raised central venous pressure above 10 cm. of water. The formula proposed as the result of this study was: the central venous pressure in centimeters of water equals the azygos vein width in millimeters × 1.4 minus 3, but the 95 per cent confidence limits for central venous pressure were ± 7 cm. from this predicted value. The tabular relationship of the width of the azygos vein in millimeters to the predicted central venous pressure is shown in Table 11–2.

An excellent drawing showing in cross section the arch of the azygos vein as it joins the superior vena cava forming the visualized knob is shown in Figure 11–15 (Tori and Garusi).

Failure of the superior part of the inferior vena cava to develop normally, with consequent continuation of the inferior vena cava as the azygos vein, is a diagnosis that can be rendered accurately with present methods of cardiac catheterization and angiocardiography. Its importance lies in the fact that half of the cases of azygos-cava anomaly also have an abnormality of abdominal situs that includes foregut, midgut, and colon malrotation. There is also a high order of association of this azygos-cava anomaly with asplenism-cyanotic and lethal heart disease, symmetry of organs, and other anomalies such as bilateral superior vena cava (Pacofsky and Wolfel).

Changes in Size and Configuration of the Mediastinum Normally. Ordinarily, the mediastinum is quite mobile, changing inspiration and expiration (Fig. 11–16). The mediastinum varies in the thoracic cage. Also, the mediastinum changes its shape in inspiration and expiration (Fig. 11–16). The mediastinum varies in size and configuration with body build, being long and thin in the asthenic individual, and short and stocky in the sthenic per-

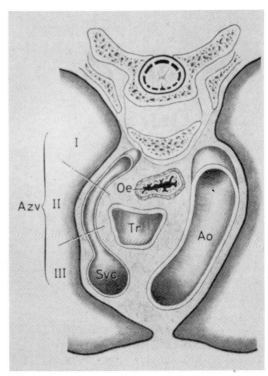

Figure 11–15. Drawing (modified from Andreassi) of a transverse section of thorax at the level of the fourth dorsal vertebral illustrates how the arch describes a medially concave curve, first passing laterally from the point of origin (I, posterior segment), then in a forward direction (II, intermediate segment), and, finally, turning inward and downward (III, terminal segment). (Ao, aorta; Azv, azygos vein; Oe, oesophagus; Svc, superior vena cava; Tr, trachea.) (From Tori, G., and Garusi, G. F.: Amer. J. Roentgenol., *87*:238, 1962.)

son. The mediastinum also changes as the individual grows, as is illustrated in Figure 11–16.

Paramediastinal Recesses. There are several so-called weak spots of the mediastinum, where protrusion may more readily occur from one side of the chest to the other. There is one situated anteriorly in the region of the shrunken thymus gland. Another weak spot exists where the esophagus and aorta are slightly separated in the lower posterior mediastinum; herniation of lung almost invariably occurs from right to left in this situation. The third is situated in the upper posterior mediastinum where the two pleural surfaces are in almost complete contact (between T3 and T5 and the esophagus in this area).

A detailed knowledge of the pleural reflections, especially around the azygos vein, is useful in the evaluation of many abnormalities of the cardiovascular system and also the right side of the mediastinum posterior to the hilus (Heitzman et al.) (Fig. 11–13). A deep inspiratory effort or a Valsalva maneuver will force lung into the mediastinal recesses and against pathologic pro-

TABLE 11–2 PREDICTED CENTRAL VENOUS PRESSURE*

Width of Azygos Vein (mm.)	Estimated Central Venous Pressure (to nearest cm.)	95 Per Cent Confidence Limits (to nearest cm.)
4	3	0–10
6	5	0–12
8	8	1–15
10	11	4–18
12	14	7–21
14	17	10–24
16	19	12–26
18	22	15–29
20	25	18–32
22	28	21–35
24	31	24–38
26	33	26–40
28	36	29–43

*From Preger, L., Hooper, T. I., Steinbach, H. L., and Hoffman, J. I. E.: Width of azygos vein related to central venous pressure. Radiology, *93*:521–523, 1969.

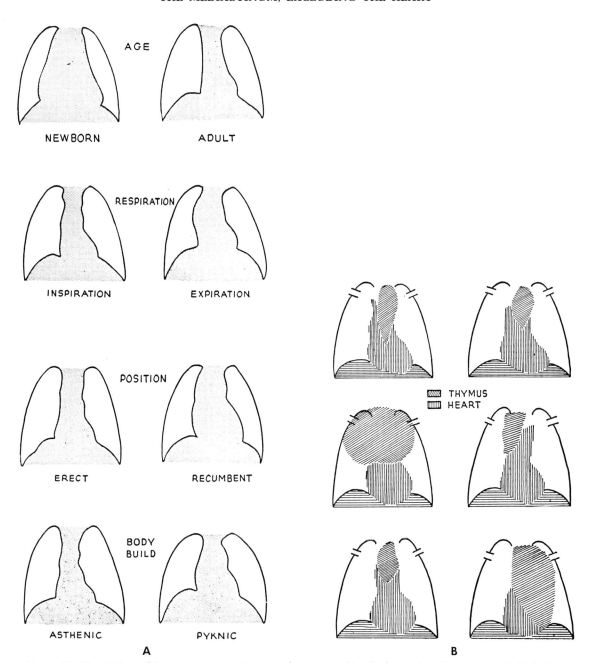

Figure 11–16.   *A.* Normal factors causing variation in the supracardiac shadow and cardiac contour. *B.* Variations in size and position of supracardiac thymic shadow in the infant.

cesses that may distort these recesses. If the mediastinum is mobile, which it usually is normally, these recesses can be accentuated by placing the patient on his side, or minimized by placing the patient supine. Thus, evaluation of enlarged mediastinal lymph nodes, left atrial enlargement, posterior mediastinal

masses, herniation of lung, or massive right pleural effusions may be significantly aided with this knowledge.

Thoracic Duct.   The relationships of the thoracic duct are illustrated in Figure 11–17. It arises in the abdomen from the cisterna chyli on the first and second lumbar vertebrae, enters the

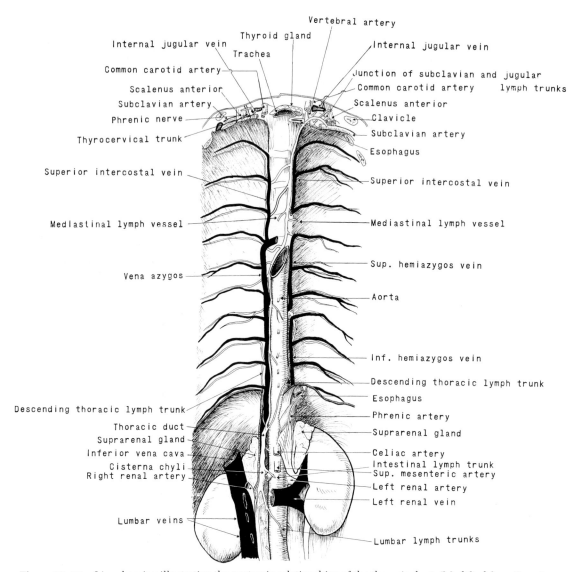

Figure 11–17. Line drawing illustrating the anatomic relationships of the thoracic duct. (Modified from Cunningham's Textbook of Anatomy, 6th ed. London, Oxford University Press, 1931.)

posterior mediastinum along with the aorta on its right, and continues upward in the posterior mediastinum between the descending aorta and azygos vein, posterior to the esophagus. At T5 level, it crosses to the left of the median plane and extends through the superior mediastinum, along the left border of the esophagus. In the root of the neck it arches behind the left carotid sheath, travels downward and in front of the subclavian artery, and terminates in the upper end of the left innominate vein. It has numerous valves and many tributaries, and varies considerably in course and termination. The thoracic duct can be visualized radiographically.

Mediastinal Lymph Nodes. The numerous mediastinal lymph nodes are liberally distributed along the internal mammary vessels, in juxtavertebral loci, and in foci adjoining the diaphragm anteriorly and lateral to the pericardial sac (Fig. 11–18). As shown in Chapter 10, they are nestled among the large vessels, both arteries and veins, and are found adjacent to the lower esophagus and descending aorta, and at bifurcations of the trachea and bronchi in both hili and lungs. Although normally not visible, they have great significance in inflammatory and neoplastic disease.

The right paratracheal lymph node chain represents a prin-

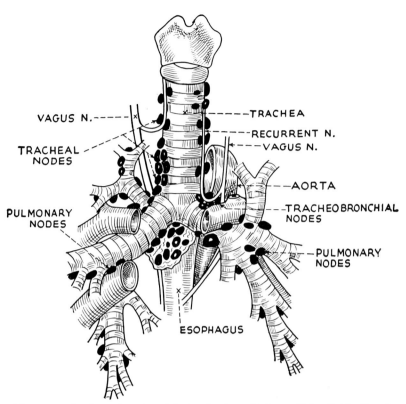

Figure 11–18.   Lymph nodes of the tracheobronchial tree. (After Sukienikow.)

cipal drainage area for the entire right lung and a major portion of the left (Rouviere and Valette; McCort and Robbins). Thus, the careful analysis and identification of each shadow of this region on the chest radiograph is imperative.

The *lymphatic drainage of the esophagus* also has great significance, since usually it occurs in longitudinal pathways in submucous and muscular lymphatic networks, extending from the internal jugular chain through the paratracheal nodal group and the posterior mediastinal nodes into the nodes of the cardia and lesser curvatures of the stomach. Careful observation of metastases from neoplasms of the esophagus corroborates the early spread of these lesions to subdiaphragmatic sites.

The Thymus

Basic Anatomy.   The thymus is a bilobed structure, largest in the child and regressing after puberty so that in the aged adult it becomes so intermingled with adjoining mediastinal parenchyma that it is difficult to ascertain its true shape or boundary. Its largest absolute size occurs during adolescence (Anson).

In the newborn it ranges in size from 4 to 6 cm. in length, 1.2 to 4.0 cm. in thickness. The gland lies mainly between the two anterior mediastinal pleural margins, but may extend superiorly into the neck as far as the lower pole of the thyroid gland. It is situated beneath the manubrium and upper part of the body of the sternum and their adjoining costal cartilages, approximately to the level of the fourth cartilage.

In the infant it is found in the superior and anterior mediastinum, and although it is largest in young adolescents, being almost three times its birth weight at that time, it is not as apparent on roentgenograms of the chest as it is in the infant, in view of the relative size and position of adjoining structures.

Thymic Patterns in the Newborn (Tausend and Stern).   The pattern of the thymus in the newborn is extremely variable. In a study involving some 1020 frontal chest roentgenograms obtained from infants born consecutively, no prominence was found on either side in 517, or approximately 50 per cent. In 276, the prominence was on the right side, and in 75 it occurred on the left side.

The frequently described "sail sign," a triangular prominence of the superior mediastinal image (Fig. 11–19 *a* and *d*), was encountered in less than 5 per cent of the thymic prominences.

An undulating contour of the lateral margin of the thymus, presumably caused by indentations by the anterior rib segments, was found rather frequently (Fig. 11–19 *d, e,* and *f*). Figure 11–19 *d* shows the scalloped margin as well as the sail sign. Even a cervical thymus gland may be encountered on occasion (Moseley and Som). Apparently the lumen of the trachea is seldom if ever compressed or displaced by a prominent thymus, regardless of its size or situation. On rare occasions there are radiolucent areas within the prominent thymus, suggesting the presence of fatty tissue (Fig. 11–19 *g*). The thymus gland decreases in size under stress and with the administration of steroid hormones (Tausend and Stern).

Thymic Angiography.   The arteries supplying the thymus are derived from the internal mammary and from the superior and inferior thyroid arteries. Technically, selective internal mammary arteriography is involved, and this requires bilateral selective catheterization.

On the other hand, normal thymic venography is apparently more feasible; two of the normal thymic venous patterns are illustrated in Figure 11–20. As shown in these diagrams, drainage occurs from the thymic region into the superior vena cava and the left innominate vein, and indirect drainage of the inferior thyroidal vein flows into the thymus and thereafter into thymic venous tributaries. The main thymic vein, the vein of Keynes, drains into the left innominate vein, 1 to 2 cm. from its junction with the superior vena cava (Yune and Klatte). Arteriography of the thymus gland has been accomplished by both selective subclavian and internal mammary angiography (Boijsen and Reuther).

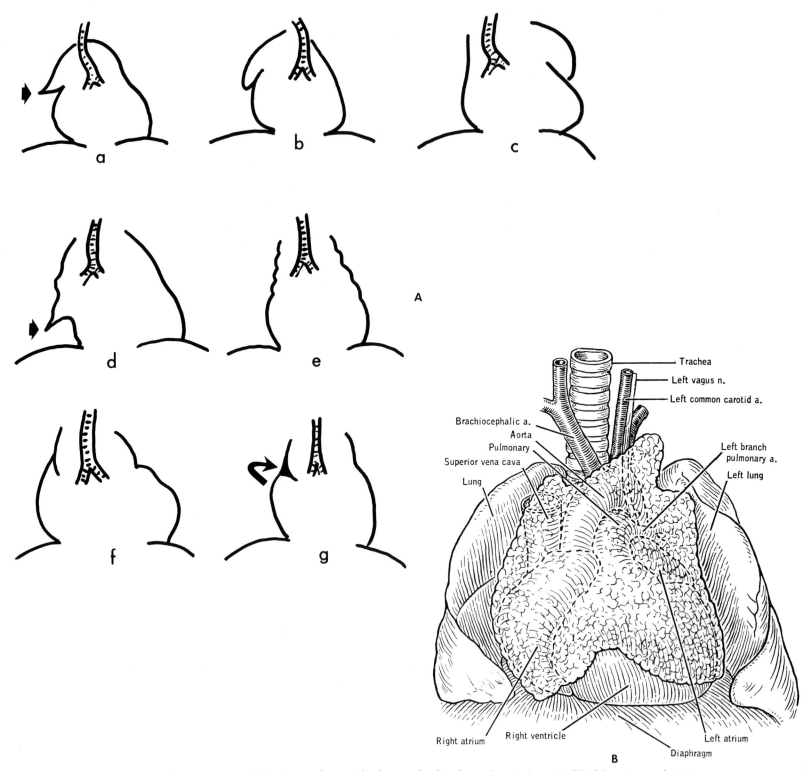

Figure 11–19. *A.* Variations in shape of the thymus gland in the newborn infant. (Modified from Tausend, M. E., and Stern, W. Z.: Amer. J. Roentgenol., 95:125–130, 1965.) *B.* Thymus of a full-term stillborn infant to show its relation to subjacent structures in the superior and anterior mediastinum prior to inflation of the lungs. Right and left lungs have been retracted laterally. (From Anson, B. J. (ed.): Morris' Human Anatomy, 12th ed. Copyright © 1966 by McGraw-Hill, Inc. Used by permission of McGraw-Hill Book Company.)

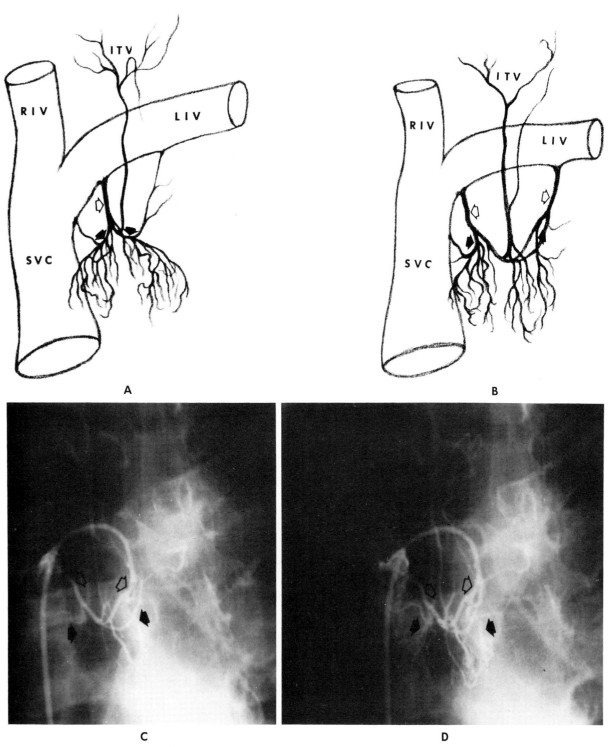

Figure 11–20. *A.* Normal thymic venous pattern as described by Kreel, showing main thymic vein of Keynes (open arrow) and lateral thymic veins (solid arrows). (LIV) left innominate vein; (ITV) inferior thyroidal vein; (RIV) right innominate vein; (SVC) superior vena cava. *B.* Variations of the normal thymic venous pattern. Diagram shows right and left limbs of the main thymic vein arcade (open arrows) and lateral thymic veins (solid arrows). (LIV) left innominate vein; (ITV) inferior thyroidal vein; (RIV) right innominate vein; (SVC) superior vena cava. *C.* Normal thymic venogram (early phase). *D.* Normal thymic venogram (late phase). The catheter tip is in the left side limb of the arcade. (From Yune, H. Y., and Klatte, E. C.: Radiology, *96:*521–526, 1970.)

Mediastinal "Stripes": The Pulmonary Ligament

Inferior Pulmonary Ligament. The inferior pulmonary ligament (Fig. 11–21) is a fibrous sheath connecting the visceral pleura on the medial surface of the lower lobe of each lung to the parietal pleura covering the mediastinum. It is actually composed of a double layer of pleura extending in a sheetlike manner from the inferior margin of the pulmonary hilus to the diaphragm, and loosely attaching the medial surface of the lung to the mediastinum. It tends to divide the anterior and posterior parts of the mediastinum below the root of the lung into compartments (Rabinowitz and Wolf). It assumes a triangular shape when the lung is displaced away from the mediastinum from any cause, and hence, has been referred to as the "triangular ligament." The apex of this triangle is situated inferior to the root of the lung, below the inferior pulmonary veins, and extends to the diaphragm with a bare area on the diaphragm between the two leaves of the ligament. Occasionally, the ligament does not reach the diaphragm and terminates in a free falciform border (Rabinowitz and Wolf) (Fig. 11–21 B). In normal subjects it is not visualized roentgenographically, but it does influence the radio-logic appearance of a number of pathologic entities such as pneumothorax, mediastinal pleural effusions, and pulmonary atelectasis. It also must be considered in surgery of this portion of the chest.

Patterns of Pleural Reflections of the Left Superior Mediastinum (Blank and Castellino). A chain of anterior mediastinal lymph nodes lies along the distribution of the phrenic and vagus nerves called the "left prevascular nodes" (Fig. 11–22 A). These nodes lie along the anterior and superior convexities of the aortic arch and continue anterior to the left carotid artery. They are somewhat lateral to the left paratracheal lymph nodes, and hence are important from the standpoint of potential distortion of the mediastinal silhouette when they become enlarged. The five basic contours for the pleural reflection of the left superior mediastinum in this location are shown in Figure 11–22 B (from Blank and Castellino). Two reflections of the pleura are identifiable: reflection A is apparently due to the pleural reflection "over the undivided portion of the pulmonary artery and is separated from this vessel by connective tissue." The relationships of the main pulmonary artery to the left cardiac margin are basic to the appearance of reflection A, although this reflection also covers fat and lymph nodes in the mediastinum.

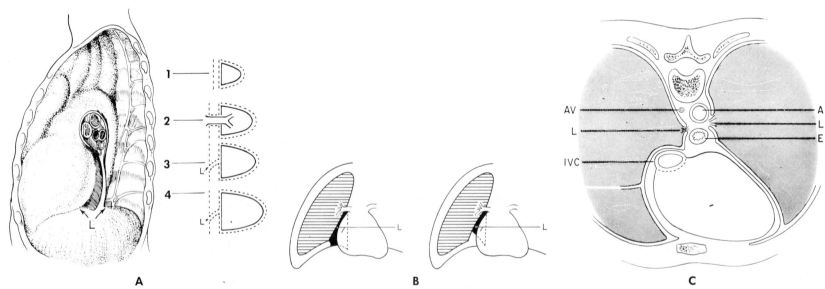

A   B   C

Figure 11–21. *A.* Diagrammatic view of the left side of the mediastinum. The pulmonary ligament (L) extends downward and backward from the hilus to the dome of the diaphragm. It has been cut along its attachment to the lung.

The side drawings are cross sections through various levels of the hemithorax to demonstrate the relationship of the visceral and mediastinal pleurae (dotted lines) to the lung and the pulmonary ligament at several levels. Above the hilus (1), the visceral and mediastinal pleurae are completely separated and the lung lies free within the thorax. The pleura that surrounds the hilus (2) is connected to both the visceral and mediastinal portions. The pulmonary ligament (3, 4) is composed of a double layer of pleura that bridges the visceral and mediastinal pleurae and attaches the lung to the mediastinum.

B. Schematic drawings to demonstrate the triangular configuration of the pulmonary ligament (L). The lung is shown retracted away from the mediastinum so that the ligament is stretched out as a sheet. The dotted lines represent the retrocardiac extension of the ligament. In the first drawing, the ligament is fully developed and its inferior margin is attached to the diaphragm. In the second drawing, the ligament fails to reach the diaphragm and ends inferiorly in a free falciform border.

C. Schematic cross section of the chest shows the relationship of the pulmonary ligaments to the mediastinal structures. Pulmonary ligament (L); aorta (A); esophagus (E); inferior vena cava (IVC); azygos vein (AV). (From Rabinowitz, J. G., and Wolf, B. S.: Radiology, *87*:1013–1020, 1966.)

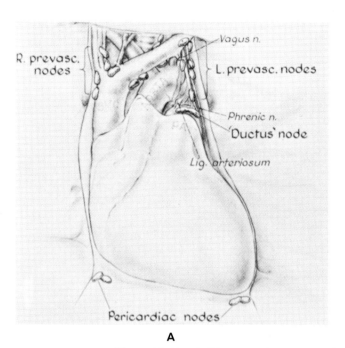

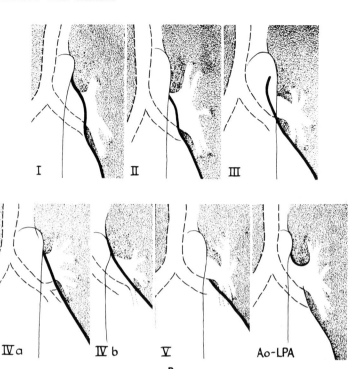

A

B

Figure 11–22. *A.* Diagrammatic representation of left and right prevascular chains of the anterior mediastinal lymph nodes. *B.* Diagrammatic representation of "reflections A and B." The heavy line in panels I–IVb represents the appearance of the pleural reflections between the aortic arch and "left heart border." "Reflection A" represents that portion extending from the aortic arch to the level of the left main bronchus. Five variations are shown.

Type I. A double curve with the lower portion convex, and the cephalad portion concave to the left (23%).

Type II. A single curve convex to the left (8%).

Type III. A line with the lower portion straight and the cephalad portion concave to the left (5%).

Type IV. A straight or slightly concave line which either intersects with (IVa – 14%) or forms a tangent passing slightly lateral to (IVb – 2%) the aortic arch.

Type V. No continuous border seen (48%).

Panel labeled Ao-LPA represents the appearance of "reflection B," indicated by heavy line extending from aortic arch and merging with the upper border of the left pulmonary artery. This reflection is present in only 38% of cases. When present, it may coexist with "reflection A" (36%) or be seen alone (64%).

In older persons the uncoiled descending thoracic aorta projects lateral to the mediastinal pleural reflections and must not be mistaken for them. Portions of transverse processes or posterior rib ends should not be confused with these reflections. Other abnormalities such as congenital cardiovascular anomalies, abnormal accumulations of fat, and primary mediastinal tumors will also produce changes in the mediastinal pleural reflections and must be considered in formulating a differential diagnosis. Finally, it must be emphasized that only the predominant recurring patterns have been presented here. (From Blank, N., and Castellino, R. A.: Radiology, 102:585–589, 1972.)

Reflection B is "probably due to projection of a segment of mediastinal pleura where it is not inseparably applied to the adventitia of the aorta and left pulmonary artery." It is usually concave to the left but may be straight in whole or in part. At times it is obscured by overlying ribs and transverse processes.

Posterior Mediastinal Line. The posterior mediastinal line between the right and left lungs probably has various component parts: (1) the esophageal-pleural stripe, which represents the pleural contact with the esophagus, and (2) the approximation of the right and left lung posterior to the collapsed esophagus between the esophagus and the spine.

At times the anterior mediastinal line, which represents the interface between the right and left lungs anterior to the heart and great vessels, is also superimposed on a teleroentgenogram. These lines may be identified, particularly in the high kilovoltage chest roentgenogram, and may be deflected in the event of a shift of lung from one side to the other (Fig. 11–23) (Cimmino and Snead).

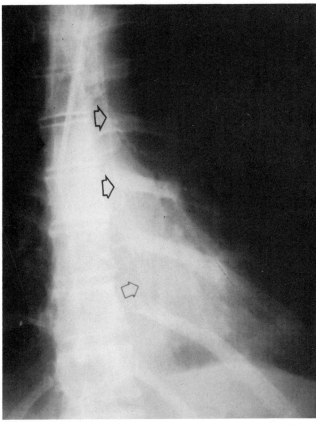

Figure 11–23. Arrows point to "posterior mediastinal stripe" shifted to left with atelectasis of left lower lobe.

RADIOLOGIC EXAMINATION OF THE MEDIASTINUM

The radiologic techniques of examination of the mediastinum include the following:

1. Posteroanterior and lateral chest roentgenograms may be made with maximal inspiration, moderate overpenetration, and barium in the esophagus (using high kilovoltage, short exposure time, and a Bucky grid).
2. Fluoroscopic examination may be used to evaluate the following parameters, especially:
   a. Pulsation—intrinsic or by impact.
   b. Abnormal response to positive intrathoracic pressure.
   c. Relationship of the movement of the mass lesion to structures within the chest: diaphragm, tracheobronchial tree, esophagus, heart, and major vessels.
   d. The relationship of the cardio-pericardial shadow to the epicardial fat (especially to exclude pericardial effusions).

3. Body section radiography. This is especially useful in:
   a. Determining the relationship of the abnormality to a specific anatomic structure.
   b. Studying the relationship of the abnormality to the vascular structures of the mediastinum.
   c. Studying the nature of calcification in the lesion, if it is present.
   d. Studying the nature of fat within the lesion, if it is present.
4. Angiography. This is especially useful in:
   a. Determining the relationship of the abnormality to opacified vascular structures such as the heart, aorta, major vessels arising from the aorta including the internal mammary (Boijsen and Reuter), and pulmonary arteries and veins.
   b. Studying the great veins leading into the heart (venacavography).
   c. Studying the azygos venous system (azygography). This may be done by intraosseous injection of the contrast agent or by selective catheterization.
5. Bronchography may indicate widening, narrowness, or filling defects in the air passages.
6. Myelograms may demonstrate the status of the subarachnoid space and indicate whether the mediastinal lesion is related to the spine or spinal cord.
7. Pneumomediastinography (Sumerling and Irvine). In this technique, the gas is introduced into the fascial planes of the mediastinum by a number of different routes. Tomography coupled with this technique is especially helpful in certain cases. This method is useful for:
   a. Ascertaining the exact relationship of a lesion to the adjoining structures.
   b. Helping to determine resectability of a lesion in the mediastinum, or of bronchogenic carcinoma.
8. Diagnostic pneumothorax and pneumoperitoneum may be used to localize the suspected lesion in relation to these potential spaces; they are especially helpful in studying herniation from the abdomen into the thoracic cage. These procedures must be performed with great care, in order to avoid a tension pneumothorax and its deleterious symptoms.
9. Radioisotopic techniques:
   a. Blood pool scans.
   b. Radioisotopic angiograms.
   c. Study of pericardial effusions.
   d. Localization of some tumors: thymoma, thyroid, and occasionally, lymph node enlargements.

Fluoroscopy and Routine Film Studies of the Chest. These have already been considered in Chapter 10. It should be emphasized that the examination of the mediastinum requires good delineation of the esophagus with barium contrast, which may be accomplished with either thick or thin barium. Air contrast has at times been used for a similar purpose. Because the mediastinum includes the esophagus, heart, and major blood vessels, it is difficult to separate the anatomic investigation of the mediastinum from these other entities. This is arbitrarily being done here for ease of description. The anatomy of the esophagus proper will be described with the anatomy of the alimentary tract (Chapter 13), and anatomy of the heart will be described in Chapter 12 in conjunction with the cardiovascular system. Other modes of investigation are distributed as follows: *angiography,* see Chapter 12; *bronchography,* see Chapter 10; *myelography,* see Chapter 9.

Pneumomediastinography. Pneumomediastinography has been utilized as a diagnostic tool since 1936 (Condorelli). Various methods for inducing pneumomediastinum have been described: (1) the retro- or transsternal method (Condorelli); (2) the suprasternal notch method (Hare and Mackay); and (3) the presacral technique utilized for retroperitoneal air insufflation (Palubinskas and Hodson).

For a more complete bibliography and details regarding pneumomediastinography the student is referred to Oliva's review of this subject. A large number of approaches have been suggested but in actual practice only five are frequently employed:

1. *Retrosternal access* (Fig. 11–24 *A*) was originally suggested by Condorelli in 1934. In this procedure a needle is advanced through the suprasternal notch and then along the posterior wall of the sternum for a distance of 4 centimeters, making certain continuously that the needle is not situated in a vessel. During the continued insufflation, the pressure varies between minus 5 and plus 5 cc. of water. Ordinarily one utilizes 300 to 400 milliliters of gas.

2. *Transtracheal access* (Fig. 11–24 *B*) was also suggested by Condorelli et al. in 1949. This approach allows better visualization of the posterior mediastinum; the anterior mediastinum is seen only after a large amount of gas has been utilized.

3. *Retroperitoneal access* was first suggested by Ruiz-Rivas in 1950. It is accomplished by a simultaneous injection into both the anterior and posterior mediastina, using the technique of pneumoretroperitoneography by the precoccygeal route into the retroperitoneal spaces and from there into the mediastina.

4. Other *direct pathways* are employed, either through the sternum, next to the sternum, or beneath the xiphoid. A pretracheal pathway may also be used.

5. *Indirect approaches* through the back have also been utilized. These have the advantages of more constant visualization of both the anterior and posterior mediastina.

Tomography is essential to success. Tomograms which have been supplied to us by Sumerling are reproduced with the further advantage of Logetronic printing. It is readily apparent that large anatomic structures may be seen, including the thoracic aorta, trachea, superior vena cava, thymus, pulmonary artery, chambers of the heart such as the right ventricle and left

atrium in margin, azygos vein, left innominate vein, right innominate vein, left carotid artery, left subclavian artery, thyroid (particularly when enlarged), right and left bronchi, pulmonary vein, and paramediastinal pleura. The gas apparently surrounds the organs, which are otherwise without contrast of their own, rendering them visible through the delineation of their margins. Unfortunately, superimposition of shadows makes the tomographic technique essential in both frontal and lateral views as shown.

With special equipment, axiotransverse tomography may also be employed, but relatively little experience with this technique has been reported (Oliva).

The procedure is generally well tolerated by the patient, although too large amounts of gas can induce a feeling of retrosternal pressure and produce pain similar to angina, but this disappears in a very short time. The appearance of subcutaneous emphysema in the supraclavicular and neck area and even dysphagia is not of significant concern. In the presence of cardiac failure, the retrosternal approach can lead to the perforation of an enlarged blood vessel, but this can be detected by good technique. The transtracheal approach can lead to the perforation of the esophagus, but ordinarily this is not followed by any serious sequelae. The precoccygeal approach is practically without danger, although significant subcutaneous emphysema, scrotal emphysema, and even perforation of the rectum may occur. It is probable that pneumomediastinography is closely akin to surgical mediastinoscopy and is an alternative method for the observation and demonstration of vessels, bronchi, lymph nodes, and tumors of the mediastinum (Fig. 11–24).

It must be emphasized further, however, that with a completely obstructed mediastinum the capacity of this area of the anatomy is virtually zero and hence, the technique can be used to distinguish a benign noninfiltrating tumor from a severely infiltrating one. Needless to say also, the transtracheal technique is contraindicated in the presence of an acute infectious process of the respiratory organs.

The transsternal technique has been utilized either directly through the bone or through the manubriosternal junction. The procedure is best done under fluoroscopic control; carbon dioxide, air, or nitrous oxide is usually employed. Because nitrous oxide and carbon dioxide are absorbed very rapidly, the first injection may be made with these gases to determine whether or not the injection is proceeding well, and thereafter air may be utilized. Image amplifier fluoroscopic control is extremely helpful.

If dissection of the gas into the mediastinum proceeds normally, 300 to 500 cc. of the gas may be employed.

Stringent precautions must be taken against the possibility of gas embolism. The examination is contraindicated in patients with a bleeding diathesis.

In the *anteroposterior view* the gas outlines the following anatomic structures in different tomographic levels: the left innominate vein, superior vena cava, azygos vein in the right tracheobronchial angle, aorta, innominate artery, left carotid artery, and left subclavian artery. Ordinarily, dissection of the gas occurs around the main pulmonary artery and aortic arch, outlining the aortic window. The outer walls of the trachea and bronchi are often outlined as far as the primary divisions. In some cases, the ligamentum arteriosum can be identified. With appropriate tomography the thymus in the adult may also be seen in the anteroposterior projection as two thin shadows on either side of the midline. The right lobe of the thymus is closely related to the superior vena cava (Fig. 11–24).

Lateral tomograms are particularly useful for outlining the thymus. The external surface of the heart and the esophagus may also be demonstrated. In the adult, the gas diffuses into the neck, and anteroposterior tomograms will clearly delineate the lobes of the thyroid gland (Fig. 11–24).

The *potential spaces of the mediastinum in the newborn* are indicated in Figure 11–25 *A* and *B*. The anterior mediastinum extends to the left of the midline adjacent to the anterior chest wall, and separation of the anterior mediastinum from the middle mediastinum occurs at its posterolateral borders by the apposition of pericardium to mediastinal pleura. Air in the anterior mediastinum is limited superiorly by the superior sternopericardial ligament. This forms the superior attachment of pericardium to the upper sternum, and the thymus is said to lie above this ligament. If the air does not rise above this ligament the typical sail sign on the chest roentgenogram with pneumomediastinum is not obtained in the newborn (Franken). A pneumomediastinum may dissect along the fibrous layer of prevertebral fascia, perivisceral fascia, esophageal fascia, and even parietal and visceral pericardial fascia, as shown in Figure 11–26 *A* and *B*. Under these cir-

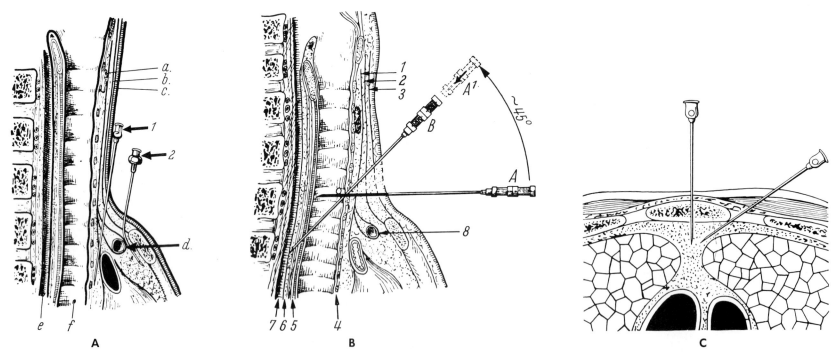

Figure 11–24. *A.* Direct approach for the introduction of the gas according to Condorelli: (1) Pretracheal access (posterior mediastinum); (2) Retrosternal access (anterior mediastinum): *a.* deep part of the middle cervical fascia, *b.* superficial part of the middle cervical fascia, *c.* superficial cervical fascia, *d.* left brachiocervical venous trunk, *e.* esophagus, *f.* trachea. (From Condorelli, L., Truchetti, A., and Pidone, G.: Ann. Radiol. Diag., *23:*33, 1951.) *B.* Transtracheal approach for the introduction of air into the posterior mediastinum according to Condorelli: (A) Position of the needle for the perforation of the skin and the anterior tracheal wall. (B) Position of the needle for the perforation of the posterior tracheal wall. (1) Deep part of the middle cervical fascia; (2) superficial part of the middle cervical fascia; (3) superficial cervical fascia; (4) anterior wall of the trachea; (5) posterior wall of the trachea; (6) areolar, loose connective tissue between trachea and esophagus; (7) esophagus; (8) left brachiocervical venous trunk. (From Cocchi, U.: Pneumoretroperitoneum and Pneumomediastinum. Georg Thieme Verlag, Stuttgart, 1957.) *C.* Schematic drawing of the transsternal and parasternal approaches according to Sansone (anterior pneumomediastinum). (From Sansone, G.: Minerva Pediat., *3:*293, 1951.)

Figure 11–24 continued on the opposite page.

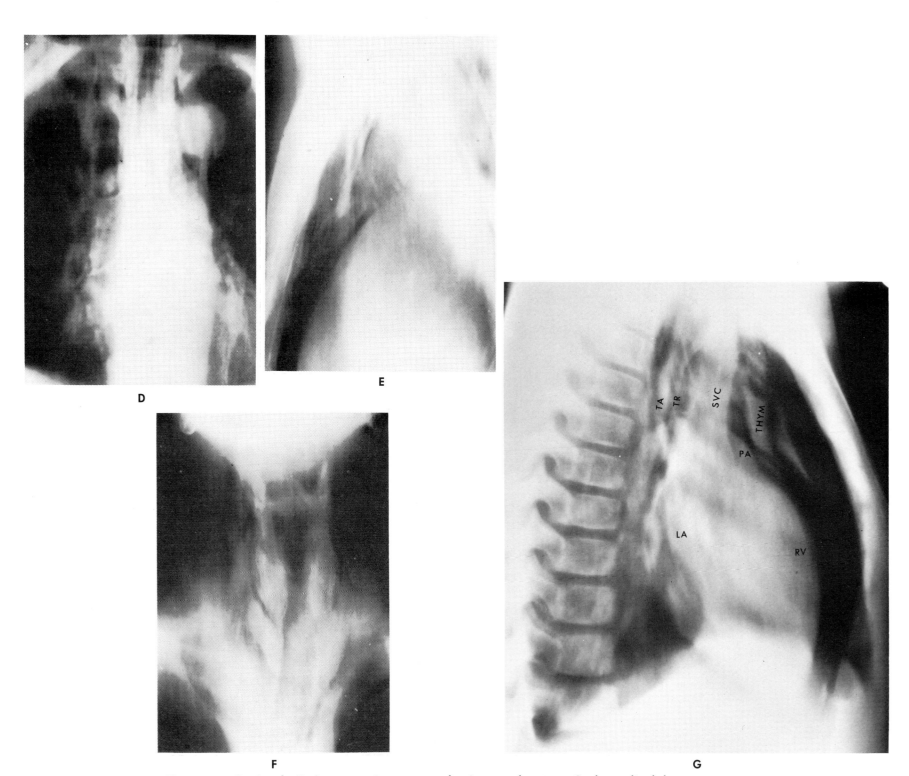

Figure 11–24 *Continued. D.* Anteroposterior tomogram showing normal anatomy. Gas has outlined the aorta, main pulmonary artery, ligamentum arteriosum, azygos vein, left subclavian artery and superior vena cava. Gas also diffused around the trachea and main bronchi, outlining their walls. *E.* Lateral tomogram showing the two lobes of the thymus outlined by gas in the anterior mediastinum. The trachea, esophagus, left innominate vein, and superior vena cava are also seen. Gas has diffused between the right ventricular outflow tract and the aorta. *F.* Anteroposterior tomogram of the cervical region shows the two lobes of the thyroid gland outlined by gas immediately below the larynx. (From Sumerling, M. D., and Irvine, W. J.: Amer. J. Roentgenol., 98:451–460, 1966.) *G.* Lateral view of pneumomediastinum in a child, demonstrating the thymus (THYM); superior vena cava (SVC); trachea (TR); thoracic aorta (TA); left atrium (LA); right ventricle (RV); and pulmonary artery (PA). (Courtesy of Dr. M. D. Sumerling.)

Figure 11–24 continued on the following page.

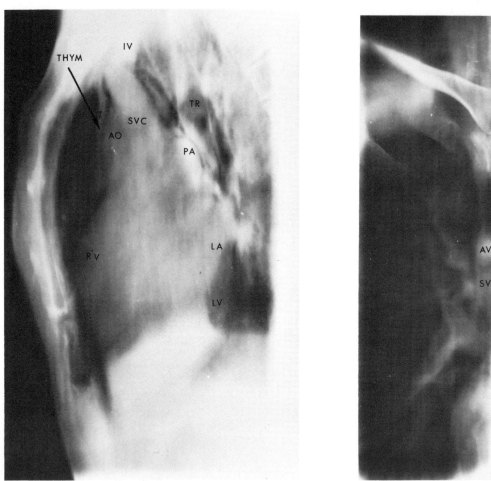

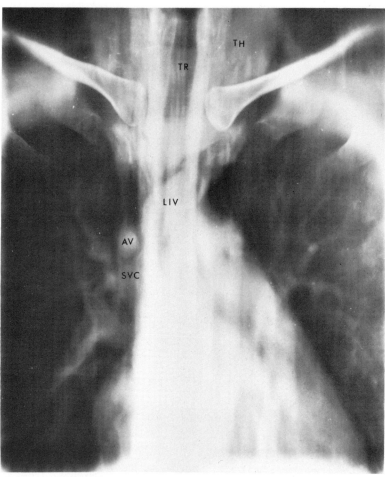

H   I

Figure 11–24 *Continued.* *H.* Lateral view of pneumomediastinum in an adult, showing the thymus (THYM) to be much smaller and the anterior mediastinal clear space much more noticeable than it is in a child. Other structures visualized in this study are the aorta (AO); superior vena cava (SVC); innominate vein (IV); pulmonary artery (PA); and, as previously, the trachea, left atrium, left ventricle, and right ventricle. *I.* Representative frontal view which shows the thyroid (TH); trachea (TR); left innominate vein (LIV); azygos vein or knob (AV); and superior vena cava (SVC). (Courtesy of Dr. M. D. Sumerling.)

Figure 11–24 continued on the opposite page.

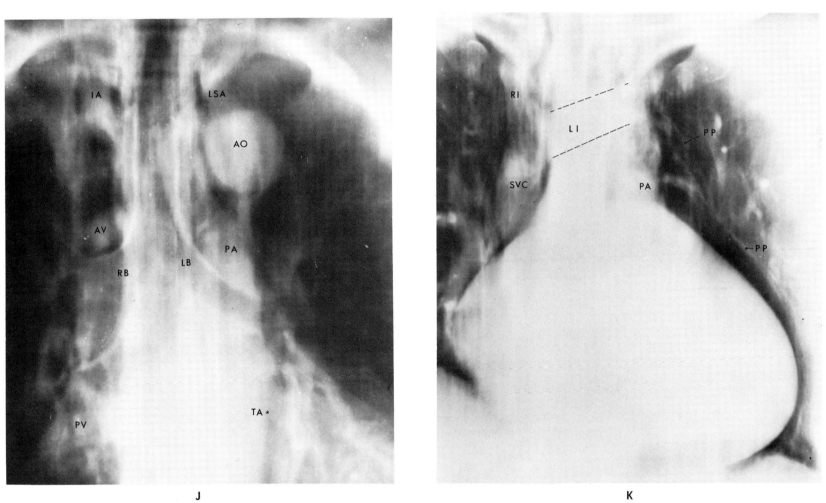

J   K

Figure 11–24 *Continued.   J.* Frontal view of an older individual showing a much more prominent aorta (AO); left subclavian artery (LSA); thoracic aorta (TA); pulmonary vein (PV); right and left bronchi (RB and LB); and right innominate artery (IA). *K.* A left innominate vein (LI) draining into the superior vena cava (SVC). A right innominate vein (RI) is also present. The paramediastinal pleura (PP) is also shown quite clearly, particularly along the left cardiac margin. (Courtesy of Dr. M. D. Sumerling.)

Figure 11–24 continued on the following page.

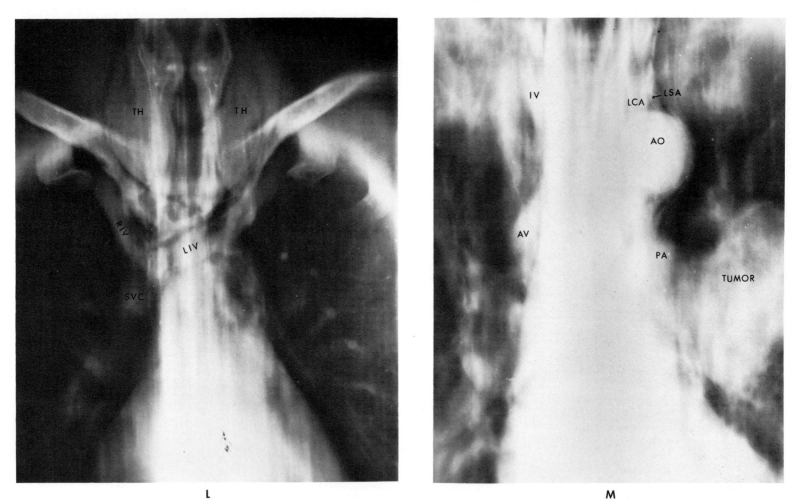

L   M

Figure 11–24 *Continued.* *L.* Somewhat similar structures are shown but the thyroid (TH) is shown to be significantly enlarged. *M.* A tumor is noted in the left lung, but additionally one can see a separation between the left subclavian artery (LSA) and the left common carotid artery (LCA). Other structures are much the same as those previously shown. (Courtesy of Dr. M. D. Sumerling.)

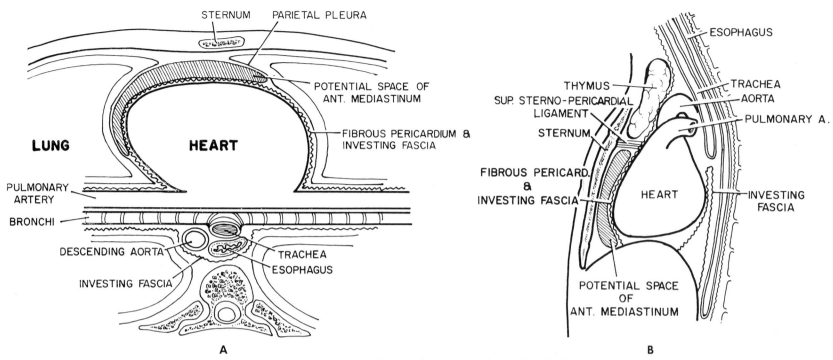

Figure 11–25. *A.* Diagrammatic cross section of the mediastinum at the level of the lung hilus. The fascia surrounding the pulmonary vessels is continuous with the fibrous pericardium and the investing fascia of the trachea and great vessels. The anterior mediastinum is anterior to this fascia. Because of the levoposition of the heart, more potential space is available to the left of midline. Air collecting in this region could therefore displace the heart posteriorly and to the right. *B.* Diagrammatic sagittal section of the mediastinum in the midline. The superior sterno-pericardial ligament limits the superior extent of the anterior mediastinum, and the thymus lies above this ligament. (From Franken, E. A., Jr.: Amer. J. Roentgenol., *109*:252–260, 1970.)

cumstances, air may be shown to dissect into peribronchial tissues from the hilar region. These mediastinal fascial planes constitute a "highway connecting the lung to the mediastinum" (Marchand).

Venography of the Azygos and Vertebral Veins. Opacification of the vertebral and azygos veins has been accomplished by femoral vein injection with simultaneous inferior caval compression (Anderson). Thirty to 35 cubic centimeters of a suitable contrast agent such as Hypaque or Renografin are injected simultaneously into both femoral veins after pressure has been applied tightly against the patient's abdomen with a plastic plate and a "football air bladder."

The vertebral veins and azygos system may also be demonstrated by intraosseous venography (Fischgold et al.). This is accomplished by injecting the contrast agent directly into a spinous process of the thoracic vertebrae or the posterior segment of the last rib. Three to four films are obtained during and after the injection. It is also possible to opacify the azygos system by retrograde injection through a catheter inserted through the superior vena cava (Ranniger; Stauffer et al.).

Abrams has studied the lumbar and azygos system by ciné

techniques. In this instance a catheter is passed from the femoral vein into the inferior vena cava and then into a third, fourth, or fifth lumbar vein. Thirty cc. of 76 per cent Renografin are then injected in 5 seconds if both this vein and an ascending lumbar vein reached from a left common iliac vein are injected. A diagrammatic representation of the azygos venous system so visualized and examples of its appearance at the upper thoracic level and via osseous vertebral venography are shown in Figure 11–27. Numerous variations, implications, and applications may be shown, and the reader is referred to Abrams and a comprehensive reference for this purpose.

Investigation of the Thoracic Duct (Rosenberger and Abrams). Various techniques have been devised for study of the thoracic duct in the living. Retrograde injection of contrast agent has been used in patients with advanced neoplastic disease (Bierman et al.; Brzek et al.). Operative injection of the thoracic duct at the time of surgery has also been tried. Lymphangiography affords an excellent opportunity for study of the thoracic duct. The technique for this procedure has already been described in relation to the lymphatics of the lower extremity, and it will be referred to again in the study of the lymphatics and lymph nodes

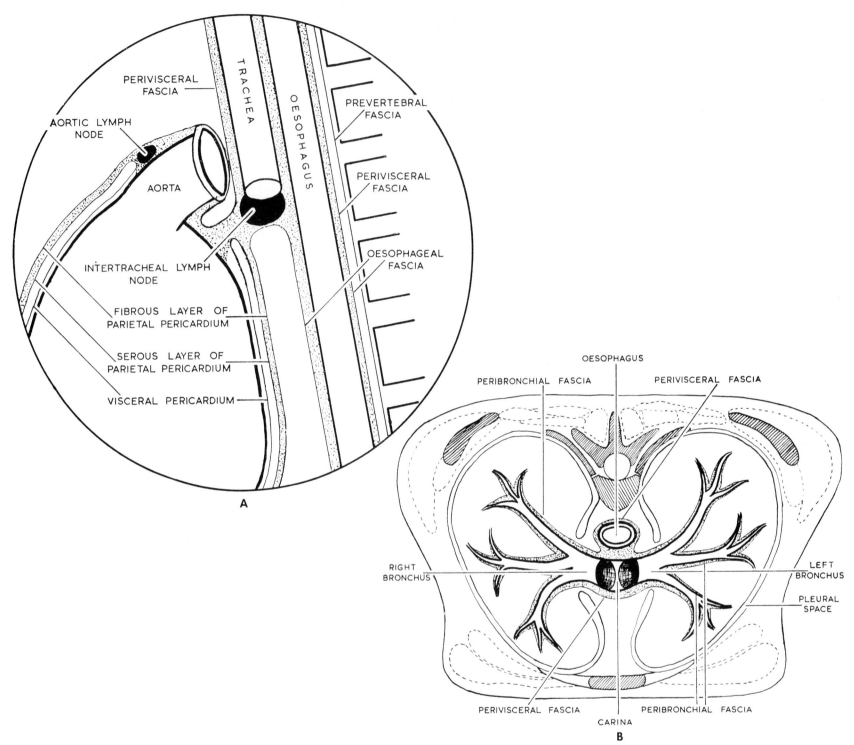

Figure 11–26.   *A*. Diagram showing the distribution of the perivisceral fascia at the bifurcation of the trachea and the relation of the intertracheal and aortic glands to the serous layers of the pericardium. The stippled area represents the subfascial connective tissue plane. *B*. Transverse section through the thorax. Diagram showing the manner in which the perivisceral fascia is prolonged around the right and left bronchi into the lung substance to form the peribronchial fascia. The stippled area represents the subfascial plane, occupied by connective tissue and in which lie the bronchial vessels and the pulmonary lymphatics. (From Marchand, P.: Thorax, 6:359–368, 1951.)

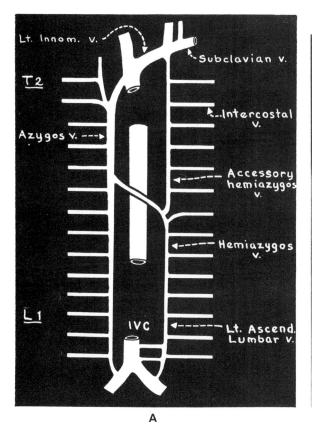

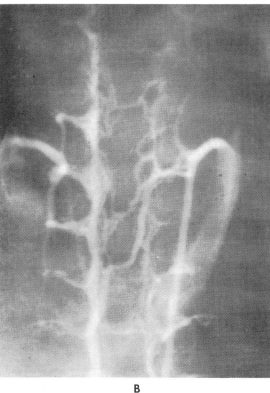

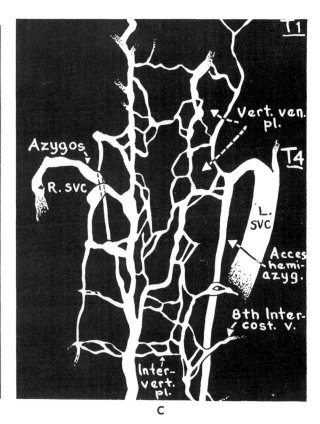

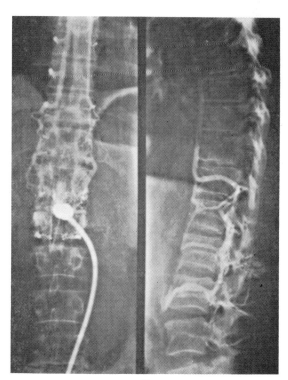

Figure 11–27. *A.* Diagrammatic representation of the azygos venous system. The segmental lumbar veins are joined to each other by a longitudinal vessel, the ascending lumbar vein. The right ascending lumbar vein as it enters the thorax becomes the azygos vein, and the left ascending lumbar vein is continuous with the hemiazygos vein. The hemiazygos vein crosses in front of the vertebral column at the level of the eighth or ninth thoracic vertebra to join the azygos vein. The accessory hemiazygos vein is continuous with the hemiazygos, receives the upper thoracic veins on the left, and joins the left superior intercostal vein above.

B and *C.* The vertebral veins at the upper thoracic level. The vertebral venous plexuses are opacified following the injection of the opaque medium into the left saphenous vein. The primitive paired arrangement of both the azygos and the superior vena cava veins is preserved, the accessory hemiazygos emptying into the left superior vena cava and the azygos emptying into the right superior vena cava. The medial portions of the intercostal veins are opacified. (R.SVC, right superior vena cava; L.SVC, left superior vena cava.)

D. Osseous vertebral venography. The opaque medium is injected into the spinous process and rapidly fills the paravertebral plexuses and the azygos system. (Courtesy of Dr. Franz P. Lessman, Roswell Park Memorial Institute, Buffalo, N.Y.) (Reproduced from Abrams, H. L.: Angiography, 2d ed. Boston, Little, Brown & Co., 1971.)

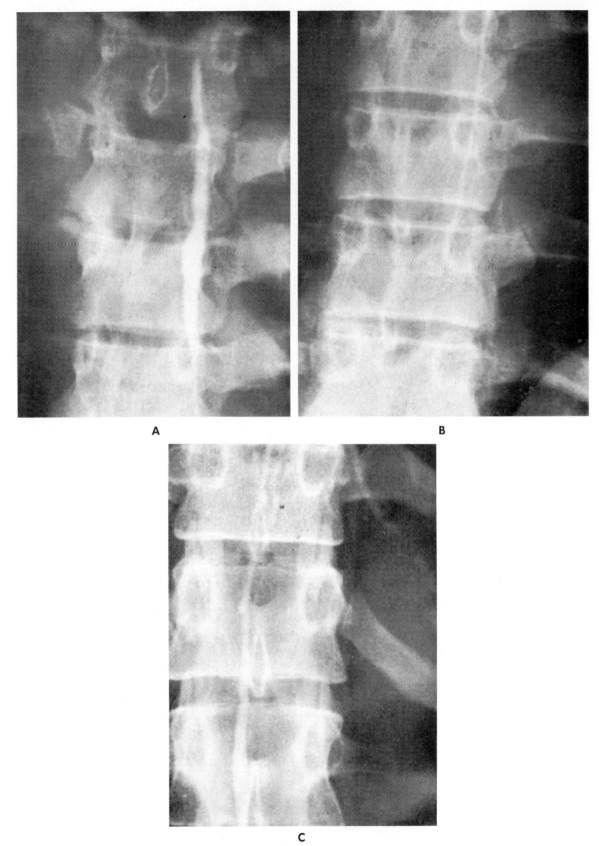

Figure 11–28. *See opposite page for legend.*

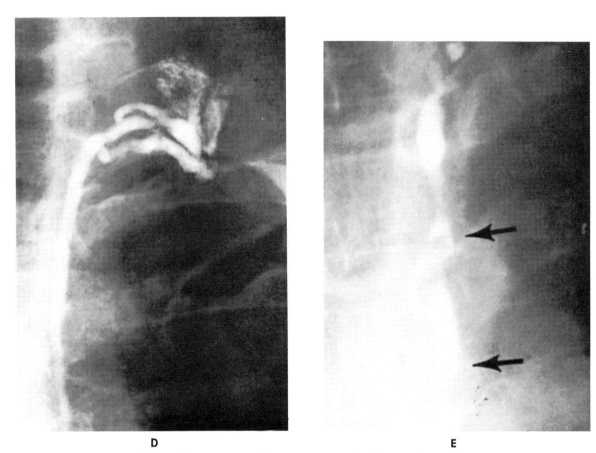

D   E

Figure 11–28. The thoracic duct. *A.* Upper thoracic segment. The thoracic duct lies anterior to the thoracic spine on its left side, immediately adjacent to the descending aorta. Above the left main-stem bronchus it parallels the course of the trachea. *B.* Mid-thoracic portion. The duct in its lower portion moves toward the midline, again following the course of the aorta. *C.* Caudal segment of the thoracic duct. The lowest portion of the duct overlies the first lumbar vertebra. It is now to the right of the midline. Its most caudal segment is continuous with the cisterna chyli. As it extends cephalad over the eleventh and twelfth thoracic vertebrae, it begins to move to the left and reaches the left of the midline at the interspace between the tenth and eleventh thoracic vertebrae. *D.* The thoracic duct, cephalic segment. The upper one-third of the duct resembles an inverted J. Notice that it becomes three separate channels just prior to its entry into the junction of the internal jugular and left subclavian veins. A few supraclavicular lymph nodes are filled with contrast agent. *E.* Valves in the thoracic duct. Valves can usually be visualized in the thoracic duct and may vary in number from two to thirteen. They are bicuspid and quite variable in size. The maximum observed diameter of a valve was 6 mm. (From Abrams, H. L.: Angiography, 2d ed. Boston, Little, Brown & Co., 1971.)

of the abdominal region. In brief review, this procedure involves the injection of a vital stain into the web space between the great toe and the second toe, surgical dissection of the subcutaneous lymphatic in this region, and insertion of a very fine catheter tip into the lymphatic. Next, a contrast agent such as Ethiodol in 3 to 5 cc. quantities is injected, and films of the lower extremities, the abdomen, and the chest are routinely taken 1 to 2 hours after the injection. Films are obtained as required in anteroposterior, lateral, and oblique projections (for a comprehensive review of this technique see Fuchs).

As noted previously, the thoracic duct is a continuation of the cisterna chyli from its abdominal segment into the thorax, enter-

ing the thorax through the aortic hiatus of the diaphragm. A representative illustration is shown in Figure 11–28. As visualized by Rosenberger and Abrams, the maximum diameter of the thoracic duct varied between 1 and 7 mm., and no difference in distribution of size was detected by them with or without mediastinal masses. Valves in the thoracic duct were noted in most cases (Fig. 11–28 *E*), and the maximum observed diameter of a valve was 6 mm. Multiple thoracic channels were observed in a number of cases, and variations of normal were not unusual. The roentgen signs of normality and abnormality were carefully documented by Rosenberger and Abrams.

REFERENCES

Abrams, H. L.: The vertebral and azygos veins. *In* Abrams, H. L. (ed.): Angiography. Second edition. Vol. 1. Boston, Little, Brown & Co., 1971.

Anderson, R. K.: Diodrast studies of the vertebral and cranial venous systems. J. Neurosurg., *8*:411, 1951.

Anson, B. (ed.): Morris' Human Anatomy. 12th edition. New York, McGraw-Hill, 1966.

Bierman, H. R., Byron, R. L., Jr., Kelly, K. H., Gilfillan, R. S., White, L. P., Freeman, N. E., and Petrakis, N. L.: The characteristics of thoracic duct lymph in man. J. Clin. Invest., *32*:637, 1953.

Blank, N., and Castellino, R. A.: Patterns of pleural reflections of the left superior mediastinum. Radiology, *102*:585–589, 1972.

Boijsen, E., and Reuter, S. R.: Subclavian and internal mammary angiography in the evaluation of anterior mediastinal masses. Amer. J. Roentgenol., *98*:447–450, 1966.

Brzek, V., Kren, V., and Bartos, V.: Retrograde lymphographie des ductus thoracicus. Fortschr. Roentgenstr., *102*:125–131, 1965.

Cimmino, C. V., and Snead, L. O.: The posterior mediastinal line on chest roentgenograms. Radiology, *84*:516–518, 1965.

Condorelli, L.: Il pneumo-mediastino artificiale; ricerche anatomiche preliminari. Tecnica delle iniezioni nelle loggie mediastiniche anteriore e posteriore. Minerva Medica, *1*:81–86, 1936.

Doyle, F. H., Read, A. E., and Evans, K. T.: The mediastinum in portal hypertension. Clin. Radiol., *12*:114–129, 1961.

Felson, B.: Letter from the editor. Sem. in Roentgenol., *2*:323, 1967.

Fischgold, H., Adam, H., Ecoiffier, J., and Piequet, J.: Opacification des plexus rachidiens et des veines azygos voie osseusse. J. Radiol. et Électrol., *33*:37, 1952.

Fleischner, F. G., and Udis, S. W.: Dilatation of the azygos vein: a roentgen sign of venous engorgement. Amer. J. Roentgenol., *67*:509, 1952.

Franken, E. A., Jr.: Pneumomediastinum in the newborn. Amer. J. Roentgenol., *109*:252–260, 1970.

Fuchs, W. A.: Technique in complications of lymphangiography. *In* Abrams, H. L. (ed.): Angiography. Second edition. Boston, Little, Brown & Co., 1971.

Hare, W. S. C., and Mackay, I. R.: Radiological assessment of the thymic size in myasthenia gravis and systemic lupus erythematosus. Lancet, *1*:746–748, 1963.

Heitzman, E. R., Scrivani, J. V., Martino, J., and Moro, J.: The azygos vein and its pleural reflections. II. Applications in the radiological diagnosis of mediastinal abnormalities. Radiology, *101*:259–266, 1971.

Hughes, D. L., Hanafee, W. N., and O'Loughlin, B. J.: Diagnostic pneumomediastinum. Radiology, *12*: 1962.

Issard, H. J., Bergelson, V. D., and Foreman, J.: Mediastinal pneumography. Amer. J. Roentgenol., *75*:771–778, 1956.

Keats, T. E., Lipscomb, G. E., and Betts, C. S., III: Mensuration of the arch of the azygos vein and its application to the study of cardiopulmonary disease. Radiology, *90*:990–994, 1968.

Knutsson, F.: The mediastinal pleura. Acta Radiol., *43*:265–275, 1955.

Kreel, L., Blendis, L. M., and Piercy, J. C.: Pneumomediastinography by trans-sternal method. Clin. Radiol., *15*:219–223, 1964.

McCort, J. J., and Robbins, L. L.: Roentgen diagnosis of intrathoracic lymph-node metastases in carcinoma of the lung. Radiology, *57*:339–359, 1951.

Marchand, P.: The anatomy and applied anatomy of the mediastinal fascia. Thorax, *6*:359–368, 1951.

Moseley, J. E., and Som, M.: Cervical thymus gland. J. Mt. Sinai Hospital, *21*:289–295, 1954–55.

Oliva, L. E.: Pneumomediastinography. *In* Rigler, L. G. (ed.): Roentgen Diagnosis. Vol. 1, General Principles and Methods. Second American edition. New York and London, Grune & Stratton, 1968.

Pacofsky, K. B., and Wolfel, D. A.: Azygos continuation of the inferior vena cava. Amer. J. Roentgenol., *113*:362–365, 1971.

Palubinskas, A. J., and Hodson, C. J.: Transintervertebral retroperitoneal gas insufflation. Radiology, *70*:851–854, 1958.

Preger, L., Hooper, T. I., Steinbach, H. L., and Hoffman, J. I. E.: Width of azygos vein related to central venous pressure. Radiology, *93*:521–523, 1969.

Rabinowitz, J. G., and Wolf, B. S.: Roentgen significance of the pulmonary ligament. Radiology, *87*:1013–1020, 1966.

Ranniger, K.: Retrograde azygography. Radiology, *90*:1097, 1968.

Rosenberger, A., and Abrams, H. L.: The thoracic duct. *In* Abrams, H. L. (ed.): Angiography. Second edition. Boston, Little, Brown & Co., 1971.

Rouviere, H., and Valette, G.: Physiologie du Systeme Lymphatique. Paris, Masson et Cie, 1937.

Ruiz-Rivas, M.: Generalized subserous emphysema with a single puncture. Amer. J. Roentgenol., *64*:723–739, 1950.

Stauffer, H. M., LaBree, J. W., and Adams, F. H.: Normally situated arch of azygos vein; roentgenologic identification and catheterization. Amer. J. Roentgenol., *66*:353, 1951.

Stranahan, A., Alley, R. D., Kousel, H. W., and Reeve, T. S.: Operative thoracic ductography. J. Thoracic Surg., *31*:183, 1956.

Sumerling, M. D., and Irvine, W. J.: Pneumomediastinography. Amer. J. Roentgenol., *98*:451–460, 1966.

Swart, B.: The width of the azygos vein as a roentgen diagnostic criterion of pathological collateral circulation. Fortschr. Roentgenstrahl., *91*:415–444, 1959.

Tausend, M. E., and Stern, W. Z.: Thymic patterns in the newborn. Amer. J. Roentgenol., *95*:125–130, 1965.

Tori, G., and Garusi, G. F.: The azygos vein. Amer. J. Roentgenol., *87*:235–247, 1962.

Vallebona, A.: Transverse stratigraphy of the mediastinum. Stratigrafia, *2*:73–89, 1957.

Wishart, D. L.: Normal azygos vein width in children. Radiology, *104*:115–118, 1972.

Yune, H. Y., and Klatte, E. C.: Thymic venography. Radiology, *96*:521–526, 1970.

12

The Heart and Major Blood Vessels

BASIC ANATOMY OF THE CARDIOVASCULAR SYSTEM

Introduction. The heart, its major blood vessels, and the blood contained within these structures are all of the same order of density, and hence any studies of the heart without contrast media in the blood must necessarily be contour studies.

These studies, therefore, presuppose a knowledge of the normal positions of the various cardiac chambers, so that they can be placed in proper position for study; they also are based upon a knowledge of the normal contours of these chambers when in these various degrees of obliquity.

The Heart. The heart is enclosed within the pericardium, and normally there is only a thin layer of fluid between the inner layer of pericardium and the epicardium of the heart. The heart is obliquely situated in the chest so that about one-third of it is situated on the right and about two-thirds on the left of the median plane (Fig. 12–1).

The heart contains four chambers—two atria and two ventricles. The atria are separated from the ventricles by the *coronary sulcus*. The groove which separates the two atria is barely visible on the posterior surface, and is hidden from view on the anterior surface by the pulmonary artery and the aorta. There are two grooves separating the ventricles—the *anterior longitudinal sulcus* near the left border of the heart, and the *posterior longitudinal sulcus* on the diaphragmatic surface of the heart. The base of the heart is the upper posterior and right aspect of the heart, while the apex is rounded and extends inferiorly and to the left (Fig. 12–2).

The right atrium is slightly larger than the left and forms the upper right margin of the heart (Fig. 12–3). It has a principal cavity and a smaller anterior pouch called the auricle. The superior and inferior venae cavae open into the right atrium, as does also the coronary sinus (Fig. 12–4). These channels return the blood from the upper and lower parts of the body and the heart musculature respectively.

Situated in the lower part of the septum between the right and left atria is the fossa ovalis, an oval depression that corresponds with the foramen ovale of the fetus.

692

The left atrium, like the right, contains a principal cavity and an auricle. There are four pulmonary veins (Fig. 12–5) that open into the upper part of the posterior surface of the left atrium. The left atrium forms the greater part of the posterior surface of the heart and the base of the heart. It is in close proximity with the esophagus in this sector, and any enlargement of the left atrium must necessarily displace the esophagus posteriorly, and usually to the right (Figs. 12–6, 12–7). (Also see cross-section diagrams of mediastinum in Chapter 11.).

The right ventricle forms the larger part of the anterior (or sternocostal) surface of the heart, and it also forms a small portion of the diaphragmatic surface. Its upper and left portion forms

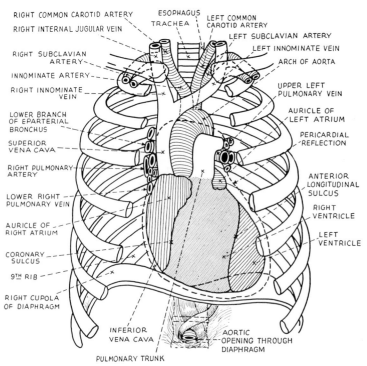

Figure 12–1. Projections of the heart in the thoracic cage with lung and rib structures removed. Frontal projection.

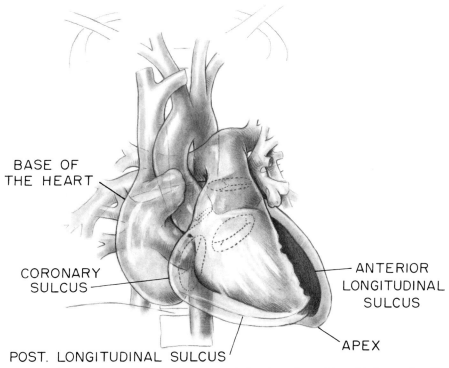

BASE OF
THE HEART

CORONARY
SULCUS

ANTERIOR
LONGITUDINAL
SULCUS

APEX

POST. LONGITUDINAL SULCUS

Figure 12–2. Frontal view of a normal heart (transparent) showing relationships of inflow and outflow tracts to chambers. (After Schad, N., et al.: Differential Diagnosis of Congenital Heart Disease. New York, Grune & Stratton, 1966.)

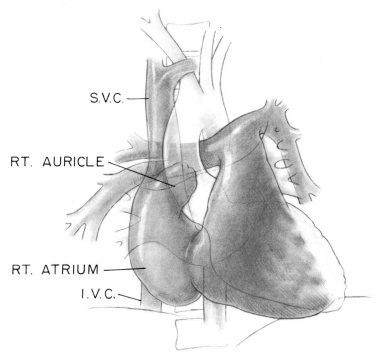

S.V.C.

RT. AURICLE

RT. ATRIUM

I.V.C.

Figure 12–3. Frontal view of the heart showing the relationship of inflow and outflow tracts to the right cardiac chambers. (After Schad, N., et al.: Differential Diagnosis of Congenital Heart Disease. New York, Grune & Stratton, 1966.)

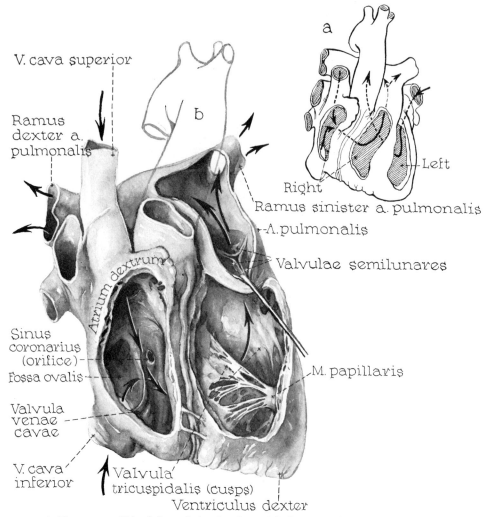

Figure 12–4. A. The course of blood through the chambers of the heart. B. The arterial "side" of the heart. (From Anson, B. J.: An Atlas of Human Anatomy. Philadelphia, W. B. Saunders Co., 1968.)

a conical pouch called the conus arteriosus or pulmonary conus. The wall of the right ventricle is thinner than that of the left, bearing a ratio of about 1 to 3 to the latter. The opening of the pulmonary artery is situated at the uppermost part of the conus arteriosus, above and to the left of the right atrioventricular opening (Figs. 12-4, 12-8, 12-9).

The left ventricle forms much of the left cardiac border below the coronary sulcus, and a considerable part of the diaphragmatic surface of the heart. The left atrioventricular orifice is below and to the left of the orifice connecting with the aorta (Fig. 12-10).

There are four series of valves regulating blood flow between the chambers of the heart and great vessels, situated between left atrium and left ventricle (mitral valves), left ventricle and aorta (aortic valves), right atrium and right ventricle (tricuspid valves), and right ventricle and pulmonary artery (pulmonary valves) (Fig. 12-11). There are three cusps (Fig. 12-12) to each of the above valves, with the exception of the mitral valve, which has only two. The tricuspid and mitral valves are attached by means of narrow bands (chordae tendineae) to the papillary muscles of the ventricular walls.

The Cardiac Cycle (Fig. 12-12). The heart normally pulsates regularly by contraction at a rate of approximately 60 to 80 times per minute. Its wave of contraction is known as systole and its period of rest as diastole. The atrial systole normally precedes

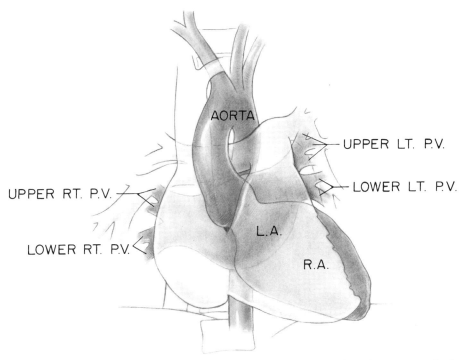

Figure 12-5. Frontal view of the heart showing the relationship of inflow and outflow tracts to the left cardiac chambers. (After Schad, N., et al.: Differential Diagnosis of Congenital Heart Disease. New York, Grune & Stratton, 1966.)

the ventricular. When the ventricles contract, the bicuspid and tricuspid valves close, preventing the regress of the blood from the ventricles back to the atria, and as the pressure rises, the pulmonary and aortic valves open and allow the flow of the blood into the pulmonary artery and the aorta. When the ventricular con-

traction ceases, these latter valves close. During the period of rest, the blood from the systemic and pulmonary veins flows into the atria.

The technique of cardiac catheterization and selective angio-cardiography will be reviewed subsequently. The diagnostic pro-

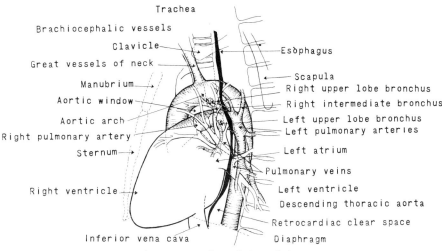

Figure 12-6. Lateral view of chest.

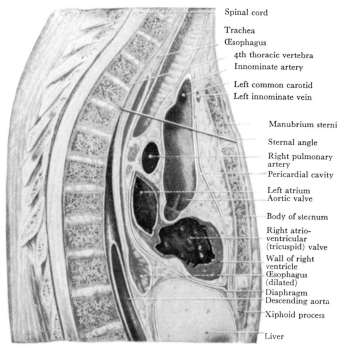

Spinal cord

Trachea

Œsophagus

4th thoracic vertebra

Innominate artery

Left common carotid

Left innominate vein

Manubrium sterni

Sternal angle

Right pulmonary artery

Pericardial cavity

Left atrium

Aortic valve

Body of sternum

Right atrio-ventricular (tricuspid) valve

Wall of right ventricle

Œsophagus (dilated)

Diaphragm

Descending aorta

Xiphoid process

Liver

Figure 12-7. Sagittal section of thorax of an old man. The upper border of manubrium sterni and the bifurcation of trachea are lower than in a young adult. The thick black line is the artificial boundary that separates the superior mediastinum from the other three. (From Cunningham's Manual of Practical Anatomy, 12th ed., Vol. 2. London, Oxford University Press, 1958.)

outside the scope of this text (see Kory et al. for a brief interpretive summary).

Fluoroscopically, the pulsations in the various portions of the heart vary somewhat in their appearance and sequence, the contractions being most forceful in the region of the left ventricular apex posteriorly (best seen in the left anterior oblique projection). The sequence and character of the pulsations, as well as the rhythm, require close study, since variations from the normal pattern are of considerable significance.

The Aorta. The aorta arises from within the cardiac silhouette in a sheath shared with the pulmonary artery. The *ascending* aorta begins on a level with the third intercostal space along the left sternal margin and ascends posterior to the sternum as far as the superior border of the right costosternal articulation or sternal angle. This segment is 5 to 5.5 cm. in length usually and 28 to 30 mm. in diameter. There is a dilatation of the aorta near its point of origin caused by the three *aortic sinuses*, one to the right and one to the left, and a third posteriorly (Fig. 12-13). The *right and left coronary arteries* arise from the superior borders of the right and left aortic sinuses.

The *arch of the aorta* lies in the superior mediastinum posterior to the manubrium, covered by an attachment of fibrous pericardium. It begins at the second right costal cartilage and curves superiorly, dorsally, and to the left and then caudally

cedures performed under radiologic control permit sampling of blood and pressure measurements in the various chambers of the heart, aorta, and pulmonary arteries proximally and distally. These measurements permit the estimation of valvular abnormalities as well as cardiac output determinations.

Figure 12-12 presents graphically the normal percentage of oxygen saturation and oxygen volume, and pressure ranges in heart chambers and great vessels. Pressure tracings are shown in relation to the electrocardiogram both in the right and left heart, with inclusion also of aortic and pulmonary pressure determinations.

In the pulmonary wedge position, 97 to 99 per cent saturated blood can be withdrawn from the wedged catheter, approximating the values of pulmonary venous blood. Note that the phasic pressures in the right atrium, left atrium, and pulmonary artery wedge position have the same overall characteristics. There are small differences in amplitude and timing of the various phases.

The level of peak systolic pressure of the left ventricle is approximately five times that in the right, but the phasic pressures in the right and left ventricles are very similar in contour. A detailed discussion of these curves, phases, and interpretation is

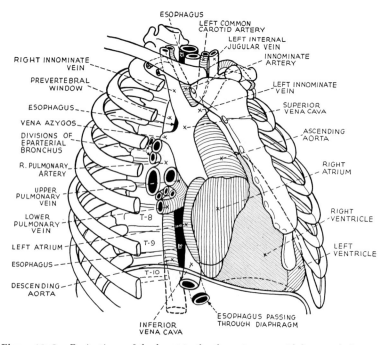

Figure 12-8. Projections of the heart in the thoracic cage with lung and rib structures removed. Right anterior oblique projection.

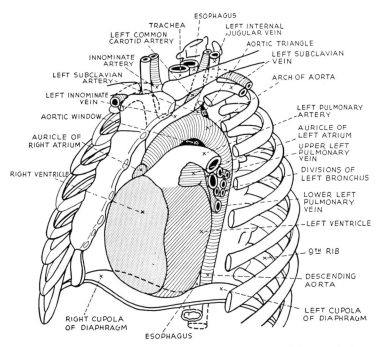

Figure 12-9. Projections of the heart in the thoracic cage with lung and rib structures removed. Left anterior oblique projection.

Variations in the main branches of the arch of the aorta, along with their statistical incidence, are indicated in Figures 12-14 and 12-15.

Anomalously, the right aortic arch may persist, resulting in a complete reversal of the branches and structures of the aortic arch. This may occur with or without a situs inversus of all of the viscera, and occurs in approximately 20 per cent of those individuals who have a tetralogy of Fallot. Also, the distal portion of the right aortic arch may persist, an anomaly that is associated with the disappearance of some or all of the proximal part. This abnormality may result in the right subclavian artery appearing to originate from the descending thoracic aorta. In these instances, the right subclavian artery passes to the right, dorsal to the trachea and esophagus, and making an esophageal impression. Other abnormalities are described with congenital anomalies in roentgenologic texts dealing with the abnormal.

The usual branches of the aortic arch are: the *brachiocephalic*, the *left common carotid*, and the *left subclavian arteries.* These supply the head and neck, superior limbs, and part of the thoracic wall (Fig. 12-16). A *thyroidea ima artery* may arise from the arch between the brachiocephalic and left common carotid arteries. (The brachiocephalic trunk and subclavian vessels have been described in relation to the upper extremity.)

along the left side of the vertebral column to a level between the fourth and fifth thoracic vertebrae, where it continues as the *descending thoracic aorta.* It arches across the right pulmonary artery and left bronchus. The aortic arch lies to the left of the trachea and esophagus.

Just beyond the origin of the left subclavian artery, the aorta narrows somewhat and is called the *isthmus,* this segment extending to the point of origin of the *ligamentum arteriosum.* The latter structure is attached to the concavity of the arch approximately opposite the third thoracic vertebra. The proximal arch of the aorta usually has a diameter of approximately 28 mm., but it diminishes in size beyond the subclavian to an average of 23 mm. When this measurement exceeds 37 mm., the aorta can be considered dilated or aneurysmal. The thymus overlies the arch of the aorta between the pleural cavities anteriorly.

Within the concavity of the arch of the aorta are the following structures: the *right pulmonary artery,* the *bifurcation of the pulmonary trunk,* the *left bronchus,* the *ligamentum arteriosum,* the *left recurrent laryngeal nerves,* the *superficial cardiac plexus,* and several *bronchial lymph nodes.*

Dorsal to the arch of the aorta are the following structures: the *superior vena cava, trachea, esophagus, thoracic duct, deep cardiac plexus,* and *left retrolaryngeal nerve.* The *left brachiocephalic vein* is superior and somewhat ventral. The chief three branches of the arch of the aorta arise along its cephalic border.

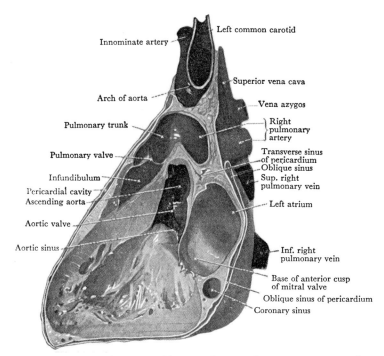

Figure 12-10. Sagittal section of heart and pericardium. (From Cunningham's Manual of Practical Anatomy, 12th ed., Vol. 2., London, Oxford University Press, 1958.)

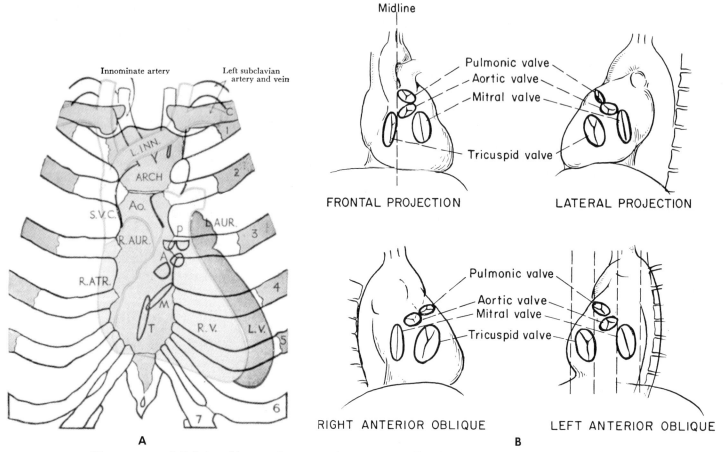

PROJECTION OF CARDIAC VALVES
IN ROUTINE POSITIONS IN RADIOGRAPHY

Figure 12–11. *A.* Relation of heart and great vessels to anterior wall of thorax. (1 to 7) Ribs and costal cartilages, (A) aortic orifice, (Ao) ascending aorta, (C) clavicle, (L.V.) left ventricle, (M) mitral orifice, (P) pulmonary orifice, (R.V.) right ventricle, (S.V.C.) superior vena cava, (T) tricuspid orifice. (From Cunningham's Manual of Practical Anatomy, 12th ed., Vol. 2. London, Oxford University Press, 1958.) *B.* Cardiac valves in routine radiographic projections.

The *common carotid arteries* ascend into the neck and are different on each side. They are 8 to 12 cm. long, extending from the sternoclavicular articulation to the superior border of the thyroid cartilage (Fig. 12–16). At the level of the fourth cervical vertebra they divide into internal and external carotid arteries. The common carotid arteries are contained in a common sheath with *the internal jugular vein* and the *vagus nerve* on each side. At the sternoclavicular joint the jugular vein lies ventrolateral to the artery, but as it ascends it becomes dorsolateral. The common carotid artery is unbranched except at its termination and does not diminish in size as it ascends in the neck, but there is a slight

dilatation for approximately 1 cm. at its bifurcation which provides for the *carotid sinus*, part of a mechanism that regulates blood pressure.

The collateral circulation of the common carotid and subclavian arteries is shown diagrammatically in Figure 12–17.

The *external carotid artery* is distributed to the anterior part of the neck, the pharynx, the tongue, oral cavity, face, temporal and infratemporal fossae, nasal cavity, and the greater part of the scalp and cranial meninges (Fig. 12–16 *B*).

There is some variability in the point of origin of the external carotid artery, but it arises at the superior border of the thyroid cartilage or the fourth cervical level in about two-thirds of the cases. It may, however, arise at the third cervical level or at the superior margin of the fifth cervical vertebra. It generally terminates posterior to the neck of the mandible, dividing into two main branches: the *maxillary* and *superficial temporal arteries.* Eight independent branches arising from the external carotid may usually be counted, given off in the following order: *superior thyroid, ascending pharyngeal, lingual, facial, occipital, posterior auricular, superficial temporal,* and *maxillary.* The *sternocleidomastoid artery* is also an independent branch. These major branches are indicated in Figure 12–16 B.

Returning to the distal portion of the arch of the aorta at the point of origin of the ligamentum arteriosum, a very slight dilatation of the aorta may occur, sometimes referred to as the *"ductus diverticulum"* (Fig. 12–18). Beyond this there may be in infants, a further slight fusiform dilatation, which His has called the *aortic spindle.* This structure may persist into adult life. In the adult, the site of insertion of the ligamentum arteriosum may appear on aortography as a very slight irregularity.

The *descending aorta* follows a downward course to the left of the vertebral column giving off numerous small branches, most of them intercostal arteries. The small *bronchial arteries* and

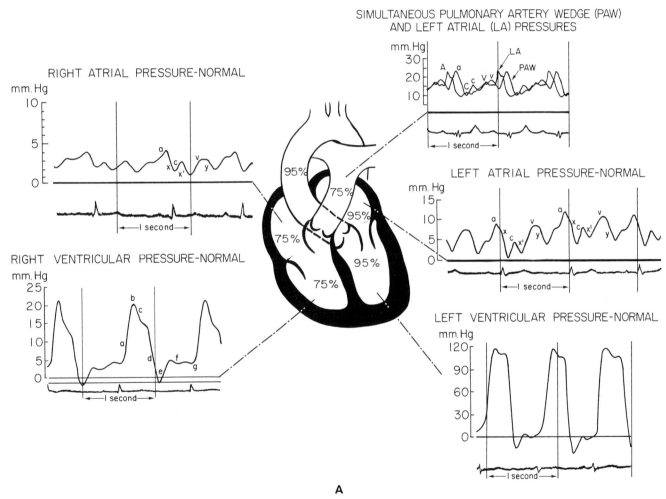

A

Figure 12–12. *A.* Diagram of the heart and its major blood vessels indicating the related pressure curves obtained from the right atrium, the right ventricle, and simultaneously from the pulmonary artery and left atrium, as well as normal pressure curves for the left atrium and left ventricle. The average oxygen saturation in the right atrium, right ventricle, pulmonary artery, left atrium, left ventricle, and aorta are also indicated.

Figure 12–12 continued on the following page.

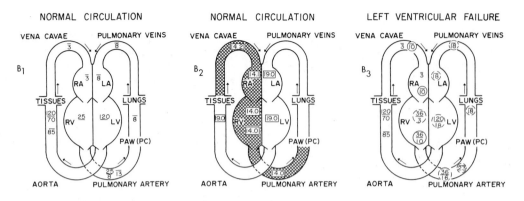

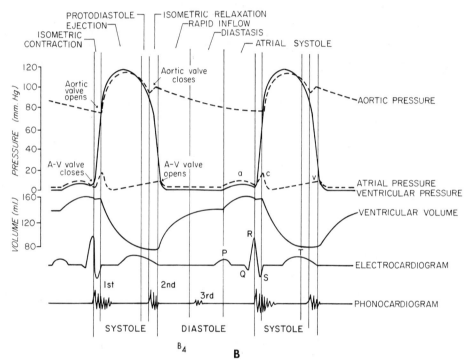

Figure 12–12 *Continued.* *B1.* Schematic diagram of the normal circulation showing representative mean pressures in millimeters of mercury in the various heart chambers, great vessels and pulmonary artery wedge (PAW). (RA) Right atrium, (RV) right ventricle, (LA) left atrium, (LV) left ventricle, (PC) pulmonary capillary.

B2. Diagram of the normal circulation showing representative values for oxygen content of the blood expressed in volumes per cent in the various heart chambers and major vessels. The cross-hatched area represents venous blood. (Abbreviations as previously indicated.)

B3. The figures encircled by interrupted lines are representative pressure values which may be recorded in the presence of left ventricular failure. Those figures encircled by solid lines are representative pressure values for right ventricular failure. (*B1, B2,* and *B3* redrawn from: Kory, R. C., Tsagaris, T. J., and Bustamante, R. A.: A Primer of Cardiac Catheterization. 1965. Courtesy of Charles C Thomas, Publisher, Springfield, Ill.)

B4. Correlation of the dynamic acoustic and electrical events of the cardiac cycle: this figure provides simultaneous recording of left atrial, left ventricular, and aortic pressures together with the electrocardiogram and phonocardiogram. (LV) left ventricle, (LA) left atrium. The numbers 1, 2, and 3 refer to the first, second, and third heart sounds respectively. (Redrawn from Guyton, A. C.: Textbook of Medical Physiology, 4th ed. Philadelphia, W. B. Saunders Co., 1971.)

Figure 12–12 continued on the opposite page.

Figure 12–12 *Continued.* *C.* Calculations of mitral and aortic valve areas, intracardiac pressures, oxygen content variation between right heart vessels and chambers, average oxygen contents and saturations in various heart chambers and vessels, and representative oxygen content evaluation in left to right shunts. (From Kory, R. C., Tsagaris, T. J., and Bustamante, R. A.: A Primer of Cardiac Catheterization, 1965. Courtesy of Charles C Thomas, Publisher, Springfield, Illinois.)

A. Calculation of Mitral Valve Area

The formula in general use for calculation of mitral valve area[47] is:

$$\text{MITRAL VALVE AREA, cm.}^2 = \frac{\text{Mitral valve flow (ml./sec.)}}{31\sqrt{\text{Diastolic gradient across the mitral valve}}}$$

$$\text{where: Mitral valve flow} = \frac{\text{Cardiac output (ml./min.)}}{\text{Diastolic filling period (sec./min.)}}$$

$$\begin{array}{l}\text{Diastolic filling} \\ \text{period} \\ \text{(sec./min.)}\end{array} = \begin{array}{l}\text{diastolic period} \\ \text{per beat} \\ \text{(sec./beat)}\end{array} \times \begin{array}{l}\text{heart rate} \\ \text{(beats/min.)}\end{array}$$

$$\begin{array}{l}\text{Diastolic gradient} \\ \text{across the mitral} \\ \text{valve (mm. Hg)}\end{array} = \begin{array}{l}\text{left atrial} \\ \text{mean pressure} \\ \text{(mm. Hg)}\end{array} \text{minus} \begin{array}{l}\text{left ventricular} \\ \text{mean diastolic} \\ \text{pressure (mm. Hg.)}\end{array}$$

and 31 = empirical constant

The *normal mitral valve area* is 4.5 cm.² Clinical disability is present with mitral valve areas of 1.0 cm.² or less (Lewis et al.).

B. Calculation of Aortic Valve Area

The formula in general use for calculation of aortic valve area is:

$$\begin{array}{l}\text{AORTIC VALVE} \\ \text{AREA, cm.}^2\end{array} = \frac{\text{Aortic valve flow (ml./sec.)}}{44.5\sqrt{\text{Systolic pressure gradient across the aortic valve}}}$$

$$\begin{array}{l}\text{where: Aortic valve flow} \\ \text{(ml./sec.)}\end{array} = \frac{\text{Cardiac output (ml./min.)}}{\text{Systolic ejection period (sec./min.)}}$$

$$\begin{array}{l}\text{Systolic ejection period} \\ \text{(sec./min.)}\end{array} = \begin{array}{l}\text{Systolic ejection period} \\ \text{per beat} \\ \text{(sec./beat)}\end{array} \times \begin{array}{l}\text{Heart rate} \\ \text{(beats/min.)}\end{array}$$

$$\begin{array}{l}\text{Systolic pressure} \\ \text{gradient across} \\ \text{the aortic valve} \\ \text{(mm. Hg)}\end{array} = \begin{array}{l}\text{left ventricular} \\ \text{mean systolic} \\ \text{pressure} \\ \text{(mm. Hg)}\end{array} \text{minus} \begin{array}{l}\text{aortic} \\ \text{mean systolic} \\ \text{pressure} \\ \text{(mm. Hg)}\end{array}$$

and 44.5 = gravity acceleration factor

The *normal aortic valve* area is 3-4 cm.² Clinical disability is generally present when the valve area is 0.75 cm.² or less (Wood) and is always present with a valve area of 0.5 cm.² or less (Gorlin et al.).

The formulas for calculation of the tricuspid and pulmonary valve areas are similar to the formulas for calculating the mitral and aortic valve areas, respectively, but are rarely used clinically.

Similar formulas can be used for estimating the size of a patent ductus arteriosus or the size of defects in the atrial or ventricular septa.

SHUNT FLOW

A central circulatory shunt is defined as an abnormal communication between the pulmonary and systemic circulations connecting either of the two pairs of cardiac chambers or the great vessels.[50] Shunting of blood may occur from left to right, right to left, or may be bidirectional.

A. OXYGEN METHOD FOR DETECTION OF SHUNTS

The determination of O_2 content in blood samples drawn at different levels within the heart and great vessels aids in determining the presence, direction, and volume of central circulatory shunts.

The average normal values for the O_2 content and saturation in the various chambers of the heart and great vessels are shown in Table 12C.

TABLE 12C
AVERAGE O_2 CONTENTS AND SATURATIONS IN VARIOUS HEART CHAMBERS AND VESSELS

	O_2 Content vol. %	O_2 Saturation
SUPERIOR VENA CAVA (SVC)	14 (±1)	70%
INFERIOR VENA CAVA (IVC)	16 (±1)	80%
RIGHT ATRIUM (RA)	15 (±1)	75%
PULMONARY ARTERY (PA)	15.2 (±1)	75%
RIGHT VENTRICLE (RV)	15.2 (±1)	75%
BRACHIAL ARTERY (BA)	19.0 (±1)	95%+

There is moderate variation in venous oxygen content from chamber to chamber even in patients without shunts. The limits of this variation which may occur normally are indicated in Table 12B (Gorlin).

TABLE 12A
INTRACARDIAC PRESSURES — NORMAL RESTING VALUES

	Pressure in mm. Hg.		
Site of Measurement	Systolic	Diastolic	Mean
Right atrium (RA)	*	*	< 5
Right ventricle (RV)	< 30	< 5 (End-diastolic)	**
Pulmonary Artery (PA)	< 30	< 10	< 20
***Pulmonary Artery Wedge (PAW)	*	*	< 12
Left atrium (LA)	*	*	< 12
Left ventricle (LV)	120	< 10 (End-diastolic)	**
Aorta (Ao)	120	70	95

*Since the pressures in the right and left atria are comparatively low and since the systolic and diastolic levels are subject to wide respiratory fluctuation, only the mean atrial pressures are commonly reported in cardiac catheterization studies.

**Since systolic pressures in the ventricles are related to ventricular ejection and diastolic pressures to ventricular filling, *mean* ventricular pressure values have no physiologic meaning and are not reported.

***The pulmonary artery wedge (PAW) pressure, also termed the pulmonary "capillary" pressure, is obtained by "wedging" the catheter into a small branch of the pulmonary artery. This pressure is essentially the same as the pressure in the left atrium (LA).

TABLE 12B
MAXIMAL NORMAL LIMIT OF O_2 CONTENT VARIATION BETWEEN RIGHT HEART CHAMBERS AND VESSELS

	Maximal Increase in O_2 Content Over the Proximal Chamber
PA (between PA and RV)	0.5 vol. %
RV (between RV and RA)	0.9 vol. %
RA (between RA and SVC)	1.9 vol. %

If the increase in oxygen content of blood in a particular chamber exceeds that of the more proximal chamber by more than the value listed, a left-to-right shunt at that chamber or great vessel level is probably present. Thus, if the O_2 content of the right ventricle exceeds the O_2 content of the right atrium by more than 0.9 vol. %, a ventricular septal defect with a left-to-right shunt is likely. However, when the shunt is small (less than 25% of the systemic flow), this method may not be sensitive enough to detect the presence of such a shunt.

Examples of commonly encountered left-to-right shunts with representative O_2 content values are shown in Table 12D.

TABLE 12D
REPRESENTATIVE O_2 CONTENT VALUES IN LEFT-TO-RIGHT SHUNTS

	O_2 Content (vol. %)		
	Atrial Septal Defect (ASD)	Ventricular Septal Defect (VSD)	Patent Ductus Arteriosus (PDA)
BRACHIAL ARTERY (BA)	20	20	20
PULMONARY ARTERY (PA)	17	17	17
RIGHT VENTRICLE (RV)	17	17	14
RIGHT ATRIUM (RA)	17	14	14
SUPERIOR VENA CAVA (SVC)	14	14	14

C

Figure 12–12 *Continued. See opposite page for legend.*

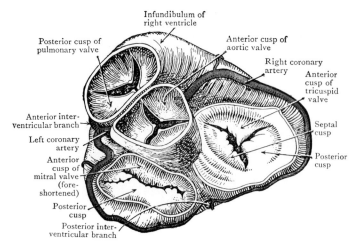

Figure 12–13. Base of ventricular part of the heart, showing arterial orifices and their valves, aortic sinuses and origin of the coronary arteries. (From Cunningham's Manual of Practical Anatomy, 12th ed., Vol. 2. London, Oxford University Press, 1958.)

esophageal branches also arise from this segment of the aorta (the bronchial arteries are described in Chapter 11 and the esophageal blood vessels will be described in conjunction with the alimentary tract in Chapter 13).

The descending thoracic aorta passes from the left side of the vertebral column, becoming more medial in its descent, and finally lies immediately in front of the vertebral column at the level of the diaphragm. It is related anteriorly to the root of the left lung, pericardium, esophagus, and diaphragm. On its right side lie the azygos vein and thoracic duct and on the left are situated the left pleura and lung. It ends at the lower border of the twelfth thoracic vertebra, where it pierces the diaphragm and continues as the abdominal aorta.

Pulmonary Artery (Fig. 12–19 *A, B, C*).   The pulmonary artery is a short, wide artery about 5 cm. in length, extending from the conus arteriosus upward and backward and passing in front of and then to the left of the ascending aorta. Under the aortic arch it divides into right and left branches.

The entire artery is contained within the pericardium. On each side of its origin is the auricle of the corresponding side and a coronary artery.

The right branch of the pulmonary artery is longer than the left and passes horizontally to the right under and posterior to the ascending aorta and superior vena cava, and anterior to the right bronchus, to the root of the right lung where it divides into two branches. These follow the course of the right main stem bronchus rather closely as indicated in Chapter 10.

The left branch of the pulmonary artery passes horizontally in front of the descending aorta and left bronchus to the root of the left lung, where it likewise divides into two main branches, one for each lobe of the lung. It is connected with the distal concavity of the arch of the aorta by the ligamentum arteriosum. On the left of the latter structure is the left recurrent nerve. The other branches of the left pulmonary artery have been previously described in connection with the blood supply of the lungs (Chapter 10).

In frontal perspective, the pulmonary artery and occasionally its left branch constitute part of the left cardiac-pericardial silhouette (Fig. 12–19 *A*). In the right anterior oblique projection it is the right pulmonary artery that is seen almost in its entirety and the left pulmonary artery appears considerably foreshortened. The left pulmonary artery is seen to best advantage in the left anterior oblique projection (Fig. 12–19 *B*). The lateral view provides an excellent study of the pulmonary outflow tract, including the infundibulum and pulmonary conus. These form a considerable portion of the superior part of the anterior cardiac border (Fig. 12–19 *C*).

The branches of the pulmonary artery conform closely to the bronchial ramifications in both lungs. To identify the bronchi is to identify the normal pulmonary arterial distribution.

Pulmonary Veins (Fig. 12–20).   There are usually two pulmonary veins on each side, each about 15 mm. long; occasionally there may be three on the right. Each vein enters the left atrium of the heart. The *right superior pulmonary vein* lies dorsal to the superior vena cava; the *left pulmonary veins* lie ventral to the thoracic aorta. Pulmonary veins within the lung lie in segmental septae, unlike the arteries, and therefore drain adjacent bronchopulmonary segments (see Chapter 10).

The two pulmonary veins on the right side drain areas as follows: the *right superior pulmonary vein* drains the right upper and middle lobe; the lower lobe is drained by the *right inferior pulmonary vein.* The *left pulmonary veins* are paired, one for each lobe. The left veins enter the left atrium ventral to those of the right.

Right Pulmonary Artery Measurements (Chang).   The normal upper limits for the inspiratory measurement of the right descending pulmonary artery of normal male adults was shown to have a maximum measurement of 16 mm. Measurements of 17 mm. or more may be regarded as abnormal. In the adult female, the comparable measurement was 15 mm., with an indication that 16 mm. or more is abnormal.

During inspiration, when the intra-alveolar pressure falls, the size of the right descending pulmonary artery increases, and during expiration the vessel's size decreases owing to compression. There is a 1 to 2 mm. difference between inspiratory and expiratory measurements (2 mm. difference was noted in 69 per cent of cases).

Other measurements are shown in Figure 12–21. The 16.3 mm. measurement indicates the sum of the diameters of the apical vein of the right upper lobe at the level of the right upper

(Text continued on p. 708.)

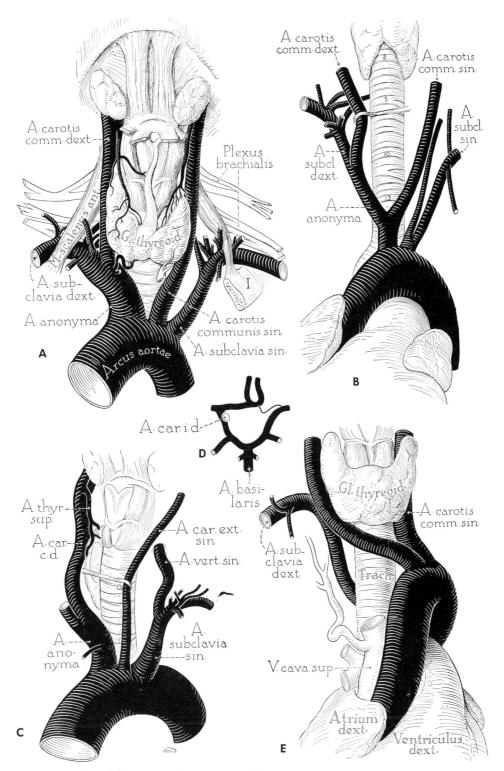

Figure 12–14. Branches of the aortic arch. Variation in the pattern of origin. *A.* Regular schema. *B.* Left common carotid from the innominate. *C.* Absence of left internal carotid artery. *D.* Form of the arterial circle (of Willis) in the same specimen. *E.* Retroesophageal right subclavian artery. (From Anson, B. J.: An Atlas of Human Anatomy. Philadelphia, W. B. Saunders Co., 1963.)

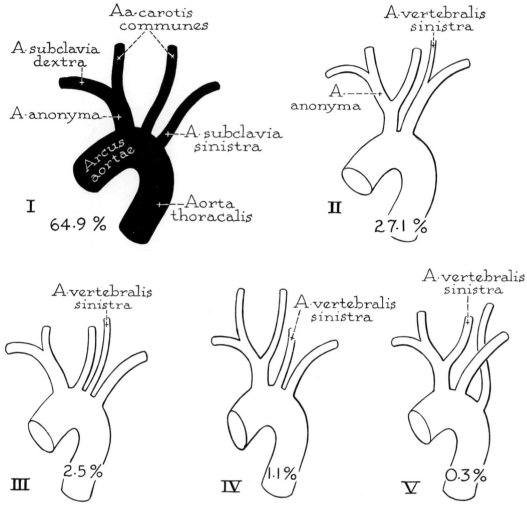

Figure 12–15. Types of branching of the aortic arch encountered in 1000 adult cadavers. I. The arrangement regarded as "normal" for man is actually encountered more frequently than all other types combined. In specimens of this variety, three branches leave the arch in the following succession, from the specimen's right to left: innominate (with right common carotid and right subclavian as derivatives); left common carotid; left subclavian. II. An arrangement distinguished by reduction in the number of stems to two, both common carotid arteries arising from the innominate. III. Here the distinguishing feature is increase, not reduction, in the number of derived branches. The left vertebral artery (usually arising from the subclavian) is the additional vessel. IV. Differing from the preceding variety, the feature is replacement, the left vertebral artery (not the left common carotid, as in Type I) being the second stem in right-to-left succession. Both common carotid arteries arise from a common stem, as they do in examples of Type II. V. In this departure from the anatomic norm, the left vertebral artery arises from the innominate, and the order of the left common carotid and left subclavian arteries is reversed.

VI to VIII (facing page). Three patterns similar in respect to the position of origin of the right subclavian artery; the latter vessel arises as the last branch of the aortic arch, reaching the right upper extremity by passing dorsal to the esophagus. In respect to the origin of the other branches, the types differ. IX. A bi-innominate sequence, in which paired vessels (in turn having matching main branches) are the only derivatives of the aortic arch. X and XI. In both these varieties the left vertebral artery arises from an aortic trunk from which the left subclavian is also derived. However, in Type X a regular innominate artery is present (as in Type I), whereas in Type XI the "innominate" (with regular branches) arises from an aortic trunk shared with the common carotid. XII. Here, as in Type III, an extra vessel arises from the arch between the innominate and the left subclavian, but the added derivative is the *a. thyreoidea ima* instead of the *a. vertebralis*. XIII. Unification is the distinguishing feature of this departure from the typical scheme of branching; the usual branches (see Type I) take origin from the aortic arch through a single trunk as an intermediary vessel. XIV. An infrequent variety with all branches derived from a common stem (as in

(Legend is continued on the opposite page.)

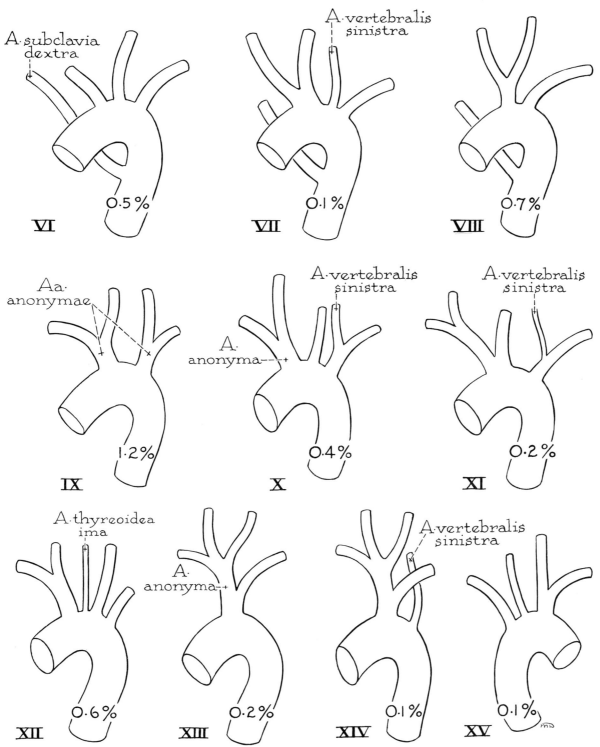

Figure 12–15 *Continued.*
Type XIII) with the exception of the left vertebral, which arises from the arch to the right of the common stem. XV. In this rare variety, in which the arch passes in a reversed direction from heart to thoracic aorta, the branches maintain a normal succession in relation to the body itself; however, their position on the aortic arch itself is as a mirror-image of the "standard" scheme of derivation. (From Anson, B. J.: An Atlas of Human Anatomy. Philadelphia, W. B. Saunders Co., 1963.)

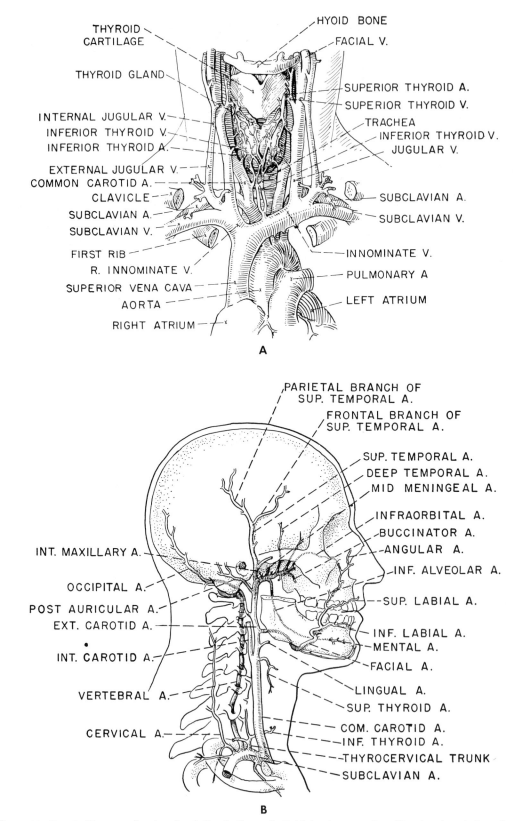

Figure 12–16. *A.* Diagram of major circulation in the neck. *B.* Major deep arteries of head and neck, lateral view.

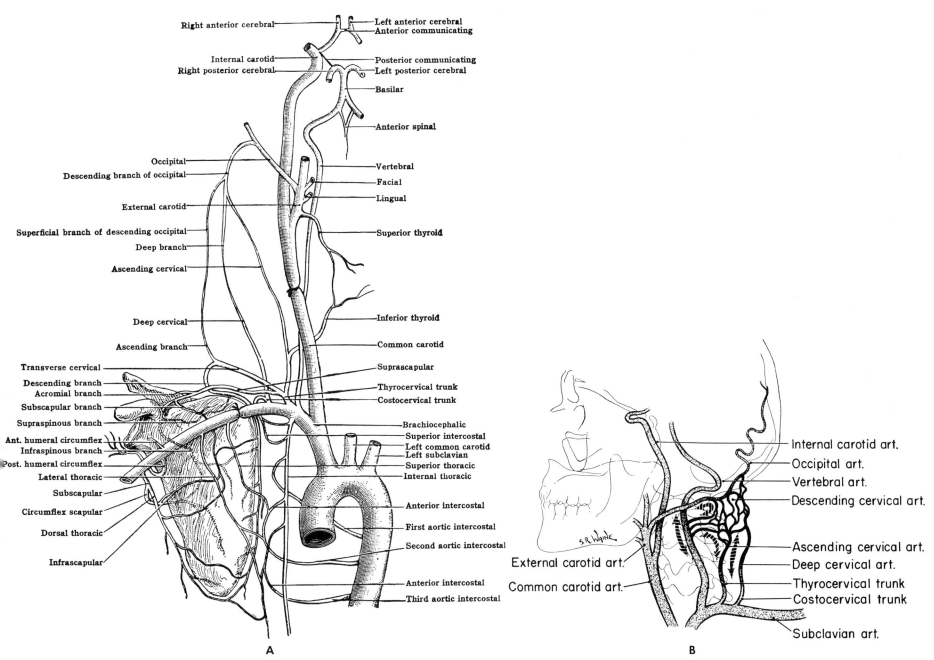

Figure 12–17. Semischematic diagram showing the potential collateral circulation of the common carotid and subclavian arteries. (From Anson, B. J. (ed.): Morris' Human Anatomy, 12th ed. Copyright © 1966 by McGraw-Hill, Inc. Used by permission of McGraw-Hill Book Company.) *B.* The "cervical arterial collateral network" which joins the carotid, subclavian, and vertebral arteries. (From Bosniak, M. A.: Amer. J. Roentgenol., 91:1222, 1964.)

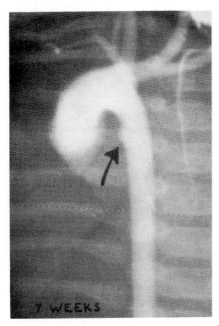

Figure 12–18. Normal aorta. Seven weeks. The aortic arch and its great branches are clearly defined. The silhouette of the arch and the descending aorta resembles an inverted J. A localized bulge at the site of the ligamentum arteriosum (*arrow*) is present. This corresponds to the "ductus diverticulum," or "infundibulum" of the ductus. (From Abrams, H. L.: Angiography, 2nd ed., Vol. 1. Boston, Little, Brown & Co., 1971.)

lobe bronchus and the posterior segmental vein of the right upper lobe at the point at which it is crossed by the anterior segmental artery. The 18.1 mm. measurement is the sum of the diameters of the superior and inferior basal veins of the right lower lobe measured 1 cm. from their junction (Lavendar et al.).

Mean measurements of arterial diameters with standard deviations as related to age and body area in children are given in the adjoining figure (Fig. 12–22).

Various Factors Influencing Cardiac Contour
(Fig. 12–23)

Constitutional Features. The general contour of the chest cavity is closely related to the contours of the organs contained therein. Thus, it has been demonstrated in anatomic sections that the outline of the circumference of the heart is closely related to the form of the circumference of the chest. In a circular chest, the cardiac contour tends to be circular also; in an ovoid chest, it tends to be ovoid.

If one arbitrarily divides the population into three groups—the asthenic or long, slender type, the pyknic or short, stocky type, and the athletic or muscular, well-proportioned group—the following cardiac contours will be characteristic:

In the asthenic group, the mediastinum as a whole is long and narrow, the diaphragm is low, and the cardiac silhouette

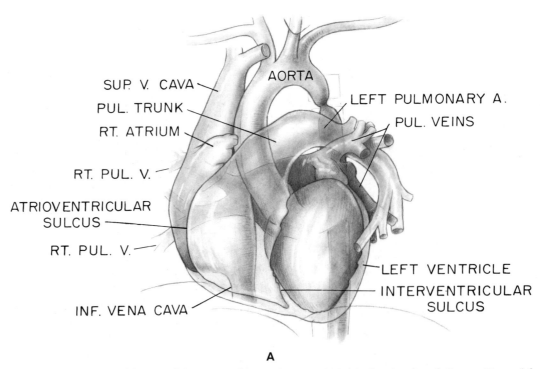

A

Figure 12–19. *A.* Normal heart in left anterior oblique view, rotation 30°, showing the relative positions of the major vessels and the inflow and outflow tracts by translucency of overlying chambers.

Figure 12–19 continued on the opposite page.

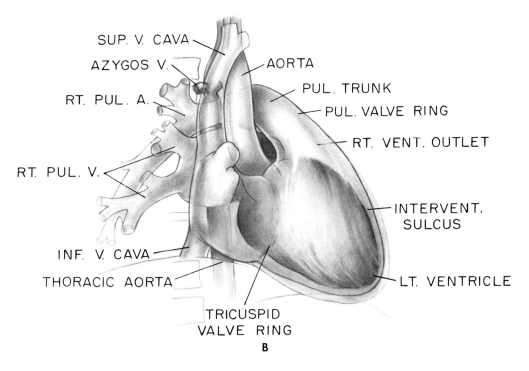

B

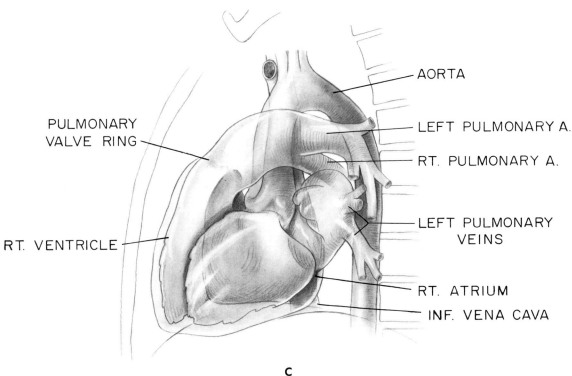

C

Figure 12–19 *Continued.* *B.* Normal heart in right anterior oblique projection, rotation 60°, showing the relationship of inflow and outflow tracts to the chambers of the heart by translucency of the chambers. *C.* Lateral view of a normal heart showing inflow and outflow tracts to the ventricles and atria. (*A–C* modified from Schad, N., et al.: Differential Diagnosis of Congenital Heart Disease. New York, Grune & Stratton, 1966.)

Figure 12–19 continued on the following page.

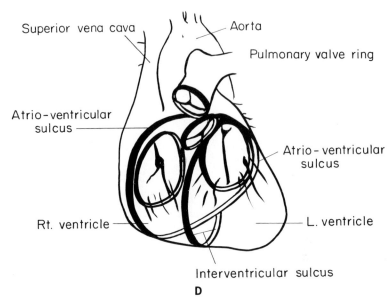

D

Figure 12–19 *Continued.* D. Slight normal left anterior oblique radiograph of the heart showing the relative positions of the pulmonary valve ring, the aortic valve ring, the tricuspid valve ring, and the mitral valve ring, with respect to the aorta, pulmonary artery, and left and right ventricles.

tends to be long, narrow, and rather straight up and down. Only the pulmonic shadow tends to be prominent. Extreme examples of this group are called "pendulous hearts," which indeed is most descriptive.

In the pyknic individual, the mediastinal shadow as a whole tends to be short and wide. The diaphragm is high, and the convexity of all the cardiac contours is marked. The heart appears diminished in height and somewhat boot-shaped, and is pushed upward and transversely by the high diaphragm. This type is indicated as horizontal or transverse.

In the athletic and sthenic individual, heart size tends to be at the upper limits of normal, and cardiac contour approaches the median group type.

Age (Fig. 12–24). Age is an important factor conditioning the relative size and shape of the heart and contiguous mediastinal structures. In younger individuals the cardiac shadow tends to be more globular and to reveal less differentiation than in the adult. In the newborn, the transverse diameter is very long in comparison with the diameter of the chest. The right side of the heart is larger than the left, and the atria and auricular appendages are large in comparison with the ventricles. The right border of the heart is therefore curved and the aortic knob cannot be differentiated.

Figure 12–20. Line diagram showing the relationship of the major ramifications of the tracheobronchial tree, pulmonary artery, and pulmonary veins to one another.

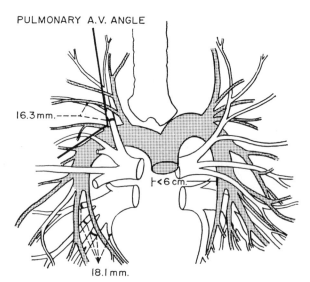

Figure 12–21. The pulmonary arteriovenous angle, which becomes more obtuse with passive hyperemia of the lungs. Also shown are several measurements which are occasionally quoted in the literature (after Logue et al.). The measurement 16.3 mm. indicates the sum of the diameters of the apical vein of the right upper lobe at the level of the right upper lobe bronchus, and the posterior segmental vein of the right upper lobe at the point at which it is crossed by the anterior segmental artery. The 18.1 mm. is the sum of the diameters of the superior and inferior basal veins of the right lower lobe measured 1 cm. from their junction. (From Lavender, J. P., and Doppman, J.: Brit. J. Radiol., 35:303–313, 1962.)

MEAN MEASUREMENTS OF ARTERIAL DIAMETERS WITH STANDARD DEVIATIONS AS RELATED TO AGE AND BODY AREA

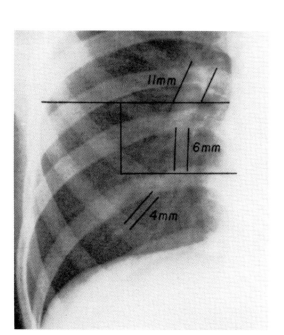

Age (yr.)	Primary Branch			Secondary Branch			Tertiary Branch		
	No.	Mean (mm.)	Standard Deviation (mm.)	No.	Mean (mm.)	Standard Deviation (mm.)	No.	Mean (mm.)	Standard Deviation (mm.)
0– 2	25*	6.1	1.2	25*	2.7	0.9	25	1.5	0.5
2– 4	16	7.3	1.0	16	4.0	0.6	16	2.2	0.4
4– 6	25	8.4	1.0	25	4.3	0.7	25	2.4	0.6
6– 8	49	9.1	1.1	49	4.5	0.7	49	2.5	0.4
8–10	26	9.1	0.7	26	4.7	0.7	26	2.8	0.5
10–12	39	10.0	1.1	39	5.0	1.1	39	3.0	0.5
12–14	28	10.6	1.0	28	5.6	1.1	28	3.0	0.6
Total	208								
Area (m²)									
0.21–0.4	11	5.8	1.0	9	3.1	1.6	11	1.4	0.4
0.41–0.6	9	6.5	1.4	8	3.5	1.1	9	1.8	0.6
0.61–0.8	18	8.3	0.8	18	4.0	0.7	18	2.3	0.5
0.81–1.00	23	9.6	1.2	23	4.8	0.7	23	2.5	0.5
1.01–1.20	17	10.0	1.1	17	5.1	0.7	17	2.8	0.6
1.21–1.40	14	10.3	1.3	14	5.1	0.4	14	3.0	0.7
Total	92								

* Out of 60 normal infant chest roentgenograms only 25 could be measured.

Figure 12–22. Division of the right lower lobe into three areas with the arterial diameters shown in each area. (From Leinbach, L. B.: Amer. J. Roentgenol., 89:996, 1963.)

During the last half of the first year, the long axis of the heart tends to rotate and descend slightly in the thorax, and the thymic shadow begins to regress. A rather definitive cardiac shadow is established between the sixth and the eighth year, but there is a relative prominence of the pulmonary artery (and conus) on the left in the frontal projection that persists in a variable degree throughout adolescence, and does not completely disappear until the early twenties.

As age increases, there is a gradual diminution of the size of the base of the heart and a tendency to increasing prominence of the aortic knob and superior vena cava shadows. The cardiac and retrocardiac structures change their relationships slightly, as shown in Figure 12–25. When arteriosclerosis of the aorta is present, there is usually a tendency toward elongation and redundancy of the entire thoracic aorta, but particularly of the aortic arch.

Cardiac Cycle. The size and shape of the cardiac silhouette varies in accordance with systole and diastole. Cardiac measure-

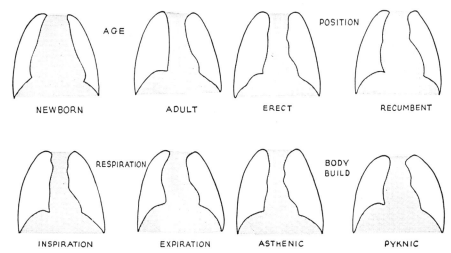

Figure 12–23. Normal factors causing variation in the supracardiac shadow and cardiac contour.

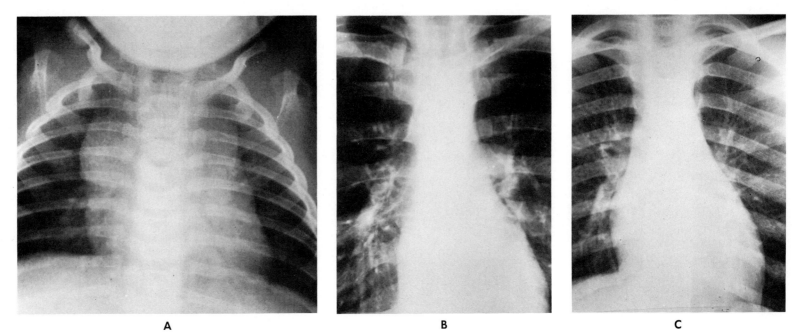

Figure 12-24.   Heart and mediastinum in respect to age. *A.* Infant 4 months of age. *B.* Child 6 years of age. *C.* Normal adult, erect inspiration performing a Valsalva maneuver. *D.* Heart, mediastinum, and chest in a patient of asthenic build, showing the heart to be rather pendulous in contour.

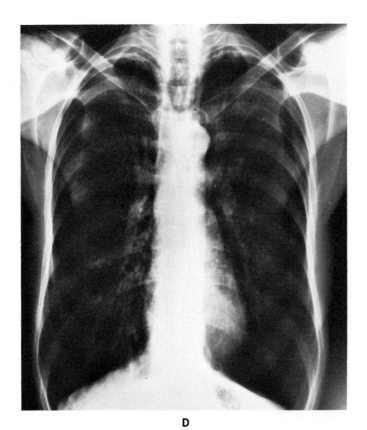

D

ments in systole and diastole were carefully made by Gammill et al., who postulated that maximum and minimum sizes of the heart with respect to the cardiac cycle would be more useful in evaluating cardiac size than the single chest roentgenogram exposed at random during the cardiac cycle. However, 52 per cent of their patients showed changes of 0.3 cm. or less and 41 per cent showed alterations of 0.4 to 0.9 cm. in the two phases of the cardiac cycle. In 7 per cent, the variation was between 1.0 cm. and 1.7 cm. Their patients also showed changes in frontal area as well as in other measurements proposed.

This difference in cardiac size and shape tends to be greater with contraction rates below 60 per minute.

For a most accurate assay, the cardiac configuration and size must be studied in identical phases of the cardiac cycle; when such accuracy is lacking, due allowance must be made for this variable factor.

Body Position (Fig. 12-25). There are quite definite changes in the cardiovascular silhouette in the different positions of the body. The change from the erect to the recumbent position causes a broadening of the cardiac silhouette, particularly at its base. The area of the cardiac shadow increases in proportion to increase in diameter and the broad diameter. These changes are probably secondary to the changes in position of the sternum, ribs, and diaphragm.

In the lateral prone position, the mediastinal structures tend to shift toward the lowermost side with the force of gravity. The lower leaf of the diaphragm ascends and increases its respiratory

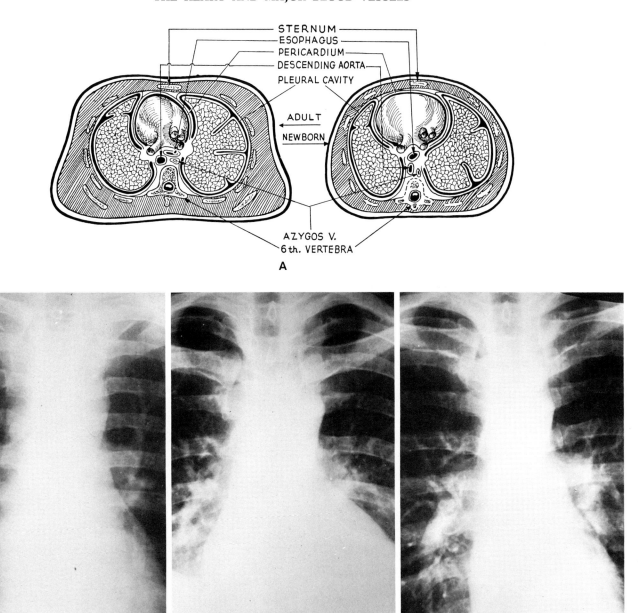

Figure 12–25. *A.* Differences in infantile and adult posterior mediastinal relationships. (Modified from Caffey.) *B.* Heart and mediastinum in a patient supine in full inspiration. *C.* Heart and mediastinum in same patient, erect during expiration. *D.* Heart and mediastinum in same patient erect in full inspiration and Valsalva maneuver.

excursions, while the uppermost leaf descends. The mediastinal shadow tends to return to the midline on deep inspiration against the forces of gravity. This movement with deep inspiration is greatest in asthenic persons.

Respiration. During ordinary quiet or tidal respiration, no significant changes in the cardiac silhouette are noted. However, with forced inspiration, changes are produced depending upon whether breathing is predominantly costal or diaphragmatic. In the diaphragmatic type, there is a slight caudal shift of the heart that is ordinarily not observed in the costal type of forced inspiration. There is a tendency for the left heart border to move medially, and the left contour is less curved. The vascular basilar shadows are elongated. The retrosternal and retrocardiac shadows are increased in radiolucency.

In forced expiration, the cardiac shadow rises and is somewhat displaced to the left. The cardiac base appears wider and shortened, and the retrosternal and retrocardiac shadows are diminished in radiolucency. When the Valsalva experiment is performed by closing the glottis at the end of full inspiration and forcing expiration, there is a slow decrease in the size of the entire cardiac silhouette, probably related to the increased intrathoracic pressure. A slowing of the heart rate occurs in some, while in others the rate increases.

The position of the diaphragm will affect cardiac size and contour significantly, not only with respect to respiration but also with regard to: (1) abdominal distention or other intraabdominal or subdiaphragmatic disease, (2) unilateral elevation from any cause, and (3) the presence or absence of increased intrathoracic tension.

Valsalva Maneuver. If the glottis is closed after deep inspiration and positive pressure is maintained against the closed glottis, cardiac size gradually diminishes for several cardiac cycles. This is called a "positive pressure study" and has been suggested as a means of differentiating compressible vascular structures from noncompressible mass lesions in the chest (Whitley and Martin; see Chapter 10).

Thoracic Deformities. Thoracic deformities alter the position of the heart as well as its size and contour. For example, dorsal lordosis, funnel chest, or pectus excavatum may produce a rotation of the heart toward the left or a flattened appearance with displacement posteriorly; kyphoscoliosis produces a rotation of the heart toward the side opposite the scoliosis.

Intrathoracic Pulmonary or Pleural Pathologic Processes. These very often affect cardiac size and contour.

Pregnancy (Fig. 12–26). In pregnancy the diaphragm is elevated and hypervolemia occurs, with a tendency toward increased cardiac size. The lungs show an increased vascularity, caused by engorgement of the breasts that imparts an increased haziness to both lung bases.

Microcardia. The heart may be small (microcardia) in association with malnutrition from any cause. A "microcardia" has been reported in patients with widespread carcinomatosis, lymphoma, ulcerative colitis, scleroderma, hepatoma, and anorexia nervosa (Altemus).

BASIC RADIOLOGIC METHODS OF CARDIAC STUDY

Role of Radiologic Examination of the Heart. It is important first to consider the part that the radiologic examination plays in the total clinical examination of the heart. Our basic physical diagnostic armamentarium consists of *inspection* to determine normal and abnormal pulsations, vascular distention, and cyanosis; *percussion* to determine mediastinal size; *palpation* to verify further facts noted above as well as the detection of palpable thrills; and *auscultation* for study of cardiac and mediastinal sounds.

The radiographic examination of the heart gives more accu-

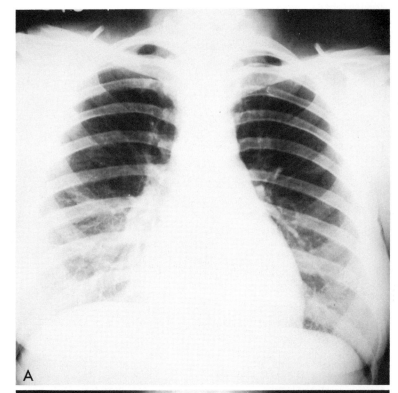
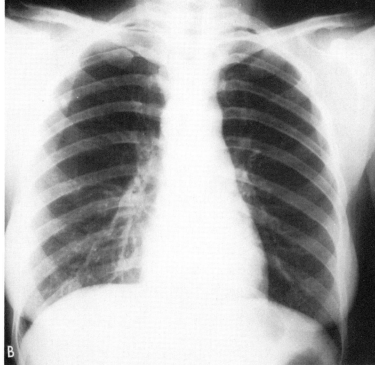

Figure 12–26. Posteroanterior views of the chest showing changes in heart size and lung appearance as the result of pregnancy. *A.* Near term pregnancy. *B.* Approximately 1 year after delivery.

rate data regarding cardiac size, contour, and pulsations than any of the above methods, *but it can never be a substitute for auscultation, for the determination of palpable thrills, and for the detection of cyanosis.* Thus the cardiac roentgenologic examination is a very useful adjunct in the total examination but it must not be regarded as independent of all other means of study.

Radiologic Methods Used in the Roentgen Cardiac Examination

1. **The Posteroanterior (PA) Teleroentgenograms of the Chest** (6 foot target-to-film distance), preferably with barium outlining the esophagus (Fig. 12–27).

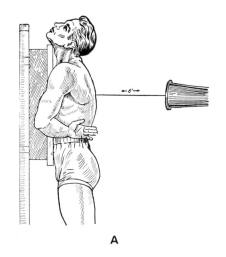

A

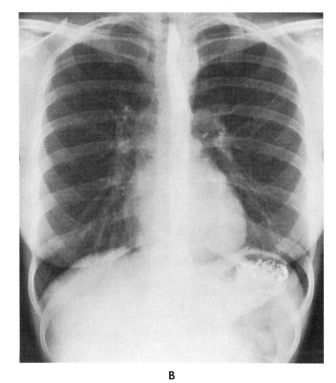

B

Figure 12–27 Cardiac esophagram, posteroanterior projection. *A.* Position of patient. *B.* Radiograph (female). *C.* Labeled tracing of *B.*

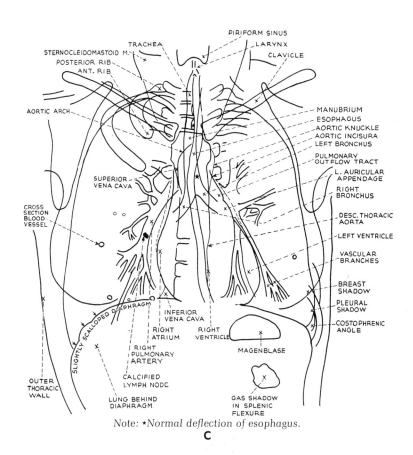

Note: *Normal deflection of esophagus.*

C

Points of Practical Interest With Reference to Figure 12-27

1. The exact course of the esophagus in this projection is noteworthy. At the base of the neck there is a slight deflection toward the left so that the esophageal projection falls behind the left sternoclavicular joint in a perfectly centered film. Thereafter it courses to the right at the level of the transverse portion of the arch of the aorta. From this position, there is a slight gradual deflection toward the left so that the diaphragm is penetrated to the left of the midline. An enlargement in any of the contiguous structures will alter this course perceptibly.

2. It is also important to trace the aortic shadow as it courses to the left of the middle, with its left margin ordinarily separate and distinct from the paraspinous shadow. This is a straight line normally below the level of the arch of the aorta; abnormally, it becomes convex, or S-shaped with elongation of the aorta.

3. The position of the "left" ventricular apex with reference to the left hemidiaphragm is important. This portion of the cardiac silhouette is not always due to the left ventricle, but may be related to the right ventricle, particularly in congenital heart disease.

2. The Left and Right Anterior Oblique Films of the Chest,
also with barium outlining the esophagus, and usually following fluoroscopy (Figs. 12–28 and 12–29).

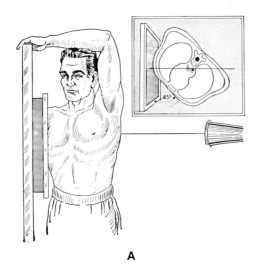

A

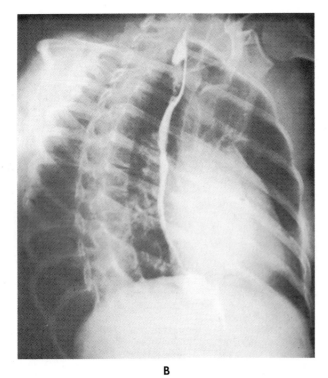

B

Figure 12–28. Cardiac esophagram, right anterior oblique projection. (There is a minimal enlargement of the left atrium in this case, purposely chosen to show its position.) A. Position of patient. B. Radiograph. C. Labeled tracing of B.

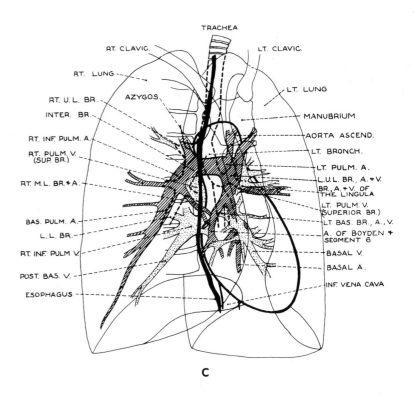

C

Points of Practical Interest With Reference to Figure 12–28

1. The relative convexity of the pulmonary sector is noteworthy. This area becomes concave in many (but not all) cases of pulmonic or infundibular stenosis; or it may increase in prominence with dilatation of the pulmonary artery.
2. When the heart enlarges diffusely, the esophagus is often displaced posteriorly —but this type of displacement is not sharply localized to the region of the left atrium. For this reason, the region of the left atrium as it impinges on the esophagus must be known accurately by the student. Once this is established, the differential diagnosis becomes less difficult.
3. Air shadows in the esophagus may produce some confusion in interpretation. These are frequent and normal, except possibly when excessive.

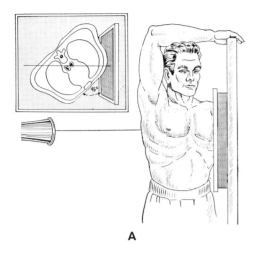

A

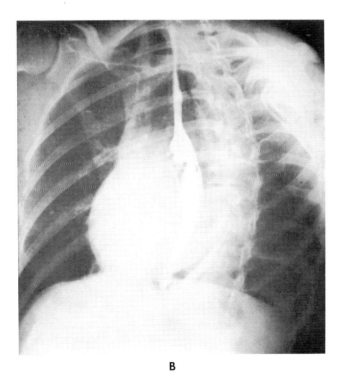

B

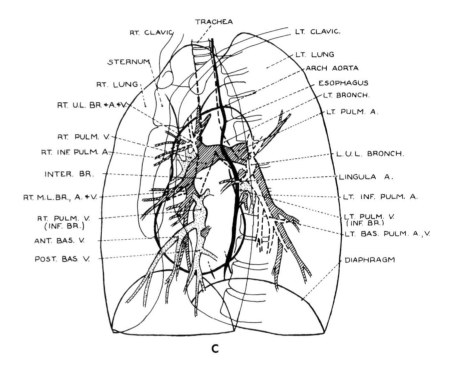

C

Figure 12–29. Cardiac esophagram, left anterior oblique projection. *A.* Position of patient. *B.* Radiograph. *C.* Labeled tracing of *B.*

Points of Practical Interest With Reference to Figure 12–29

1. The student should learn to identify the following anatomic areas of the cardiac silhouette particularly, in this view: right and left ventricle; arch of aorta; left atrium; and the position of the aortic and mitral valves. The relative prominence of each of these areas should be noted.
2. The trachea and its bifurcation can be clearly identified in this projection. Position and contour description will help detect such abnormalities as narrowness, deflection, compression, and filling defects.

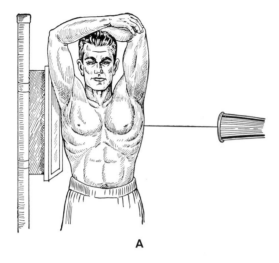

A

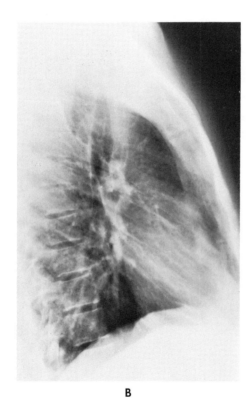

B

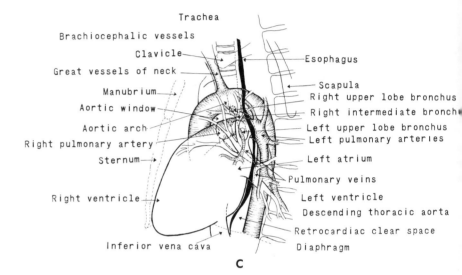

C

Figure 12–30. Lateral view of the chest with barium in the esophagus. *A.* Position of patient. *B.* Radiograph. *C.* Labeled tracing of *B.*

Points of Practical Interest With Reference to Figure 12–30

1. The following areas are of particular interest and value for identification:
   (a) The relationship of the right ventricle to the posterior margin of the sternum. With enlargement of the right ventricle, its shadow "rises" higher on the sternum.
   (b) The degree of clarity of the anterior mediastinal clear space.
   (c) The relationship of the left ventricle posteriorly to the shadow of the inferior vena cava. This will allow early and accurate detection of enlargement of the left ventricle.
   (d) The relationship of the esophagus to the left atrium.
   (e) The relative prominence of the pulmonary arteries. This requires considerable experience, but is very valuable from the standpoint of detecting abnormalities of lymph node origin, or tumor masses.

3. **A Lateral Film of the Chest with Esophagram** (Fig. 12–30).

4. **A PA or AP Teleroentgenogram of the Chest in the Recumbent Position** for comparison with the erect film, if pericardial fluid is suspected (Fig. 12–31). Other special procedures such as kymography, angiocardiography, cardiac catheterization, orthodiagraphy, and retrograde aortography are considered outside the scope of this text.

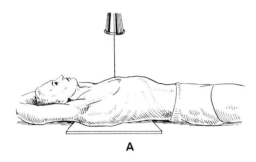

A

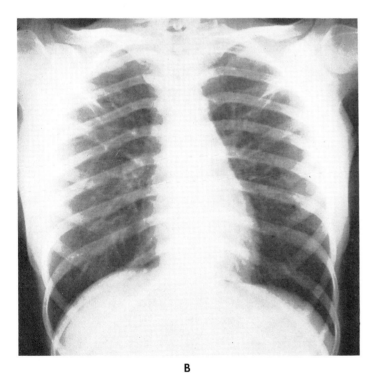

B

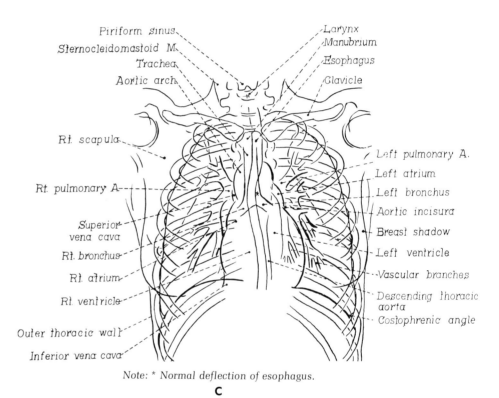

Note: * Normal deflection of esophagus.

C

Figure 12–31. Anteroposterior recumbent study of chest. *A.* Position of patient. *B.* Radiograph. *C.* Labeled tracing of *B.*

Points of Practical Interest With Reference to Figure 12–31

1. Although it is difficult to obtain a view of the upper lung fields in this projection because of the shadows of the scapulae, considerable improvement will result if the patient crosses his arms above his head, thus rotating the scapulae outward.
2. The clavicles, on the other hand, are projected above the lung apices sufficiently so that this area of the lungs may be more clearly shown.
3. The analysis of the cardiac silhouette is not as favorable in this projection in the adult, because of the straightening of the left margin and broadening of the base.

5. **Fluoroscopy.** Fluoroscopy with image amplification should precede the film studies. The following outline is recommended.

The Heart and Mediastinal Structures are Studied in the Frontal Projection. (1) The pulsations along the left cardiac border are investigated and the radiologist proceeds around the periphery of the mediastinum, studying carefully the pulsations of the pulmonary arteries, aorta, and right atrium. (2) The cardiac position is carefully noted, both in inspiration and expiration, and changes with respiration are detected.

The Patient is Thereafter Turned in the Right Anterior Oblique Position. (1) Once again the cardiac contour and pulsations are carefully noted. The pulsations in the apex of the left ventricle are particularly important, since this area is prone to suffer from coronary vascular impairment. (2) The pulmonary outflow tract is observed, since this projection is particularly suited for this purpose. (3) The anterior margin of the ascending aorta is then studied. (4) Thereafter the posterior mediastinal space is viewed. Normally this space is clear, because it is occupied by structures of lesser opacity such as the esophagus, aorta, and veins. The prominence of the left atrium in relation to the posterior mediastinum is particularly noteworthy. Its relationship to the esophagus (barium-filled) is particularly important.

The Patient is Then Turned in the Left Anterior Oblique Position. (1) In this position the posterior basilar portion of the left ventricle is studied. The pulsations here are usually of greater amplitude than elsewhere. Some concept of left ventricular size can be obtained from the fact that in the 45 degree obliquity the left ventricle normally clears the spine. (2) The anterior margin of the heart in this projection is formed by the right ventricle usually. A fairly straight line is formed by the anterior margin of the right ventricle and the ascending aorta in this projection. Any unusual convexities, either in the right ventricle or in the ascending aorta, are of pathologic significance. (3) This position affords the most accurate means of studying the arch of the aorta in relation to the left pulmonary artery, which lies beneath it. There is ordinarily a clear space known as the "aortic window" between the aortic arch and the pulmonary artery. Any enlargement of a contiguous structure will cause its obliteration.

Size of Fluoroscopic Field. By carefully restricting the size of the fluoroscopic field, the cardiac shadow is surveyed for any areas of calcification and hyperlucency. (1) Care must be exercised to insure that the calcification is projected within the heart in every view and pulsates synchronously with the heart, since calcified mediastinal lymph nodes can cause occasional confusion. (2) The heart normally does not contain calcification, but the following cardiopericardial structures may contain calcium abnormally (Fig. 12–32): (a) the pericardium, (b) the coronary vessels, (c) the myocardium, (d) the endocardium, (e) the papil-

lary muscles, (f) the cardiac valves (Fig. 12–33), and (g) the rings at the base of the cardiac valves and the aortic sinus of Valsalva.

The position of the cardiac valves in various projections is indicated in Figure 12–33. Calcified valves may be differentiated by their characteristic "dance," which is synchronous with the cardiac pulsations. The motion is jerky and steplike.

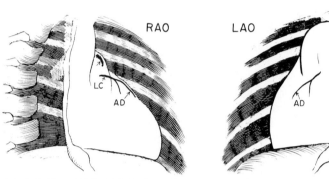

CALCIFIED LEFT CORONARY A.   CALCIFIED LEFT CORONARY A.

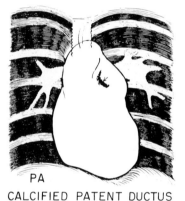

CALCIFIED PATENT DUCTUS

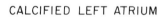

CALCIFIED LEFT ATRIUM   CALCIFIED LEFT ATRIUM

A

Figure 12–32. A, B, and C. Cardiopericardial structures which may contain calcium as depicted radiographically.

Figure 12–32 continued on the opposite page.

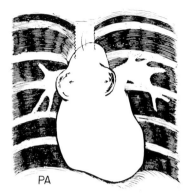

CALCIFIED SINUS OF VALSALVA
ANEURYSM

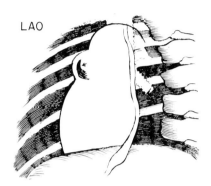

CALCIFIED SINUS OF VALSALVA

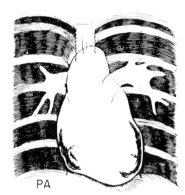

CALCIFIED PERICARDIUM

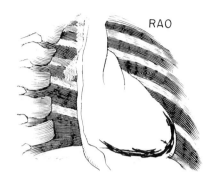

CALCIFIED PERICARDIUM
WITH CONSTRICTIVE PERICARDITIS

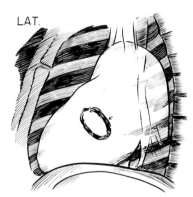

CALCIFIED MITRAL RING

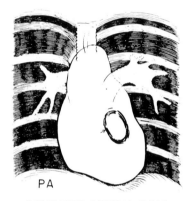

CALCIFIED MITRAL RING

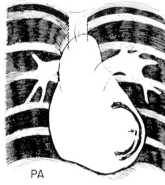

CALCIFIED
MYOCARDIAL INFARCT

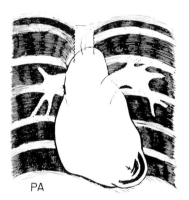

CALCIFIED
LEFT VENTRICULAR ANEURYSM

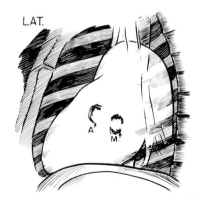

CALCIFIED MITRAL VALVE
CALCIFIED AORTIC VALVE

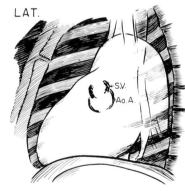

CALCIFIED SINUS OF VALSALVA
CALCIFIED AORTIC ANNULUS

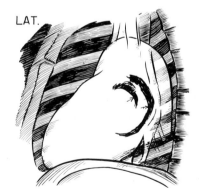

CALCIFIED LEFT ATRIUM
WITH CALCIFIED THROMBUS

B

C

Figure 12–32 *Continued.*

PROJECTION OF CARDIAC VALVES
IN ROUTINE POSITIONS IN RADIOGRAPHY

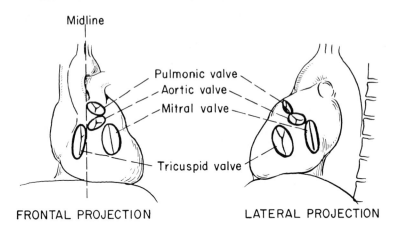

Midline

Pulmonic valve
Aortic valve
Mitral valve

Tricuspid valve

FRONTAL PROJECTION   LATERAL PROJECTION

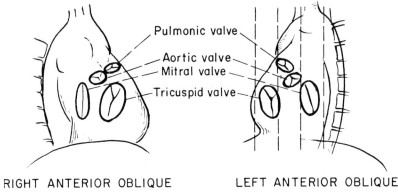

Pulmonic valve

Aortic valve
Mitral valve
Tricuspid valve

RIGHT ANTERIOR OBLIQUE   LEFT ANTERIOR OBLIQUE

Figure 12–33.

Aortic sinus of Valsalva calcification is best seen in the lateral view. It is identified by its calcified origin near the left coronary artery and is projected near the anterior wall of the ascending aorta into the base of the heart. The appearance resembles a parentheses when there are two portions calcified, or a comma when only one is calcified.

The motion as visualized cinefluoroscopically conforms to the pulsation of the ascending aorta, and the calcification is contiguous with the ascending aorta in all projections (Levitan and Reilly).

Fluoroscopy with image amplification and cineradiography has proved to be of great value in the detection of cardiac or intracardiac calcifications, even when the more conventional procedures fail.

(3) *Under image amplification, the epicardial fat can often be seen. Pericardial effusion* outside this fat layer may thereby often be differentiated from other causes of cardiopericardial enlargement.

A barium swallow should always be part of the fluoroscopic and radiographic study of the heart, with good delineation of the esophagus in all projections. Since the esophagus is so closely applied to the descending aorta on the one hand and the posterior cardiac structures on the other, changes in the course of the esophagus are of considerable value in the interpretation of cardiovascular and aortic anatomy.

The patient is then lowered into a recumbent position and a study of the mediastinum is repeated as described earlier in the frontal and oblique projections, noting carefully the changes that occur with change in body position.

The cardiac valves in the living person are farther to the right and nearer to the midline than might be expected from anatomic textbooks which are based upon cadaver studies. Moreover, since calcified valves are themselves pathologic and are frequently associated with cardiac hypertrophy and dilatation, a study of cardiac valves in such subjects can hardly be compared with normal studies on human cadavers.

The demonstration on roentgenograms requires a very small focal spot, extremely rapid exposure, and coning down over the valve area in the proper degree of obliquity as determined fluoroscopically.

PLAIN FILM ROUTINE STUDIES OF HEART (USING BARIUM IN THE ESOPHAGUS)

1. **The 6 Foot Posteroanterior View of the Heart with Barium in the Esophagus.** The various parts demonstrated in silhouette along the right margin of the central mediastinal shadow are as follows (Fig. 12–27): the inferior vena cava, in the right cardiophrenic angle; the right atrium, forming the major portion of the right cardiac shadow; the ascending portion of the arch of the aorta; and the superior vena cava, extending above and to the right of the latter. The anatomic parts contributing to the left side of the shadow are as follows (from above downward): the aortic knob, which forms a knucklelike shadow superiorly; the aortic incisura, which is the notch between the aortic knob and the pulmonary artery below it; the left auricular appendage, which may protrude very slightly below the pulmonary artery; and the large sweeping convex shadow below this, which extends down to the diaphragm. There is frequently a less dense shadow in the vicinity of the left ventricular apex caused by the pericardial fat pad, which has a triangular appearance and should not enter into the computation of the cardiac size.

The esophagus after it descends into the thorax lies in close proximity with the aorta. It has various impressions upon it, and the uppermost indentation is that produced by the arch of the aorta, which displaces the esophagus to the right and posteriorly.

Normally, in this projection, the esophagus descends straight downward, and any deviation is significant from the standpoint of cardiac chamber enlargement. A study of the esophagus in this view is therefore of value in detection of such abnormalities as rightsided aorta, left atrial enlargement, and abnormalities of the descending thoracic aorta.

This 6 foot film of the heart is also called a teleroentgenogram and is obtained for evaluation of cardiac size and contour in the posteroanterior projection. Actually, this is usually the routine chest film obtained in most clinics. As indicated in Chapter 1, distortion and magnification are two major problems in radiography that to a great extent can be obviated if a long film-to-target distance is utilized. The degree of magnification and distortion will vary in accordance with the relative distances of the anatomic part and the tube target from the film. A 6 foot film-to-target distance has been found to be practicable, and for all ordinary adult chests the magnification is no greater than 5 to 10 per cent. Since this study is usually combined with a study of the lung fields, an extremely short exposure is employed, about one-tenth to one-twentieth of a second (or even less). A short exposure of this type will usually portray the heart in some phase between systole and diastole, and hence allowance must be made for such differences as may occur in the various phases of the cardiac cycle, which may be 1 cm. or more. The cardiac size will also vary somewhat in the different phases of respiration, being smallest in deep sustained inspiration.

The pericardium, which invests the entire heart and is attached to the diaphragm below and the base of the major vessels above, ordinarily does not cast a shadow of its own, and is normally not distinguishable.

2. **The Right Anterior Oblique View with Esophagram.** In this position the patient is rotated so that his right side is in contact with the cassette, and he is rotated away from the cassette approximately 45 degrees (Fig. 12–28). The esophagus occupies the space between the descending aorta and the posterior margin of the cardiac shadow, and there is a slight undulation of the esophagus produced by the impression of certain structures upon it. We depend upon the esophagus to delineate most accurately the retrocardiac structures. The uppermost impression upon the esophagus after it enters the thorax is that produced by the arch of the aorta as it displaces the esophagus to the right and posteriorly. Just below this indentation, another slight posterior impression is frequently produced by the left atrium. This impression is virtually absent normally, and an impression beyond a minimal degree (such as is illustrated in Fig. 12–28) is indicative of left atrial enlargement, a most significant finding. The right atrium forms the lowermost slight convexity in the cardiac outline posteriorly in this projection.

The retrocardiac space is ordinarily fairly large, and when encroached upon is likewise an indication of abnormality.

The descending thoracic aorta overlaps the anterior margin

of the thoracic spine in its descent, and, significantly, the esophagus descends in practically the same sheath as the aorta. Elongation and tortuosity of the aorta therefore have a definite bearing on the appearance of the esophagus.

The trachea and left bronchus can be identified as a straight air shadow above the shadow of the left atrium, and just above the left atrium, the pulmonary artery can usually be seen as a circular opaque shadow (seen end-on).

Between the left atrial impression and that of the aorta, there is frequently a lesser impression produced by the bronchial bifurcation.

The anterior border of this central mediastinal shadow permits delineation of the following structures: the ascending portion of the arch of the aorta seen superiorly; usually a small notch between this shadow and that of the pulmonary conus, which has a slight anterior convexity; seen below this shadow is that of the left ventricle or right ventricle depending upon the degree of rotation of the patient. This view forms a valuable one for visualization of the anterior apical area of the left ventricle (frequently involved by infarction) and the main pulmonary artery (frequently involved in congenital heart disease).

3. **The Left Anterior Oblique View with Barium in the Esophagus.** In this position, the patient is rotated 45 degrees with the left anterior shoulder against the cassette (Fig. 12–29). When sufficiently rotated, the left ventricle just barely clears the anterior margin of the thoracic spine. This is the posterior basilar portion of the left ventricle. Above this lies the left atrium. The arch of the aorta is seen in its entirety. The anterior margin of the silhouette is formed inferiorly by the right ventricle (this is the only view in which the right ventricle is adequately and definitely seen), and above this by the right atrium. The tracheal bifurcation is seen very clearly in this projection. The left pulmonary artery is seen in the clear space above the left atrium, and that portion beneath the arch of the aorta is known as the aortic window.

The aortic triangle is frequently identified above the arch of the aorta, bounded by the arch of the aorta below, the dorsal spine posteriorly, and the left subclavian artery anteriorly. The latter can be faintly identified branching from the aortic arch.

In this projection, the esophagus is normally not diverted from a relatively straight course. Deviations, if they occur, are of pathologic significance.

4. **The Anteroposterior Recumbent Study of the Cardiopericardial Shadow** (Fig. 12–31). There is a normal change in shape of the cardiopericardial shadow that accompanies a change in posture from the erect to the recumbent position. This has been previously described and is due to the upward shift of the diaphragm. In the presence of fluid in the pericardial space in excess of about 300 cc., this change in shape becomes most pronounced when the pericardial fluid shifts from the lower portion of the space to the base of the heart. This produces a marked widening of the base of the heart.

These recumbent studies are also sometimes necessary if the patient cannot stand erect.

In any case, the film-target distance should be carefully stated so that adjustment can be made for distortion and magnification. (The method of determination of magnification will be described in conjunction with pelvicephalometry in Chapter 17.)

5. **The Lateral View of the Chest with Barium in the Esophagus** (Fig. 12–30). The lateral view of the chest with barium in the esophagus is a valuable adjunct in the study of the heart, particularly in the following circumstances:

(a) It allows the radiologist another perspective for study of the relationship of the esophagus to the left atrium. The course of the esophagus is normally straight. Indentation in the region of the left atrium is usually an indication of enlargement of this chamber.

(b) The right ventricle is seen in silhouette anteriorly, and when enlarged encroaches upon the anterior mediastinal clear space. The right ventricle in this perspective usually forms a smooth convexity anteriorly from its junction with the shadow of the aorta, gradually meeting the anterior chest wall in the vicinity of the xiphoid process of the sternum inferiorly. Its junction

with the chest wall above this level is usually an indication of chamber enlargement. This is particularly true in congenital heart disease.

(c) The pulmonary arteries form an ovoid structure identifiable below the arch of the aorta. These can be evaluated for size and differentiated from other mediastinal structures that may on occasion be enlarged, such as mediastinal lymph nodes.

(d) The ascending portion of the aorta and arch of the aorta can be fully evaluated as to size and contour.

(e) The relationship of the left ventricle posteriorly projected over the shadow of the inferior vena cava shadow is of importance in evaluating the size of the left ventricle (Fig. 12–34). Ordinarily the shadow of the inferior vena cava is seen about 5 to 18 mm. behind that of the adjoining left ventricular shadow. With enlargement of the latter chamber, particularly in association with mitral insufficiency, the left ventricle protrudes beyond 18 mm. posteriorly. Such enlargement of the left ventricle is not apt to occur with relatively pure mitral stenosis.

(f) In attempting differentiation of diffuse cardiac enlargement from pericardial effusion, a careful study of the pulsations of the heart *posteriorly* in this projection may be very helpful. These

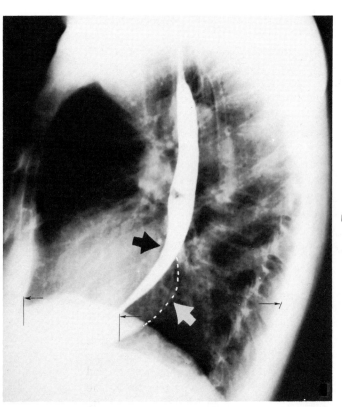

LV   Left ventricle
IVC   Inferior vena cava
LD   Left hemidiaphragm
RD   Right hemidiaphragm

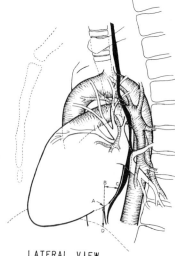

LATERAL VIEW

Eyler et al.:Radiology 73:56,1959.
    Mitral insuff. A > 15 mm.
    Mitral stenosis A < 15 mm.
Keats and Rudhe:Radiology 83:616,
                             1964.
    Atrial secundum defect
        IVC partially
            free of heart shadow.
    Ventricular septal defect
        IVC is over mass of
            heart with large shunt.

Point A = crossing of inferior
             vena cava & left ventricle.

Point B is 2 cm. cephalad to A.
Line BC parallels plane of
             dorsal vertebrae.
Line AD is vertical distance to
             left hemidiaphragm.
Left ventricular enlargement
        Present when BC >18 mm.
Left ventricular hypertrophy
        Suspect when AD < 0.75 cm.

A   B

Figure 12–34.   A and B. Important measurements on lateral view of the heart.

may be more accurately ascertained with the aid of kymograms. With pericardial effusion, pulsations in this area are usually completely lacking, whereas with diffuse cardiac enlargement some degree of pulsation is usually manifest here.

DETERMINATION OF CARDIAC ENLARGEMENT (Fig. 12–35)

Definition of the "Normal" Sized Heart. It can be assumed that the majority of a large population is normal, and the problem of determining the "normal" sized heart on a radiograph becomes one of correlating various cardiac measurements with any other bodily factors that allow a high statistical correlation in the majority of the population. In statistical terms, this is called a "high correlation coefficient." It is thus possible to determine how many chances (per hundred) the individual heart has of being within normal limits. In the individual case, this statistical approach

may cause inaccuracy, but in the consideration of a large group it is a satisfactory means of assay. *We must be cognizant of the fact that the boundary between the normal and the abnormal is an arbitrary one, based upon statistical correlation alone.*

Introduction. Increase in cardiac size is the most consistent indication of cardiac disease. Cardiac mensuration is an accurate method for determination of cardiac enlargement; correlation with actual cardiac weight, however, is not very satisfactory, since the element of dilatation in respect to enlargement cannot be accurately evaluated separately from cardiac hypertrophy.

Greatest accuracy and best correlation is obtained by the determination of relative cardiac volume. Ungerleider and Gubner's frontal area method is also included for reference.

Measurements are made directly on teleroentgenograms of the chest obtained in suspended respiration at a 6 foot target-to-film distance. The cardiac image is magnified to approximately 5 per cent. The most frequent and useful measurements obtained from the teleroentgenograms are (Fig. 12–36):

(Text continued on page 729.)

CARDIAC MENSURATION

1. UNGERLEIDER AND GUBNER NOMOGRAM METHOD
(FOR INDIVIDUALS 56-80" HT.; 95-300 # WT.)

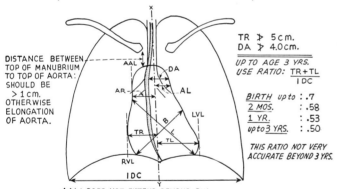

TR ⟩ 5 cm.
DA ⟩ 4.0 cm.

UP TO AGE 3 YRS.
USE RATIO: $\frac{TR+TL}{IDC}$

BIRTH up to : .7
2 MOS. : .58
1 YR. : .53
up to 3 YRS. : .50

THIS RATIO NOT VERY ACCURATE BEYOND 3 YRS.

DISTANCE BETWEEN TOP OF MANUBRIUM TO TOP OF AORTA: SHOULD BE >1 cm. OTHERWISE ELONGATION OF AORTA.

AAL: DOES NOT EXTEND BEYOND RVL.
RVL: DOES NOT EXTEND BEYOND MEDIAL 1/3 of DIAPHRAGM.
LVL: DOES NOT EXTEND BEYOND MEDIAL 1/2 of DIAPHRAGM.

1. $A = \frac{\pi}{4} L \times B = .7854 \times L \times B$
2. GREATEST TRANSVERSE DIAMETER (GTD) OF HEART: TR+TL
3. COMPARE MEASURED AND CALCULATED VALUES FOR A and GTD WITH VALUES ANTICIPATED FROM BODY HEIGHT AND WEIGHT. NORMAL RANGE IS VALUE ANTICIPATED ± 10%
4. MEASURED AORTIC VALUE : AR+AL
   ANTICIPATED AORTIC VALUE:

CHART VALUE	
−1 mm.	+1 mm.
For each 3 YRS. <43 YRS.	For each 3 YRS. >43 YRS.

2. USE SIMILAR MEYER'S TABLES FOR CHILDREN 3-16 YRS. OF AGE
EXCEPT A = .68 × L × B.

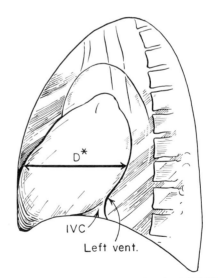

LATERAL VIEW OF NORMAL HEART

*D = Greatest anterior-posterior measurement of heart

A

Figure 12–35. *A. Left,* Cardiac mensuration by the Ungerleider and Gubner technique. *Right,* lateral view of the normal heart showing the method of obtaining D, the greatest anteroposterior measurement of the heart in calculation of cardiac volume.

Figure 12–35 continued on the following page.

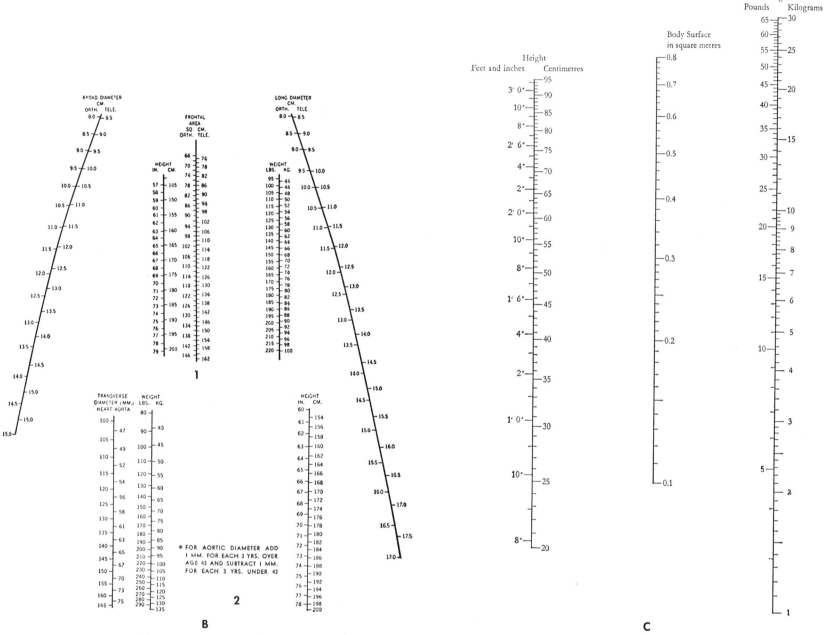

Figure 12–35 *Continued. B.* (1) Nomogram showing the frontal area of the heart predicted from height and weight, and actual area obtained from the measured long and broad diameters (for both orthodiagrams and telerentgenograms). Values exceeding 10 per cent above predicted values are abnormal. (2) Nomogram showing the predicted transverse diameter from height and weight, and diameter of the aorta. For the aortic diameter add 1 mm. for each 3 years over age 43 and subtract 1 mm. for each 3 years under 43.

Figure 12–35 continued on the opposite page.

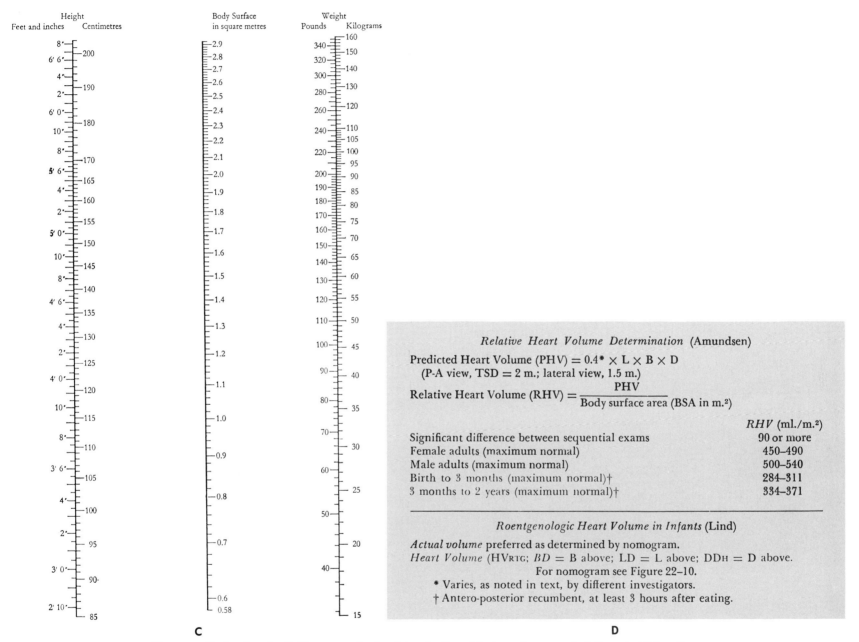

Height
Feet and inches   Centimetres

Body Surface
in square metres

Weight
Pounds   Kilograms

C

D

Relative Heart Volume Determination (Amundsen)

Predicted Heart Volume (PHV) = 0.4* × L × B × D
(P-A view, TSD = 2 m.; lateral view, 1.5 m.)

$$\text{Relative Heart Volume (RHV)} = \frac{\text{PHV}}{\text{Body surface area}} \text{ (BSA in m.}^2)$$

	RHV (ml./m.²)
Significant difference between sequential exams	90 or more
Female adults (maximum normal)	450–490
Male adults (maximum normal)	500–540
Birth to 3 months (maximum normal)†	284–311
3 months to 2 years (maximum normal)†	334–371

Roentgenologic Heart Volume in Infants (Lind)

Actual volume preferred as determined by nomogram.
Heart Volume (HVRTG; *BD* = B above; LD = L above; DDн = D above.
For nomogram see Figure 22–10.
* Varies, as noted in text, by different investigators.
† Antero-posterior recumbent, at least 3 hours after eating.

Figure 12–35 *Continued.* C. Nomogram for the determination of body surface area of adults and children (by Du Bois). *Key:* The body surface area is given by the point of intersection with the middle scale of a straight line joining height and weight. D. Summary of concepts of relative heart volume determination and roentgenologic heart volume in infants according to Amundsen and Lind respectively. Mannheimer's values for children are presented in Table 12–1.

Figure 12–35 continued on the following page.

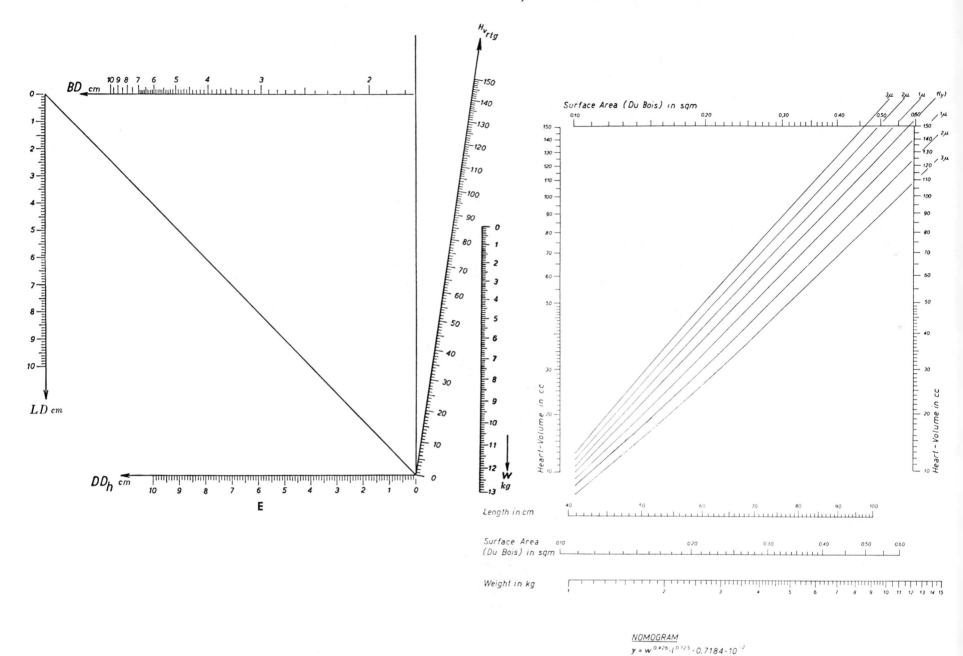

NOMOGRAM

$$y = w^{0.426} \cdot l^{0.725} \cdot 0.7184 \cdot 10^{-2}$$

$$H_v = 289.42\,y - 19.06 \qquad \textbf{F}$$

Figure 12–35 *Continued.* E. Nomogram for roentgenologic heart volume in infants. *Key to nomogram:* A line is drawn connecting DD_h and BD. A second line is drawn from LD to the point of intersection of the line between DD_h and BD with the diagonal; this is continued until it cuts the vertical line with no scale. This latter point is joined by a straight line to the weight scale (in kilograms). The point of intersection of this line with the Hv_{rtg} scale indicates the roentgenologic heart volume. F. Nomogram for predicted heart volume and comparison with the roentgenologic heart volume in infants. *Key to nomogram:* The surface area is read at the point at which a straight line connecting weight and length intersects the surface-area scale. From this point of intersection a line is drawn to the same point on the opposite surface-area scale. The intersection of the vertical line and the regression line [F(Y)] represents the predicted heart volume read on the heart-volume scale. A line is drawn from the point on the heart-volume scale representing the roentgenologic heart volume to the same point on the opposite scale. The intersection of this line with the vertical line from the surface-area scale indicates the position of the roentgenologic heart volume, within the standard deviation limits (mμ), that is, the relationship between the roentgenologic and predicted heart volume.

Figure 12–35 continued on the opposite page.

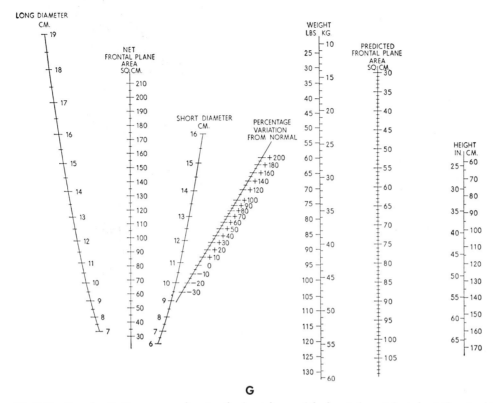

G

Figure 12–35 *Continued.* G. Nomograms showing the frontal area of the hearts from 6-foot chest films in children between the ages of 3 and 16 years inclusive. (From Meyer, R. R., in Radiology, 53:363–370, 1949.) The long and short diameters are obtained as previously described and the net frontal plane area is obtained from the nomogram portion reading "net frontal plane area." Next, the predicted frontal plane area is obtained from the nomogram by placing a straight edge between the appropriate body weight and height. When the ruler is placed so that it connects the values for "net" and "predicted frontal plane area," the "percentage variation from normal" is read off the sloping center scale at the point intersected by the ruler.

Transverse Diameter (TR + TL). This is the sum of the maximum projections of the right and left borders of the heart from the midline.

Long Diameter (L). This is the distance between the left ventricular apex and the small notch on the right border of the heart between the right atrium and the superior vena cava.

Broad Diameter (B). This is the greatest diameter of the cardiac shadow perpendicular to the long diameter. Occasionally, it is necessary to extend the right cardiac margin inferiorly in its natural curvature to delineate the lower margin of this diameter.

Anteroposterior Diameter (D). This is the greatest antero-posterior dimension of the cardiac silhouette on the lateral view.

Aortic Arch Diameter (AR + AL). This is the sum of the maximum extensions to the right and to the left of the aortic shadow from the midline as projected above the base of the heart. When the esophagus is also delineated, the maximum extension to the left of the aortic shadow in relation to the lateral margin of the esophagus is a measure of the diameter of the descending limb of the arch of the aorta. Normally, this measurement may vary between 1.8 and 3.8 cm.; a measurement greater than 4 cm. is abnormal. These measurements have no correction for magnification, and do not take into account the 3 mm. thickness of tissue between the lumen of the esophagus and the aorta.

DETERMINATION OF RELATIVE CARDIAC VOLUME (Amundsen)

The physical factors employed are (1) a target-to-film distance on frontal view of 2 meters, and (2) a target-to-film distance on lateral view of 1.5 meters.

Basic Formula. Volume = K × L × B × D (Fig. 12–35), where K = 0.42 (standard deviation 7.4 per cent) based on 45 cases, comparing calculated value with autopsy-determined value.

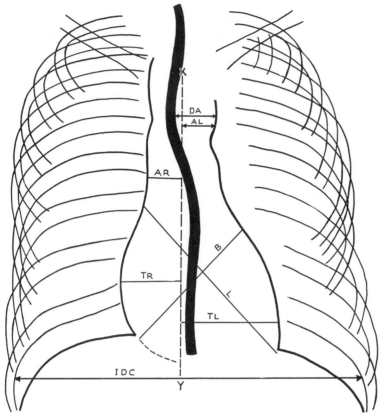

Figure 12–36. Diagram of teleroentgenograms of heart showing most frequent and useful cardiac measurements obtained therefrom: (*TR*) Maximum projection of the right cardiac border from the midline, (*TL*) maximum projection of the left cardiac border from the midline, (*TR* plus *TL*) the greatest transverse diameter of the heart, (*L*) the long diameter of the heart which extends from the junction of the cardiac silhouette and vascular pedicle on the right to the apex on the left, omitting consideration of the fat pad frequently seen in this location, (*B*) the broad diameter of the heart, which is the greatest diameter of the cardiac shadow perpendicular to the long diameter. It may be necessary to extend the lower right heart border in its natural curve, (*XY*) the midline in a perfectly straight PA projection (falls over spinous processes of dorsal spine), (*AR*) the maximum extension to the right of the vascular pedicle from the midline. (Note: The vascular pedicle shadow usually includes superior vena cava as well as aorta.) (*AL*) The maximum extension to the left of the vascular pedicle from the midline, (*AR* plus *AL*) the aortic arch diameter, (*DA*) the measurement of the descending aorta which represents the distance from the left margin of the esophagus to the outermost left margin of the aortic knob, (*IDC*) the greatest internal diameter of the chest.

Relative heart volume is defined as the volume per square meter of surface area using the DuBois nomograms for calculation of surface area from body height and weight. Thus, the formula for *relative heart volume* is:

$$\frac{0.42 \times L \times B \times D}{\text{Body surface area in square meters}}$$

A difference of 90 ml. per square meter or more between two successive examinations of the same patient indicates a significant change in relative heart volume.

The mean volume per square meter for adult males is 420 ± 40 cc., and for adult females it is 370 ± 40 cc. The second or third standard deviation indicates a suspicion of cardiomegaly, and above this limit there is only a 3 per cent chance of a normal heart size.

The second to third standard deviation above the mean is:

Female adults	450–490 ml. per sq. m.
Male adults	500–540 ml. per sq. m.
Birth to 3 months	284–311 ml. per sq. m.
3 months to 2 years	334–371 ml. per sq. m.

In infants, Lind's technique calls for carefully centered anteroposterior *supine* films.

Nomograms for the determination of body surface area of children and adults are appended for use.

Transverse Diameter of the Aorta.   Measurements AR and AL are added together (Fig. 12–35 *E*). Ungerleider and Gubner's nomogram for predicting aortic diameter is used, corrected as follows: (1) 1 mm. is added for each 3 years over the age of 43, and (2) 1 mm. is subtracted for each 3 years under the age of 43.

Since the *relative heart volume* is more accurate than the frontal area of the heart, we no longer employ the nomogram for *cardiac frontal area*.

Normal Heart Volumes in Children (Table 12–1; Fig. 12–35 *C*).   These values may be utilized along with those of Amundsen and Lind.

Relative heart volume calculation is now considered the method of choice for daily practice for both children and adults.

TABLE 12–1   NORMAL HEART VOLUMES IN CHILDREN*

Age	Volume per Square Meter of Body Surface (Relative Heart Volume)	Standard Error of the Mean
0–30 days	196	22.6
30–90 days	217.8	33.9
90–360 days	282	35.8
1–2 years	295	30.4
2–4 years	304	41.5
4–7 years	310	36.2
7–9 years	324	28.6
9–12 years	348	33.6
12–14 years	369	53.8
14–16 years	398	61.9

*Adapted from Mannheimer, in Keats, T. E., and Enge, I. P.: Radiology, *85*:850, 1965.

Frontal Cardiac Area. This may be determined with a fair degree of accuracy in accordance with the formula:

$$A = \pi/4 \; L \times B$$

where A is the frontal area, and L and B are the long and broad diameters respectively. The frontal area of the heart provides a reasonably accurate concept of cardiac size, although relative heart volume is considered more accurate.

The frontal cardiac area may be determined by utilization of nomograms as shown in Figure 12–35 B-1 for adults, and Figure 12–35 B for children.

The bodily factors most frequently employed for correlation are body height, weight, surface area, age, and sex. Weight is a better criterion than height but fails in the presence of obesity. Height is therefore a valuable criterion to compensate for this failure. Height groups are also found to be better criteria than age groups in children.

The correlation coefficient of body surface area with cardiac frontal area has been found to be as high as 0.84 to 0.92 (1.0 being perfect). Since the surface area equals $0.425 \; W \times 0.725 \; H \times 71.84$ (where W and H are the weight and height respectively), there is a sufficiently high correlation between surface area and the product of height and weight to use the latter as a substitute for surface area.

The greatest internal diameter of the chest has a poor correlation with cardiac frontal area.

The right and left cardiac margins must be delineated as separate and distinct from the pericardial fat pads in the cardiophrenic angles (Fig. 12–37).

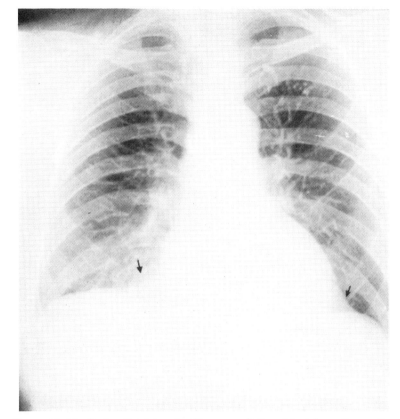

Figure 12–37. Pericardial fat pads. These are distinguished from the cardiac margins in both the right and left cardiophrenic angles.

RADIOGRAPHIC CARDIAC CONTOUR CHANGES IN RELATION TO SPECIFIC CHAMBER ENLARGEMENT

Introduction. As a matter of principle we have not included abnormalities of anatomy, but, in this region we shall demonstrate cardiac contour changes when specific chambers are enlarged to emphasize some of the normal roentgenographic anatomy.

Left Ventricle. Contour changes with left ventricular enlargement are indicated in Fig. 12–38. The left ventricular contour is rounded, extends farther laterally, and in the left lateral view is displaced posterior to the reflection of the inferior vena cava by a distance of 18 mm. or more, when measurements are made as demonstrated in the illustration. In the left anterior oblique view, the left ventricle usually overlaps the spine more than 1 cm. in the 45 degree obliquity. *Patients with a giant left atrium, a deformity of the left hemidiaphragm, a markedly enlarged right ventricle, or depression of the sternum (pectus excava-*

tum) cannot be evaluated by this method (Dinsmore et al.; Hoffman and Rigler).

Right Ventricle (Fig. 12–39). In infants, when the right ventricle is enlarged, it is projected above the left ventricular apex, imparting a squared appearance to this left margin near the diaphragm—the so-called "coeur en sabot" (wooden shoe) shape. In frontal view either no changes may be detected, or the right atrium may be displaced somewhat toward the right. The best view for detection of right ventricular enlargement is the straight lateral, in which an encroachment can be noted on the anterior and superior mediastinal clear space as the enlarged right ventricle "climbs the sternum" on its internal aspect.

Left Atrial Enlargement (Fig. 12–40). In the frontal projection, the right cardiac border assumes a double-contoured appearance because of the projection of the right margin of the left atrium toward it. The esophagus is usually displaced toward the right but occasionally toward the left, depending upon any associated aortic elongation that may be present and affecting the esophagus. There is a prominence of the left auricular appendage,

HYPERTROPHY AND DILATATION
LEFT VENTRICLE

POSTERO-ANTERIOR

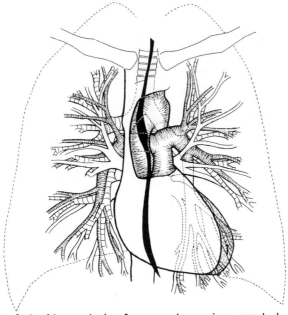

1. Left ventricular contour is rounded,
   extends farther laterally, and
   left diaphragm is depressed;
   rounding due to hypertrophy,
   distension to left due to
   dilatation.

A

LEFT ANTERIOR OBLIQUE

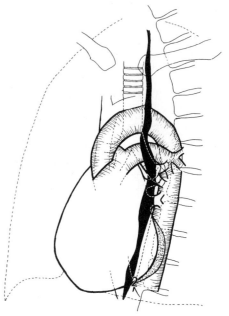

2. Left ventricle extends beyond
   retrocardiac space and cannot
   "clear the spine" readily;
   is rounded.

B

Figure 12–38. Diagrams showing changes in appearance of cardiac contour with left ventricular hypertrophy and dilatation.

Figure 12–38 continued on the opposite page.

producing an extra "hump" beneath the pulmonary sector, and it contributes to the convexity of the left cardiac margin. The left bronchus may be slightly displaced upward.

In the right anterior oblique as well as the right or left lateral views, the esophagus is displaced posteriorly in the region of the left atrium. A notch may be detected in the contour at the interatrial groove along the posterior margin of the heart. In the left anterior oblique view, the aortic window is usually obliterated by the enlarged left atrium or its appendage.

Also in the lateral view, the trachea, the right bronchus, and the left bronchus are normally in line with one another. The major bronchi appear tapered.

If, in the lateral view, the left upper lobe bronchus is displaced posteriorly, it is a good indication of left atrial enlargement and is sometimes a more sensitive indicator than displacement of the esophagus posteriorly (Lane and Whalen).

Right Atrial Enlargement (Fig. 12–41). Isolated right atrial enlargement is rare. It usually accompanies a diffuse or right ventricular enlargement. In the frontal view, the right cardiac margin may extend toward the right, but this is not a reliable sign (Klatte et al.). The most reliable indicators are revealed by the following methods:

1. Study of the heart fluoroscopically in the left anterior oblique view, in at least 45 degrees obliquity. Right atrial pulsations can be readily distinguished from those of the right ventricle on the right border of the heart. If the right atrium occupies 50 per cent or more of this border, right atrial enlargement is almost certainly present.

2. On film studies, the left anterior oblique and lateral views are most accurate. Here, when the right atrium is enlarged, the right auricular appendage produces a squared appearance of the right cardiac border.

LATERAL

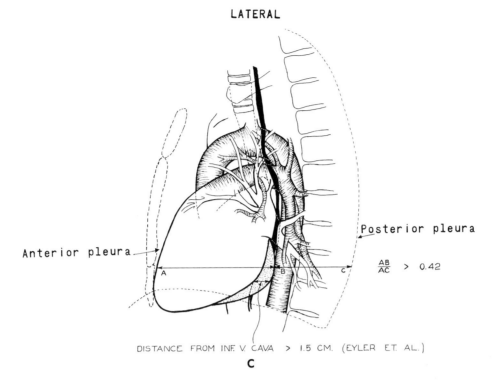

Anterior pleura

Posterior pleura

$\frac{AB}{AC} > 0.42$

DISTANCE FROM INF. V. CAVA > 1.5 CM. (EYLER ET. AL.)

C

RIGHT ANTERIOR OBLIQUE

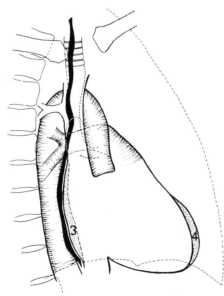

4. Anterior apical portion of heart extends farther anteriorly.

Heart intersects left leaf of diaphragm.

3. Heart as a whole is displaced posteriorly and comes close to spine.

LEFT VENTRICULAR HYPERTROPHY

D

Figure 12-38 Continued.

RIGHT VENTRICLE HYPERTROPHY AND DILATATION.

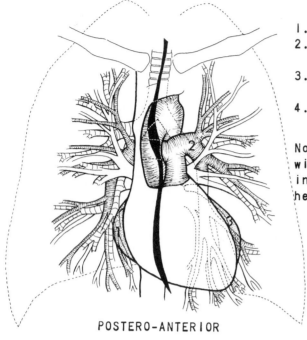

1. Enlarged right atrium.
2. Enlargement and dilatation of pulmonary arteries.
3. Increased convexity in left pulmonary sector.
4. Right ventricle bulges convexly on anterior aspect.

Note: "Wooden shoe" shape associated with right ventricular hypertrophy in tetralogy of Fallot not included here.

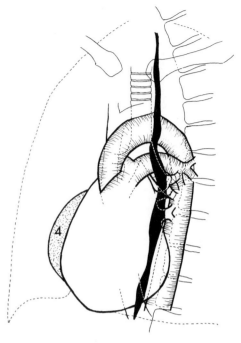

POSTERO-ANTERIOR
A

LEFT ANTERIOR OBLIQUE
B

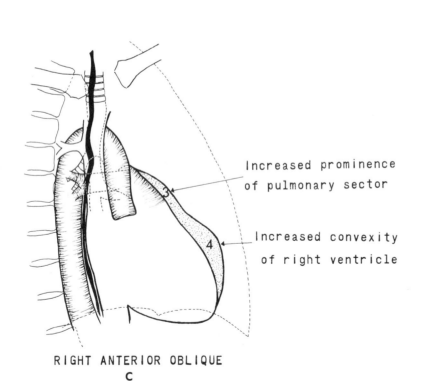

Increased prominence of pulmonary sector

Increased convexity of right ventricle

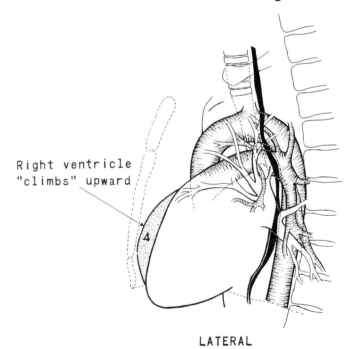

Right ventricle "climbs" upward

RIGHT ANTERIOR OBLIQUE
C

LATERAL

Right ventricle enlargement and encroachment on mediastinal clear space
D

Figure 12–39.   Diagrams showing cardiac contour changes with right ventricular hypertrophy and dilatation in the various conventional views.

In the lateral view, the right atrium, when markedly enlarged, protrudes posterior to the esophagus. This, however, is not a reliable sign by itself and is valid only when the right atrium is judged to be enlarged in the left anterior oblique view. (The left ventricle, when enlarged, also protrudes behind the esophageal shadow in the lateral projection, and the left anterior oblique view is necessary to distinguish this possibility.)

The right hemidiaphragm may be elevated, with right-sided cardiac dilatation and failure because of an engorged liver.

Aorta.   In the frontal projection, there is no convexity to the right of the vascular pedicle at the base of the heart. The aortic knob falls 1 to 2 cm. below the clavicles, and the measurement of the descending limb of the arch of the aorta does not exceed 3.8 cm., or 4 cm. in markedly sthenic individuals. In the left anterior oblique projection, the anterior margin of the ascending limb of the arch of the aorta forms a smooth continuous convexity with the anterior border of the right ventricle. The aortic window is well preserved.

Main Pulmonary Artery.   The pulmonary artery is best visualized in the right anterior oblique projection, and normally is not visualized in the other projections to good advantage. It forms a continuous straight line, or a slightly convex curve anteriorly above the left ventricular margin when the patient is rotated 45 degrees. Abnormality of the conus is also best reflected in this segment but may also be demonstrated by secondary enlargement or distortion and increased pulsations of the pulmonary arteries. For a more complete description and illustration of aortic and pulmonary artery abnormalities, the reader is referred to our companion texts, Analysis of Roentgen Signs and Roentgen Signs in Clinical Practice.

SPECIAL STUDIES OF THE HEART AND MAJOR BLOOD VESSELS

Newer advances in surgery of the heart and peripheral vascular system have necessitated great accuracy in depiction of cardiac abnormalities in diagnostic studies. Special techniques in cardiac radiology, and the greater collaborative efforts of radiologist, cardiologist, and physiologist, have helped greatly in the achievement of this aim. The most important of these special cardioradiologic techniques are: (1) venous angiocardiography, (2) selective angiocardiography, (3) aortography, (4) peripheral arteriography, (5) azygography, (6) venography, and (7) lymphangiography.

However, before delving into these special contrast studies, a few comments in relation to orthodiagraphy and kymography are in order.

Orthodiagraphy.   An orthodiagram is an outline drawing of the heart made on a celluloid cover or transparent paper placed over the fluoroscopic screen while moving the screen and x-ray tube independently, so that only the central ray is employed to record every point on the cardiac border. Since only the central ray is employed, the complete absence of divergent beams eliminates the element of magnification. Also, it is possible to plot the points in a given phase of the cardiac cycle and in a given respiratory phase also, eliminating these variables as well. It is very time-consuming and requires a specially constructed independently moving fluoroscopic screen and x-ray tube; *the advantages gained are not usually sufficiently great to warrant the performance of this procedure or the hazards of radiation exposure to patient and physician.*

Magnification of Teleroentgenograms and the Fallacy of Comparison of Orthodiagrams with Teleroentgenograms.   In orthodiagraphy the central ray is employed in a designated phase of respiration and cardiac cycle. Teleroentgenography, on the other hand, is a 6 foot projection of the heart in suspended inspiration in no definite phase of the cardiac cycle. Even at 6 feet a certain amount of magnification (approximately 5 per cent) is inevitable, depending upon the distance of the heart from the film on the one hand, and the distance of the heart from the tube-target on the other. Differences of cardiac measurements in systole and diastole will impose an additional 5 to 10 per cent variation. Differences produced by body habitus and phase of respiration, as well as body position, impose additional necessary corrections. (Apparatus is available, however, by means of which a roentgenogram of the heart in any phase of the cardiac cycle can be obtained by triggering the x-ray exposure during any desired phase of the electrocardiogram.)

The complexity of this comparison can be seen immediately, and it is readily apparent that no actual constant arithmetical factor can be given between orthodiagraphy and teleroentgenography.

Kymography (Boone et al.) (Fig. 12–42).   The conventional multiple-slit kymograph consists of a sheet of lead in which multiple parallel slits about 1 mm. wide have been cut about 1 cm. apart. This is placed over a cassette, and the lead sheet is made to move the distance between the slits (1 cm.) during three to five cardiac systoles. As the slits descend, an outline of the pulsations of each portion of the cardiac outline is obtained. The peaks represent diastole and the valleys systole. The configuration of the contractions can be studied, and abnormalities in pulsations recorded for future reference and comparison. However, respiratory changes, the changes in contour with the rotary movement of the heart, and the neutralization effects of one chamber on another all make this method of recording pulsations rather inaccurate. A more accurate method has been advocated (Boone et al.) which employs the current in a photoelectric cell as the recording medium of the pulsation. The cardiac pulsations at a given point will interrupt the passage of a fine x-ray beam through the chest at

LEFT ATRIAL ENLARGEMENT

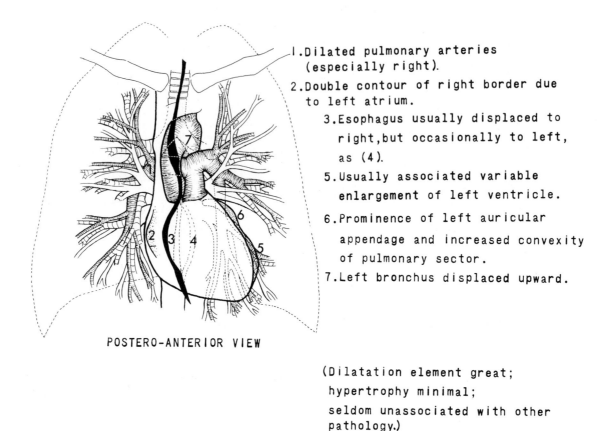

1. Dilated pulmonary arteries (especially right).

2. Double contour of right border due to left atrium.

3. Esophagus usually displaced to right, but occasionally to left, as (4).

5. Usually associated variable enlargement of left ventricle.

6. Prominence of left auricular appendage and increased convexity of pulmonary sector.

7. Left bronchus displaced upward.

POSTERO-ANTERIOR VIEW

(Dilatation element great; hypertrophy minimal; seldom unassociated with other pathology.)

A

Figure 12–40. Diagrams illustrating cardiac contour changes with left atrial enlargement in the conventional projections.

Figure 12–40 continued on the opposite page.

this point, and this variation in the intensity of the x-ray beam after it has passed through the body is recorded by means of a photoelectric cell. Records can be obtained which are indicative of abnormality at given points in the cardiac outline, but here, too, the torsion of the heart with pulsations and the respiratory effect will modify the curve obtained, and thus produce inaccuracies.

Application of Special Contrast Studies to a Study of the Heart and Major Blood Vessels (Venous Angiocardiograms). In 1938, Robb and Steinberg described a method for visualization of the cardiac chambers and major blood vessels leading from the heart, by means of the rapid injection of a relatively large quantity (50 cc.) of double concentration (70 per cent) Diodrast into a vein of the arm or leg. This method of examination was called "cardioangiography."

Originally, their method required timing the films in accordance with the major and lesser circulation times which were ob-

tained prior to the Diodrast injection. More recently, apparatus has been devised which permits obtaining films at very rapid intervals, up to 12 per second with 16 or 35 mm. movie films with very high frame frequencies per second (24 to 60 being most frequently employed). This allows the production of sequential films for twelve or more seconds after the injection depending on the "program selection." With the aid of such apparatus, it is unnecessary to time the exposures with great accuracy, so long as a sufficient number of exposures is obtained while the dye is passing through the right side of the heart, and then the left side of the heart and aorta. Simultaneous or near simultaneous films may be obtained in two planes perpendicular to one another.

It is essential in this method of examination that a large bulk of the dye (up to 50 cc.) be injected very rapidly (in 2 seconds or less), so that the concentration of the dye in the blood will be sufficiently high to produce a good contrast not only in the right side

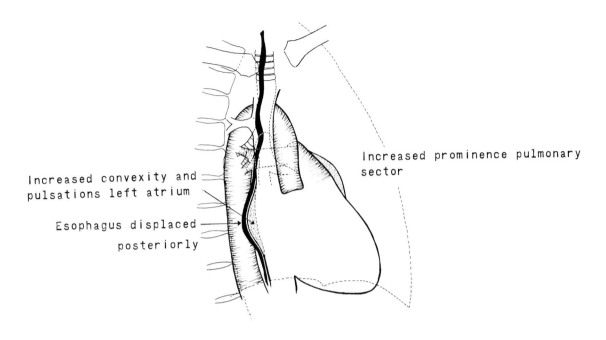

Increased convexity and
pulsations left atrium

Esophagus displaced
posteriorly

Increased prominence pulmonary
sector

RIGHT ANTERIOR OBLIQUE
B

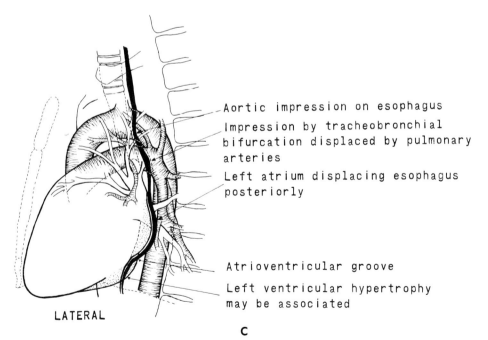

Aortic impression on esophagus

Impression by tracheobronchial
bifurcation displaced by pulmonary
arteries

Left atrium displacing esophagus
posteriorly

Atrioventricular groove

Left ventricular hypertrophy
may be associated

LATERAL

C

Figure 12–40 Continued.

RIGHT ATRIAL ENLARGEMENT

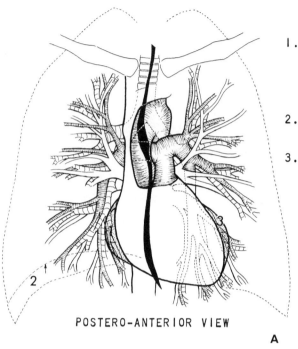

1. Extension to right of right atrial border, with increased convexity. Occasionally enlarged right ventricle does this.
2. Elevated diaphragm from enlarged liver.
3. Usually left-sided heart enlargement, since mitral and aortic valvular disease are associated with tricuspid.

POSTERO-ANTERIOR VIEW

A

"Squaring off" of right atrial appendage

Right atrial margin comprises 50% or more of entire right cardiac margin, judged by studying pulsations

LEFT ANTERIOR OBLIQUE

B

Figure 12-41. Diagrams showing cardiac contour changes which may be present with right atrial enlargement.

Figure 12-41 continued on the opposite page.

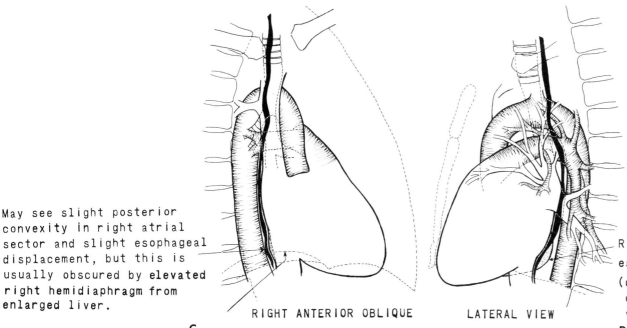

May see slight posterior convexity in right atrial sector and slight esophageal displacement, but this is usually obscured by elevated right hemidiaphragm from enlarged liver.

RIGHT ANTERIOR OBLIQUE

C

LATERAL VIEW

Right atrium protrudes behind esophagus - (compare with right anterior oblique view to exclude left ventricle)

D

Figure 12-41 *Continued.*

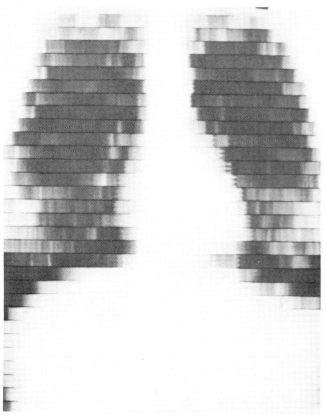

Figure 12-42. Posteroanterior kymogram.

of the heart, but also in the left. For this reason a special syringe with a large bore and a large bore needle (12 gauge) must be employed. It is sometimes advisable in children to expose a vein in the ankle and insert the needle under direct visualization. Special automatic pressure injectors have also been devised for this purpose. At best, the concentration of the dye in the left side of the heart under normal conditions allows only a moderate intensification and visualization of the anatomy.

In normal individuals, the superior vena cava and the right atrium are visualized in 1 to 1½ seconds; the right ventricle and pulmonary arteries in 3 to 5 seconds (Fig. 12–43); and the left atrium, left ventricle, and aorta in 6 to 10 seconds following the beginning of the injection period.

On the right side (Fig. 12–43 *A*), the following structures can be identified: the *superior vena cava and its tributaries* (which may be referred to as the inflow tract); *the right atrial and ventricular cavities and walls;* the *auricular appendage;* the *tricuspid valve;* the *trabeculae;* the *ventricular septum;* the *pulmonic valve;* and the *pulmonary artery with its subdivisions.*

The space between the right border of the contrast-filled atrium and the right border of the cardiac silhouette represents the free wall of the right atrium, which normally measures 2 to 3 mm. in diameter. When this space is increased, pericardial effusion is indicated.

The right atrial appendage or auricle extends cephalad and medially from the upper portion of the right atrium, overlapping to some extent the inflow tract. The *tricuspid valve* is in an

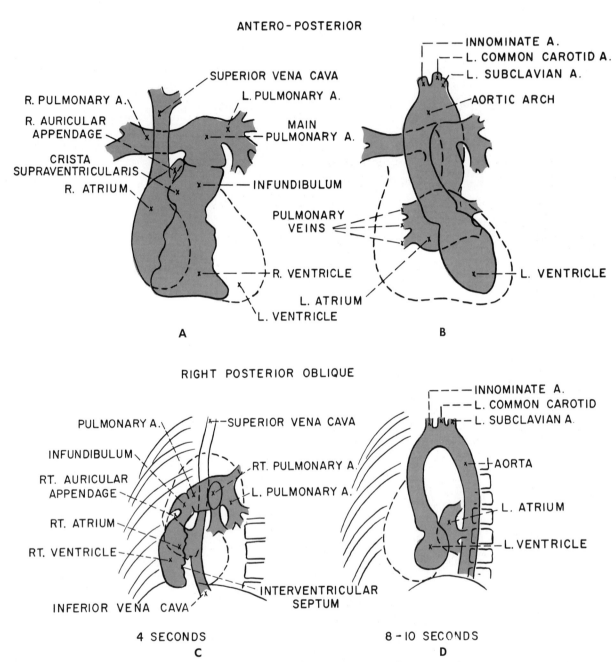

Figure 12–43. A and B. Major structures visualized in venous angiocardiograms in the anteroposterior projection. A. Lesser circulation phase. B. Greater circulation phase. C and D. Major structures visualized in venous angiocardiograms in the right posterior oblique projection. C. Lesser circulation phase. D. Greater circulation phase.

Figure 12–43 continued on the opposite page.

LEFT POSTERIOR OBLIQUE

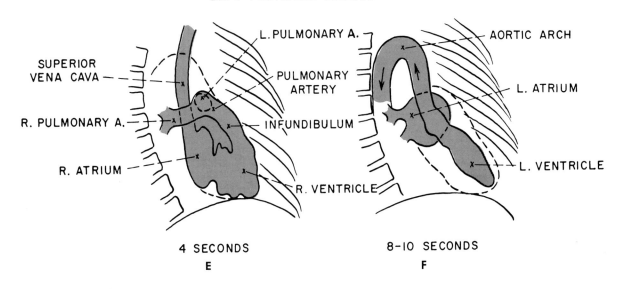

4 SECONDS
E

8-10 SECONDS
F

RIGHT LATERAL

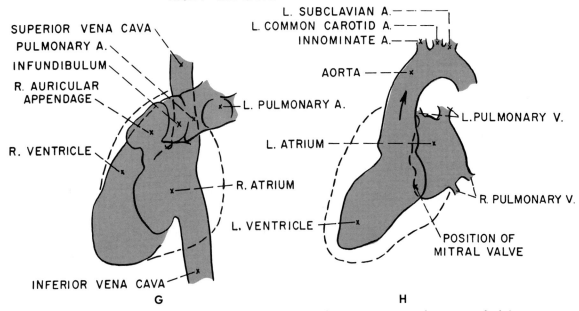

G

H

Figure 12-43 *Continued. E* and *F.* Major structures visualized in venous angiocardiograms in the left posterior oblique projection. *E.* Lesser circulation phase. *F.* Greater circulation phase. *G* and *H.* Major structures visualized in venous angiocardiograms in the right lateral projection. *G.* Lesser circulation phase. *H.* Greater circulation phase.

oblique plane between the right atrium and right ventricle and may be represented as an ellipse (Fig. 12-44). The inferior margin of the *tricuspid annulus* is adjacent to the junction of the *inferior vena cava* and *right atrium.* The *coronary sinus* is situated in this same region. (This similarity in position may give rise to confusion in catheterization, because the catheter may enter the coronary sinus and advance into the great cardiac vein rather than upward into the outflow tract of the right ventricle.) The atrium and ventricle tend to lie over one another in the immediate vicinity of the tricuspid annulus.

The *right ventricle* is a chamber roughly triangular in shape, divided into two component parts: (1) a large trabeculated inflow

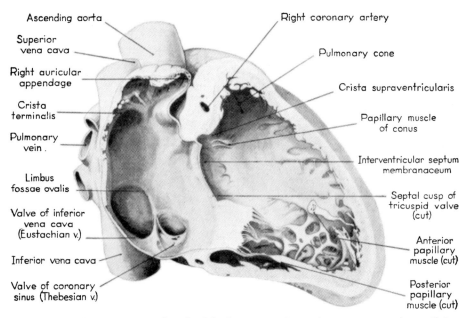

Ascending aorta

Superior
vena cava

Right auricular
appendage

Crista
terminalis

Pulmonary
vein

Limbus
fossae ovalis

Valve of inferior
vena cava
(Eustachian v.)

Inferior vena cava

Valve of coronary
sinus (Thebesian v.)

Right coronary artery

Pulmonary cone

Crista supraventricularis

Papillary muscle
of conus

Interventricular septum
membranaceum

Septal cusp of
tricuspid valve
(cut)

Anterior
papillary
muscle (cut)

Posterior
papillary
muscle (cut)

Figure 12-44 Right side of the heart opened in a plane approximately parallel to the septa, to show the interior of the right atrium and the right ventricle. A segment of the septal leaflet of the tricuspid valve has been cut away to expose more fully the region of the membranous portion of the interventricular septum. (From Gould, S. E. 1959. Pathology of the Heart, 2d ed. Courtesy of Charles C Thomas, Publisher, Springfield, Illinois.)

portion communicating with the right atrium, and (2) a tubular upper portion representing the *outflow tract*. The right border of the inflow portion is formed by the *tricuspid valve,* whereas the left border is formed by the *interventricular septum*. The right border of the outflow tract is formed by a sheet of muscle extending from the tricuspid to the pulmonic valve lying in front of the aorta; it is a localized prominence in this muscle that is called the *crista supraventricularis.* The *pulmonic valve,* when normal, is not easily identified in the frontal view and is best seen in oblique or lateral projections. The *pulmonary trunk* is visualized cephalad to the pulmonic valve and branches almost immediately into *right and left pulmonary arteries.* The right pulmonary artery courses in a direct horizontal direction to the right and is clearly identified in this projection; the left pulmonary artery is directed posteriorly and is foreshortened. It is best demonstrated in a left lateral or steep left anterior oblique view. Contrast agent may remain in the superior vena cava or in the right atrium, obscuring the right pulmonary artery.

In the *lateral projection* (Fig. 12–44) the right atrium is projected posterior to the right ventricle, and the posterior margin of the right atrium is clearly identified. The anterior margin of the right atrium is formed by the tricuspid valve and

annulus of this valve that forms a boundary between the right atrium and the right ventricle. The atrial appendage rises cephalad to the tricuspid valve, extending anteriorly and superiorly and overlapping the pulmonic valve very slightly. The ostium of the coronary sinus lies in the inferior portion of the atrium just in front of the entrance of the inferior vena cava. It curves posteriorly from the superior vena cava and can be recognized in this way.

Because of the interference by the right atrial appendage, the *right ventricle* is best studied by selective angiocardiography. The inflow portion of the right ventricle lies in front of the tricuspid valve, with the crista supraventricularis situated just superior and anterior to the tricuspid annulus. It marks the inferior margin of the infundibulum—the outflow portion of the right ventricle. The outflow portion is readily identified as a tubular sector leading directly to the pulmonic valve. The valve cusps are readily identified in the lateral view. This view is also best for identifying an *infundibular stenosis,* a common congenital anomaly. The left pulmonary artery is clearly identified in the lateral view as it courses posteriorly, but the right pulmonary artery is too foreshortened in this view to be accurately seen.

On the left side (Fig. 12–43 B), the following components may be seen: the *pulmonary veins;* the *left atrial and ventricular cavities and walls;* the *auricular appendage;* the *aortic valve;* and the *entire thoracic aorta* with its main branches.

In *frontal projection,* the left heart is first identified by detecting the left atrium, which lies just above and to the right of the left ventricle. The two superior pulmonary veins enter the uppermost portion of the left atrium, whereas the inferior pulmonary veins can be identified below them forming a horizontal V-shaped structure that extends on each side of the circular left atrium. The left atrial appendage has a hooklike contour extending upward and to the left and overlying the left superior pulmonary vein. The left ventricle, for the most part, can be identified below the level of the mitral valve as well as the aortic valve. It is oval in shape with its apex pointing downward and to the left. Generally, the *trabeculation of the left ventricular cavity is much finer than that of the right ventricle* and hence, one can identify right and left ventricles by the trabecular architecture—an important differentiation in certain congenital heart conditions. The superior margin of the annulus of the mitral valve is continuous with that of the aortic ring and is usually not well identified in frontal view. The membranous portion of the interventricular septum cannot be delineated on angiocardiograms, but it lies beneath the anterior portion of the posterior cusp of the aortic valve, a small part of the adjacent right cusp, and the commissure between the two. In frontal projection the right cusp is seen *en face;* the left cusp forms the left border of the aortic valve, whereas the noncoronary cusp forms the right border. The right coronary artery can often be identified faintly in angiocardiograms but it is best identified by selective angiography (to be discussed subsequently). It arises from the midportion of the aortic valve, whereas the left coronary artery originates from the left border of the aortic valve. The entire right border of the left ventricle is formed by the interventricular septum, the upper part being membranous and the remainder being muscular.

In some anomalous conditions it is important to recall that the tricuspid valve attachment reaches almost to the aortic valve and actually crosses the membranous septum.

In the *lateral view* (Fig. 12–45) the left atrium is projected posterior to the left ventricle. The anterior margin of this chamber is formed by the mitral valve. The left atrial appendage arises above the mitral valve and extends anteriorly and cephalad to the sinuses of Valsalva. The posterior border of the atrial cavity is a free wall of the atrium, and the pulmonary veins enter its superior and middle portions. The mitral valve forms the posterior boundary of the left ventricle and its upper margin extends to the aortic valve in the region of the commissure between the left (coronary) and posterior (noncoronary) cusps. The left ventricular cavity extends inferiorly and anteriorly from the mitral valve and aortic sinuses; its entire anterior margin is formed by the interventricular septum. In lateral view, the right coronary cusp of the aortic valve forms the anterior border of the valve; the left and posterior cusps are projected obliquely, posteriorly, with the posterior noncoronary cusp lower than the left cusp (coronary). The membranous portion of the interventricular septum lies directly below the commissure between the right and noncoronary cusp.

The right coronary artery may occasionally be identified on angiocardiograms but is best visualized in selective angiocardiography or selective coronary arteriograms. The right coronary artery arises from the upper portion of the right sinus of Valsalva; the left coronary artery is foreshortened in this lateral view.

When the right ventricle is enlarged, the sulcus between the ventricle and right atrium is displaced anteriorly. This in turn will displace the position of the coronary artery.

The tricuspid valve lies anterior to the mitral valve.

The supraventricular crest lies directly in front of the right sinus of Valsalva.

The wall thickness of the right ventricle may at times be measurable – 2 to 3 mm. The left ventricular wall, *smoother than that of the right,* usually measures between 7 and 10 mm. in thickness.

The *arch of the aorta* is demonstrable as it extends anteriorly and upward, and then arches posteriorly and to the left. It descends down the left side of the thoracic spine and in the posterior mediastinal space as a tubular structure approximately 3.5 cm. in diameter. The wall thickness of the aorta is usually in the order of 3 mm.

The *innominate, left common carotid, and left subclavian arteries* can occasionally be distinguished as they branch from the arch of the aorta along its anterior aspect.

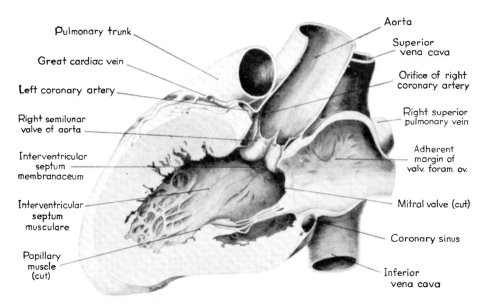

Figure 12–45. Left side of the heart opened in a plane approximately parallel to the septa, to show the interior of the left atrium and left ventricle. A segment of the anterior leaflet of the mitral valve has been cut away to expose more fully the region of the membranous portion of the interventricular septum and the aortic orifice. (From Gould, S. E. 1959. Pathology of the Heart, 2d ed. Courtesy of Charles C Thomas, Publisher, Springfield, Illinois.)

The *aortic triangle* is likewise delineated. It is bounded anteriorly by the left subclavian artery, posteriorly by the spine, and inferiorly by the arch of the aorta.

CATHETERIZATION OF THE HEART

Cardiac Catheterization. In view of the great technical advances made by cardiac surgeons in relation to open heart surgery and repair of defects, the roentgen examination of the heart and its inflow and outflow tracts has become much more exacting. The surgeon must know the answers to many questions, such as the size and extent of a defect or stenosis, the degree of overriding of the aorta, and the appearance of the pulmonary arteries, veins, and systemic arteries.

In recent years, the technique of cardiac catheterization has been increasingly applied and developed in this direction. Passing a catheter into the right heart and then sequentially into the pulmonary artery provides the physician with the following opportunities: (1) blood samples may be obtained from any of these areas or all of them, and *gas analysis* may be performed on the samples to determine the site of shunt formation; (2) the *volume of blood shunting* may be calculated; (3) *pulmonary blood flow* may be readily calculated; (4) *pressures* in the various chambers may be recorded and evaluated in relation to the dynamics of the cardiac circulation (see Chapter 11); (5) if the catheter takes an *abnormal route,* a defect may be recognized directly—for example, a patent interatrial septum; (6) at the end of these procedures, one may selectively inject into any region a quantity of opaque media under sufficient pressure to visualize carefully a given area without too much interference from adjoining areas. This latter technique is called "selective angiocardiography," in contrast to the previously described venous angiocardiography.

Selective Angiocardiography. There are different types of catheters used for this purpose, each with its own advocates. A mechanical pressure device for the injection must usually be employed to provide a satisfactory jet of contrast media within $1/2$ to 1 second. A number of these are available commercially, varying in complexity and cost from several hundred dollars to several thousand. Injection directly into the right ventricle is by far the most common procedure, and the injection is followed by serial films taken as rapidly as 12 per second (simultaneously in two planes), or by 16 or 35 mm. cineradiographs for cinema depiction. Care must be exercised to locate the catheter tip accurately, lest the injection be made into a coronary vein.

The projection planes most frequently employed are the straight frontal (anteroposterior), right posterior oblique, and lateral. Usually, a simultaneous biplane technique is desirable.

Most of the catheters now used by angiographers, with the exception of expensive preshaped molded varieties, are supplied in long rolls and are custom-made for a particular use, being discarded after one use. Usually they are radiopaque in order to facilitate manipulation and guidance under fluoroscopic control, with image amplification. Generally, polyethylene catheters seem to change the least when made radiopaque; the lead oxide incorporated into polyethylene in Kifa tubing was one of the earliest materials used for this purpose. (Lead is now prohibited from such use.) Radiopaque polyethylene catheters are available from many manufacturers and are supplied in rolls of 10 to 20 feet, color-coded according to their size.

Most catheters are inserted percutaneously by the Seldinger technique. As shown in Figure 12–46, this involves the initial insertion of a special type of needle through both walls of the artery and gradual retraction of the tip of the cannula into the arterial lumen after withdrawal of the needle insert. A guidewire is then passed through the cannula into the artery, and the cannula is removed over the guidewire. A catheter is then gently rotated over the guidewire into the lumen of the artery. To accomplish this, the catheter must be carefully tapered by heating it with the guidewire still in place. With the guidewire in place the catheter is then bent into its desired curve and immersed in hot water (over 140 degrees F.), after which it is immediately plunged into cold water so that the shaping is permanent. Side holes are usually provided in the catheter, as close to the end hole as possible to concentrate the bolus, yet to avoid a jet stream. The side holes, appropriately placed, help prevent recoil of the catheter out of the vessel during injection of the contrast material.

The proximal end of the catheter is usually equipped with a special adapter attached to a Luer-lock stopcock. Catheters, of course, must be thoroughly tested to avoid leakage around the stopcock or connector. Various catheter-manipulating devices that allow for ease of insertion into the desired blood vessels are also commercially available.

Some catheters used for angiocardiography are inserted directly into surgically exposed arteries or veins, making end holes unnecessary. Absence of the end hole decreases the chance of intramural injection into a cardiac chamber. One such commer-

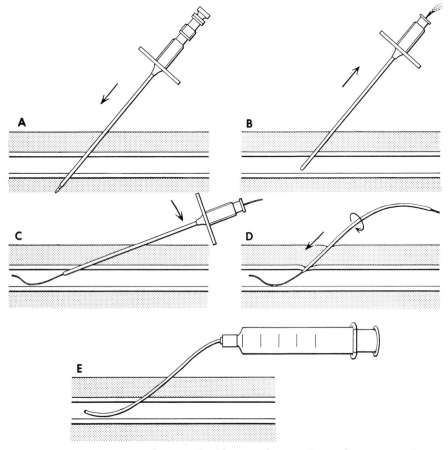

Figure 12–46. Application of Seldinger technique of arterial puncture. *A.* Puncture of both walls of the vessel. *B.* Retraction of tip of cannula into arterial lumen after withdrawal of needle insert. *C.* Passage of guidewire through cannula into artery. *D.* Passage of smoothly tapered catheter tip over guidewire into artery; gentle rotation of the catheter facilitates the entry. *E.* Catheter in lumen of artery after withdrawal of guidewire. (From Curry, J. L., and Howland, W. J.: Arteriography. Philadelphia, W. B. Saunders Co., 1966.)

cially available device is the Lehman ventriculography catheter, made of woven Dacron (or Teflon) with thin walls and a closed distal tip, and four side holes 4 cm. from the tip. The Rodriquez-Alvarez catheter has thin walls of smooth nylon reinforced with woven Dacron, and six openings arranged in three opposing pairs within the first centimeter of the tip. (For a more detailed discussion of catheters see Bierman.)

Injection rates in various portions of the heart or major blood vessels vary in order to obtain most satisfactory visualization. For example, selective coronary arteriography is performed at injection rates of 4 cc. per second approximately, with hand injections. Aortography or angiocardiography requires larger injection volumes in short periods of time. Whereas 8 to 10 cc. per second is adequate within a cardiac chamber, aortography requires injection rates of up to 40 or 50 cc. per second. These high rates require mechanical injectors, which are now commercially available so that the desired rate of injection and timing can be very accurately controlled.

Much has been written concerning other aspects of this highly specialized technique, for example, the advantages of large film studies as opposed to ciné film studies. With the ciné technique, it is now possible to expose several hundred frames in 1 second, if desired. Each has its proponents, and its advantages and disadvantages. A radiology study group under the aegis of an intersociety commission for heart disease resources formulated guidelines for optimal equipment for a catheterization-angiocardiography laboratory, and the reader is referred to their preliminary report for greater detail regarding the organization and space required for the laboratory, and specific equipment, electrical power, and physiologic monitors necessary (Abrams). (Detailed chapters devoted to this equipment as well as to catheters, injectors, and other aspects of angiography are also available in this text.)

Various contrast media have been suggested for selective angiocardiography; the agents usually used are Renografin (meglumine diatrizoate), Hypaque (sodium diatrizoate), and iothalamate (Jacobson and Paulin).

Apart from coronary arteriography (which will be discussed subsequently), selective angiocardiography in relation to the heart and major vessels at this writing includes the passage of a catheter into the right atrium, right ventricle, pulmonary artery, right and left pulmonary artery branches, through the foramen ovale into the left atrium, and through the mitral valve into the left ventricle. Catheters are also passed backward from the arm or leg into the ascending aorta, the sinuses of Valsalva, and through the aortic valve into the left ventricle.

In view of the complexity of this procedure, radiation exposure must be kept to an absolute minimum. An accurate record of fluoroscopic time, physical factors employed, and films made during all procedures should allow the radiologist to estimate the approximate radiation dosage to the patient. The gonads and all other body areas not required for diagnosis should be carefully protected from the primary beam and, as far as possible, from external scatter as well.

Several other techniques for catheterization of the left chambers of the heart are also available: (1) retrograde catheterization of the left ventricle from a peripheral artery; (2) direct puncture of the left chambers of the heart by a transthoracic needle; (3) transbronchial needle puncture of the left atrium; and (4) catheterization of the left atrium and ventricle by a transseptal needle and overlying catheter. Transbronchial and direct transthoracic cardiac puncture are seldom employed because the placement of a large-bore catheter into the left heart is difficult and risky with these techniques, and they do not allow easy positioning of the patient for repeated injections of the contrast agent. Generally, for left ventricular catheterization, retro-aortic catheterization via the femoral artery using a Seldinger technique is preferred. However, complications of transseptal puncture for left heart catheterization are few (Bell). This technique is diagrammatically illustrated in Figure 12–47.

Representative Angiocardiograms. Representative angiocardiograms are shown in Figure 12–48. With *right heart visualization,* there is rapid sequential filling of the superior vena cava, right atrium, and right auricular appendage. The tricuspid valve region is identified between the right atrium and right ventricle, and thereafter filling of the infundibulum and pulmonary artery and its major branches is shown. In the *lateral view* (Fig. 12–48 G-K), the right auricular appendage overlaps the pulmonary artery, although usually the pulmonary valve can be identified as an umbrella-shaped structure just above the projection of the right atrial appendage. Note that during atrial systole, the atrial ventricular border shifts dorsally. The crista terminalis presses into the lumen, resembling a membrane.

On *left heart visualization,* the left ventricle, mitral valve (Fig. 12–49), and left atrium appear as shown. The superior and inferior right pulmonary veins are clearly in evidence, whereas those on the left are somewhat obscured. The left auricular appendage is seen projected just above the left ventricle to the left of the midline. The aorta may thereafter be visualized. The aortic sinuses and valves as well as the coronary arteries may also be visualized following selective catheterization of the left ventricle.

In *lateral view* these structures may once again be identified and the thickness of the left ventricle readily measured.

Gross differences between the normal child and adult are shown in Figure 12–50. In frontal perspective in the adult the cardiac chambers are more horizontally disposed, with a much tighter U-shaped curve of the right heart. In the left heart, the axes of both the inflow and outflow tracts lie in a more horizontal plane in infants and children than in adults.

In venous angiography when injection is made in both arms, the entire venous inflow tract to the heart is excellently visualized (Fig. 12–51).

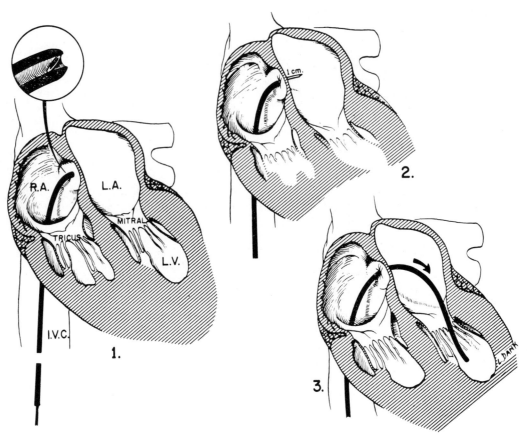

Figure 12–47. Diagrammatic representation of transseptal puncture with catherization of left atrium and left ventricle by the overlying catheter. (1) Proper positioning of needle and catheter for septal puncture, (2) septal puncture by the needle, and (3) catheterization of left ventricle by the overlying catheter. (From Schobinger, R. A., and Ruzicka, F. F., Jr.: Vascular Roentgenology. New York, The Macmillan Company, 1964.)

CORONARY ARTERIOGRAPHY AND VENOGRAPHY

Basic Anatomy. Two coronary arteries supply the heart. The *left coronary* originates from the left aortic sinus at the level of the free edge of the valve cusp. Its short common stem bifurcates or trifurcates about 0.5 to 2 cm. from its origin (Fig. 12–52). The *anterior interventricular or descending branch* courses downward in the anterior interventricular groove just to the right of the apex of the heart, and may ascend a short distance up the posterior interventricular groove. There are branches to the adjacent anterior right ventricular wall and septal branches, supplying the anterior two-thirds of the apical portion of the septum. The

anteroapical portions of the left ventricle ordinarily have several branches. The second branch of the left coronary artery, the *circumflex*, runs in the left atrioventricular sulcus, giving off branches to the upper lateral left ventricular wall and left atrium. When there is a third branch of the left coronary artery, it originates between the anterior interventricular and circumflex branches and supplies the left ventricle.

The *right coronary artery* arises from the right anterior sinus of Valsalva (aortic sinus) and courses along the right atrioventricular sulcus. It rounds the acute margin of the right ventricle to reach the crux (junction of the posterior interventricular sulcus and the posterior atrioventricular groove). It gives off branches to the anterior right ventricular wall; the branch along the acute

(Text continued on page 750.)

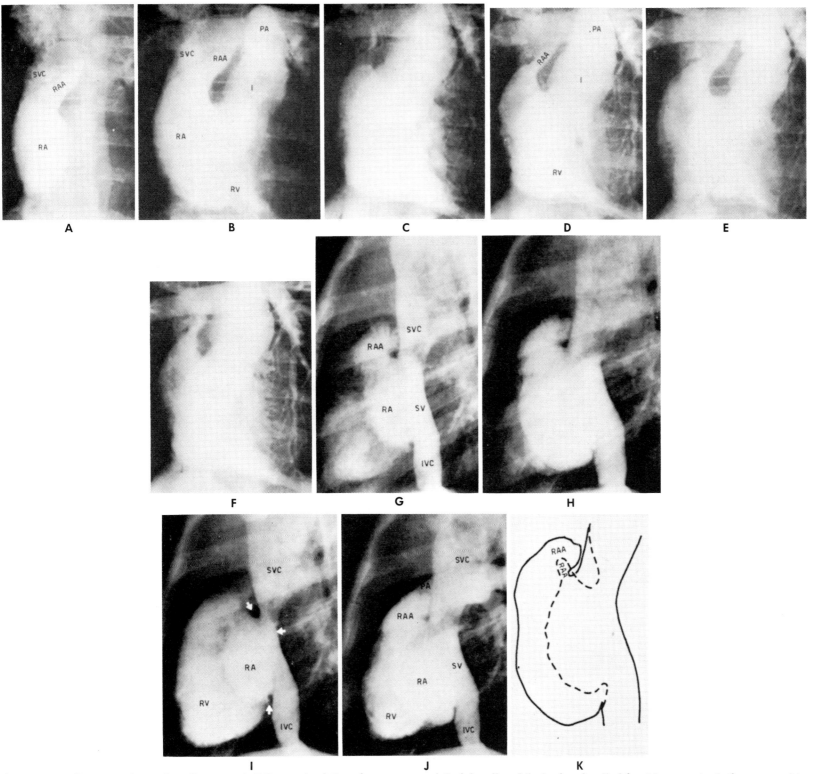

Figure 12–48. Representative angiocardiograms. *A–F*. Lesser circulation phase, frontal projection. Right auricular appendage lies directly to the right of the infundibulum and the right ventricle and lower part of the pulmonary artery which, consequently, in lateral projection, are overlapped by the appendage. (AO) Aorta, (I) infundibulum, (IVC) inferior vena cava, (LA) left atrium, (LV) left ventricle, (PA) pulmonary artery, (RA) right atrium, (RAA) right auricular appendage, (RV) right ventricle, (SV) sinus venosus, (SVC) superior vena cava. *G–K*. Lesser circulation phase, lateral projection. During atrial systole, the atrioventricular border is shifted dorsally, while the dorsal wall of the atrium remains in the same position. The crista terminalis presses into the lumen like a membrane (*I*, lower arrow). Sphincter mechanism of the venae cavae is clearly visible. *K*. Collective picture of appearance of atrium in late diastole (solid line) and late systole (broken line). (From Diagnosis of Congenital Heart Disease, 2d ed., by Kjellberg, Sven R., et al. Copyright © 1959 by Year Book Medical Publishers, Inc., Chicago. Used by permission.)

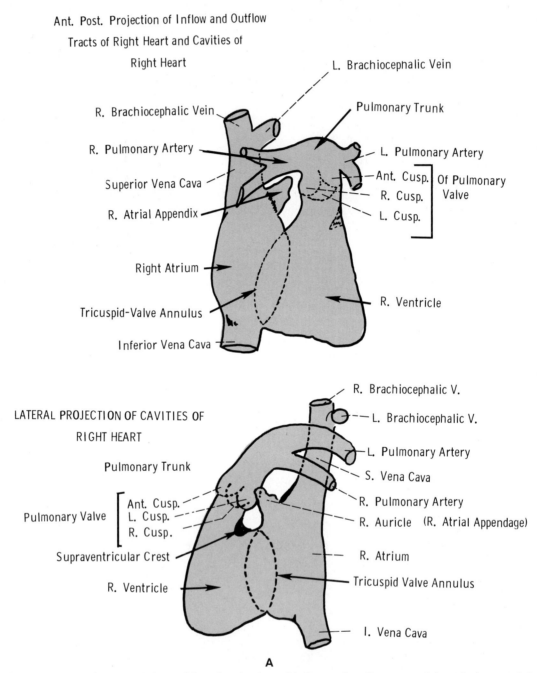

Ant. Post. Projection of Inflow and Outflow
Tracts of Right Heart and Cavities of
Right Heart

L. Brachiocephalic Vein

R. Brachiocephalic Vein

Pulmonary Trunk

R. Pulmonary Artery

L. Pulmonary Artery

Superior Vena Cava

Ant. Cusp.

R. Cusp.   Of Pulmonary Valve

L. Cusp.

R. Atrial Appendix

Right Atrium

R. Ventricle

Tricuspid-Valve Annulus

Inferior Vena Cava

LATERAL PROJECTION OF CAVITIES OF
RIGHT HEART

R. Brachiocephalic V.

L. Brachiocephalic V.

Pulmonary Trunk

L. Pulmonary Artery

S. Vena Cava

R. Pulmonary Artery

Pulmonary Valve
Ant. Cusp.
L. Cusp.
R. Cusp.

R. Auricle (R. Atrial Appendage)

Supraventricular Crest

R. Atrium

Tricuspid Valve Annulus

R. Ventricle

I. Vena Cava

A

Figure 12–49.   *A.* Anteroposterior and lateral projections of inflow and outflow tracts of the right heart and the cavities of the right heart, also showing the relative positions of the cusps of the pulmonary valve.

Figure 12-49 continued on the opposite page.

Ant. Post. Projection Left Heart and Aorta
as seen in Angiography

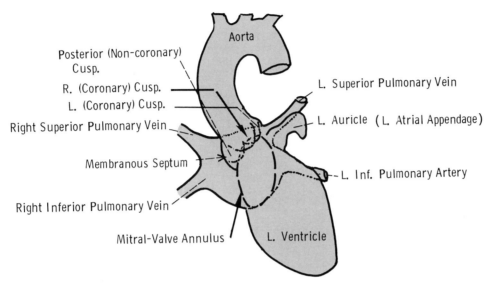

Lateral Projection of Cavities of Left Heart

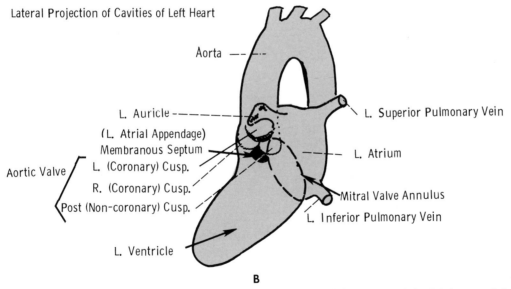

B

Figure 12–49 *Continued.* B. Anteroposterior and lateral projections of the cavities of the left heart and the outflow tracts, also showing the relative positions of the cusps of the aortic valves.

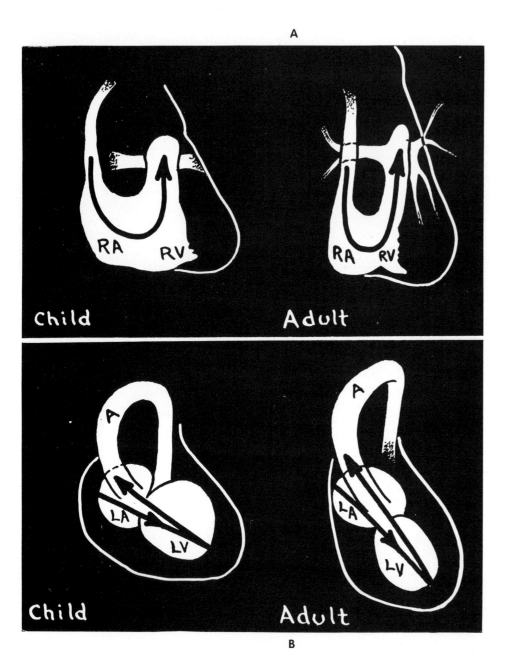

Figure 12-50. *A.* Semidiagrammatic tracings of the normal right heart as seen in representative frontal angiocardiograms of children and adults. Note the more horizontal relationships of the cardiac chambers in the child, and the much tighter "U"-shaped curve of the right heart in the adult. This difference reflects the change from a relatively transverse position of the heart in infancy and childhood to a more vertical position in adult life, and parallels the changing configuration of the thoracic cage. *B.* Semidiagrammatic tracings from angiocardiograms of the normal left heart and aorta in children and adults. Frontal projection. The axes of both the inflow and outflow tracts of the left ventricle lie in a more horizontal position in infants and children than in adults. This reflects the transverse position of the heart and the relatively greater horizontal diameter of the chest in the early years. (From Abrams and Kaplan: Angiocardiographic Interpretation in Congenital Heart Disease, Charles C Thomas.)

margin of the heart and another supplying the posterior interventricular branch are usually well developed. The posterior papillary muscle of the left ventricle usually has a dual supply from both the left and the right coronary arteries. One branch, which originates from the right coronary artery, ascends along the anteromedial wall of the right atrium and supplies the *superior vena caval branch or nodal artery*, posterior and to the left of the superior vena caval ostium. It then rounds this ostium to the sinoatrial node.

Variations in the branching pattern of the coronary artery are frequent. In about two-thirds of the cases, the right coronary artery is dominant, crossing the crux and supplying part of the left ventricular wall and the ventricular septum. In 15 per cent of cases the left coronary artery is dominant and its circumflex branch crosses the crux, supplying the posterior interventricular branch and all of the left ventricle, the ventricular septum, and part of the right ventricle. In 18 per cent of cases both coronary arteries reach the crux and this is the so-called "balanced coronary arterial pattern" (Netter). In about 40 per cent of cases, a large anterior atrial branch of the left coronary artery courses toward the superior vena cava rather than the anterior atrial branch of the right coronary artery. It is also quite common for the first, second, and even third branches of the right coronary artery to originate independently from the right aortic sinus rather than from the right coronary artery proper.

Oblique projections of the right and left coronary arteries are shown diagrammatically in Figure 12-53.

The two largest veins are the *great cardiac vein* in the anterior interventricular groove along with the left coronary artery, and the *middle cardiac vein* in the posterior interventricular groove, along with the posterior interventricular branch of the right coronary artery. There may also be a large *posterior left ventricular vein* as well. Small valves may be present in each of these larger veins. The oblique vein of the left atrium enters the coronary sinus near its junction with the great cardiac vein and it does not have a valve. The small cardiac vein may enter the coronary sinus as shown (Fig. 12-54), or it may enter the right atrium independently. There are anterior cardiac veins that do almost always enter the right atrium independently. As shown in the illustration, there are veins in the inferior interventricular groove and the atrioventricular groove along the right border that appear to flow into the small cardiac vein and thence into the coronary sinus. Small veins situated in the atrial septum and ventricular walls that enter the cardiac chambers directly are called the *Thebesian* veins.

Coronary Arteriography

Brief Review of Technique. (For greater detail see Abrams and Adams, and Judkins.) This procedure requires the skilled

(Text continued on page 754.)

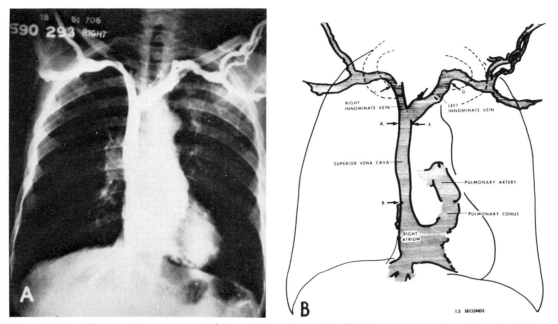

Figure 12–51. The superior vena cava and innominate veins as visualized by venous angiocardiography. (From Roberts, D. J., Jr., Dotter, C. T., and Steinberg, I.: Am. J. Roentgenol., 66:341–352, 1951.)

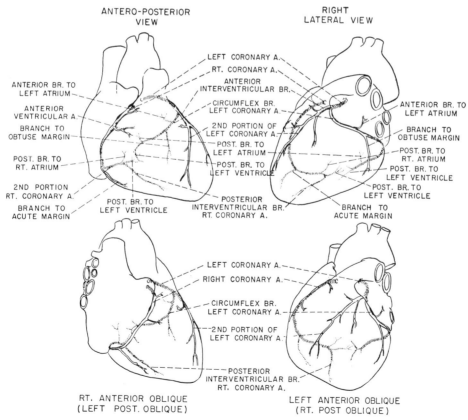

Figure 12–52. Diagram of coronary circulation as might be seen in frontal, lateral and oblique projections. (Modified from Guglielmo and Guttadauro: Acta Radiol., Supp. 97, 1952.)

RIGHT CORONARY ARTERY LEFT ANTERIOR OBLIQUE

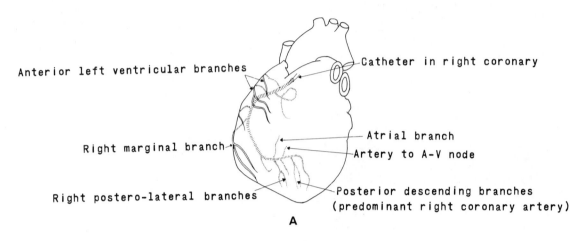

LEFT CORONARY ARTERY —— RIGHT ANTERIOR OBLIQUE

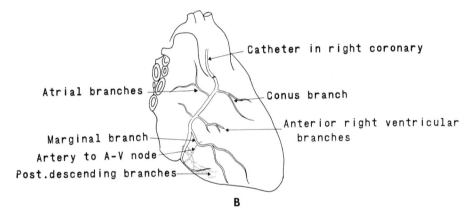

LEFT CORONARY ARTERY   LEFT ANTERIOR OBLIQUE

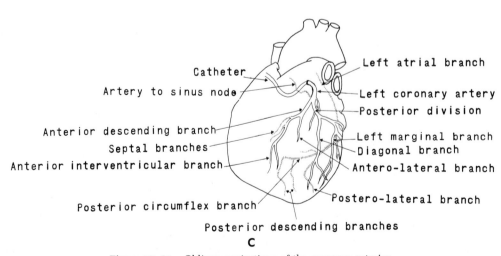

Figure 12–53. Oblique projections of the coronary arteries.

Figure 12–53 continued on the opposite page.

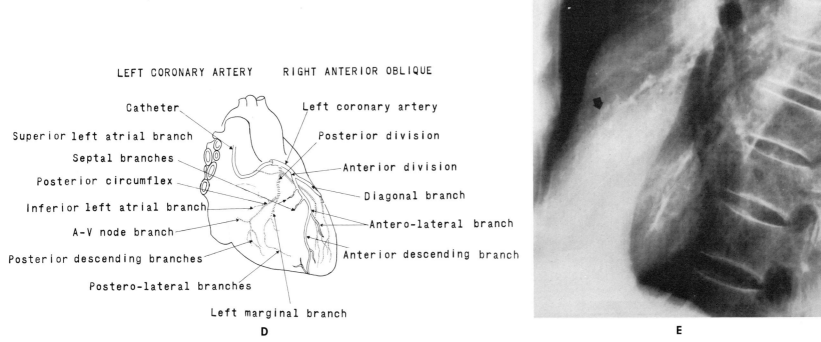

Figure 12–53 *Continued.*   *D.* Right anterior oblique projection of left coronary artery. *E.* Calcification in coronary arteries seen on plain film.

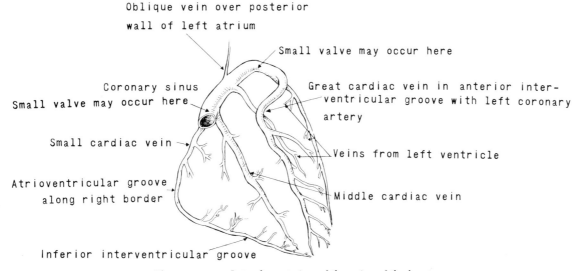

Figure 12–54.   Lateral erect view of the veins of the heart.

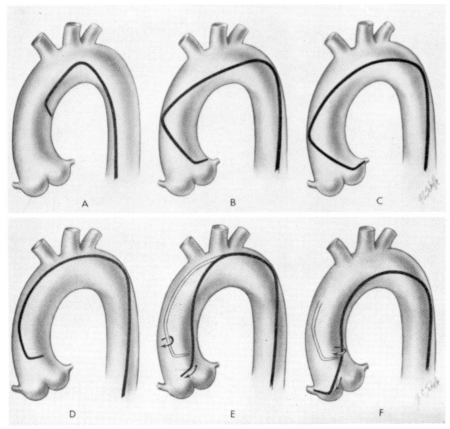

Figure 12–55. *A, B,* and *C.* Diagrammatic illustrations of left coronary catheterization. *D, E,* and *F.* Diagrammatic illustrations of right coronary catheterization (see text). (From Judkins, M. P.: Radiol. Clin. N. Amer., 6:467–492, December, 1968.)

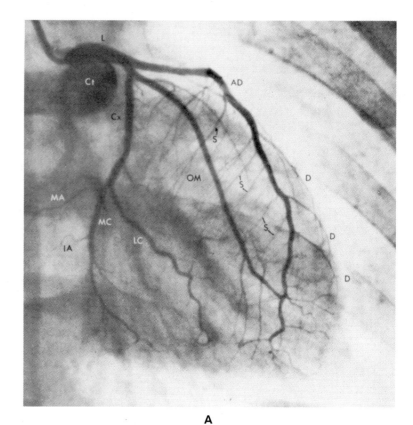

A

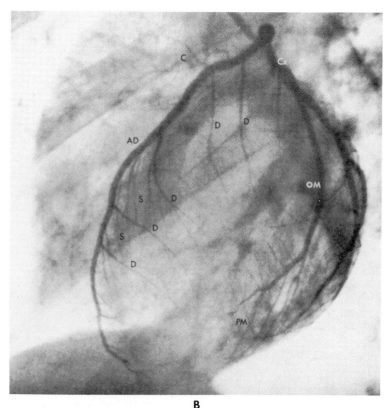

B

Figure 12–56. *See opposite page for legend.*

collaboration of radiologists and cardiologists, each with a thorough knowledge of the cardiac pharmacology. The two basic techniques for coronary artery visualization involve: (1) the introduction of a catheter into a supravalvular site with a forceful injection, which allows visualization of the coronary arteries as they leave the aortic sinuses; and (2) selective coronary arteriography whereby a catheter is inserted into the ostium of each coronary artery in sequence for injection. There are a number of modifications of the selective approach: (a) by a cutdown technique over the brachial artery and the insertion of a single catheter into each coronary artery sequentially; or (b) a percutaneous femoral approach involving insertion of a specially shaped catheter into each coronary ostium separately. In this latter approach usually the catheter is separately shaped for each of the two insertions. Each technique has its proponents, but some would prefer a technique that obviates the need for performing a

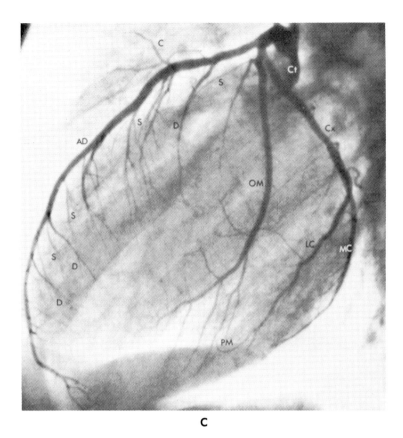

C

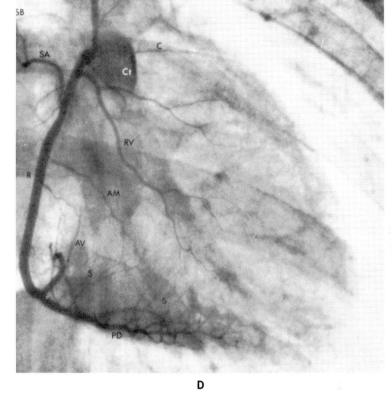

D

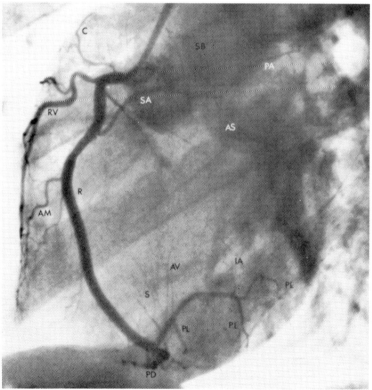

E

Figure 12–56. *A–C.* High-resolution normal left selective coronary arteriography. *A.* Right anterior oblique 20°. *B.* Left anterior oblique 70°. *C.* Lateral. Contrast agent injections of each coronary artery are filmed in three projections by both cinéfluorography and high-resolution serial techniques. These three projections were selected because they uncover and give dimension to all parts of the coronary tree. In each, the heart is projected free of the spine.

Legend: L, Left main; AD, anterior descending; D, diagonal; S, septal; C, conus branches; Cx, circumflex; OM, obtuse marginal; LC, lateral circumflex; MC, medial circumflex; AC, atrial circumflex; MA, middle arterial; IA, inferior atrial; PM, papillary muscle artery; Ct, contrast material in the sinus of Valsalva.

D–F. High-resolution normal right selective coronary arteriography. *D.* Right anterior oblique 20°. *E.* Left anterior oblique 70°.

Legend: R, Right main; C, conus branch; RV, right ventricular artery; SA, sinus node artery; SB, sinus node branch; PA, posterior atrial branch; AS, atrial septal branch; AM, acute marginal; PD, posterior descending; AV, atrioventricular node artery; PL, posterior lateral arteries; MA, middle atrial; IA, inferior atrial; S, septal; Ct, contrast material in the sinus of Valsalva. (*A–F* from Judkins, M. P.: Radiol. Clin. N. Amer., 6:467–492, December, 1968.)

Figure 12–56 continued on the following page.

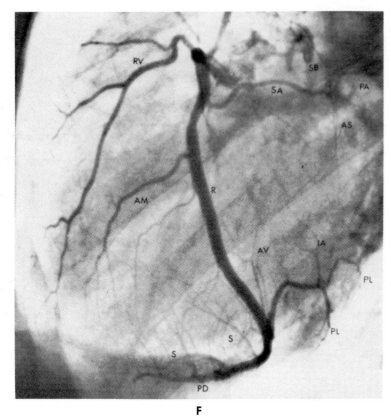

F

Figure 12-56 *Continued.* F. Lateral film in high-resolution normal right selective coronary arteriography. See full legend on page 755.

cutdown over any artery, particulary the small caliber brachial artery with its associated difficulties of catheter manipulation. Many different injection devices have been described for use with selective coronary arteriography. Many, however, require a manual injection of small volumes (4 to 8 ml.) of contrast agent into each coronary artery.

Serialographic rapid film technique or coronary cinéangiography may be employed. Left ventricular cinéangiography should probably be an integral part of coronary arteriography so that ventricular contractility may be assessed prior to the visualization of the coronary arteries. It should be emphasized that experienced personnel, careful monitoring of cardiac rhythm, and "adequate facilities for immediate resuscitation and cardioversion, and prompt surgical intervention in the event of vascular occlusion or hemorrhage are mandatory to keep a low incidence of complications. Under ideal conditions the risk should be no greater than that of thoracic aortography or other intracardiovascular diagnostic procedures" (Abrams and Adams) (Fig. 12-55).

Select Coronary Arteriograms for Demonstation of Anatomy. Normal left and right selective coronary arteriograms, with important branches labeled, are indicated in Figure 12-56. Some variations of normal are illustrated in Figure 12-57. Numerous other variations could be described (Levin and Baltaxe). Also, numerous anastomoses of the coronary arteries are described, with preferential pathways of collateral flow. These are illustrated in Figures 12-58 and 12-59.

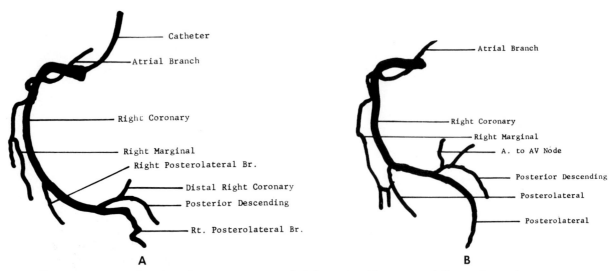

A   **B**

Figure 12-57. *A* and *B.* The right coronary artery in the left anterior oblique in two different phases of respiration.

Figure 12-57 continued on the opposite page.

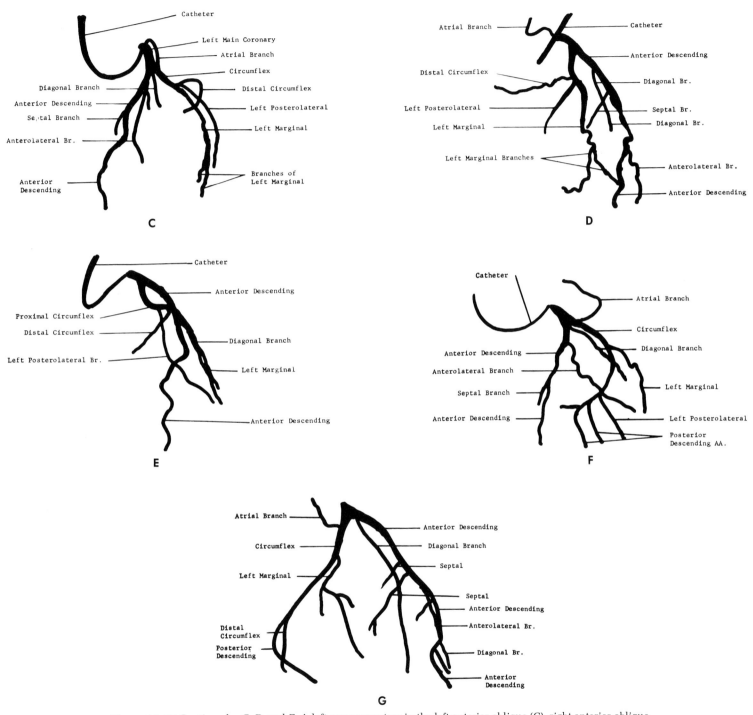

Figure 12–57 *Continued.*   C, D, and E. A left coronary artery in the left anterior oblique (C), right anterior oblique (D), and posteroanterior projections (E).
   F and G. A left coronary artery in the left (F) and right (G) anterior oblique projections. (From Sewell, W. H.: Amer. J. Roentgenol., 97:359–368, 1966.)

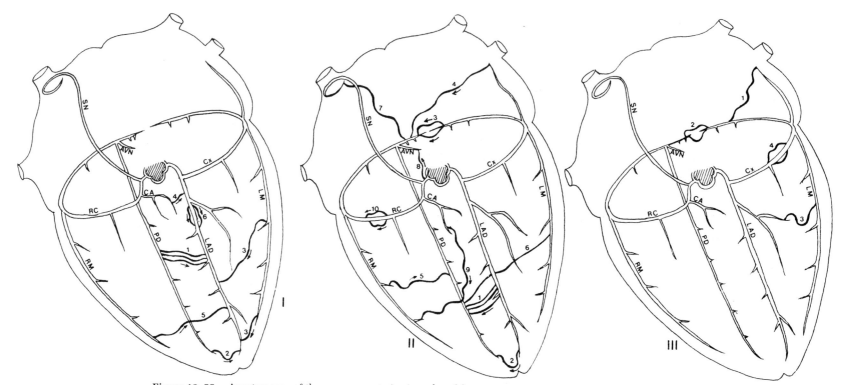

Figure 12–58.   Anastomoses of the coronary arteries in order of frequency.

I. Left Anterior Descending Artery: (1) septal anastomoses, (2) anastomoses over the apex, (3) left marginal anastomoses to the LAD, (4) Vieussen's circle, (5) right marginal anastomoses to the LAD, (6) intracoronary anastomoses.

II. Right Coronary Artery: (1) septal anastomoses, (2) apical anastomoses, (3) left circumflex anastomoses with distal RC, (4) atrial circumflex anastomoses with distal RC, (5) right marginal anastomoses with posterior descending, (6) left marginal anastomoses with posterior descending, (7) sinus node artery anastomoses with distal RC, (8) Kugel's artery, (9) conus artery anastomoses with the right marginal branches, (10) intracoronary anastomoses across occlusion.

III. Left Circumflex Artery: (1) anastomoses from the left atrial circumflex to the circumflex, (2) anastomoses from the right coronary artery to the left circumflex, (3) diagonals over left margins to the left circumflex, (4) intracoronary anastomoses bridging the occlusion.

(LC) left main coronary artery; (Cx) left circumflex artery; (RC) right coronary artery; (AVN) atrioventricular node artery; (LAD) left anterior descending artery; (LM) left marginal artery of the obtuse angle; (RM) right marginal artery of the acute angle; (SN) sinus node artery; (CA) conus artery. (From Jochem, et al.: Amer. J. Roentgenol., *116*:60, 1972.)

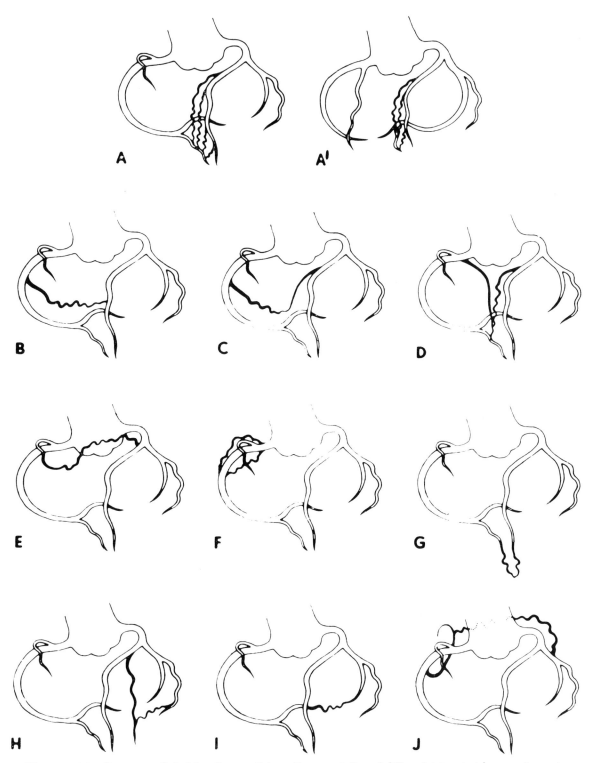

Figure 12–59. Coronary collateral pathways. Schematic presentation of different interarterial connections. *A.* Septal collaterals. *A'.* Same collaterals as in *A* with a more prominent left circumflex artery. *B.* Epicardial collaterals of right ventricular wall. *C.* Collateral in moderator band. *D.* Collateral in crista supraventricularis. *E.* Epicardial collateral of the pulmonary conus. *F.* Direct by-passing collateral. *G.* Epicardial collateral at apex. *H.* Collateral in left ventricular wall. *I.* Collateral in atrioventricular sulcus. *J.* Collateral in atrial wall. (From Paulin, S.: Investigative Radiol., 2:147–159, 1967.)

REFERENCES

Abrams, H. L.: Angiography, Vol. 1. Second edition. Boston, Little, Brown & Co., pp. 119–122, 1971.

Abrams, H. L., and Adams, D. F.: Coronary arteriography. *In* Abrams, H. L. (ed.): Angiography. Second edition. Boston, Little, Brown & Co., 1971.

Altemus, L. R.: Malnutrition with microcardia. Amer. J. Roentgenol., *99*:674–680, 1967.

Amundsen, P.: The diagnostic value of conventional radiological examination of the heart in adults. Acta Radiol. (Suppl.), *181*:1–87, 1959.

Anson, B. J.: Atlas of Human Anatomy. Philadelphia, W. B. Saunders Co., 1963.

Bell, A. L. L.: Catheterization of the left heart by transeptal needle and overlying catheter. *In* Schobinger, R. A., and Ruzicka, F. F. (eds.): Vascular Roentgenology. New York, Macmillan, 1964.

Bierman, H. R.: Selective Arterial Catheterization, Springfield, Ill., Charles C Thomas, 1969.

Boone, B. R., Chamberlain, W. E., Gilbeck, F. G., and Henny, G. C.: Interpreting the electrokymogram of heart and great vessel motion. Amer. Heart. J., *34*:560–681, 1947.

Bosniak, M. A.: An analysis of some anatomic-roentgenologic aspects of the brachiocephalic vessels. Amer. J. Roentgenol., *91*:1222–1231, 1964.

Boyden, E. A.: Segmental Anatomy of the Lungs: A Study of the Patterns of the Segmental Bronchi and Related Pulmonary Vessels. New York, McGraw Hill Book Co., 1955.

Chang, C. H. J.: Right pulmonary artery measurements. Amer. J. Roentgenol., *87*:929–935, 1962.

Cunningham, D. J.: Manual of Practical Anatomy, Vol. 2. 12th edition. London, Oxford University Press, 1958.

Dinsmore, R. E., Goodman, D. J., and Sanders, C. A.: Some pitfalls in evaluation of cardiac chamber enlargement on chest roentgenograms. Radiology, *87*:267–273, 1966.

Gammill, S. L., Krebs, C., Meyers, P. et al.: Cardiac measurements in systole and diastole. Radiology, *94*:115–119, 1970.

Gorlin, R.: Normal variations in venous oxygen content. *In* Warren, V. J. (ed.): Methods in Medical Research. Vol. 7. Chicago, Year Book Medical Publishers, 1958.

Gorlin, R., McMillan, I. K. R., Medd, W. E., Matthews, M. D., and Daley, R.: Dynamics of the circulation in aortic valvular disease. Amer. J. Med., *18*:855, 1955.

His, quoted in Abrams, H. L.: Angiography. Second edition. Boston, Little, Brown & Co., 1971.

Hoffman, R. B., and Rigler, L. G.: Evaluation of left ventricular enlargement in the lateral projection of the chest. Radiology, *85*:93–100, 1965.

Jacobson, B., and Paulin, S.: Experience with different contrast media in coronary angiography. Acta Radiol. (Suppl.), *270*:103, 1967.

James, T. N.: Anatomy of the Coronary Arteries. New York, Paul B. Hoeber, Inc., 1961.

Jochem, W., Soto, B., Karp, R. B., et al.: Radiographic anatomy of the coronary collateral circulation. Amer. J. Roentgenol., *116*:50–61, 1972. fig. 9.

Judkins, M. P.: Percutaneous transfemoral selective coronary arteriography. Radiol. Clin. N. Amer., *6*:467–492, December, 1968.

Klatte, E. C., Tampas, J. P., and Campbell, J. A.: Evaluation of right atrial size. Radiology, *81*:48–55, 1963.

Lane, E. J., Jr., and Whalen, J. P.: A new sign of left atrial enlargement: posterior displacement of the left bronchial tree. Radiology, *93*:279–284, 1969.

Lavender, J. P., and Doppman, J.: The hilum in pulmonary venous hypertension. Brit. J. Radiol., *35*:303–313, 1962.

Leinbach, L. B.: Normal pulmonary arteries in children. Amer. J. Roentgenol., *89*:995–998, 1963.

Levin, D. C., and Baltaxe, H. A.: Posterior descending coronary artery. Amer. J. Roentgenol., *116*:41–49, 1972.

Levitan, L. H., and Reilly, H. F., Jr.: Aortic sinus of Valsalva calcification: a roentgen sign on the lateral chest film. Radiology, *87*:1074–1075, 1966.

Lewis, B. M., Gorlin, R., Haussay, H. E. J., Haynes, F. W., and Dexter, L.: Clinical and physiological correlation in patients with mitral stenosis. Amer. Heart J., *43*:2, 1952.

Lind, J.: Heart volume in normal infants. Acta Radiol., (Suppl.), *82*:3–127, 1950.

Meschan, I.: Analysis of Roentgen Signs. Philadelphia, W. B. Saunders Co., 1973.

Michelson, E., and Salik, J. O.: The vascular pattern of the lung as seen on routine and tomographic studies. Radiology, *73*:511–526, 1959.

Netter, F. H.: Ciba Collection of Medical Illustrations, Vol. 5. Ciba Pharmaceutical Company, Division of Ciba-Geigy Corporation, 1969.

Paulin, S.: Coronary angiography: technical, anatomic and clinical studies. Acta Radiol. (Suppl.), *233*:5–215, 1964.

Paulin, S.: Interarterial coronary anastomoses in relation to arterial obstruction demonstrated in coronary arteriography. Invest. Radiol., *2*:147–159, 1967.

Robb, G. P., and Steinberg, I.: Practical method of visualization of chambers of the heart, the pulmonary circulation, and the great blood vessels in man. J. Clin. Invest., *17*:507, 1938; Amer. J. Roentgenol., *41*:1–17, 1939.

Sewell, W. H.: Roentgenologic anatomy of human coronary arteries. Amer. J. Roentgenol., *97*:359–366, 1966.

Ungerleider, H. E., and Gubner, R.: Evaluation of heart size measurements. Amer. Heart J., *24*:494–510, 1942.

VonHayek, H.: The Human Lung. New York, Hafner Publishing Co., Inc., 1960.

Wilson, W. J., Lee, G. B., and Amplatz, K.: Selective coronary arteriography. Amer. J. Roentgenol., *100*:332–340, 1967.

Wood, P.: Aortic stenosis. Amer. J. Cardiol., *1*:553, 1958.

13

The Upper Alimentary Tract

PRINCIPLES INVOLVED IN STUDY OF THE ALIMENTARY TRACT

The walls of the alimentary tract are intermediate in radiographic density, and hence require some type of contrast material for detection by means of x-rays. Normally, there is a variable amount of gas in the stomach and colon that permits a relatively gross and inadequate visualization of these structures. In the normal adult, gas in the small intestine is considered abnormal and the introduction of contrast material into the small intestine is therefore essential.

Although negative contrast may be employed in the visualization of the gastrointestinal tract, it is usually supplementary to the more significant positive contrast with radiopaque media.

Since the physiology and function of the gastrointestinal tract are readily altered by so many factors such as hypotonicity or hypertonicity, alkalinity, acidity, proteins, fats, carbohydrates, amino acids, and any slight mechanical irritation, it is essential for any opaque contrast medium to be physiologically inert.

The most commonly used medium thus employed in present-day radiography of the gastrointestinal tract is barium sulfate in water suspension, although bismuth salts, radioactive Umbrathor and barium sulfate in isotonic saline, "buttermilk," or other commercial suspensions are also employed by some, or used on special occasions. In certain patients, in whom obstruction by barium mixtures may occur, organic soluble iodides are utilized by intubation techniques. In infants or other patients in whom aspiration is a potential danger, small quantities of iodized oil are helpful, at least until it is certain that aspiration is not taking place. Iodized oil is a poor contrast agent beyond the esophagus because it distorts the normal physiologic pattern.

On certain occasions, it is advantageous to use so-called double contrast in which gas is introduced after administering the barium suspension. The gas and barium suspension are thus mixed and are helpful in outlining polyps and small tumors. The gas employed may be air, carbon dioxide, or a mixture of both, as when ginger ale, carbonated water or Seidlitz powder are introduced into the stomach.

The usual radiologic methods include: (1) fluoroscopy, (2) spotfilm radiography, (3) routine radiography in certain positions; any or all of the usual erect, recumbent, supine, prone, lateral or oblique positions are employed.

Other methods of radiologic study of the upper alimentary tract include *hypotonic duodenography, angiography,* and *endoscopic pancreatocholangiography,* as well as other pararadiologic procedures not included in this text, such as ultrasonography and radioisotopic scanning procedures.

Parietography—the demonstration of the walls of the gastrointestinal tract by filling the peritoneal cavity and the lumen of the studied organ simultaneously with air or gas—is a further refinement of the air constrast technique. This may be especially helpful when combined with tomography.

In many of these methods, *pharmacoradiography,* or the injection of drugs in order to influence the radiologic examination, may be employed.

There are two major principles involved in the radiologic anatomy of the gastrointestinal tract:

1. We are examining a dynamic, moving, functioning system of organs. They are not static. Their structure must at all times be considered along with their function, and the two aspects are inseparable.

2. When the lumen of a hollow organ is filled with contrast substance, we can visualize the inner lining with accuracy, but the wall of the organ outside the innermost lining can be studied only indirectly as it affects the lumen or the mucosa. It is conceivable that considerable abnormality may exist outside the lumen within the wall of the organ, which may not be reflected in the mucosal pattern.

(Parietography, does, however, permit visualization of the outer walls of the gastrointestinal tract simultaneously with the lumen of the studied organ, particularly when combined with tomography.)

762

THE MOUTH AND OROPHARYNX

The mouth and oropharynx are so readily examined by direct inspection and palpation that it is not usual to employ the radiograph except for demonstration of hidden structures.

In a direct lateral view (Fig. 13–1), the air within the mouth and pharynx permits a contrast visualization of the tongue surface, the hard and soft palate, and the nasopharynx and oropharynx.

Special views of the salivary glands may be obtained after the injection of iodized water soluble contrast agents into the ducts. Soft tissue studies of the floor of the mouth or the cheek are also feasible.

Brief mention of the radiography of the teeth has already been made (see Chapter 6), and will not be further discussed in this text.

Soft Tissue Study of the Mouth and Pharynx by Lateral Projection. This projection is identical with that employed for a lateral view of the cervical spine, except that technical factors are varied slightly to emphasize the soft tissues rather than the skeletal structure (see Chapters 9 and 10).

The structures demonstrated in profile are: the tongue and floor of the mouth, the hard and soft palate and uvula, the vallecula at the base of the tongue and the pyriform sinuses on either side, the nasopharynx above the palate with turbinates and eustachian orifice, the lymphoid structures in the nasopharynx, and the epiglottis. The laryngeal structures seen in this projection have been previously described (Chapter 10).

The width of the soft tissues projected under the sphenoid is considerably narrower in the adult than in the child, owing to the markedly enlarged lymphoid apparatus in the child after 3 to 6 months of age. This view affords a ready means of investigating these lymphoid and adenoid structures (Chapter 10).

The width of the retro-oropharyngeal soft tissues in the child is also considerably greater than it is in the adult when these structures are compared with the retrolaryngeal soft tissues between the larynx and the cervical spine. Thus in the newborn and infant, the ratio of the retro-oropharyngeal soft tissues to the retrolaryngeal soft tissues is approximately 1 to 1, while in the adult it is usually in the order of 1 to 3. These measurements are of value in the detection of space-occupying lesions such as inflammations and tumors in these locations, which by direct inspection are difficult to evaluate because they may be posterior to the visible mucosa, or because the patient may be unable to open his mouth. (See Chapter 10.)

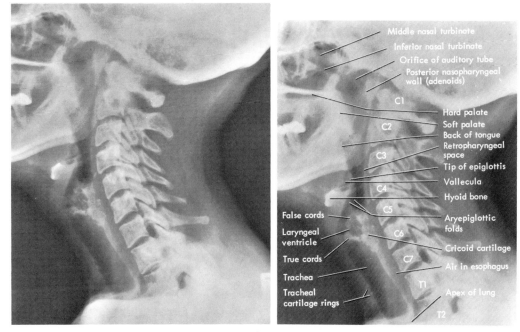

Figure 13–1. Lateral soft tissue film of neck.

Soft Tissue Radiography of the Floor of the Mouth with the Aid of the Occlusal Type Dental Film. By placing an occlusal type dental film in the mouth (Fig. 13–2) and directing the x-ray beam perpendicular to it, the soft tissues of the submandibular area are penetrated, as well as the mandible. These soft tissues are not visualized in sufficient detail to distinguish the various anatomic structures such as the salivary glands and ducts, lymph nodes, and tongue, but this method of examination does afford a ready means of investigating abnormal calcareous deposits in these structures. Hence an understanding of the normal appearance of this projection is essential.

Soft Tissue Radiography of the Cheek. This can be performed in a similar manner by placing an occlusal film on the inside of the cheek. Care must be exercised to place the film sufficiently posterior to obtain a visualization of as much of Stenson's duct as possible, since occasionally calcareous deposits in this location may lead to obstructive inflammation and symptoms.

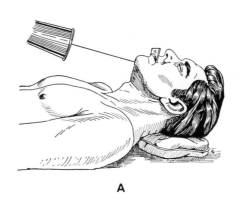

A

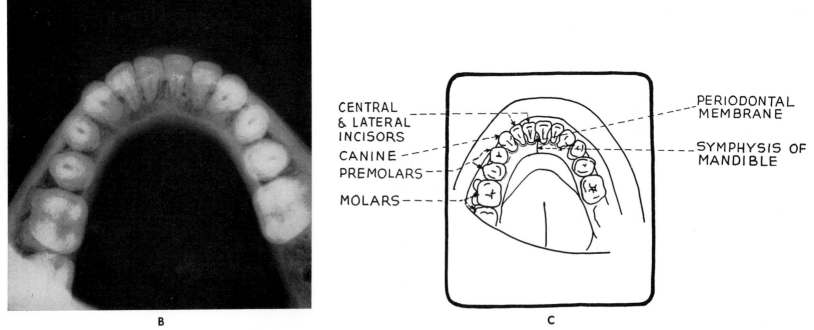

B   C

Figure 13–2. Occlusal type dental film of floor of mouth. *A.* Position of patient. *B.* Radiograph. *C.* Labeled tracing of *B.*

Radiography of the Hard Palate. Apart from the lateral projection previously described, the hard palate may be visualized by means of an occlusal film in the mouth as illustrated in Figure 13–3. There are considerable differences in density in the various portions of the hard palate owing to the presence of the aerated sinuses, the alveolar process, and the bony nasal septum, all of which overlie the palate. This variation in density is important in interpretation of the osseous structure of the hard palate.

The incisive foramen and the major palatine foramen can usually be identified. Frequently, the midline suture as well as the transverse palatine suture can also be noted.

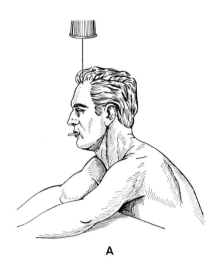

A

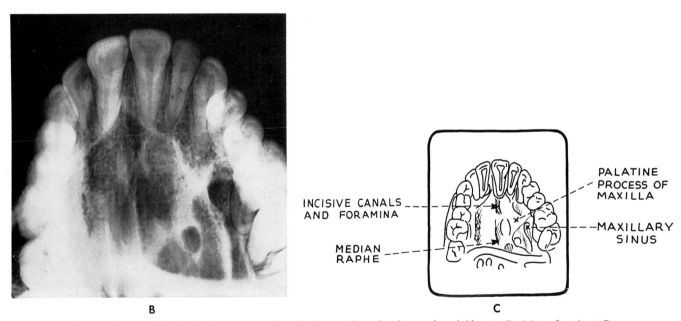

B

C

INCISIVE CANALS AND FORAMINA

MEDIAN RAPHE

PALATINE PROCESS OF MAXILLA

MAXILLARY SINUS

Figure 13–3. Method of radiography of hard palate with occlusal type dental film. *A.* Position of patient. *B.* Radiograph. *C.* Labeled tracing of *B.*

THE SALIVARY GLANDS

Normal Anatomy. There are three salivary glands, each with a separate duct or ducts opening into the mouth: the parotid, the submaxillary, and the sublingual.

The parotid gland is the largest of these and lies on the side of the face, below and in front of the ear, bounded by the zygoma above, the sternomastoid muscle behind, and the ramus of the mandible in front. Approximately one-quarter or one-third of the gland is usually deep to the posterior margin of the mandible and extends almost to the pharyngeal wall, being separated from the latter by the branches of the carotid artery, several veins and nerves, and small muscles. Actually, the anterior surface of the gland is wrapped around the posterior margin of the ramus of the mandible. The parotid duct (or Stensen's duct) runs across the masseter muscle superficially, accompanied by branches of the facial nerve. At the anterior margin of the masseter muscle, it turns sharply inward, pierces the buccinator muscle, and opens into the vestibule of the oral cavity on a small papilla opposite the second upper molar tooth. It is approximately 6 cm. in length.

The submaxillary gland lies in the submaxillary triangle on either side of the neck. This gland lies under cover of the body of the mandible for the most part, in its submaxillary fossa. There are a few small lymph nodes embedded in the substance of the gland, and the external maxillary artery runs through its superior and posterior portion. The submaxillary duct (Wharton's duct) runs forward, inward, and upward to open into the floor of the mouth, in a papilla on the plica sublingualis close to the frenulum of the tongue. This duct is about 5 cm. in length.

The sublingual gland is the smallest of the salivary glands, and is more deeply situated. It lies under the mucosa of the floor of the mouth, just posterior to the symphysis and in the sublingual fossa of the medial surface of the mandible. It has approximately 12 separate excretory ducts which open on the plica sublingualis, for the most part, but one or two of them may open into the submaxillary duct. This latter point is important from the standpoint of sialography, since one of the ducts opening into the submaxillary duct may be injected by error, and the submaxillary gland visualized instead of the sublingual.

Radiographic Technique of Examination. The salivary glands may be examined by means of plain radiographs, or after the injection of contrast media into the salivary duct. Plain radiographs are of value only when a calculus is suspected. In other instances, contrast studies are necessary.

With regard to *plain radiographs,* the following studies may be performed:

1. For parotid calculi, a lateral view (in stereoscopic projection preferably) is taken, centering over the gland, with the neck extended and the mouth open.

2. For submaxillary and sublingual calculi, a stereoscopic lateral view is obtained with the mouth closed, and usually it is best to incline the x-ray tube slightly cephalad to prevent superimposition of the two rami of the mandible. Also a view of the floor of the mouth is obtained with the aid of an occlusal type dental film as previously described.

Sialograms are defined as the radiographic demonstration of the salivary ducts and alveoli by the injection of contrast media. The technique is as follows (Chisholm et al.; Park and Mason):

The duct may be dilated with olive-tipped lacrimal probes. A sterile polyethylene catheter is thereafter inserted with a wire stylus for rigidity for a distance of 3 to 4 cm.

The contrast medium usually employed is a diatrizoate such as Hypaque or Renografin. It may be injected directly or by means of a glass reservoir positioned 70 cm. above the patient's head. If direct injection is employed, the injection is continued until definite pain is experienced by the patient. In the second technique (Park and Mason, 1966), underfilling seldom occurs because the film is taken while the contrast medium is still flowing and the pressure is therefore maintained. Moreover, overfilling rarely occurs because of the almost constant pressure. Usually 1 to 2 cc. of the contrast agent is adequate.

Films are obtained in the anteroposterior, lateral, or lateral-oblique positions (Fig. 13–4) at the completion of the filling phase. The polyethylene catheter may be plugged while the films are checked for adequacy. These films are then followed by a secretory film taken 5 minutes after the completion of the filling phase. To insure rapid expulsion of the contrast medium, salivary flow is stimulated by a few drops of lemon juice or by sucking on a lemon for 1 minute, after which the patient rinses his mouth. Normally, the gland should be empty within 5 minutes, although a faint "acinar" cloud may persist for up to 24 hours.

The emptying phase is considered as important as the "filling phase" to be described.

The Normal Filling Phase Sialogram. The appearance of the normal sialogram simulates the skeletal structure of a leaf (Fig. 13–4).

The parotid duct is somewhat narrower than the submaxillary, angulating sharply as it leaves the masseter muscle and passing obliquely through the buccinator muscle. There is usually a large forked branch from the parotid duct directed superiorly, called the "socia parotidis," but otherwise the branching ducts tend to join the main duct almost at right angles.

The secondary ductules of the submaxillary duct are less regular than those of the parotid, but are otherwise very similar.

The sublingual gland has numerous excretory ducts, and ordinarily only a small segment of the gland is visualized by a single injection. Occasionally, as mentioned earlier, a portion of the sublingual gland may be visualized after injecting the submaxillary duct, since the sublingual excretory duct may empty into the submaxillary duct rather than into the mouth.

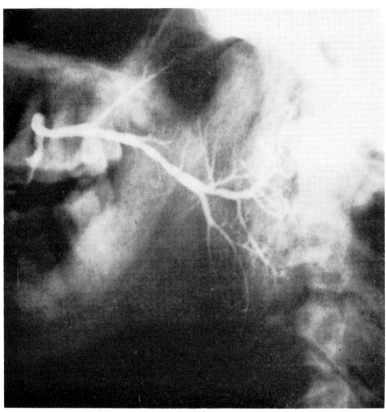

Figure 13-4. Normal sialogram of the parotid gland. (Courtesy Dr. L. B. Morettin, Galveston, Texas.)

ROENTGENOLOGIC CONSIDERATIONS OF THE HYOID APPARATUS

Basic Anatomy (Porrath). The hyoid bone is suspended in the anterior portion of the neck above the larynx, beneath the mandible, and anterior to the epiglottis. It is connected inferiorly by broad membranous bands to the thyroid cartilages of the larynx, and by other broad ligamentous sheaths to the epiglottis. It is suspended from the styloid processes by two ligaments, the stylohyoid ligaments, which may be variably ossified. The stylohyoid ligaments attach to the lesser horns of the hyoid bone, which consists of a body and two pairs of processes, the greater and lesser horns (Fig. 13-5).

There is a synovial articulation between the lesser and greater horns of the hyoid bone, and a synchondrosis of the greater horn with the body of the hyoid bone. The synovial articulations are subject to all diseases of synovia, such as rheumatoid arthritis.

Roentgen Appearance. In the lateral view (Fig. 13-6), the body of the hyoid bone is parallel to the body of the mandible and to the thyroid cartilages.

The stylohyoid ligaments extending from the free tips of the styloid process to the lesser horns vary considerably in degree of ossification as well as in length and width.

The paired lesser horns of the hyoid are small and conical and are united to the body of the hyoid by fibrous tissue and occasionally a synovial joint. As pointed out previously, the lesser horns articulate with the greater horns by means of a synovial joint.

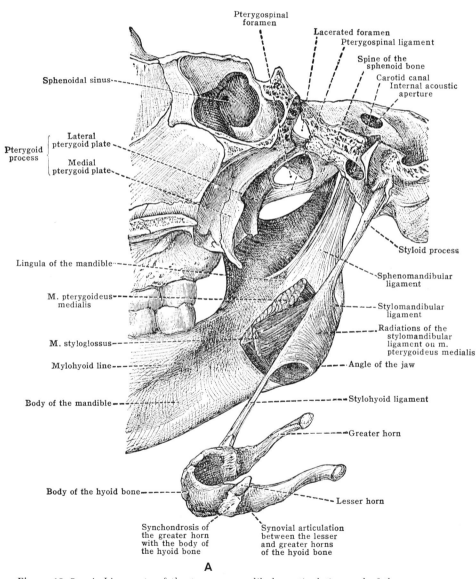

A

Figure 13-5. A. Ligaments of the temporomandibular articulation and of the hyoid bone; medial view. (After Toldt.) (From Anson, B. J. (ed.): Morris' Human Anatomy, 12th ed. Copyright © 1966 by McGraw-Hill, Inc. Used by permission of McGraw-Hill Book Company.)

Figure 13-5 continued on the following page.

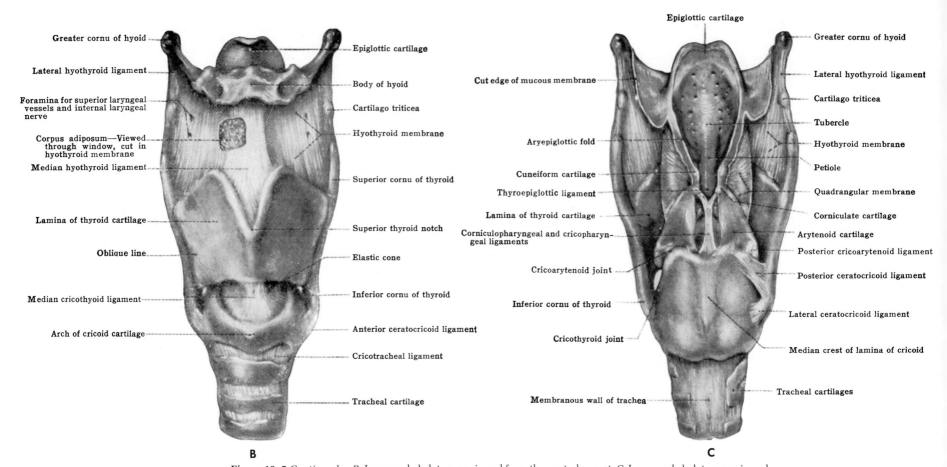

B   C

Figure 13–5 *Continued. B.* Laryngeal skeleton, as viewed from the ventral aspect. *C.* Laryngeal skeleton, as viewed from the dorsal aspect. (From Anson, B. J. (ed.): Morris' Human Anatomy, 12th ed. Copyright © 1966 by McGraw-Hill, Inc. Used by permission of McGraw-Hill Book Company.)

Figure 13–5 continued on the opposite page.

The posterior surface of the hyoid is parallel to the epiglottis and is separated from it by the hyothyroid membrane and loose areolar tissue. Several bursae may be interposed between the membrane and the bone in these regions.

The recognition of hyoid fractures as well as anomalies of this bone require a good appreciation of the normal roentgen anatomy (Porrath).

THE ESOPHAGUS

Gross Anatomy and Relationships of the Esophagus. The esophagus extends from the pharynx at the inferior border of the cricoid cartilage to the cardiac orifice of the stomach opposite the eleventh thoracic vertebra. Its course is in the midline anterior to the vertebral column, but it deviates to the left at the base of the neck for a short distance. At about the level of the seventh thoracic vertebra it passes slowly to the left and anteriorly to reach the esophageal orifice of the diaphragm, and it maintains this direction until it reaches the stomach.

Its length varies between 25 and 30 cm., and its breadth between 12 mm. and 30 or more mm. in its distended state.

In cross section it usually appears as a flattened tube, or a tube with a stellate lumen.

There are certain anatomic relationships of the esophagus (Fig. 13–7) which are of definite importance:

In the neck it is loosely connected by areolar tissue with the posterior aspect of the trachea. It is possible, however, for an abnormal structure such as aberrant thyroid tissue to lie between the trachea and esophagus, and hence it is important to obtain a lateral visualization of the base of the neck with barium in the esophagus when studying the thyroid gland.

In the thorax, the trachea lies anterior to the esophagus as far as the fifth thoracic vertebra near which the trachea bifurcates.

The *arch of the aorta,* passing back to reach the vertebral column, crosses to the left side of the esophagus, causing a *slight deviation of the esophagus to the right.*

The *thoracic aorta* lies first to the left of the esophagus, then posterior to it, and finally, both posterior and to the right of it.

Immediately *below the level of the bifurcation of the trachea,* the esophagus is *crossed by the left bronchus,* and in the rest of its

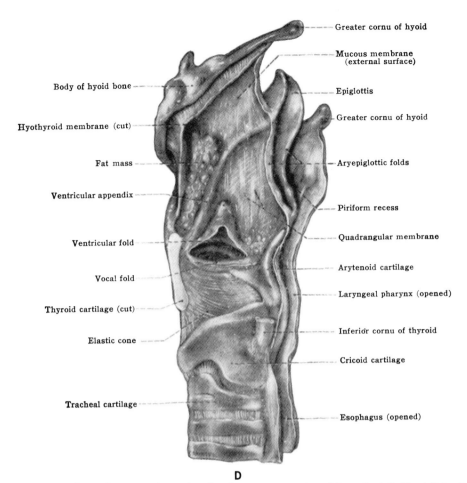

Greater cornu of hyoid

Mucous membrane (external surface)

Body of hyoid bone

Epiglottis

Greater cornu of hyoid

Hyothyroid membrane (cut)

Fat mass

Aryepiglottic folds

Ventricular appendix

Piriform recess

Ventricular fold

Quadrangular membrane

Arytenoid cartilage

Vocal fold

Laryngeal pharynx (opened)

Thyroid cartilage (cut)

Inferior cornu of thyroid

Elastic cone

Cricoid cartilage

Tracheal cartilage

Esophagus (opened)

D

Figure 13–5 *Continued.* *D.* Larynx and certain related structures as viewed from the left. The left lamina of the thyroid cartilage has been removed and the laryngeal ventricle opened. All muscles have been removed and the hyothyroid membrane partially cut away. (Anson, B. J. (ed.): Morris' Human Anatomy, 12th ed. Copyright © 1966 by McGraw-Hill, Inc. Used by permission of McGraw-Hill Book Company.)

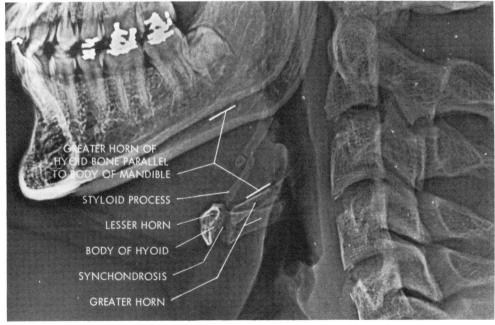

GREATER HORN OF HYOID BONE PARALLEL TO BODY OF MANDIBLE

STYLOID PROCESS

LESSER HORN

BODY OF HYOID

SYNCHONDROSIS

GREATER HORN

Figure 13–6. Xeroradiograph of the hyoid bone in the lateral view, with parts labeled.

769

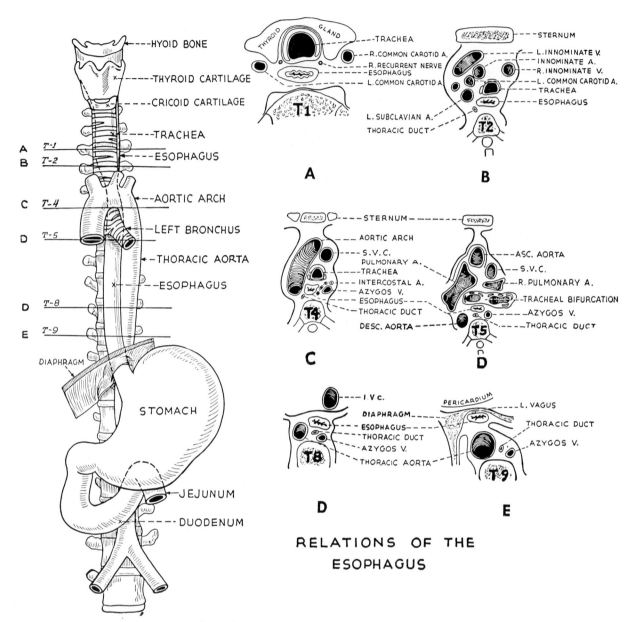

Figure 13-7. Relationship of esophagus to contiguous structures at various levels.

thoracic course it *lies close to the posterior surface of the pericardium.*

In this location it is situated in the posterior mediastinum, and is *separated from the vertebral column by the azygos vein, thoracic duct, and lower thoracic aorta.* It is in *close proximity with the left atrium,* and any enlargement of the latter structure is reflected in displacement of the esophagus posteriorly and to the right (Fig. 13-8).

The two *vagus nerves* descend to the esophagus after forming the anterior and posterior pulmonary plexuses, and unite with the sympathetic branches to form the anterior and posterior esophageal plexuses. The left vagus then winds anteriorly and the right posteriorly, and the two vagi descend in the esophageal sheath through the diaphragm to reach the stomach.

The esophagus is connected with the *esophageal orifice of the diaphragm* by strong fibrous tissue throughout its circumference,

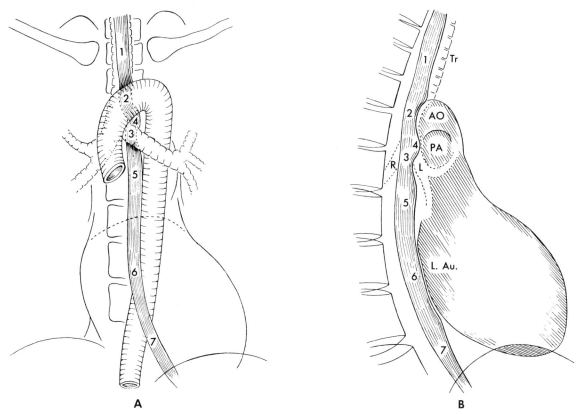

Figure 13-8. Segments of the esophagus. *A.* The segments of the thoracic esophagus (anteroposterior view): (1) paratracheal segment, (2) aortic segment, (3) bronchial segment, (4) interaorticobronchial triangle, (5) interbronchial segment, (6) retrocardiac segment, (7) epiphrenic segment.

B. The segments of the esophagus (right anterior oblique view). Shown are: trachea (Tr), right (R) and left (L) main bronchi, pulmonary artery (PA), left auricle (L. Au), and the different segments of the paratracheal (1), aortic (2), bronchic (3), interaorticobronchial (4), interbronchial (5), retrocardiac (6), and epiphrenic (7) esophagus. (From Brombart, M.: Roentgenology of the esophagus. *In* Margulis, A. R., and Burhenne, H. J., (eds.): Alimentary Tract Roentgenology, 2nd ed. St. Louis, C. V. Mosby Co., 1973.)

but any defects in this supportive tissue may cause hiatal protrusion of the stomach.

The *abdominal portion of the esophagus* is approximately 1 to 3 cm. in length and runs in the esophageal groove on the posterior surface of the liver.

The *phrenic ampulla* is that portion of the esophagus that lies just above the esophageal orifice of the diaphragm (Fig. 13-9). It is rather bulbous, varies in size, and causes confusion radiographically with a hiatal hernia of the stomach through the diaphragm. The esophageal ampulla appears as a segmented ovoid structure 3 to 5 cm. in length and 2 to 4 cm. in diameter, and it is separable from the stomach pattern below. The hiatal herniation of the fundus through the diaphragm has considerably more variation in size, and its rugal pattern can usually be more closely identified with that of the contiguous portion of the stomach

The esophageal vestibule is another name for the intra-abdominal portion of the esophagus. The vestibule is often situated above the diaphragm, producing a sliding hernia. The inferior esophageal sphincter and mucosal junction between esophagus and stomach are, under these circumstances, situated between the vestibule and the ampulla.

The diaphragm and its ligamentous esophageal attachments (phrenicoesophageal membrane) at the esophageal hiatus produce a valve like action called a constrictor cardiae.

Normal Points of Narrowness in the Esophagus. There are four definite constrictions in the normal esophagus (Fig. 13-8): one at its cricoid beginning, a second at the level of the aortic knob, a third opposite the crossing of the left bronchus, and the fourth at the place where it passes through the diaphragm. The lumen at the site of the upper constrictions is smaller than the

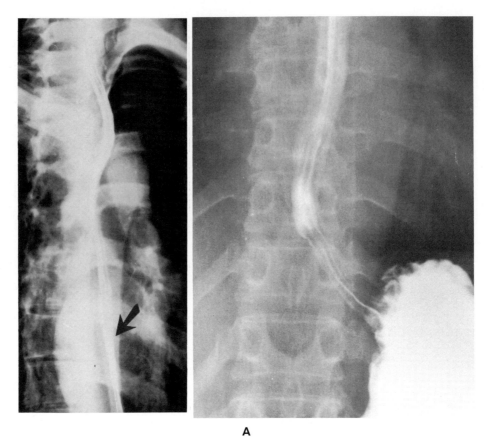

Figure 13–9. A. Rugal pattern of the esophagus.

Figure 13–9 continued on the opposite page.

fourth, and ordinarily, when a foreign body fails to pass down the esophagus, the site of obstruction occurs at one of the upper points of narrowness.

Esophageal Lip (Fig. 13–10). The esophageal lip is an indentation on the posterior aspect of the esophagus at its junction with the hypopharynx. It is postulated that this is caused by the cricopharyngeal muscle. Differential diagnosis of this formation from a foreign body or other abnormality may cause some problems. It is probable that the esophageal lip is not associated with dysphagia and is of no definite pathologic significance (Siebert et al.).

The Normal Rugal Pattern of the Esophagus. The mucous coat of the esophagus is very loosely connected with the muscular coat by the areolar tissue of the submucous layer. When the esophagus is empty, the mucous coat is thrown into a series of longitudinal folds (Fig. 13–9); otherwise it is very smooth in contrast with the mammillated gastric mucous membrane.

The longitudinal folds of the empty or partially empty esophagus impart to the radiographic picture the typical rugal pattern attributed to this organ. These consist of parallel lines throughout the esophagus which become more closely approximated as

the distal funnel end of the esophagus is reached just above the cardia (Fig. 13–11).

Abnormalities in the esophageal wall are reflected to a great extent in alteration of this normal rugal pattern, either by the appearance of abnormal folds or by the lack of folds.

The Normal Swallowing Function. The process of deglutition has been thoroughly studied by cineradiography in recent times. Briefly, the sequence of events is as follows:

1. There is a forward and upward movement of the tongue which displaces the contents of the mouth backward.

2. The soft palate is raised and the palatoglossal and palatopharyngeal muscles relax.

3. The hyoid and the lateral walls of the pharynx then rise abruptly.

4. The epiglottis deflects the food bolus into the lateral food channels and then reverts back and inferiorly to cover the laryngeal vestibule. The role of the epiglottis is secondary to the sphincteric action of the supraglottic laryngeal musculature.

5. The cricopharyngeus relaxes ahead of the advancing bolus.

6. There is a continued contraction of the muscles around the

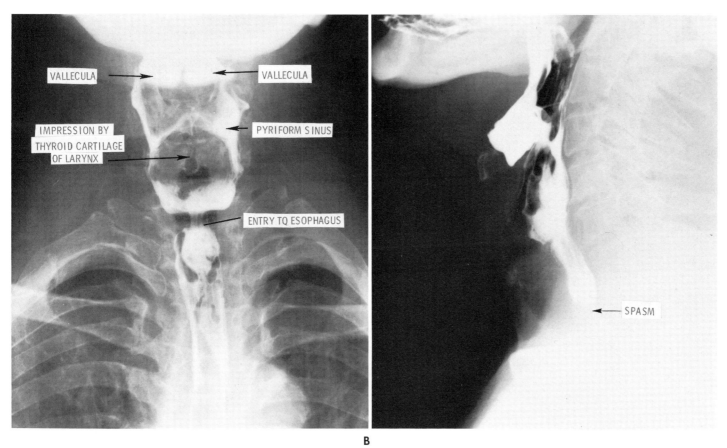

B

Figure 13–9. *Continued.* *B. Left,* Normal anteroposterior view of laryngeal and pharyngeal esophagus with barium. *Right,* Lateral view of a patient with cricopharyngeal spasm and barium accumulating in the vallecula.

Figure 13–9 continued on the following page.

mouth, and the supraglottic muscles and epiglottis prevent the food from entering the larynx. The elevation of the soft palate simultaneously approximates it to the posterior pharyngeal wall, preventing the return of the material into the mouth or nasopharynx.

7. Intrapharyngeal pressure rises with the entry of the bolus into the pharynx, but in the region of the cricopharyngeus, the high resting pressure falls abruptly on swallowing, with an equally abrupt return to high pressure after the passage of the bolus into the esophagus. Thus, the cricopharyngeus acts as a true sphincter, preventing egress of material back into the hypopharynx.

8. The tubular portion of the esophagus, by means of a peristaltic wave, transports the food bolus toward the stomach. The peristalsis begins in the posterior pharynx and is shallow in type and nonocclusive.

9. The function of the gastroesophageal segment is quite complex. There is a small pouch formed just above the esophageal hiatus, depending upon the quantity of fluid swallowed, the consistency of the fluid, the caliber of the submerged segment as defined by Wolf, and the height of intra-abdominal pressure. Pressure in the submerged segment as well as in the ampulla remains somewhat elevated, and as the peristaltic wave descends to it, the combined pressures of peristaltic and submerged pressure force the food bolus into the stomach. When the food bolus has left the ampullary region and submerged segment, the elevated pressure zone in the esophagogastric region persists so that no significant reflux is thereby permitted. These pressure relationships are illustrated in Figure 13–12.

Basic Anatomic Concepts Regarding the Lower Esophagus. Great interest and considerable confusion have arisen in relation to that segment of the esophagus just above the diaphragm and

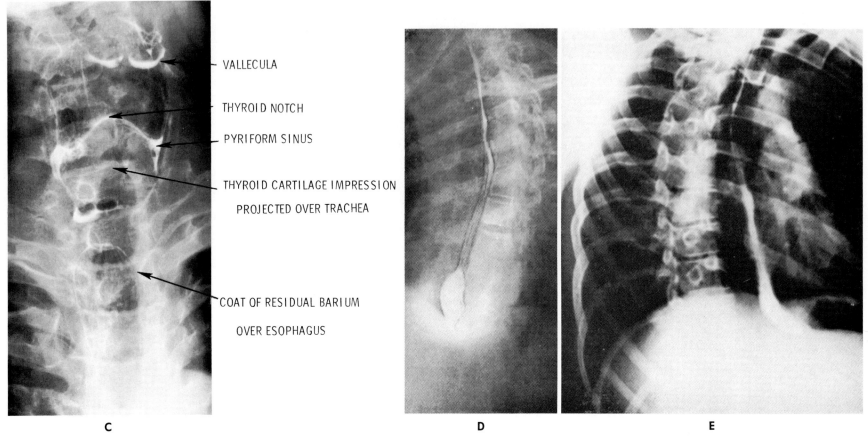

- VALLECULA
- THYROID NOTCH
- PYRIFORM SINUS
- THYROID CARTILAGE IMPRESSION
  PROJECTED OVER TRACHEA
- COAT OF RESIDUAL BARIUM
  OVER ESOPHAGUS

C   D   E

Figure 13-9 *Continued.*   C. Pharyngeal region and upper esophagus coated with a thin coat of barium. *D* and *E*. Radiograph of esophagus. *D*. Demonstrating the esophageal phrenic ampulla (intensified). *E*. Showing rugal pattern of esophagus.

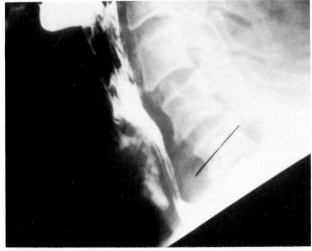

Figure 13-10.   Lateral view of the pharyngeal and upper esophagus, demonstrating an esophageal lip.

extending to the stomach (Lerche; Johnstone; Berridge; Wolf, 1973). A dynamic functional concept of the gastroesophageal junction is necessary. Fluoroscopy has shown that the junctional area between the esophagus and stomach is mobile and undergoes changes in position, shape, and architecture according to changes in body position, intra-abdominal pressure, and swallowing movements of the patient (Adler, 1962) (Fig. 13–13).

Although there is no morphologically discernible sphincter in the distal esophagus, newer manometric recording devices have made it possible to demonstrate a long-suspected sphincterlike action inherent in the function of the distal esophagus in a segment about 4 cm. in length that straddles the diaphragm at the esophageal hiatus. The resting intraluminal pressure within this segment is higher than that within the stomach. The sphincterlike action of this segment appears to be completely separate from the behavior of the diaphragm.

In an effort to clarify the terminology in respect to this area, Wolf (1970) has called the long narrow segment that is sometimes

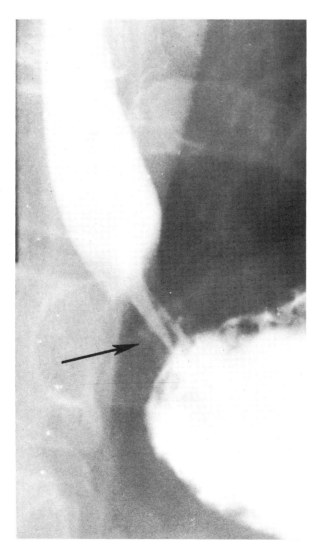

Figure 13–11. Radiograph showing normal rugal pattern of the lower esophagus.

lishing a high pressure zone to prevent reflux from the stomach to the esophagus. It is when the fundus slides above the diaphgram through a patulous hiatus to create a hiatal hernia that the function of this segment is most vulnerable and the barrier furnished by it to regurgitation and reflux may be inadequate to protect the lower esophagus from the refluxing digestive enzymes of the stomach.

The junction of the vestibule and fundus of the stomach is often demarcated by an epithelial ring which can be identified radiographically (Fig. 13–14).

With a hiatal hernia, a ring is often identified between the esophagus and herniated portion of stomach; it is called a

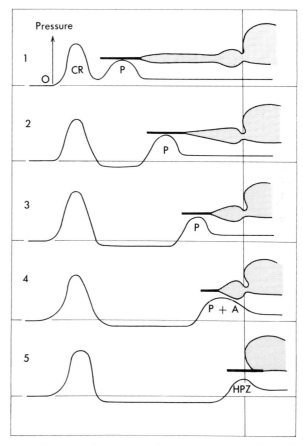

Figure 13–12. Diagrammatic representation of normal peristaltic activity of the esophagus during the act of swallowing. (1) The reconstituted resting cricopharyngeal sphincter (CR) returns to a state of elevated pressure as the stripping wave (P) enters the proximal esophagus. (2 to 5) The peristaltic stripping wave continues distally without change in the tubular configuration of the body of the esophagus. The size of the pouch formed above the hiatus depends on the quantity of fluid swallowed, the consistency of the fluid, the caliber of the submerged segment, and the height of intra-abdominal pressure. Note that in contrast to pressure in the body of the esophagus, pressure in the ampulla may rise while it still contains barium so that an elongated pressure curve (P + A) is obtained (4). With complete emptying, elevated pressure in the esophagogastric region persists, that is, the esophagogastric composite sphincter is reconstituted. (From Wolf, B. S.: Roentgenology of the esophagogastric region. *In* Margulis, A. R. and Burhenne, H. J., (eds.): Alimentary Tract Roentgenology, 2nd ed. St. Louis, C. V. Mosby Co., 1973.)

referred to as the esophageal vestibule when beneath the diaphragm the "submerged segment," and he further names "A," "B," and "C" rings (Fig. 13–13). In this terminology, the cardia (CO) is the orifice at the junction between the esophagus and the diaphragm; it is normally situated beneath the diaphragm. The A ring, originally referred to by Lerché as the inferior esophageal sphincter, is an inconstant constriction at the superior margin of the esophageal ampulla. The B ring refers to the true mucosal junction between the esophagus and the stomach when there is a hernia of the stomach above the diaphragm. The submerged segment, or C ring, is defined by the constrictor cardiae or phrenicoesophageal membrane of the diaphragm.

The submerged segment functions most effectively when a portion of the esophagus lies beneath the diaphragm (esophageal vestibule), where the diaphragmatic contraction assists in estab-

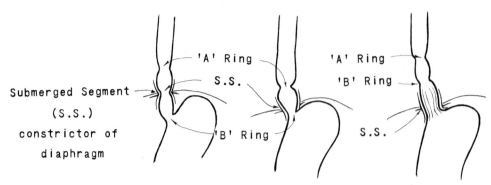

Figure 13–13. Anatomic concept of lower esophagus, modified from Wolf et al.

"Schatzki ring" or a "Templeton ring"). This is in fact a B ring. It is probably of clinical significance when its transverse measurement is less than 13 mm. (Fig. 13–15) and when there is an associated reflux to the level of the tracheal bifurcation.

Figure 13–16 illustrates what Wolf considers a variety of

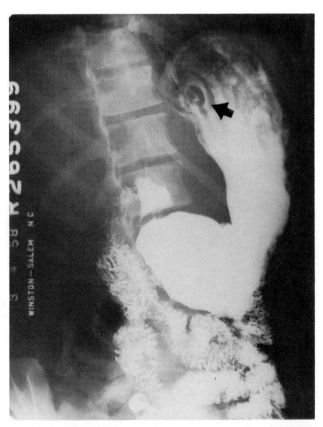

Figure 13–14. "Epithelial ring" at the cardioesophageal junction.

pressure profiles in patients with sliding hernias; they are significant only in so far as they contribute to a knowledge of the normal anatomic landmarks at this junction. One or another of the A or B rings or the submerged segment itself may act as a barrier to reflux from the stomach and as a high pressure zone. It is when no high pressure zone is functioning that symptoms of "epigastric burning" (pyrosis) are probable.

Barrett's epithelium is a *columnar epithelium* which may be found in the upper and lowermost portions of the esophagus and may represent an embryonic type of epithelium. This may, at times, be situated between the squamous epithelium and the normal simple columnar epithelium of the esophagus.

The phrenic esophageal ampulla is a physiologic dilatation of the lower esophagus which can be identified particularly when this region is distended by a bolus of food or barium. It may be seen most clearly in full inspiration. The ampulla is accentuated by a contraction or constriction of the esophagus just proximal to it.

The anatomic presence of the inferior esophageal sphincter has been demonstrated by Lerché. The narrowing produced in the esophageal appearance in this area is due in part to the contraction of the sphincter and in part to the downward pull of the phrenoesophageal membrane, the upper end of which is attached at this point.

The phrenicoesophageal membrane is the anchoring apparatus for the lower esophagus to the diaphragm. This membrane divides into an ascending portion that is attached at the level of the inferior esophageal sphincter and a descending portion that is attached to the muscular coat of the cardia of the stomach in the region of the gastroesophageal junction. The phrenicoesophageal membrane ordinarily serves as a channel for the esophagus, resisting excessive shortening or lengthening of the organ during the act of respiration. On the other hand, in deep inspiration the diaphragm constricts the lower end of the esophagus (constrictor diaphragmatis) and in expiration the area expands fully. With changes in position, there is a sliding movement of the esophagus in this area so that the relationship of the esophagus to the diaphragm actually changes with respiration.

The gastroesophageal vestibule corresponds with the abdominal portion of the esophagus or submerged segment. This has been referred to as the gastric antrum or antechamber of the stomach. When the phrenic ampulla is full, the vestibule is ordinarily empty. It is essential that the gastroesophageal vestibule be recognized so that it is not mistaken for a sliding hiatal hernia. When the vestibule is empty the longitudinal rugae are thin and parallel and resemble closely the rugal pattern of the esophagus above this level. When the vestibule is full, however, the rugae are effaced and closely resemble the rugae of the gastric fundus. Hence, serial film studies are necessary to differentiate this area accurately.

HERNIATIONS

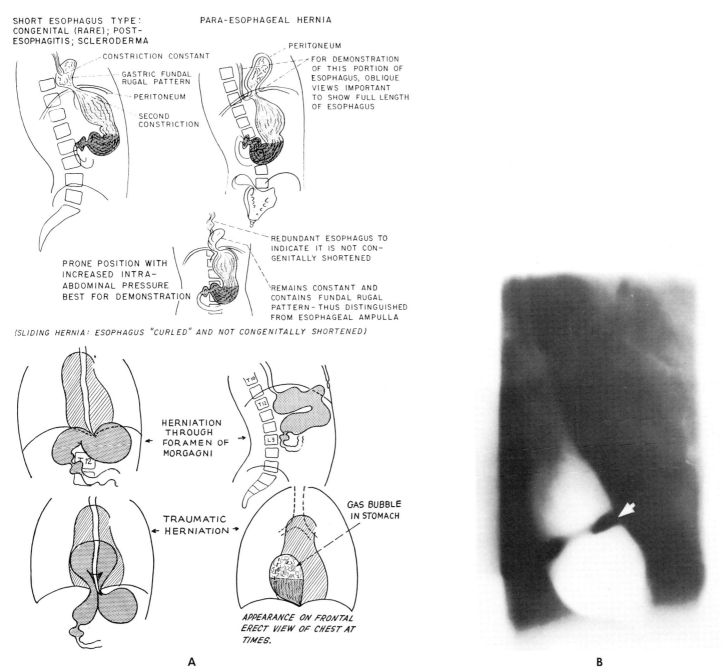

SHORT ESOPHAGUS TYPE:
CONGENITAL (RARE); POST-
ESOPHAGITIS; SCLERODERMA

PARA-ESOPHAGEAL HERNIA

CONSTRICTION CONSTANT

GASTRIC FUNDAL
RUGAL PATTERN

PERITONEUM

SECOND
CONSTRICTION

PERITONEUM

FOR DEMONSTRATION
OF THIS PORTION OF
ESOPHAGUS, OBLIQUE
VIEWS IMPORTANT
TO SHOW FULL LENGTH
OF ESOPHAGUS

PRONE POSITION WITH
INCREASED INTRA-
ABDOMINAL PRESSURE
BEST FOR DEMONSTRATION

REDUNDANT ESOPHAGUS TO
INDICATE IT IS NOT CON-
GENITALLY SHORTENED

REMAINS CONSTANT AND
CONTAINS FUNDAL RUGAL
PATTERN - THUS DISTINGUISHED
FROM ESOPHAGEAL AMPULLA

(SLIDING HERNIA: ESOPHAGUS "CURLED" AND NOT CONGENITALLY SHORTENED)

HERNIATION
THROUGH
FORAMEN OF
MORGAGNI

TRAUMATIC
HERNIATION

GAS BUBBLE
IN STOMACH

APPEARANCE ON FRONTAL
ERECT VIEW OF CHEST AT
TIMES.

A

B

Figure 13–15. A. Summary diagram illustrating herniations of the stomach through the diaphragm. B. Radiograph demonstrating Schatzki's ring.

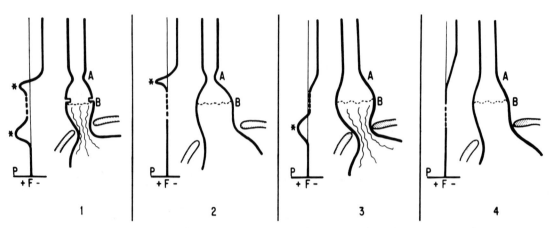

Figure 13–16. Diagram illustrating a variety of pressure profiles in patients with sliding hernias. Panels 1–4. A and B levels are indicated in each panel. F indicates fundic pressure; pressure (P) higher than F is on the plus (+) side, lower than F on the minus (−) side. Peak pressures are indicated by asterisks (*) on the pressure curves. The length of plateau region varies (dashes) depending on the size of the hernia. Panel 1 shows two peaks of resting pressure, one in the region of the A ring and another at the level of the hiatus. Panel 2 shows one peak related to the A level and a wide barium column traversing the hiatus. Panel 3 shows a single peak in the region of the hiatus with a relatively narrowed gastric channel or collar within the hiatus. Panel 4 shows no peak and a continuous wide barium channel extending from the tubular esophagus into the stomach below the diaphragm. A "B" ring is shown in Panel 1 but may or may not be present in any of these configurations. The Z line, although indicated, is not evident roentgenologically. (From Wolf, B. S.: Amer. J. Roentgenol., *110*:274, 1970.)

The constrictor cardia is at the gastroesophageal junction and ordinarily is located beneath the diaphragm at the junction of the esophageal and gastric mucosa. There is an abrupt change from the squamous epithelium of the esophagus to the columnar epithelium of the stomach at this site. At times, this epithelial line appears as an epithelial ring (Fig. 13–14) as previously illustrated.

Blood Supply of the Esophagus

Venous Drainage of the Lower Esophagus and Its Importance. The veins of the esophagus form a plexus exteriorly (Fig. 13–17). The venous drainage of the lower esophagus passes to the coronary vein of the stomach, and the latter vein empties into the portal vein. Higher up, the veins of the esophagus empty into the azygos system and thyroid veins. (See Chapter 12.)

Thus, the esophagus forms a communicating link between the portal circulation on the one hand and the systemic veins on the other, since the azygos vein empties into the superior vena cava.

Obstruction of the portal vein from any cause may, in turn, cause considerable distention of the lower esophageal veins and other tributaries of the coronary vein of the stomach. These irreg- ular distentions are spoken of as "varices," and have the appearance and the same physiologic significance as hemorrhoids in the case of the anal canal (Fig. 13–18). These veins may rupture and cause considerable embarrassment from bleeding. They produce a marked irregularity of the rugal pattern of the lower esophagus, especially when the venous pressure is increased as in the case of forced expiration. Indeed, the relative disappearance of the irregularity in deep inspiration, and reappearance with forced expiration is pathognomonic of esophageal varices.

Arterial Supply of the Esophagus. The arterial supply of the esophagus is derived from esophageal branches of the aorta (Fig. 13–19), bronchial arteries, the inferior phrenic artery, and left gastric arteries. Veins accompany these arteries, which usually number three at the most. At times, esophageal branches are received from the bronchial arteries. Ascending branches of esophageal arteries from an abnormal level are also shown.

The veins form a plexus on the outer surface of the esophagus opening into the left gastric, azygos, and thyroid veins cranially, as previously described, thus establishing a communication between portal and systemic veins.

Lymphatics in the Esophagus. The lymphatics in the esophagus arise chiefly in the mucosa and drain into the inferior deep cervical, posterior mediastinal, and superior gastric lymph nodes.

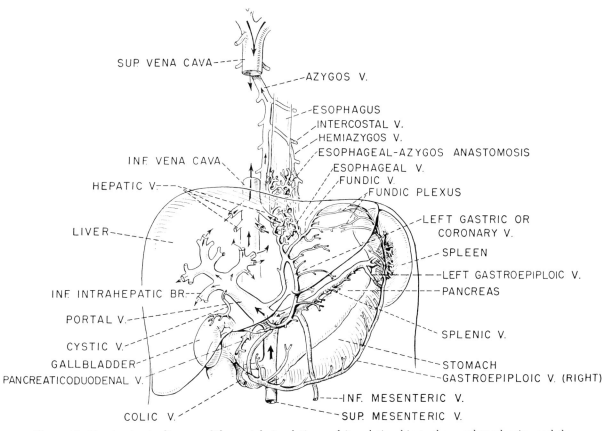

Figure 13–17. Anatomic diagram of the portal circulation and its relationship to the esophageal veins and the azygos venous system.

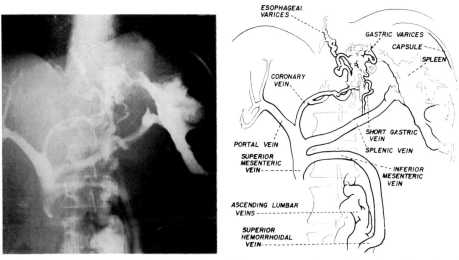

Figure 13–18. Roentgenogram at 12 seconds demonstrates coronary vein, gastric and esophageal varices. The anastomosis between the inferior mesenteric vein and superior hemorrhoid plexus is demonstrated. The latter is also seen to drain into the vertebral venous plexus. Tracing at right. (From Evans, J. A., and O'Sullivan, W. D.: Amer. J. Roentgenol. *77,* 1957.)

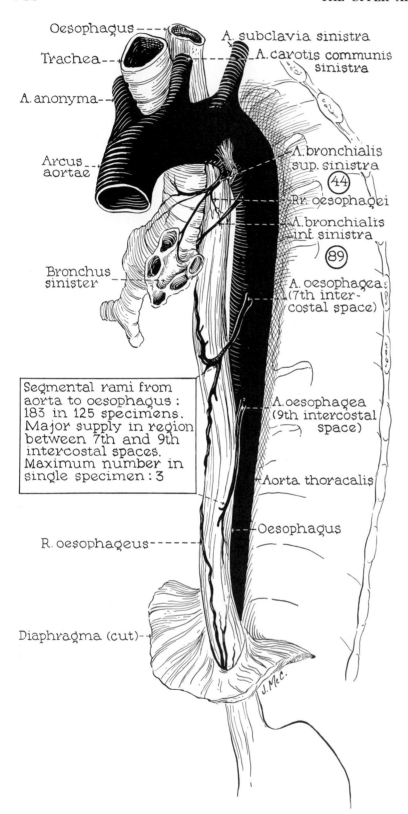

Oesophagus

Trachea

A. subclavia sinistra

A. carotis communis sinistra

A. anonyma

Arcus aortae

A. bronchialis sup. sinistra

(44)

Rr. oesophagei

A. bronchialis inf. sinistra

(89)

Bronchus sinister

A. oesophagea (7th intercostal space)

Segmental rami from aorta to oesophagus: 183 in 125 specimens. Major supply in region between 7th and 9th intercostal spaces. Maximum number in single specimen: 3

A. oesophagea (9th intercostal space)

Aorta thoracalis

Oesophagus

R. oesophageus

Diaphragma (cut)

J. McC.

Technique of Examination of the Esophagus

Fluoroscopy. The proper examination of the esophagus involves a combination of fluoroscopy and radiography, with spot film radiography in selected areas. We now consider cinefluoroscopy and radiography to be an essential part of this examination with respect to the swallowing function.

The sequence is as follows: (1) survey fluoroscopy of chest; (2) survey fluoroscopy of abdomen; (3) the swallowing of a single mouthful of thin barium is studied in frontal and oblique perspective; (4) for mucosal detail, the swallowing of thick barium paste is thereafter viewed in frontal and oblique perspectives; (5) the patient is then placed in the supine position and the study is repeated. When the patient is in the left posterior oblique, regurgitation is assayed by gravity and positive pressure (Valsalva maneuver). The water test is done in this position also.

The Trendelenburg position is utilized when a hiatal hernia is suspected.

The prone position for demonstration of a hiatal hernia with the patient straining is particularly useful and is repeated with both thick and thin barium with the patient in the right anterior oblique position. Spot films are obtained in at least two separate sequences.

Technique of the Water Test (Linsman; Crummy). The patient is supine and turned obliquely on his left side. After the fundus of the stomach is filled with barium, he is asked to drink a mouthful of water through a straw. He is asked to swallow this while his esophagogastric junction is carefully studied fluoroscopically. The bolus of water is identified by the air swallowed with the water, and the water is detected as it enters the stomach. Normally, very little of the barium is observed to reflux into the esophagus at this juncture. With a positive water test a large amount of barium is seen to reflux up the esophagus, usually above the level of the hilar vessels and frequently above the aortic arch. At such times, clearing of the esophagus is slow and several peristaltic waves are required to empty the esophagus of the regurgitated barium.

Figure 13–19. Thoracic sources of esophageal arteries, diagrammatic. The encircled numbers represent the frequency with which esophageal rami arose from the particular bronchial artery in 125 dissections. Ascending branches of esophageal arteries from abdominal level and descending branches of the segmental esophageal arteries of thoracic level are also shown. (From Anson, B. J.: An Atlas of Human Anatomy. Philadelphia, W. B. Saunders Co., 1963.)

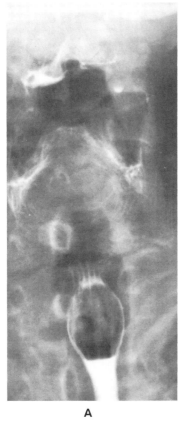
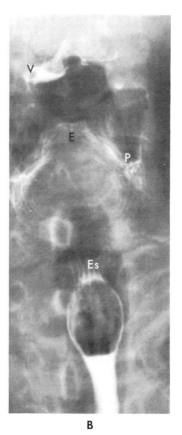

A   **B**

Figure 13–20. *A.* Anteroposterior view of neck with barium in the esophagus. *B.* Same view labeled: (V) vallecula, (E) epiglottis, (P) pyriform sinus, (Es) upper esophagus.

In studies correlating reflux of barium into the esophagus as demonstrated by the water-siphonage test of de Carvalho (Crummy), in 650 routine upper gastrointestinal studies in patients with pyrosis ("heartburn"), the following statistics were reported:

a. 10.3 per cent of the patients had reflux, and 68.6 per cent of these complained of pyrosis.

b. 89.7 per cent did not have reflux, and 3.4 per cent of these complained of pyrosis.

c. 10.1 per cent of the total group complained of pyrosis, and 69.6 per cent of these had a positive water test.

d. 30.4 per cent of those with pyrosis as a complaint showed no reflux when tested.

e. 46 of these 650 patients had hiatal herniae.

f. Of 48 per cent with pyrosis, 91 per cent had a positive water test.

g. Of 52 per cent who were asymptomatic, 91.7 per cent had a negative water test.

h. In only 14 cases did reflux occur with change of position only. All 14 had a positive water test, but only half of these had pyrosis.

Thus the water test is highly satisfactory for detection of gastroesophageal reflux, and reflux occurring under these circumstances correlates well with pyrosis, especially in patients with hiatal hernia.

Spot Film Radiography. Spot films are obtained whenever a suggestion of abnormality is seen. (Water test films and films of the lower esophagus are routine.)

Cineradiography. We now consider cineradiography (or video tape recording) an essential part of a study of the swallowing function and use it routinely, usually in the erect, supine, and prone positions.

Films Obtained. (1) Anteroposterior film study of the esophagus, including neck to diaphragm (Figs. 13–20, 13–21). (2) Right anterior oblique projection (Fig. 13–22). (3) Left anterior oblique projection (Fig. 13–23). (4) A lateral view of the neck with barium in the esophagus (Fig. 13–24).

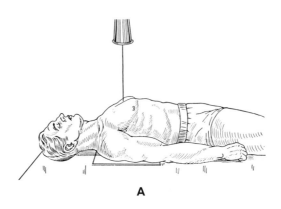

A

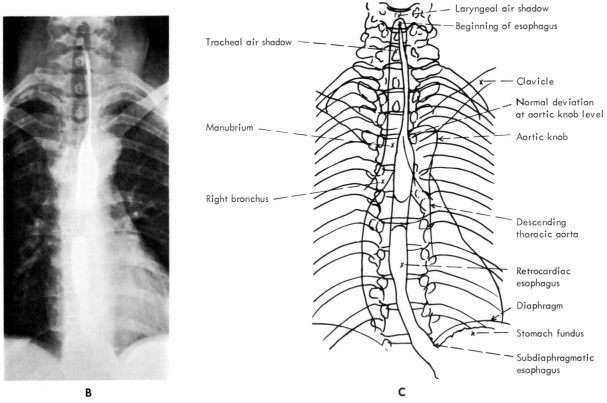

B   C

Figure 13–21.   Anteroposterior film study of esophagus. *A.* Position of patient. *B.* Radiograph. *C.* Labeled tracing of *B.*

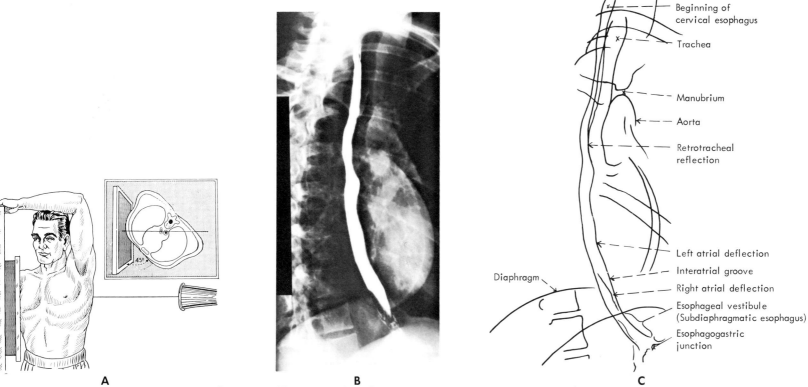

Figure 13–22. Right anterior oblique view of esophagus. *A.* Position of patient. *B.* Radiograph. *C.* Labeled tracing. (This same view is frequently taken in the recumbent position as well.)

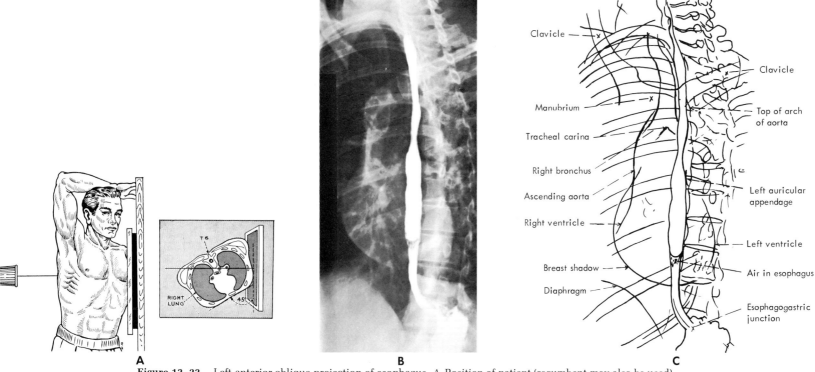

Figure 13–23. Left anterior oblique projection of esophagus. *A.* Position of patient (recumbent may also be used). *B.* Radiograph (intensified). *C.* Labeled tracing.

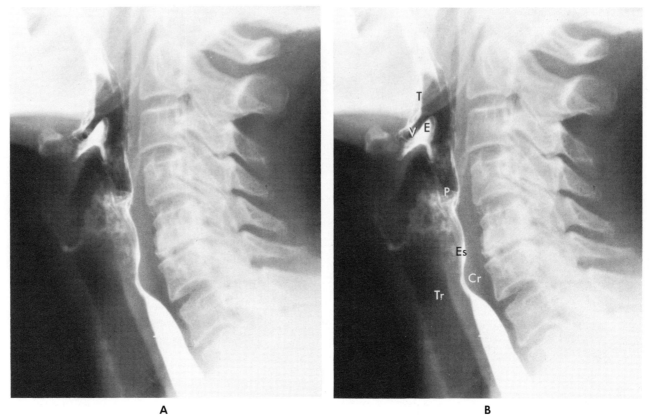

A   **B**

Figure 13-24.   *A.* Lateral roentgenogram of the neck with barium in the esophagus. *B.* Same radiograph labeled:
(T) back of tongue, (V) vallecula, (E) tip of epiglottis, (P) pyriform sinus, (Es) upper esophagus above (Cr) cricopharyngeus muscle impression, (Tr) trachea.

**Special Procedure for Suspected Swallowing of Foreign
Body.**   (1) Lateral films of the neck and chest without contrast
media. (2) Lateral film of the neck during deglutition, so that the
calcified, cartilaginous structures will be elevated, bringing into
clear relief any postcricoid foreign body. (3) Routine fluoroscopy of
the esophagus as outlined above.

It has been recommended by some that the swallowing of a
small cotton ball soaked with barium or a barium-filled gelatin
capsule be employed. If this is done, interpretation must be
carried forward with great caution since either of these may be
delayed in transit and false conclusions drawn.

A plain survey film of the abdomen prior to the introduction
of barium is advisable, as is an AP or PA film of the chest to determine whether or not the suspected foreign body has been
aspirated into the chest or swallowed into the gastrointestinal
tract below the level of the esophagus.

Routine Film Studies of the Esophagus

Anteroposterior Film Study of the Neck (Fig. 13-20).   The
cervical portion of the esophagus begins at the lower border of the

cricoid cartilage approximately at the level of the sixth cervical
vertebra. The pharyngoesophageal junction is usually closed and
the esophagus collapsed. Occasionally, however, air may be detected in this sector. Although the esophageal inlet relaxes during swallowing, it immediately contracts and tapers again af-
terwards. A peristaltic wave passing downward in unbroken
succession may be visualized in the pharynx. The esophagus is in
the midline at its origin and deviates slightly to the left in the
caudal part of the neck and cranial part of the thorax. Its rugal
pattern is longitudinal, cephalocaudad. At the base of the neck
the esophagus protrudes slightly beyond the left margin of the
trachea. The tracheal air shadow may be clearly identified in
relation to the barium-containing cervical esophagus.

Since the esophagus is relatively longer in a newborn infant
than in the adult, the cervical esophagus is farther cranial in
children, corresponding to the more cranial vertebral level of the
larynx.

In **lateral projection** (Fig. 13-24) the esophagus is immediately posterior to the trachea and separated from it by a thin fascial plane.

The Anteroposterior Film Study Below the Neck (Fig. 13-
21).   In this projection, the esophagus is tapered superiorly and

inferiorly immediately above the diaphragm, and is largely a midline structure, except where it deviates to the right by the left bronchus impression in the upper part of its course, and slightly to the left and anteriorly in the region of the diaphragm in the lower part of its course. There may be a very slight impression by the left auricular appendage, displacing the esophagus slightly to the right also. If this displacement is more than extremely slight, it is usually indicative of enlargement of the left atrium.

Right Anterior Oblique Projection (Fig. 13–25). In this projection the esophagus is rather closely applied to the spine in the neck and to the posterior margin of the pericardium in the thorax. The previously described "aortic" indentation in the region of the left bronchus is also seen to displace the esophagus slightly posteriorly. There is a slight indentation of the esophagus in the region of the left atrium, which is in a posterior position. The clear space behind the esophagus increases above the diaphragm, in view of the gradually increasing anterior course of the esophagus.

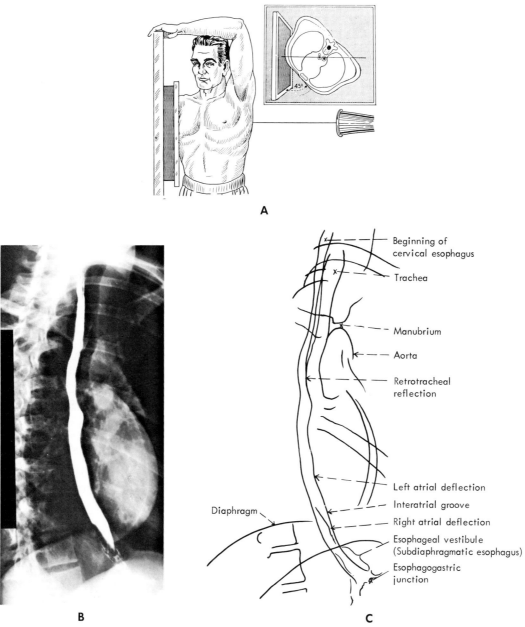

Figure 13–25. Right anterior oblique view of esophagus. *A.* Position of patient. *B.* Radiograph. *C.* Labeled tracing. (This same view is frequently taken in the recumbent position as well.)

Left Anterior Oblique Projection (Fig. 13–26). In this view, the slight posterior impression produced by the left bronchus is once again seen, but otherwise, the esophagus courses directly down to the diaphragm on the anterior aspect of the thoracic spine.

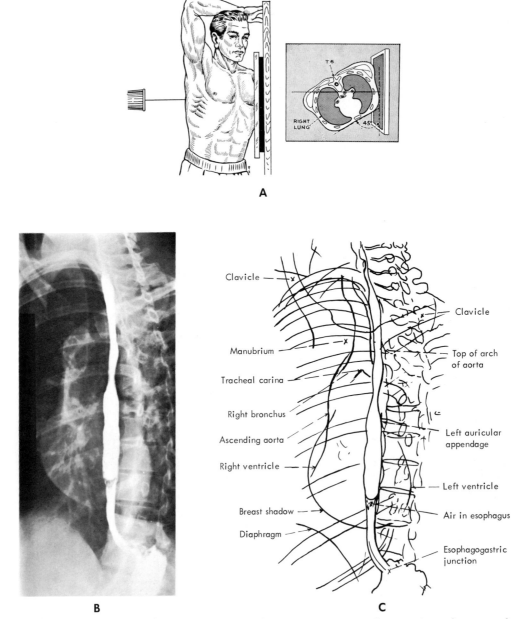

Figure 13–26. Left anterior oblique projection of esophagus. *A.* Positioning of patient (recumbent may also be used). *B.* Radiograph (intensified). *C.* Labeled tracing.

Iodized Oil Study. Iodized oil is possibly somewhat less irritating when inhaled into the trachea or bronchial tree than is the barium sulfate suspension. On the other hand, it is more expensive and somewhat more irritating to gastric mucosa.

When a patient gives a history of extreme difficulty in swallowing, followed by considerable coughing, it usually indicates that he inhales the swallowed bolus, at least in part. In such instances, an iodized oil such as Dionosil (oily) may be injected by syringe onto the back of the tongue and swallowed. The barium sulfate suspension may be used thereafter if inhalation of the Dionosil has not occurred.

This is particularly true in cases of pharyngeal palsies, pseudopharyngeal palsies, and such congenital anomalies as esophageal atresias, where there is usually a communication between the esophagus and the trachea or bronchial tree. Barium sulfate suspension may be used initially, however, if desired,

since it has been tolerated as a bronchographic agent also (Fig. 13–27).

THE STOMACH AND DUODENUM

Subdivisions of the Stomach. The stomach is arbitrarily divided into three parts: the fundus, the body, and the pyloric portion (Fig. 13–28).

The fundus is that portion of the stomach that lies above a horizontal plane through the junction of the stomach and esophagus (this latter being called the "cardiac orifice" or "cardia"), and the pyloric portion is that part that falls between the incisura angularis and the pylorus. The body is represented by the intervening portion.

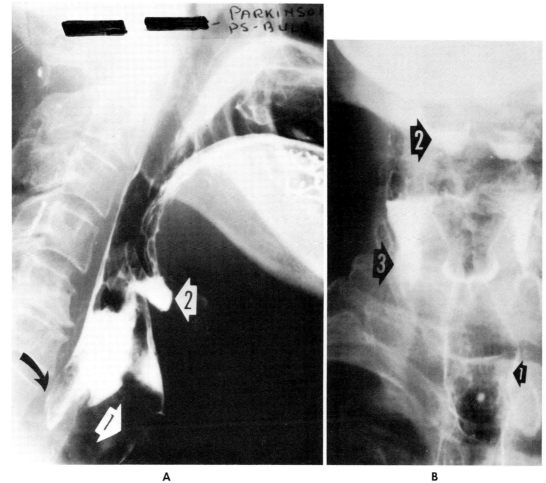

A   B

Figure 13–27. *A* and *B.* Pseudobulbar palsy in a patient with Parkinson's disease. (1) Trachea, (2) vallecula, (3) pyriform sinuses.

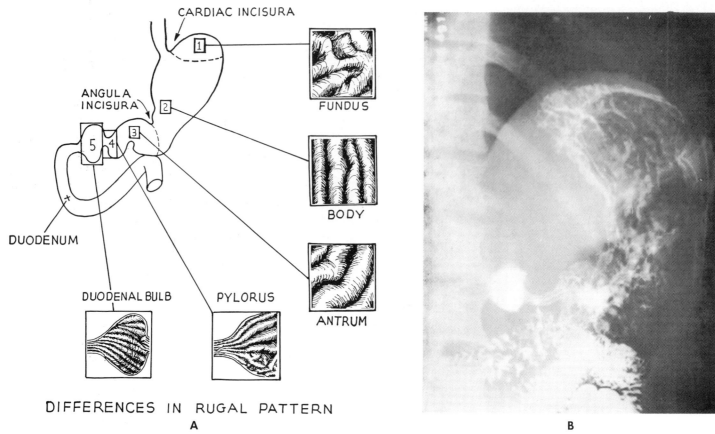

CARDIAC INCISURA

ANGULA INCISURA

DUODENUM

DUODENAL BULB

PYLORUS

FUNDUS

BODY

ANTRUM

DIFFERENCES IN RUGAL PATTERN

A

B

Figure 13-28. Stomach. *A.* Subdivisions and rugal pattern. *B.* Radiograph showing rugal pattern. (The distal portion of the pyloric antrum is in a contracted state and its rugal pattern merges imperceptibly with the pattern of the pyloric canal.)

The right wall of the cardia merges into the lesser curvature of the stomach, while the left wall is deeply notched by the cardiac incisura.

A pyloric constriction marks the junction between the stomach and duodenum. The pyloric sphincter is sharply demarcated from the duodenum, but blends imperceptibly with the thickened masculature of the pyloric antrum. The pyloric canal traverses the pyloric sphincter and is approximately 5 mm. in length. The gastric mucous membrane is continued into the duodenum without any alteration visible to the naked eye.

The greater curvature corresponds in its greater part with the attachment of the gastrosplenic and gastrocolic ligaments.

Stomach Contour Variations in Accordance with Body Build (Fig. 13-29). Gastric tone and contour normally follow the habitus of the individual closely. In the individual who is short and stocky, the stomach is usually high in position and "steerhorn" in shape, its lumen being largest above and tapering toward the pylorus. It extends more quickly toward the right. At

times, it is even horizontal in position. The incisura angularis is difficult to identify, and occasionally the pylorus is the lowermost part of the stomach.

In the sthenic individual, the eutonic stomach is J-shaped, and the body of the stomach tends to be vertical in the frontal projection and uniform in size. The lowermost part of the stomach in the erect position tends to be at the level of the iliac crests.

In asthenic individuals, the stomach tends to be hypotonic, and shaped rather like a fishhook. The greater curvature tends to sag down into the pelvis, with the greatest diameter between the incisura angularis and the adjoining greater curvature.

Each of the stomach types may occur in individuals of any body build, but in general the hypotonic stomach tends to occur more frequently in underweight individuals, whereas the steerhorn type tends to occur more frequently in the overweight. Indeed, according to a study which we have conducted, when the hypotonic stomach occurs in an overweight individual, it is almost invariably symptomatic. Likewise, a cascade stomach tends

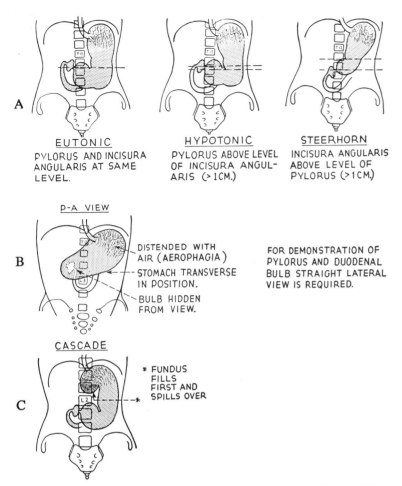

A

EUTONIC
PYLORUS AND INCISURA
ANGULARIS AT SAME
LEVEL.

HYPOTONIC
PYLORUS ABOVE LEVEL
OF INCISURA ANGUL-
ARIS (>1CM.)

STEERHORN
INCISURA ANGULARIS
ABOVE LEVEL OF
PYLORUS (>1CM.)

P-A VIEW

B

DISTENDED WITH
AIR (AEROPHAGIA)
STOMACH TRANSVERSE
IN POSITION.
BULB HIDDEN
FROM VIEW.

FOR DEMONSTRATION OF
PYLORUS AND DUODENAL
BULB STRAIGHT LATERAL
VIEW IS REQUIRED.

CASCADE

C

* FUNDUS
FILLS
FIRST AND
SPILLS OVER

Figure 13–29. Variations in stomach contour. A. In relation to body build and general stomach type. B. The infantile stomach. C. The cascade stomach.

to be symptomatic in an overweight person, whereas in normal or underweight individuals the cascade stomach is relatively asymptomatic. The symptoms are vague abdominal distress, sometimes suggestive of peptic ulcer.

The normal relationships of each type of stomach to each type of body build have been carefully worked out and tabulated as shown in Figure 13–11. Measurements can be taken as indicated and should fall within the normal range; if they are outside this normal range, the physician should be strongly suspicious of displacement of the stomach by some extrinsic lesion (see Table 13–1). A more accurate method of measurement in the left lateral erect with compression is illustrated in Figure 13–30 B.

Variations of the Stomach in Different Positions (Fig. 13–30). Gravity will influence the position of the gastric contents and the position and contour of the stomach. Thus, in the supine recumbent position, there is a tendency for the stomach to move up-

ward. At the same time, gastric contents will flow into the fundus, and the air in the stomach, which in the erect position is found in the fundus, will move anteriorly to occupy the anterior portion of the body of the stomach. Some of the air is invariably trapped in the pyloric portion also, but if there is sufficient barium suspension in the stomach, the pyloric portion and duodenal bulb will fill with it as well as with trapped air, producing a double contrast effect.

In the prone recumbent position, gravity tends to reverse these positional relationships. The barium mixture usually flows into the pyloric portion while the gas moves into the fundus. At the same time, there is a tendency for the stomach itself to move downward slightly, more closely resembling the appearance in the erect position.

In order to separate the shadows of the pyloric antrum and the duodenal bulb, it is usually necessary to place the patient in a slight right anterior oblique position. Otherwise, these structures usually overlie one another.

The lateral projection also finds wide usefulness, in that one can demonstrate positional relationships of the stomach to the pancreas and the omental bursa with greatest accuracy in this projection. The *left* lateral *standing* view is most valuable for this purpose since the relationship of the stomach to retrogastric structures is most accurately depicted thereby, particularly with compression. On the other hand, in the *right* lateral *recumbent* position, the stomach swings forward on its two areas of fixation (diaphragm and postbulbar duodenum), changing its relationship to the retrogastric structures. In this latter view, however, the pyloric antrum and body of the stomach fall anteriorly away from the level of the duodenum, producing a clearer depiction of the pylorobulbar area.

When the patient is supine, the stomach does not necessarily fall closely toward the retrogastric structures. This relationship is sometimes altered by the fact that the gas content of the stomach causes it to rise anteriorly. In our experience, therefore, a left lateral study of the stomach, obtained with a horizontal x-ray beam and the patient lying supine, is *less* valuable for study of stomach relationships to retrogastric structures than is the left lateral erection position, especially with compression.

Other Factors Which Influence Gastric Contour. Vagal stimulation increases gastric tone, whereas sympathetic stimulation decreases it. Thus, when an individual is frightened or otherwise emotionally disturbed, the stomach tends to be hypotonic. These psychic effects are usually temporary. Pathologic processes in the gastrointestinal and biliary tracts will also cause changes in gastric contour, but these are outside the scope of the present text.

The Duodenum. The duodenum is ordinarily examined simultaneously with the stomach, and it is discussed separately here for the sake of convenience only. The first part of the duodenum—the duodenal bulb—is integrated both structurally

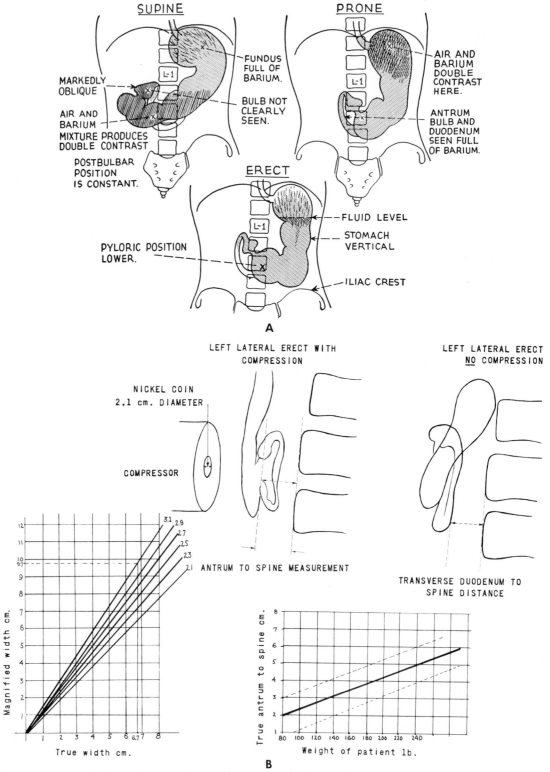

Figure 13–30. *A.* Variations in stomach contour in relation to body position. *B.* Method of measuring "retroantral" and "retroduodenal" space. The coin on the compressor allows correction for magnification (graph, lower left). The normal standards for antrum to spine are shown in the graph, lower right. (From Poole, G. J.: Radiology, *97:*71–81, 1970.)

and functionally with the pyloric antrum. The structure of the remainder of the duodenum resembles that of the small intestine.

The duodenum differs from the rest of the small intestine in several important respects:

1. It has no mesentery, and is fixed to the posterior abdominal wall for the most part.
2. The ducts of the liver, gallbladder, and pancreas open into it (at the duodenal papilla, or ampulla of Vater) in the descending part of the duodenum.
3. The duodenum contains some distinctive glands of its own, the duodenal glands of Brunner.
4. It is the shortest, widest, and most fixed portion of the small intestine.

Subdivisions. The duodenum is variably described as consisting of three or four parts (Fig. 13–31):

1. The superior portion, or duodenal bulb, which runs superiorly backward and to the right, is in direct continuity with the pylorus of the stomach. This portion has a mesentery of its own for a short distance.
2. The descending portion, which begins at the neck of the gallbladder, runs down on the posterior abdominal wall and usually ends approximately opposite the upper border of the fourth lumbar vertebra on the right of the vertebral column.
3. The inferior part is variably described as having one or two separate parts. It consists of a transverse portion, which crosses to the left of the midline, across the vena cava, aorta, and vertebral column; and an ascending portion, which ascends on the left of the vertebral column to the inferior surface of the pancreas. There it bends abruptly forward, forming the duodenojejunal flexure.

The duodenum is in the form of a U, with the superior portion more anterior than the descending part, the transverse portion coming directly forward and to the left, and the ascending portion in the same plane as the superior portion but to the left of the midline.

Gross Anatomy and Relationships of Each Subdivision of the Duodenum

THE SUPERIOR PORTION, DUODENAL BULB OR CAP. SITES OF NORMAL "FLECK" FORMATION. This first part of the duodenum is rather conical in shape, approximately 3.5 to 5 cm. in length, and

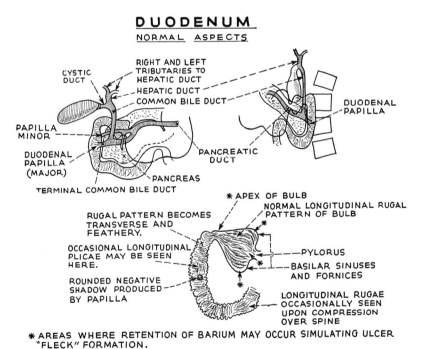

Figure 13–31. *A.* Normal relationships of the bile ducts to the duodenum, and the narrow mucosal patterns of the duodenum proper. *B.* A dissection to show the duodenum and pancreas. The right and left hepatic veins have been cut away at their points of entry into the inferior vena cava. The superior hypogastric plexus is shown in front of the sacral promontory and the sympathetic nerves which form it are seen descending across the bifurcation of the aorta, the left common iliac vein and the body of the fifth lumbar vertebra. (In this specimen the left renal artery is situated anterior to the left renal vein at the hilus of the kidney.)

3 cm. in diameter. It is described as having a base and an apex, the base forming a "stem-and-leaf" relationship with the pyloric canal (Fig. 13–32 A and B.)

As previously indicated, the rugal pattern of the bulb more closely resembles that of the pyloric antrum than the remainder of the duodenum, tending to be rather parallel, or parallel in spiral fashion from the base to apex. The contraction pattern and motor physiology of the bulb form a transition between that of the antrum and the distal duodenum.

Radiologically, a "fleck" (from the German meaning "spot") is a loculation of barium of any size from a few millimeters to 2 or more centimeters which strongly suggests a break in the normal mucosal structure and ulceration. In view of the great frequency of ulceration in this area, the detection of a fleck in this location is of extreme importance.

There are certain locations in the duodenal bulb, however, where fleck formation may be a normal variant, and these must be differentiated from the pathologic variety: (1) when the pylorus closes, there may be a dimple of mucosa at the base of the bulb in which the barium may accumulate, giving rise to the appearance of a fleck (Fig. 13–32 C); (2) the outer periphery of the base of the bulb occasionally acts as a groove, or sinus, in which barium may accumulate, and when seen in profile, gives the appearance of fleck formation at the base of the bulb; (3) the concentration of rugae at the apex of the bulb may simulate fleck formation on occasion also; (4) flecks of an inconstant variety may be simulated by peristaltic waves passing over the duodenal bulb.

The anatomic relationships of the bulb which are important are as follows (Fig. 13–33): the duodenal bulb forms the inferior boundary of the foramen epiploicum (foramen of Winslow), and hence a pathologic penetration of the bulb finds ready access into the lesser omental bursa. The hepatic artery is also in contact for a short distance with the superior margin of the bulb. Below, the bulb rests on the head and neck of the pancreas. There are several large blood vessels which come into close contact with this area (Fig. 13–33 B), and are of considerable importance from the standpoint of possible erosion of an ulcer. On the left side lie the portal vein, gastroduodenal artery (and bile duct); close to the posterior aspect is the right side of the inferior vena cava; and adjoining the inferior margin are the superior pancreaticoduodenal and the right gastroepiploic vessels (Fig. 13–34).

The common bile duct may occasionally indent the bulb, giving rise to an apparent deformity, and the gallbladder lies in close apposition with the superior and right margins of the first part of the duodenum, occasionally producing an indentation of the duodenum.

THE SECOND, OR DESCENDING PART OF THE DUODENUM. DESCRIPTION OF VILLI AND PLICAE CIRCULARES. This part of the duodenum is retroperitoneal in position with the root of the transverse mesocolon, crossing it at its middle. The head of the pancreas is in contact with its left margin (Fig. 13–35) and occasionally overlaps it both anteriorly and posteriorly, and along this margin run the branches of the pancreaticoduodenal arteries. The bile duct, after descending behind the duodenal blub, passes between the head of the pancreas and this part of the duodenum, where it joins with the pancreatic duct. The two together pierce the duodenal wall obliquely, and open by a common orifice on its inner aspect at the apex of the duodenal papilla (ampulla of Vater) medially (Fig. 13–36).

The mucous membrane of this part of the duodenum, as well

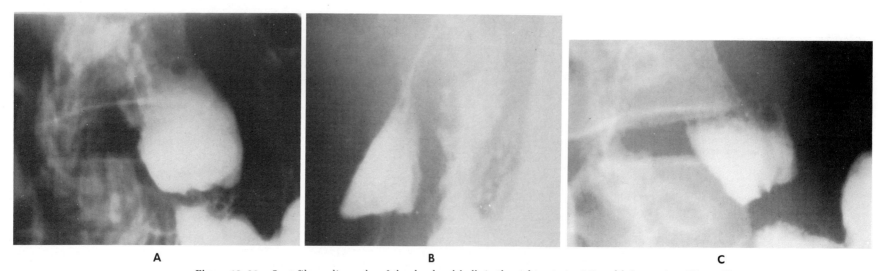

A   B   C

Figure 13–32.   Spot film radiographs of the duodenal bulb in the right anterior (A) and left anterior oblique (B) position. C. There is a "dimple" at the base of the duodenal bulb when the pylorus closes normally. The dimple simulates an ulcer niche.

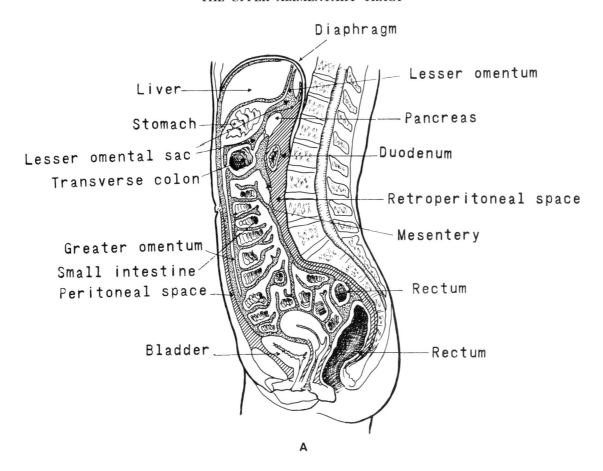

A

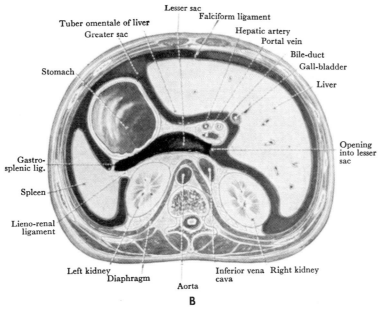

B

Figure 13–33. *A.* Sagittal diagram of abdomen showing relationships of lesser omental sac. *B.* Transverse section of abdomen to show the arrangement of peritoneum at the level of the opening into lesser sac. (From Cunningham's Manual of Practical Anatomy, 12th ed., Vol. 2. London, Oxford University Press, 1958.)

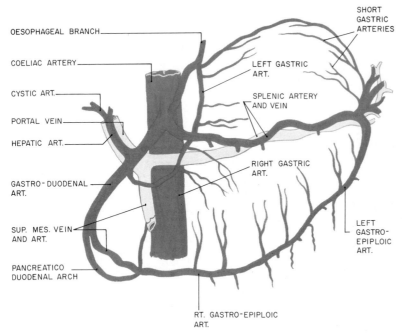

OESOPHAGEAL BRANCH

COELIAC ARTERY

CYSTIC ART.

PORTAL VEIN

HEPATIC ART.

GASTRO-DUODENAL ART.

SUP. MES. VEIN AND ART.

PANCREATICO DUODENAL ARCH

SHORT GASTRIC ARTERIES

LEFT GASTRIC ART.

SPLENIC ARTERY AND VEIN

RIGHT GASTRIC ART.

LEFT GASTRO-EPIPLOIC ART.

RT. GASTRO-EPIPLOIC ART.

Figure 13-34. Coeliac artery and its branches. (Redrawn from Cunningham's Manual of Practical Anatomy, 12th ed., Vol. 2. London, Oxford University Press, 1958.)

as all parts of the small intestine, presents a soft, velvety internal surface which is caused by the presence of the minute mucosal processes known as villi. These begin at the edge of the pyloric valve where they are quite broad, but they become narrower as they proceed down the small intestine. The only place they are not found is immediately over the solitary lymph nodules. These villi play an important part in the absorption function of the small intestine (Figs. 13-31 A and 13-38).

The mucous membrane of the small intestine is thrown into numerous folds which may to a great extent disappear upon distention, but there are permanent folds known as the plicae circulares (Fig. 13-37) or valvulae conniventes. They are crescentic folds running around the small intestine in circular fashion. They may bifurcate, and they usually project about 8 mm. into the lumen of the small intestine. *They begin in the second part of the duodenum* (Fig. 13-38), and gradually become more prominent, so that in the region of the duodenal papilla, they are very distinct and remain prominent in the rest of the duodenum. The combination of the plicae circulares and the villi imparts a feathery pattern to the duodenum and jejunum when viewed radiographically in the absence of distention, and this is the typical rugal pattern not only of the duodenum but also of the

jejunum. The absence of plicae circulares in the duodenal bulb accounts for its closer resemblance radiographically to the pyloric antrum (Fig. 13-39).

THE HORIZONTAL PORTION OF THE INFERIOR PART OF THE DUODENUM (THIRD PART). This part is somewhat concave upward, is retroperitoneal, and is crossed by the superior mesenteric vessels and the root of the mesentery near the midline. It crosses the inferior vena cava, and is closely applied to the inferior aspect of the head of the pancreas.

THE ASCENDING PORTION OF THE INFERIOR PART OF THE DUODENUM (FOURTH PART). This part lies on the aorta, the left renal vein, and occasionally also the left renal artery (Fig. 13-40 A). As previously indicated, it extends obliquely anteriorly and to the left, and its left side lies in contact with some coils of small intestine. In addition to being clothed by peritoneum anteriorly (as is the case of the second and third parts), it is also covered by peritoneum on its left side.

The duodenojejunal flexure is fixed by the musculus suspensorius (suspensory ligament) of Treitz, opposite the left side of the first or second lumbar vertebrae. This latter suspensory muscle blends with the muscular coat of the duodenum, passes upward behind the pancreas to blend partially with the celiac artery, and then is attached to the right crus of the diaphragm.

In the neighborhood of the ascending part of the duodenum, three peritoneal fossae may frequently be present (Fig. 13-40 B). Two of these, the superior and inferior duodenal fossae, are formed by slips of fibrous tissue covered by peritoneum extending from the left side of the duodenum to the peritoneal surface adjoining it, and form very small pouches directed caudad and cephalad respectively. The third, however, which is called the paraduodenal fossa, is produced by a fold of peritoneum formed by the inferior mesenteric vein as it courses along the left lateral side of the ascending part of the duodenum. The inferior mesenteric vein is accompanied in part of its course by the left colic artery. This fossa is capable of forming a hernial sac, and therefore may be of some clinical significance.

IMPORTANCE OF A STUDY OF THE DUODENAL CONTOUR. The duodenum is in a fixed position for the most part, and hence variations from its normal position become significant in the detection of space-occupying lesions in adjoining structures, such as the pancreas, lesser omental bursa, colon, gallbladder, and biliary ducts.

There is, however, a considerable variation in different individuals in the normal contour of the duodenum. To a great extent, this is correlated with body habitus. Thus in pyknic individuals with high steer-horn stomachs (Fig. 13-41 and Table 13-1) the duodenal loop appears widened; and in asthenic individuals, portions of the duodenal loop will appear to be very close to one another, and sometimes overlapping. Occasionally, there is a redundancy of the first part of the duodenum (Fig. 13-42) with a greater segment peritonealized than is ordinarily seen. In some

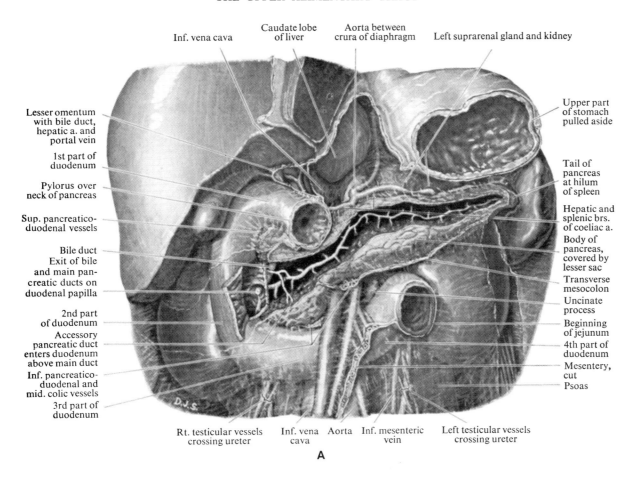

Inf. vena cava

Caudate lobe of liver

Aorta between crura of diaphragm

Left suprarenal gland and kidney

Lesser omentum with bile duct, hepatic a. and portal vein

1st part of duodenum

Pylorus over neck of pancreas

Sup. pancreatico-duodenal vessels

Bile duct
Exit of bile and main pancreatic ducts on duodenal papilla

2nd part of duodenum

Accessory pancreatic duct enters duodenum above main duct

Inf. pancreatico-duodenal and mid. colic vessels

3rd part of duodenum

Upper part of stomach pulled aside

Tail of pancreas at hilum of spleen

Hepatic and splenic brs. of coeliac a.

Body of pancreas, covered by lesser sac

Transverse mesocolon

Uncinate process

Beginning of jejunum

4th part of duodenum

Mesentery, cut

Psoas

Rt. testicular vessels crossing ureter

Inf. vena cava

Aorta

Inf. mesenteric vein

Left testicular vessels crossing ureter

A

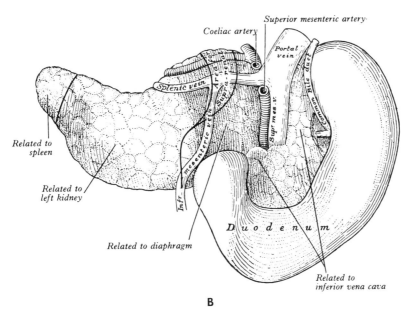

Coeliac artery

Superior mesenteric artery

Portal vein

Splenic vein

Related to spleen

Related to left kidney

Related to diaphragm

Duodenum

Related to inferior vena cava

B

Figure 13–35. *A.* Dissection of duodenum and pancreas. Transverse colon and part of stomach removed. (Reprinted by permission of Faber and Faber, Ltd., from Anatomy of the Human Body, by Lockhart, Hamilton, and Fyfer: Faber and Faber, London; J. B. Lippincott Company, Philadelphia.) *B.* Posterior aspect of the pancreas and duodenum from behind. (From Warwick, R., and Williams, P. L.: Gray's Anatomy, 35th British ed. Longman, London (for Churchill Livingstone), 1973.)

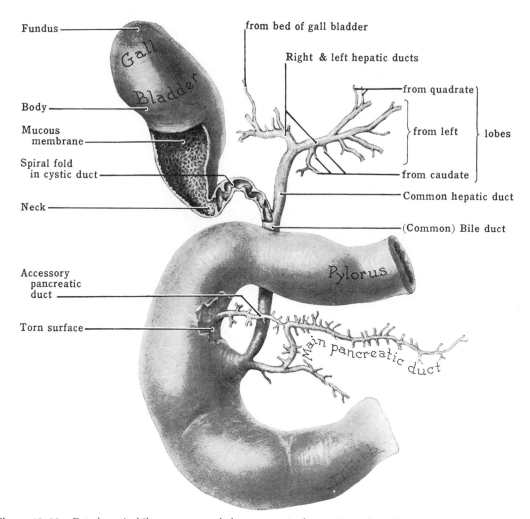

Figure 13–36. Extrahepatic bile passages and the pancreatic ducts. (Reproduced by permission from J. C. B. Grant: An Atlas of Anatomy, 5th ed. Copyright © 1962 by The Williams and Wilkins Company.)

individuals, the second part of the duodenum may be virtually lacking, and it would appear that the superior part of the duodenum connects almost directly with the horizontal part of the inferior portion of the duodenum.

These normal variations and anomalies must be constantly borne in mind when radiography of the duodenum is attempted.

Variations in the appearance of the duodenal bulb (Fig. 13–43). This is by far the most important part of the duodenum from the standpoint of incidence of abnormality. The normal bulb is usually very regular. It tends to be conical or triangular in shape, and variations from this configuration are usually of considerable significance. The apex of the bulb is usually surrounded by the feathery mucosa of the duodenum which contains plicae circulares, but the mucosal pattern of the bulb proper usually consists of fairly parallel rugae, or rugae arranged in the form of a spiral (Figs. 13–28 and 13–38).

The body habitus of the individual will to some extent cause some variation in the appearance of the bulb. In the short, squat person, the bulb tends to be small and posterior, hiding as it were behind the pyloric antrum. Occasionally also, in such people, the bulb will extend obliquely downward, especially if the stomach is high and steer-horn in type (Fig. 13–44 *A* and *B*).

Occasionally, the bulb is large and patulous in type, and tends to remain filled for a considerable period of time.

The normal rugae are ordinarily quite flexible and elastic, and can be quite readily obliterated by pressure, in contrast to the abnormal "fleck" which has already been mentioned (Fig. 13–45 *A* and *B*).

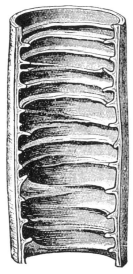

Figure 13-37. Anatomic presentation of the plicae circulares of the small intestine (jejunum). (From Cunningham's Textbook of Anatomy, 6th ed. London, Oxford University Press, 1931.)

The duodenum distal to the duodenal bulb. The second, third, and fourth portions of the duodenum have the normal feathery mucosal pattern already described. They appear as a single loop, with peristaltic waves carrying the barium around this loop.

Occasionally the duodenal papilla in the middle of the descending part of the duodenum will fill with barium or produce a small filling defect in the contour of the duodenum. This must not be interpreted as abnormal (Fig. 13-46).

There may be a slight hesitation when the barium passes the duodenojejunal junction, and usually an angulation can be detected in this region. This angle tends to be more obtuse in pyknic individuals.

Important Anatomic Relationships of the Stomach. The position of the stomach varies in different individuals, and in the same individual depending upon posture and emotional factors, as well as upon the digestive state (Figs. 13-29 and 13-30). The

The posture of the patient will also affect the appearance of the bulb. The duodenal bulb is best seen and most copiously filled when the patient is lying obliquely prone on his right side. It is least filled in the supine position.

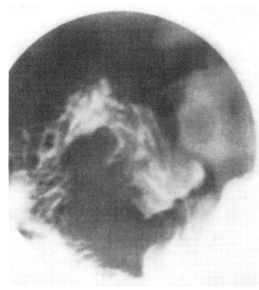

Figure 13-38. Mucosal pattern of the duodenal bulb and the change in pattern which occurs at the beginning of the second part of the duodenum.

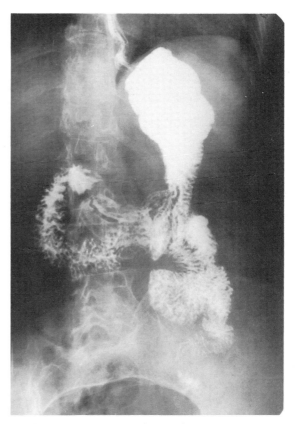

Figure 13-39. Anteroposterior view of stomach in slight left posterior oblique. Note the excellent double contrast of the distal stomach while the fundus is completely filled with barium. Note also the changes in mucosal pattern which occur more distally in the bulb and duodenum as well as in the jejunum.

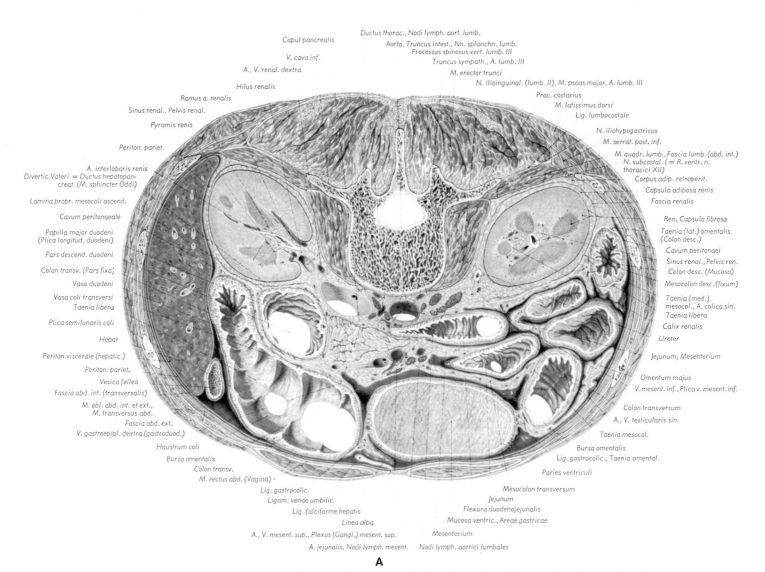

Caput pancreatis

Ductus thorac., Nodi lymph. aort. lumb.
Aorta, Truncus intest., Nn. splanchn. lumb.
Processus spinosus vert. lumb. III
Truncus sympath., A. lumb. III
M. erector trunci
N. ilioinguinal. (lumb. II), M. psoas major, A. lumb. III
Proc. costarius
M. latissimus dorsi
Lig. lumbocostale
N. iliohypogastricus
M. serrat. post. inf.
M. quadr. lumb., Fascia lumb. (abd. int.)
N. subcostal. (= R. ventr. n.
thoracici XII)
Corpus adip. retroperit.
Capsula adiposa renis
Fascia renalis
Ren, Capsula fibrosa
Taenia (lat.) omentalis
(Colon desc.)
Cavum peritonaei
Sinus renal., Pelvis ren.
Colon desc. (Mucosa)
Mesocolon desc. (fixum)
Taenia (med.)
mesocol., A. colica sin.
Taenia libera
Calix renalis
Ureter
Jejunum, Mesenterium
Omentum majus
V. mesent. inf., Plica v. mesent. inf.
Colon transversum
A., V. testicularis sin.
Taenia mesocol.
Bursa omentalis
Lig. gastrocolic., Taenia omental.
Paries ventriculi

V. cava inf.
A., V. renal. dextra
Hilus renalis
Ramus a. renalis
Sinus renal., Pelvis renal.
Pyramis renis
Periton. pariet.
A. interlobaris renis
Divertic. Vateri = Ductus hepatopan-
creat. (M. sphincter Oddi)
Lamina propr. mesocoli ascend.
Cavum peritonaeale
Papilla major duodeni
(Plica longitud. duodeni)
Pars descend. duodeni
Colon transv. (Pars fixa)
Vasa duodeni
Vasa coli transversi
Taenia libera
Plica semilunaris coli
Hepar
Periton. viscerale (hepatic.)
Periton. pariet.
Vesica fellea
Fascia abd. int. (transversalis)
M. obl. abd. int. et ext.,
M. transversus abd.
Fascia abd. ext.
V. gastroepipl. dextra (gastroduod.)
Haustrum coli
Bursa omentalis
Colon transv.
M. rectus abd. (Vagina)

Lig. gastrocolic.
Ligam. venae umbilic.
Lig. falciforme hepatis
Linea alba
A., V. mesent. sup., Plexus (Gangl.) mesent. sup.
A. jejunalis, Nodi lymph. mesent.

Mesocolon transversum
Jejunum
Flexura duodenojejunalis
Mucosa ventric., Areae gastricae
Mesenterium
Nodi lymph. aortici lumbales

A

Figure 13–40. A. Transverse section through abdomen at the level of the third lumbar vertebra. Section through spatium hepatorenale (compartment for liver, colon, duodenum, and kidneys) and spatium retrogastricum (cavum bursae oment.) of cavum peritonaei. (From Pernkopf, E.: Atlas of Topographical and Applied Human Anatomy. Vol. 2, Thorax, Abdomen, and Extremities. Philadelphia, W. B. Saunders Co., 1964.)

Figure 13–40 continued on the opposite page.

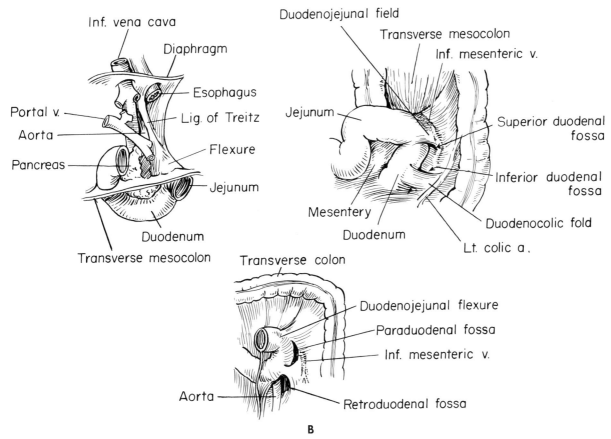

Figure 13–40 *Continued.* B. Line drawing indicating the structures involved at the duodenojejunal flexure and the duodenal fossae and folds. Note the superior duodenal fossa, the inferior duodenal fossa, and the paraduodenal fossa, and the relationship to the duodenojejunal flexure.

pylorus may lie as high as the twelfth thoracic vertebra, or as low as the upper sacrum. It may lie in the midline, or to the right or left of it. Associated with these different positions of the pylorus, there is a difference in the position of the first part of the duodenum, and its relation to the head of the pancreas. Likewise, the stomach may be high and the liver low, and vice versa, indicating no definite relation between their relative positions (Fig. 13–47).

Ordinarily, the stomach is obliquely placed in the left upper abdominal cavity (Fig. 13–48), with the fundus somewhat more lateral than the pylorus. In the lateral projection, the fundus is posterior to the liver, in apposition with the diaphragm above and behind. The body of the stomach is anterior, lying immediately under the anterior abdominal wall. The pyloric antrum extends obliquely posteriorly, superiorly, and to the right. Usually the pylorus is situated just above the head of the pancreas (Fig. 13–

48) in the posterior part of the abdomen, in a plane just anterior (1 to 2 cm.) to the plane of the second part (retroperitoneal portion) of the duodenum.

The hepatogastric and hepatoduodenal ligaments constitute the lesser omentum which is attached to the lesser curvature of the stomach and forms a part of the omental bursa—an anatomic relationship of considerable practical significance (Fig. 13–49).

The spleen lies posterior and somewhat lateral to the body of the stomach, with the gastrosplenic ligament attaching it to the greater curvature of the stomach (Fig. 13–50).

The head of the pancreas lies in the duodenal loop (Fig. 13–48), whereas the body of the pancreas lies posterior to the pyloric portion of the stomach. The tail of the pancreas usually lies just posterior to the body of the stomach, and comes into contact with the medial surface of the spleen. The pancreas forms a large part

(Text continued on page 804.)

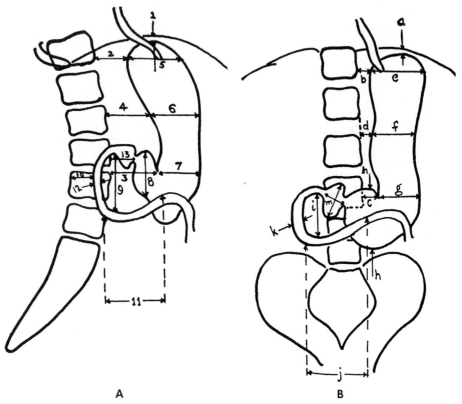

A   **B**

Figure 13–41. Lateral (*A*) and frontal (*B*) views of the stomach showing the various measurements which can be taken in an effort to associate the normal stomach with body build. (From Meschan, I., et al.: South. Med. J., *46*, 1953.)

1, Distance between top of fundus and diaphragm.
2, Cardia of stomach to anterior spine.
3, Stomach to anterior spine at level of cardia.
4, Stomach to anterior spine midway between cardia and incisura angularis.
5, Horizontal measurement of fundus at level of cardia.
6, Horizontal midway measurement of body of stomach at level of measurement 4.
7, Horizontal measurement of stomach at level of incisura angularis.
8, Maximal vertical measurement of pyloric antrum.
9, Maximal vertical internal diameter of duodenal loop.
10, Minimal measurement of outer margin of second portion of duodenum to posterior margin of vertebral bodies.
11, Maximal horizontal internal diameter of duodenal loop.
12, Maximal outer diameter of second part of duodenum.
13, Distance between pylorus and anterior margin of spine.

a, Measurement between diaphragm and top of fundus.
b, Distance between cardia and lateral margin of spine.
c, Distance between incisura angularis and lateral margin of spine.
d, Distance between stomach and lateral margin of spine midway between b and c.
e, Maximal horizontal measurement of fundus at level of cardia.
f, Midway measurement of body of stomach at level of measurement d.
g, Horizontal measurement of body of stomach at level of incisura angularis.
h, Maximal vertical measurement of pyloric antrum.
i, Maximal vertical internal diameter of duodenal loop.
j, Maximal horizontal internal diameter of duodenal loop.
k, Diameter of second part of duodenum.
m, Ratio of the measurement of base of the bulb over its height from apex to pylorus.

TABLE 13–1 RELATIONSHIPS OF STOMACH AND DUODENUM TO THE SPINE IN DIFFERENT WEIGHT AND STOMACH TYPE GROUPS (BOTH ASYMPTOMATIC AND SYMPTOMATIC SUMMATED)*

Weight Group	Stomach Type	No. of Cases	4 Rt. Lat.[a] Avg. of Medians	4 Rt. Lat.[a] Range	4 Lt. Lat.[a] Avg. of Medians	4 Lt. Lat.[a] Range	9 Rt. Lat.[a] Avg. of Medians	9 Rt. Lat.[a] Range	10 Rt. Lat.[a] Avg. of Medians	10 Rt. Lat.[a] Range	11 Rt. Lat.[a] Avg. of Medians	11 Rt. Lat.[a] Range	13 Rt. Lat.[a] Avg. of Medians	13 Rt. Lat.[a] Range
Normal	J-shape	58	5.5	1 — 8.5	4	0 — 8	6.5	4 — 9.5	3	−1 — 9	3	0 — 12.5	4	−0.5— 8
	Fish-hook	10	4	1.5— 6	3	0.5— 6.5	6	4 — 8	3	2.5— 4	5.6	3.5— 8	4.5	2.5— 9
	Cascade[b]	13	6	1 — 13	5.5	1.5— 13	6	4.5— 6	4.3	2 — 9.5	6.6	1 — 11	6	2.5— 9
	Steer-horn	9	5	0 — 11	4	1 — 13	6.5	5.5— 8	3.5	−0.5— 5	5.5	1.5— 9	5	2.5— 10
Underweight	J-shape	56	4.5	1.5— 7	2	0.5— 8	5.5	2 — 11	3	−0.5— 7	4	0 — 9	3	0.5— 6.5
	Fish-hook	21	4	0 — 7.5	2.6	−1.5— 4.5	5.5	3.5— 8	2.5	0 — 5	3	1.5— 5	2.5	1 — 4
	Cascade[b]	5	5	2 — 8	2.6	0 — 5	6	5.5— 6.5	2.5	2 — 3.5	4.5	4 — 5	3	2 — 5
	Steer-horn	3	5	4.5— 6	6.5	0.5— 7.5	8	8	4.5	2 — 6	7	6.5— 8	4	1.5— 5
Overweight	J-shape	13	5.5	1.5— 10	4	1.5— 8.5	6.5	4 — 9	3.3	2 — 7	4.5	3.5— 9	3.5	1.5— 9.5
	Fish-hook	5	5	3 — 7.5	4	0 — 5.5	5	3 — 7.5	2.5	0 — 4	4.5	2 — 9.5	4.6	3 — 6.5—
	Cascade[b]	10	5	2 — 11	5.5	0 — 9	7	4 — 9	4	1 — 7.5	5	1.5— 10	5.6	3 — 12
	Steer-horn	8	6	2.5— 9.5	4.6	2.5— 8	6	5.5— 8	4	3.5— 5.5	5	3 — 7.5	4.5	3 — 7.5—
	Total	211												

*From Meschan, I. et al.: The normal radiographic adult stomach and duodenum. South. Med. J., 46:878, 1953.
[a]Measurements are defined in Figure 13–41.
[b]Asymptomatic cascade is farther from spine than symptomatic.

DUODENAL ANOMALIES

DEFECTIVE ATTACHMENT OF DUODENAL MESENTERY

MOBILE DUODENUM

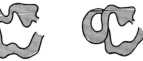

DUODENUM APPEARS INVERTED

RECUMBENT

DUODENUM HAS NORMAL APPEARANCE

ERECT

REDUNDANCY – FIRST PART

REDUNDANCY- 3rd PART

NONROTATION OF DUODENUM

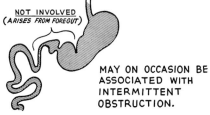

NOT INVOLVED (ARISES FROM FOREGUT)

LOWER DUODENUM CURVES TO RIGHT INSTEAD OF LEFT AND JOINS JEJUNUM IN RIGHT UPPER QUADRANT (USUALLY NONROTATION OF JEJUNUM ALSO.)

MAY ON OCCASION BE ASSOCIATED WITH INTERMITTENT OBSTRUCTION.

INVERTED DUODENUM

MAY PREDISPOSE TO PANCREATITIS DUE TO TWIST OF BILE DUCT AND REFLUX INTO PANCREAS.

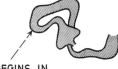

INVERSION BEGINS IN 2nd PART USUALLY.

Figure 13–42.

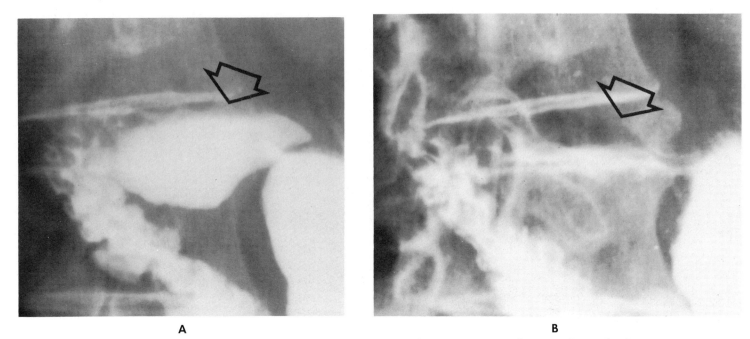

Figure 13-43. *A* and *B*. Normal duodenal bulb in two stages of contraction, *B* simulating an elongated pyloric canal.

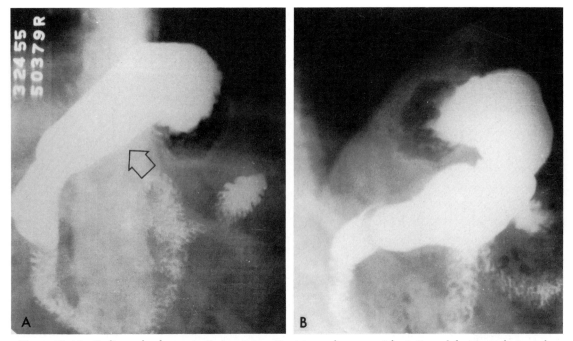

Figure 13-44. Radiographs demonstrating an intermittent type of organoaxial rotation of the stomach. In *A* the inferior margin of the stomach is concave and the stomach is situated high under the diaphragm. In *B* the stomach is in a relatively normal position. This type of rotation has also been referred to as incomplete volvulus.

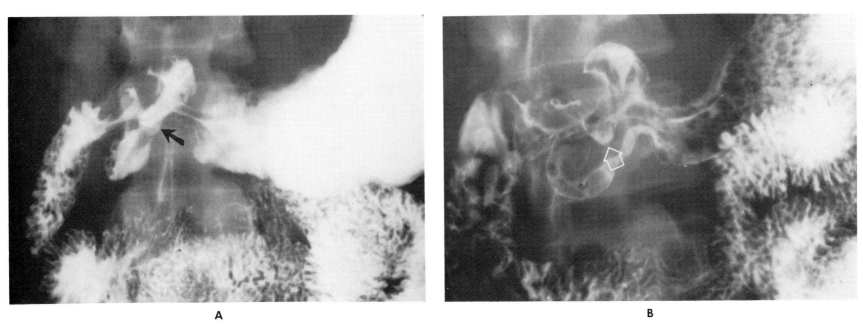

Figure 13–45. *A* and *B*. Duodenal ulcer showing the advantages of double contrast with barium and air, (*A*) erect, and (*B*) supine. Both views show the ulcer.

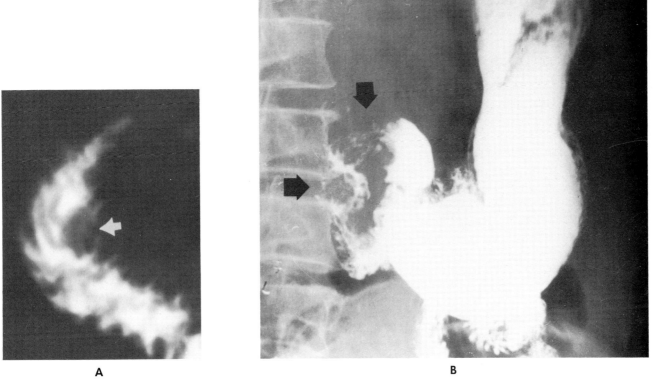

Figure 13–46. *A*. Occasional normal appearance of the major papilla indenting the second part of the duodenum. *B*. Abnormal indentations on the second part of the duodenum (for comparison with *A*). (Carcinoma of the pancreas with matted lymph nodes and a dilated common duct.)

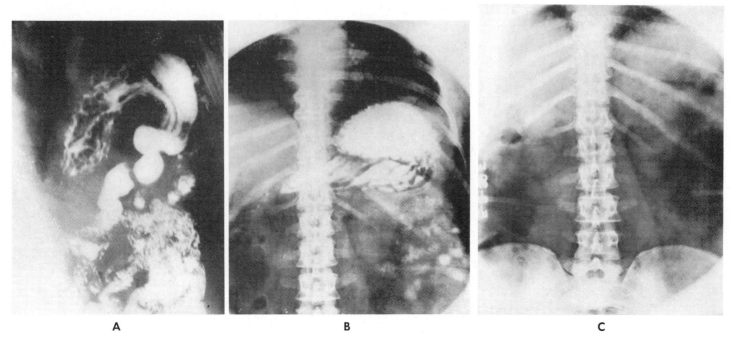

A   B   C

Figure 13-47. "Cascade" stomach. *A.* Radiograph in the right anterior oblique position. *B.* Slight cascade stomach in anteroposterior projection. *C.* Same as *B* without the barium, showing how the fundus of such a stomach may simulate a mass in the left upper quadrant. (*B* and *C* courtesy of Drs. H. L. Friedell and C. C. Dundon, University Hospitals, Cleveland, Ohio.)

of the posterior wall of the lesser omental bursa, whereas the posterior wall of the stomach forms the greater part of the anterior wall of this important "sac." Abnormalities of this bursa and the pancreas are therefore frequently reflected in pressure upon the stomach, with alteration of the normal gastric contour (Fig. 13–51).

The transverse colon is loosely connected with the greater curvature of the stomach via the greater omentum, which hangs like an apron over the entire intestinal tract. The splenic flexure of the colon is lateral to the lower greater curvature of the stomach and closely applied to the undersurface of the spleen.

In most texts dealing with gross anatomy, there is reference to the "stomach chamber" or "bed" in which the stomach is said to lie. Radiographically, the stomach usually extends more inferiorly than is indicated by the dissection of the cadavers.

When the patient lies down, the stomach moves freely about its two points of fixation, the diaphragm superiorly and the postbulbar duodenum inferiorly. In the right lateral projection, it swings anteriorly like a hammock, and is no longer closely applied to the retrogastric structures. In the right lateral position with the patient lying down, the relationship of fundus-to-body-to-antrum will vary from one patient to another, depending upon

adjoining pressure phenomena. When the patient lies on his left side, the stomach is concave toward the left, with the fundus and duodenal bulb being uppermost. Any food or barium in the stomach under these circumstances will tend to gravitate to the body of the stomach and air will rise to the fundus and duodenal bulb. Thus, the left posterior oblique, approximately 45 degrees with the patient lying supine on his left side, is particularly valuable for obtaining double contrast visualization of the fundus, antrum, and duodenal bulb (and sometimes the remainder of the duodenum as well). When the patient is in the prone position, in the right anterior oblique, the fundus of the stomach continues to retain some air, but barium contained within the stomach will gravitate to the body and antrum as well as to the duodenal bulb. When the patient is lying directly prone, there is some pressure of the spine upon the adjoining portion of the pyloric antrum and duodenal bulb. The right anterior oblique view frees the stomach from pressure against the spine and hence, is ordinarily the desired view for optimum visualization of peristalsis. The left lateral erect film offers the best opportunity to study the stomach in relation to the structures posterior to it.

To demonstrate gastroesophageal reflux, the optimum positions are as follows: first, the patient lies supine on the left side in

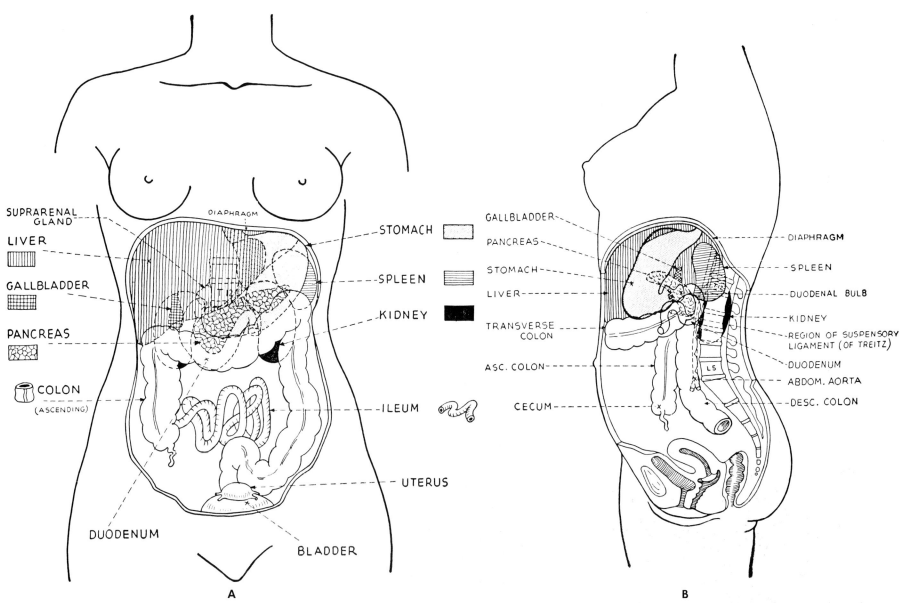

Figure 13–48.   Important anatomic relationships of the stomach. *A.* Anteroposterior view. *B.* Lateral view (right, recumbent).

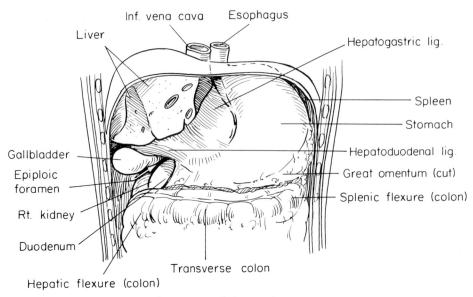

Figure 13–49. Stomach *in situ*, with hepatic ligaments, greater omentum cut.

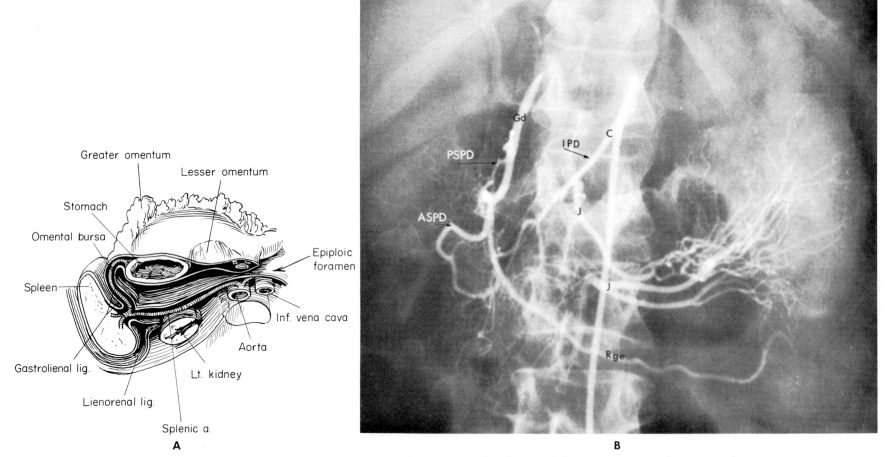

A   **B**

Figure 13–50. *A*. Cross-section showing relation of stomach, spleen, and adjoining structures to lesser omental bursa and epiploic foramen. *B*. Celiac arterial axis as related to the stomach, spleen, and greater omentum. (J) Catheter *in situ*, (Rge) right gastroepiploic artery, (C) celiac artery, (IPD) inferior anterior pancreaticoduodenal artery, (PSPD) posterior superior pancreaticoduodenal artery, (ASPD) anterior superior pancreaticoduodenal artery, the latter two making an arcade. (From Ruzicka, F. F., and Rossi, P.: Radiol. Clin. N. Amer., 8:3–29, 1970.)

Figure 13–50 continued on the opposite page.

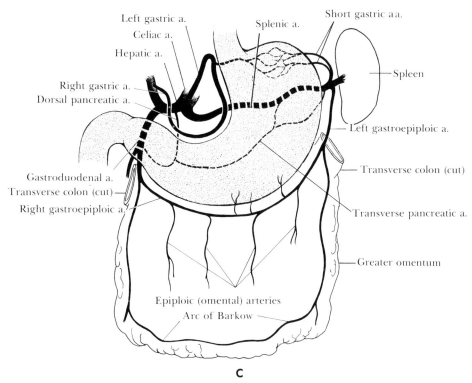

Left gastric a.
Celiac a.
Hepatic a.
Right gastric a.
Dorsal pancreatic a.
Splenic a.
Short gastric a a.
Spleen
Left gastroepiploic a.
Transverse colon (cut)
Transverse pancreatic a.
Gastroduodenal a.
Transverse colon (cut)
Right gastroepiploic a.
Greater omentum
Epiploic (omental) arteries
Arc of Barkow

C

Figure 13–50 *Continued.* C. Line drawing representative of celiac arterial axis as related to stomach and greater omentum. (Modified from Ruzicka, F. F., and Rossi, P.: Radiol. Clin. N. Amer., 8:3–29, 1970.)

a moderate Trendelenburg position; second, the patient bends forward so that the esophagus lies below the level of the fundus of the stomach. Both methods demonstrate a gastroesophageal reflux in the presence of an incompetent gastroesophageal junction.

The Rugal Pattern of Each Subdivision of the Stomach (Fig. 13–28).   When the stomach is wholly or partially empty, the muscular layers contract and throw the mucosa into numerous folds or rugae which project into the interior of the stomach. The rugae of the fundus tend to be arranged in a mosaic, which gradually becomes more regular in the body of the stomach. The mosaic appearance is more marked along the greater curvature and this pattern gradually diminishes toward the pylorus.

The rugae tend to remain parallel in a narrow segment on the lesser curvature of the stomach throughout the entire length of the stomach from the cardia to the pylorus. These longitudinal rugae form the "magenstrasse," which seems to consitute a channel for the usual descent of the food, although not invariably so.

The rugae in the pylorus are thin parallel folds. These parallel folds continue into the duodenal cap or bulb, where they either remain parallel or spiral toward the apex of the duodenal bulb.

Between the rugae, there are minute depressions caused by the openings of the small gastric glands, and minute ridges around them, giving the stomach mucosa the so-called mammillated appearance. These minute mammillae are not recognizable radiographically.

The rugal pattern of the stomach must not be thought of as completely static—it can vary in the same individual under different physiologic conditions. Thus, it will vary in accordance with the degree of vascularity of the mucosa and submucosa and also with the degree of distention of the stomach. Cold tends to make the rugae smaller and more numerous, and certain chemicals such as pilocarpine and physostigmine have the same effect, whereas atropine has the opposite effect.

However, the rugal pattern will change in certain pathologic states such as inflammation, ulceration, and neoplastic infiltration, as well as from extrinsic pressure, and the rugae thus become one of the most accurate indices which the radiologic examination of the stomach furnishes. Examination for rugal pattern constitutes one of the most important aspects of the gastrointestinal examination, if not the most important.

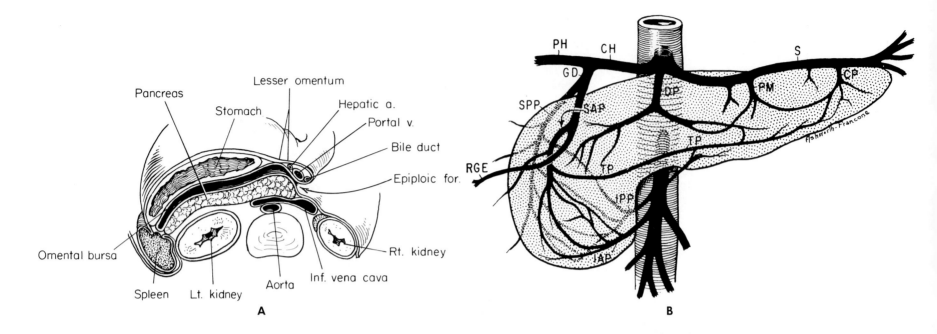

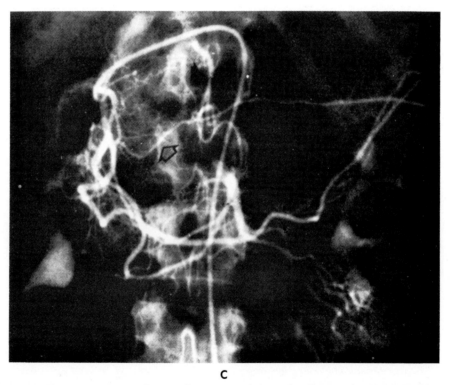

Figure 13–51. *A.* Transverse section relations of pancreas and stomach to lesser omental sac. *B.* Schematic drawing of the arterial supply to the pancreas. (CH) common hepatic, (PH) proper hepatic, (GD) gastroduodenal, (RGE) right gastroepiploic, (SAP) superior anterior pancreaticoduodenal, (SPP) superior posterior pancreaticoduodenal, (IAP) inferior anterior pancreaticoduodenal, (IPP) inferior posterior pancreaticoduodenal, (S) splenic, (DP) dorsal pancreatic, (PM) pancreatic magna, (CP) caudal pancreatic, (TP) transverse pancreatic. *C.* Superselective arteriography of the normal gastroduodenal artery with visualization of its pancreaticoduodenal branches. The transverse pancreatic (unfilled arrow), dorsal pancreatic (filled arrow), and branches of the superior mesenteric artery are filled through anastomotic vessels. (*B* and *C* from Rösch, J., and Judkins, M. P.: Seminars in Roentgenol., 3:296–309, 1968.)

Physiologic Considerations Concerning the Stomach

Gastric Glandular Secretions (Figs. 13–52 and 13–53). Gastric glandular secretions arise from (1) cardiac glands, situated in a 5 mm. zone (approximately) around the esophagogastric junction or cardia; (2) fundic glands situated for the most part throughout the remainder of the fundus and body of the stomach; and (3) pyloric glands, situated in the region of the antrum. There is no sharply demarcated boundary line in the stomach in respect to these glandular secretions. The fundic glands contain chief cells which are responsible for pepsinogen secretion; parietal cells are responsible for the secretion of hydrochloric acid as well as intrinsic factors. There are scattered argentaffin cells throughout the body and antrum, and occasionally parietal cells are also found in the antrum. In addition, the hormone gastrin is secreted by the antrum. This apparently is responsible for stimulating the activity of parietal cells.

Although mucus is found predominantly surrounding the cardiac orifice, where it is secreted by cardiac glands, and in the antrum, secreted by pyloric cells, mucous secretions are found throughout the entire stomach and arise from fundic glands as well.

In subtotal gastric resection in the treatment of persistent peptic ulcer, it is important to extirpate those portions of the stomach that are predominantly responsible for acid secretion and also the portion responsible for gastrin secretion that, if allowed to remain, will stimulate the remaining parietal cells to hyperactivity. Subtotal resections of the stomach, therefore, must include for the greatest efficiency the entire body and antrum of the stomach and possibly portions of the fundus.

Gastric and Duodenal Evacuation, Tone, and Peristalsis. Usually, from two to five simultaneous peristaltic waves are observed in the stomach, with the greatest activity occurring in the distal half. The stomach will empty its contents when the pressure in the stomach exceeds the pressure in the duodenum;

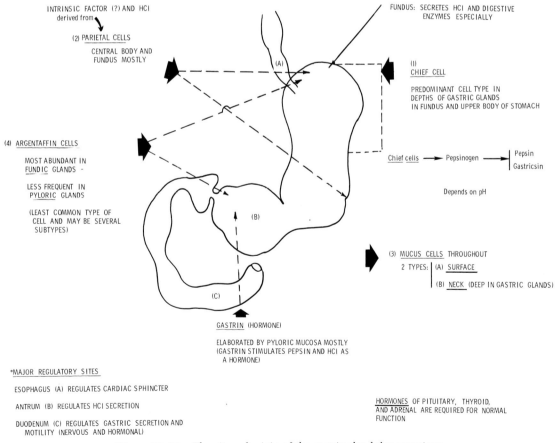

Figure 13–52. The sites of origin of the gastric glandular secretions.

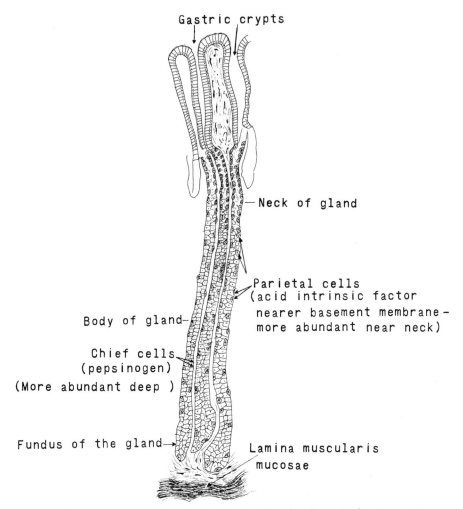

Gastric crypts

Neck of gland

Parietal cells
(acid intrinsic factor
nearer basement membrane—
more abundant near neck)

Body of gland

Chief cells
(pepsinogen)
(More abundant deep)

Fundus of the gland

Lamina muscularis
mucosae

Figure 13–53. Histology of a fundic gland. (Modified from Jordan, H. E.: A Textbook of Histology. New York, D. Appleton-Century, 1934.)

The main function of the pyloric sphincter normally is to prevent regurgitation from the duodenum into the stomach (Quigley and Meschan). The entire process of gastric evacuation is very aptly described by Quigley and Louckes as follows: "The stomach is a tolerant organ and accepts with relative indifference substances which are very hot, cold, hypertonic, or distinctly irritant. . . , and the volume which may be ingested without gastric rebellion may stretch the very elastic gastric wall almost to the point of rupture."

"The duodenum, in contrast, will only accept chyme in small quantities and after the chyme is prepared to meet rigid requirements. If chyme enters the duodenum too rapidly or is too hot or cold or contains excessive concentrations of fats, alcohol, condiments, etc., the duodenum revolts by producing nausea or vomiting or signals by a 'feed-back' mechanism to the stomach that evacuation should be retarded and the material retained by the stomach until it is made more acceptable to the duodenum. This 'feed-back' mechanism operates in a more moderate form to depress the antral peristalsis and insure the chyme of being delivered to the duodenum in moderate quantities and in a form which will be readily tolerated."

"In brief, it is the purpose of the stomach to accept almost anything that is presented to it in almost any volume, and, by bringing this material to body temperature and proper isotonicity and dilution (fats, condiments, etc.) to make it acceptable to the relatively 'intolerant' duodenum and then deliver it to the duodenum at a moderate rate."[1]

In the presence of gastric retention it must not be assumed that the obstruction is necessarily pyloric in origin. At times, inadequacy of the evacuation mechanism may result from a hypotonicity of the stomach from some undetermined cause (that is, vagotomy). It would be folly to treat such dysfunction with atropine-like drugs (Fig. 13–54).

Gastric Tone. Vagal stimulation increases gastric tone, whereas sympathetic stimulation decreases it. Thus, when a person is frightened or otherwise emotionally disturbed, the stomach tends to be hypotonic. Pathologic processes in the gastrointestinal tract elsewhere or the biliary tract may also cause changes in the stomach.

Factors Influencing Rate of Gastric Evacuation. Of practical importance are the following normal considerations:

The type of meal will alter the rate of gastric evacuation considerably. The presence of any food will depress gastrobulbar peristalsis and prolong the emptying time by about three times. This function is caused by a reflex or hormone (enterogastrone) operating from the duodenum. The presence of alkali such as sodium bicarbonate in the stomach will increase the rate of gastric evacuation. Only isotonicity, with no food substances contained in the meal, will not alter the rate of evacuation. Normally, with

regurgitation from the duodenum will occur when there is a reversal of this pressure relationship. The pyloric antrum, pylorus, and duodenal bulb tend to act as a single unit in response to various food stimuli.

After the introduction of barium into the stomach, emptying begins almost immediately, and the main bulk of the barium meal will have left the stomach in 1 to 2 hours, with no residual trace after 3 hours. Hyperacidity in the stomach will permit the retention of a coating of barium on the gastric mucosa that in itself is not an indication of abnormality. Six hour retention to any significant degree is pathologic, and it is customary to obtain a film 3 to 6 hours later for this purpose. On the other hand, retention in infants may be normal up to 8 hours after a barium meal, but anything beyond 8 hours may be interpreted as pathologic.

[1]Quigley, J. P., and Louckes, H. S.: Amer. J. Digest. Dis., 7:672–676, 1962.

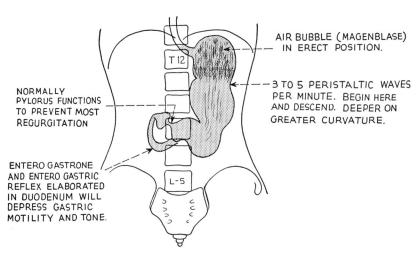

NORMALLY PYLORUS FUNCTIONS TO PREVENT MOST REGURGITATION

T 12

AIR BUBBLE (MAGENBLASE) IN ERECT POSITION.

3 TO 5 PERISTALTIC WAVES PER MINUTE. BEGIN HERE AND DESCEND. DEEPER ON GREATER CURVATURE.

ENTERO GASTRONE AND ENTERO GASTRIC REFLEX ELABORATED IN DUODENUM WILL DEPRESS GASTRIC MOTILITY AND TONE.

L-5

Figure 13–54. Diagram illustrating résumé of gastric motor physiology.

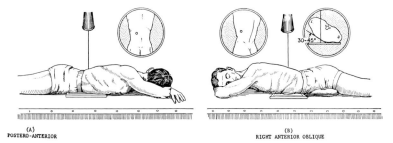

(A) POSTERO-ANTERIOR

(B) RIGHT ANTERIOR OBLIQUE

Figure 13–55. Radiographic examination of the esophagus, stomach, and duodenum.

food-free barium suspension, emptying will begin almost immediately after the introduction of the barium into the stomach, and the main bulk of the meal will have left the stomach in 1 hour, with no residual trace in 2 or 3 hours. Hypoacidity in the stomach will permit the retention of a coating of barium on the gastric mucosa, which in itself is not an indication of abnormality. Six hour retention of any significant degree in the adult, or 8 hour retention in the infant is pathologic, and it is customary to obtain a film in 6 or 8 hours for this purpose.

Cascade Stomach (Fig. 13–47). Occasionally, the posterior portion of the fundus of the stomach will fill first, and the remainder of the stomach will fill by overflow from the fundus. This is called a cascade stomach. It may be related to overdistention of the splenic flexure of the colon or to localized muscular hypertonus. Occasionally it is related to adhesions between the stomach and the diaphragm, but it cannot be properly called a normal variation under these circumstances.

Methods of Roentgenologic Study of the Stomach and Duodenum

Technique of Fluoroscopy and Spot Film Compression Radiography (Figs. 13–55, 13–56, and 13–57)

1. With the patient standing, after the initial survey of the chest and abdomen, the patient is given a cup of barium suspension containing 100 grams of barium sulfate suspended in a glassful (8 oz.) of water.

2. The manner in which the barium enters the stomach is carefully studied. Ordinarily, this first swallow of barium follows

along the "magenstrasse" on the lesser curvature of the stomach. In the presence of excessive fluid in the stomach the barium drops into the fluid like pellets in a glass of water. The lesser curvature is normally smooth below the level of the cardia and any variation is of definite significance. Spot films of the rugal pattern of the stomach are obtained at this time, particularly in the right anterior oblique, using compression if desirable (Fig. 13–57 A, B, C).

If the barium fills the duodenal bulb and spills over into the second part of the duodenum at this point, an additional spot film of the duodenal bulb is obtained (Fig. 13–57 D).

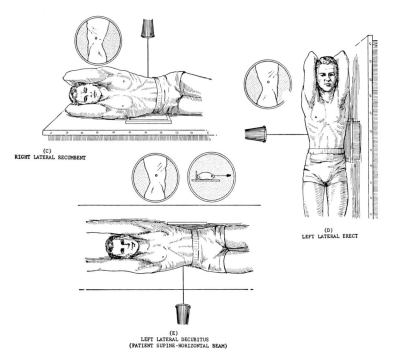

(C) RIGHT LATERAL RECUMBENT

(D) LEFT LATERAL ERECT

(E) LEFT LATERAL DECUBITUS (PATIENT SUPINE-HORIZONTAL BEAM)

Figure 13–56. Diagrams illustrating the routine positioning technique for examination of the stomach radiographically, apart from fluoroscopy.

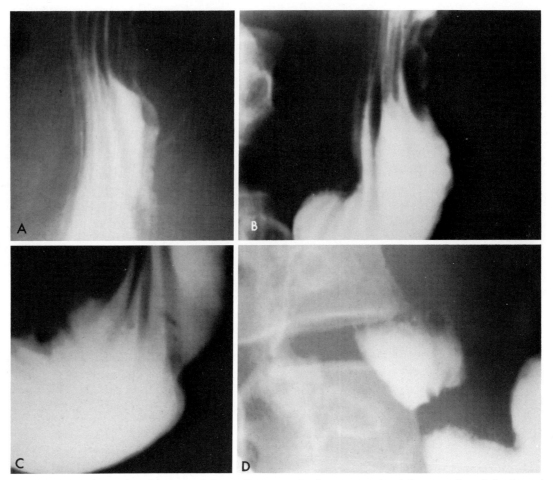

Figure 13–57. Films ordinarily obtained during fluoroscopy and routine study of the stomach and duodenum. *A.* Initial spot film of gastric rugae (body of stomach) immediately following the first swallow of barium. *B.* Second spot film showing the rugal pattern of the body and antrum. *C.* Third spot film demonstrates the lower half of the body and antrum of the stomach. *D.* Spot film showing the distal antrum, pyloric canal, and initial filling of the duodenal bulb.

Figure 13–57 continued on the opposite page.

3. Otherwise, the patient, still in the right anterior oblique, is given additional swallows of barium, and the swallowing function as well as the stomach are studied. The gastroesophageal junction and the action of the constrictor diaphragmae are particularly noted. The patient is in frontal and right anterior oblique projections at this point, and additional spot film studies of the duodenal bulb are obtained in these projections (Fig. 13–57 *E*).

4. The patient then swallows the remainder of the barium, and peristalsis and contour of the stomach and duodenum are studied in all projections. An additional spot film of the stomach or duodenal bulb in the left anterior oblique projection is obtained if necessary (Fig. 13–57 *F*).

This provides a profile study of the duodenal bulb on its anterior and posterior aspect as well as the stomach on its lesser and greater curvature.

5. The patient is then turned with his right side toward the table, arms above his head, leaning slightly in the right anterior oblique, and the tilt table is turned into the horizontal so that the patient is lying somewhat prone on his right side.

6. The gastroesophageal junction, peristalsis of the stomach, and the duodenum are then studied in this right lateral relationship. A spot film of the entire duodenal loop is obtained at this juncture (Fig. 13–57 *G*), and, if desired, an additional film of the gastroesophageal junction.

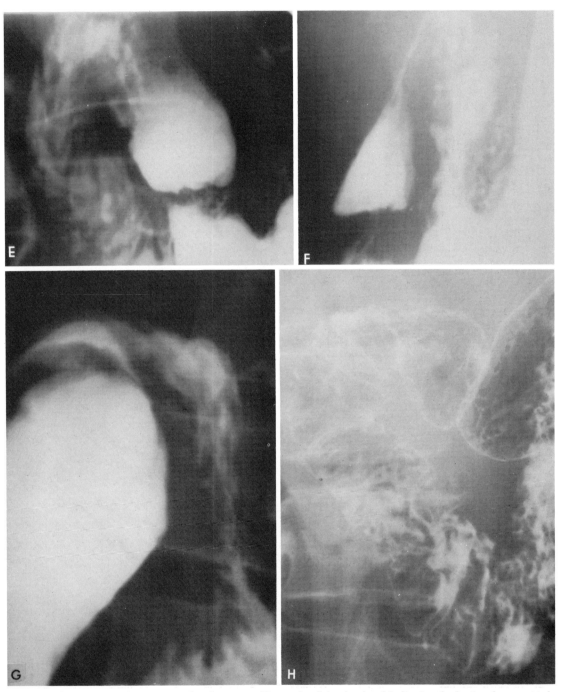

Figure 13–57 *Continued.* E. Somewhat later spot film study of the duodenal bulb after the barium has emptied from it into the second part of the duodenum (patient still in the erect position). F. Spot film study in the left anterior oblique, demonstrating the full duodenal bulb, especially in relation to its anterior and posterior margins. The apex of the bulb and second part of the duodenum are also well demonstrated. G. This film study, with the patient lying on his right side, slightly oblique toward prone, demonstrates the relationship of the stomach, the duodenum, and the duodenal bulb. H. Patient supine with right side elevated, left side down. The air rises into the duodenal bulb and second part of the duodenum, imparting to these structures a double contrast. A spot film is then obtained.

Figure 13–57 continued on the following page.

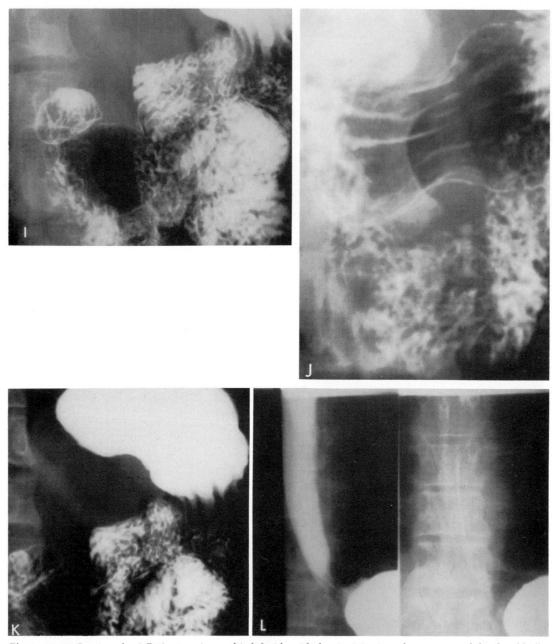

Figure 13–57 *Continued.* *I.* Patient supine on his left side with the air rising into the antrum and duodenal bulb. A full film of the stomach is then obtained. *J.* Patient supine with air occupying the body of the stomach for demonstration of double contrast visualization of the rugae of the body of the stomach. *K.* Patient supine with the barium moving by gravity into the fundus of the stomach. The full contour of the fundus of the stomach is thereby studied. *L.* Patient supine on left side. Additional swallows of barium are given and the esophagus studied both morphologically and physiologically. The patient is asked to strain with the Valsalva maneuver immediately after swallowing and then after the esophagus is emptied. The esophagus is studied for possible gastroesophageal reflux. This may be followed by a "water test" in all cases where hiatal hernia is demonstrated and where esophageal reflux is suspected.

Figure 13–57 continued on the opposite page.

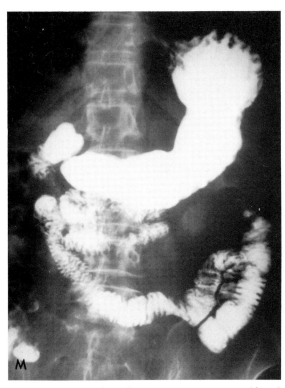

Figure 13–57 *Continued.* M. The full 14 × 17 posteroanterior film of the stomach and proximal small intestine obtained with routine Bucky technique, immediately following the fluoroscopy.

swallows of barium, the patient is encouraged to empty the contents of his mouth, and attempt an additional straining maneuver to see whether or not gastroesophageal reflux is obtained in this projection (Fig. 13–57 M).

10. Further tests for gastroesophageal reflux may be made by turning the patient into the Trendelenburg position at this time and studying regurgitation with a swallow of water. The barium normally will reflux back somewhat into the esophagus, but abnormally a considerable admixture of water with the barium rises from the stomach back into the esophagus.

11. If a hiatal hernia is noted or if esophageal varices are suspected, thick barium is then administered in order to study the rugal pattern of the lower esophagus with and without the Valsalva maneuver. Varices will impart a wormlike pattern to the lower esophageal rugae which is accentuated by the Valsalva maneuver. This accentuation is virtually pathognomonic of esophageal varices in contrast with other irregularities such as esophagitis, which produce a somewhat similar appearance.

This routine of examination of the esophagus, stomach, and duodenum is the one we have followed satisfactorily for a considerable period of time. Other routines in current use may be found in the study reported by Burhenne of 15 different institutions in the United States and Europe.

The pyloric canal is ordinarily no greater than 5 mm. in length and 5 to 8 mm. in diameter. The direction of the long axis of the pylorus, like that of the stomach, will depend upon those factors discussed under variation in gastric contour. Tone, body habitus, and emotional influences all play a part, as previously indicated. The pylorus is ordinarily centrally placed with respect to the base of the duodenal bulb; eccentricity is of pathological significance. Its appearance in relation to the duodenal bulb resembles that of a basal stem to its leaf. The rugae of the pyloric canal are quite narrow and parallel in contrast with the slightly wider rugal pattern of the antrum on the one side and the spiral pattern of the duodenal bulb on the other.

Attention is paid throughout this examination to the position, contour, pliability, and peristalsis of the stomach, and points of tenderness and masses nearby. If pancreatic disease is suspected from the clinical history, it is particularly important to study the patient in the left lateral erect position.

The importance of spot film compression radiography can hardly be overemphasized in the radiographic study of the gastrointestinal tract. Film visualization of an anatomic part is far more accurate and detailed than is fluoroscopy, and this method of film radiography has the additional advantage of compression, the patient being turned so that the desired anatomy is demonstrated. The permanent recording of a part under fluoroscopic control is possible. It has been repeatedly demonstrated that compression may bring out a defect which otherwise might escape detection.

7. The patient is next turned to the prone or the 45 degree oblique position, and peristalsis of the entire stomach and duodenum is carefully studied and spot films obtained as necessary.

8. Next, the patient is turned onto his left side at an obliquity of 45 degrees. Gas in the stomach will then rise to the pyloric antrum, duodenal bulb, and duodenum. One or two spot films of the entire duodenal loop are taken with the double contrast provided by the air entering the antrum and the duodenum (Fig. 13–57 H). Additional spot films of the stomach are obtained with this double contrast evaluation (Fig. 13–57 I and J). With the patient lying somewhat flatter on his back, the entire fundus is carefully studied since it is now filled with barium (Fig. 13–57 K).

9. In the same position (45 degrees oblique, supine, left side down), the patient is given an additional half cup of barium to swallow. The entire esophagus is then studied and spot films are obtained of the esophagogastric junction with the patient performing the Valsalva maneuver (Fig. 13–57 L). After several

Routine Films Obtained Following Fluoroscopic Study

In addition, the *routine radiographs usually obtained are:* (1) recumbent posteroanterior (prone), straight frontal projection (Fig. 13–58); (2) right anterior oblique prone (Fig. 13–59); (3) right lateral recumbent (Fig. 13–60); (4) posteroanterior full abdominal view in 4 or 6 hours for study of the extent of gastric evacuation (Fig. 13–61).

These are demonstrated in the accompanying illustrations, and the various anatomic portions labeled.

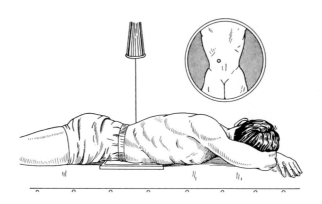

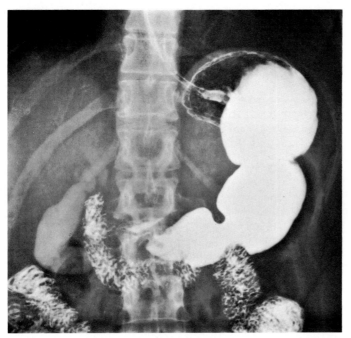

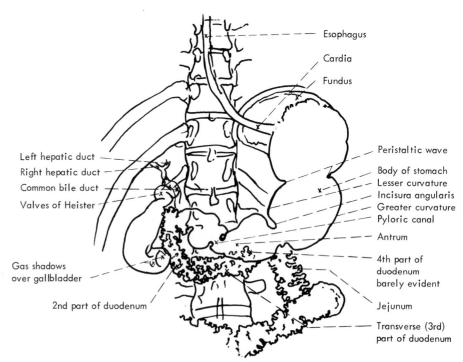

Figure 13–58. Recumbent posteroanterior projection of stomach and duodenum. (An oral cholecystogram was also obtained at this time in the film illustrated.)

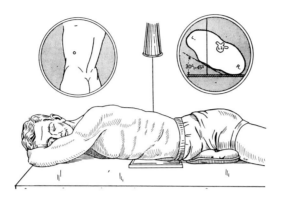

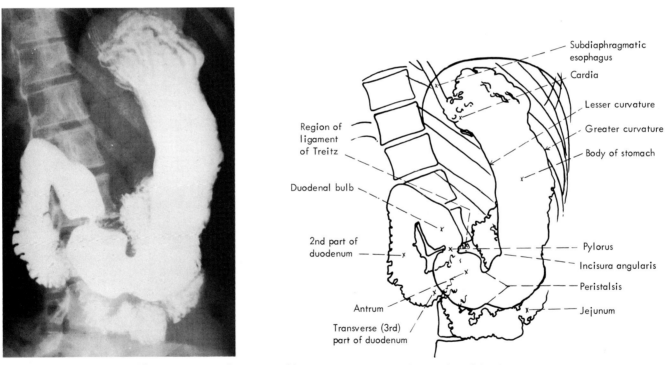

Figure 13–59. Right anterior oblique prone projection of stomach and duodenum.

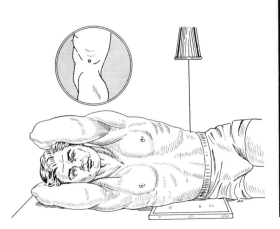

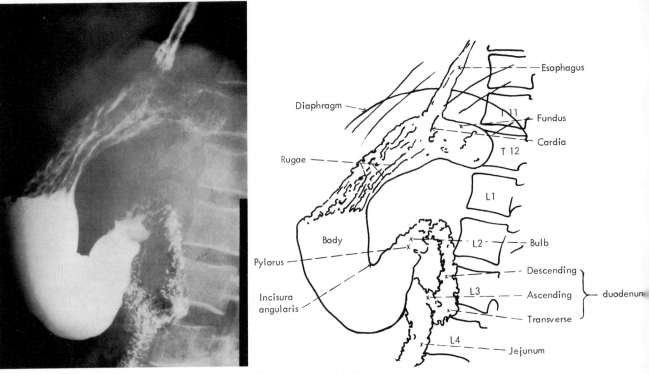

Figure 13–60. Right lateral recumbent view of stomach and duodenum.

Esophagus
Diaphragm
T 11
Fundus
Cardia
Rugae
T 12
Body
L1
Pylorus
L2 — Bulb
Incisura angularis
Descending
L3 — Ascending — duodenum
Transverse
L4
Jejunum

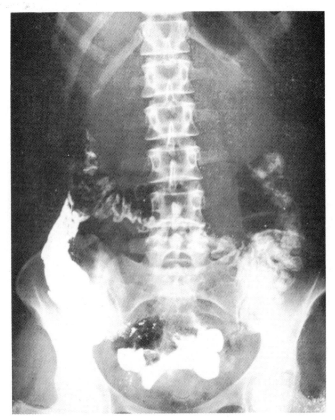

Figure 13–61. Six-hour film study of gastric evacuation.

Additional studies of the stomach and duodenum may be carried out as follows:

Left Lateral Erect Film of Stomach and Duodenum (Fig. 13–62). The left lateral erect view of the stomach and duodenum is most useful to demonstrate the exact relationship of the stomach to retrogastric structures. Anatomic detail is obscured, and hence

this film study is obtained when especially indicated by clinical history suggesting pancreatic or retrogastric disease.

Anteroposterior View of Stomach in Slight Left Posterior Oblique (Fig. 13–57 *J*). In this position, the air in the stomach rises and when admixed with the barium furnishes a double contrast visualization of the body, antrum, and bulb, and a com-

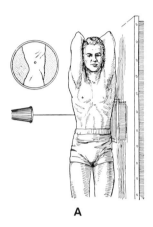

A

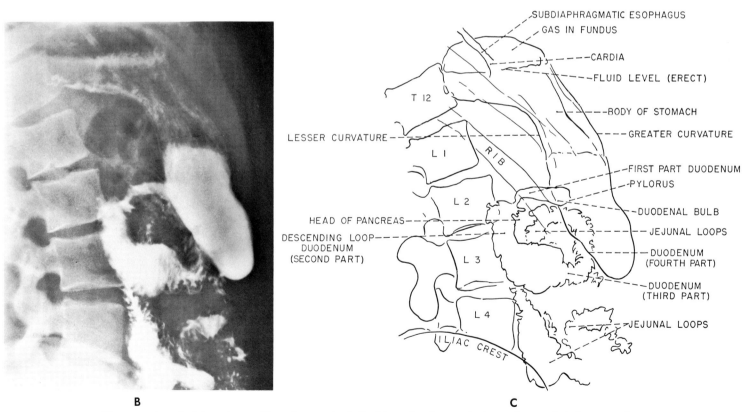

B   C

Figure 13–62. Left lateral erect film of stomach. *A.* Position of patient. *B.* Radiograph. *C.* Labeled tracing of *B.*

pletely barium-filled fundus. Filling defects and mucosal disturbances are thereby sometimes intensified in these areas.

Air Insufflation of the Stomach. Air may be introduced into the stomach as a special examination either by stomach tube, or indirectly by Seidlitz powders or a carbonated drink. The stomach should be empty for this examination. The direct introduction of air has the advantage of permitting the examination of the dry gastric mucosa, following which the addition of a small amount of barium mixture permits double contrast. The carbonated drink method has the disadvantage of diluting the barium which interferes with its coating property.

In either case the patient is first examined fluoroscopically in all projections, and films in any desired position are obtained.

Special Studies of the Stomach and Duodenum

Hypotonic Duodenography. Hypotonic duodenography refers to a barium and gas study of the duodenum after the administration of a gas-producing medication or intubation, followed immediately by an atropinelike drug. Double contrast visualization of the duodenum has proved to be of considerable value in studying both intraluminal and extraluminal disorders of this area. Thirty to 60 mg. of Pro-banthine is administered intramuscularly (or 30 mg. intravenously, adult dose) for this purpose. The barium may be injected by tube also if a duodenal tube is used for the introduction of the air. At times, it may be satisfactory to allow air to enter the duodenum from the stomach at the time the antivagal drug is administered. The patient should be in the supine left posterior oblique position. *Pro-banthine is contraindicated in patients with heart abnormalities or glaucoma. Two to five mg. of glucagon may be used instead in nondiabetic patients.*

Some advantages of double contrast in the duodenum and hypotonic duodenography are shown in Figure 13–63.

Duodenal atony occurs about 5 minutes after the intramuscular introduction of 60 mg. of Pro-banthine and lasts about 20 minutes. The subtle alteration in the pancreaticoduodenal interface has been carefully studied by this method in the normal (Ferruci et al.). The method allows: (1) differentiation of duodenal mucosal fold effacement, (2) differentiation of pathologic papillary defects from normal papilla, and (3) straightening of the contour of the duodenum. Lesions of the tail of the pancreas cannot be studied in this way (Fig. 13–64).

Utilization of Water Soluble Contrast Media for Gastrointestinal Study. Water soluble contrast media have been recommended by some (Rea; Jacobson et al.), when barium is contraindicated. This is best administered by gastric tube since it is bitter to taste. A flavoring agent may be added to make it more palatable but this may alter normal physiologic responses.

Sixty cc. of 60 per cent Hypaque or Gastrografin or 50 grams of powdered Hypaque dissolved in 75 cc. of sterile water, to which 10 drops of a wetting agent (Tween–80) have been added, are utilized as the contrast agent.

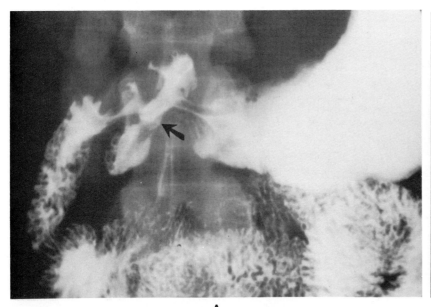
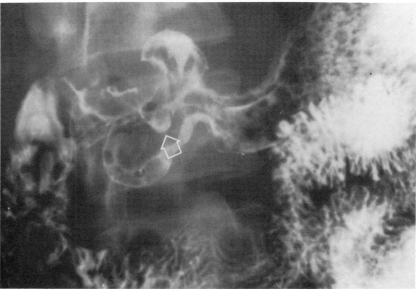

A   B

Figure 13–63. *A* and *B*. Duodenal ulcer showing the advantages of double contrast with barium and air, (*A*) erect, and (*B*) supine. Both views show the ulcer.

Figure 13–63 continued on the opposite page.

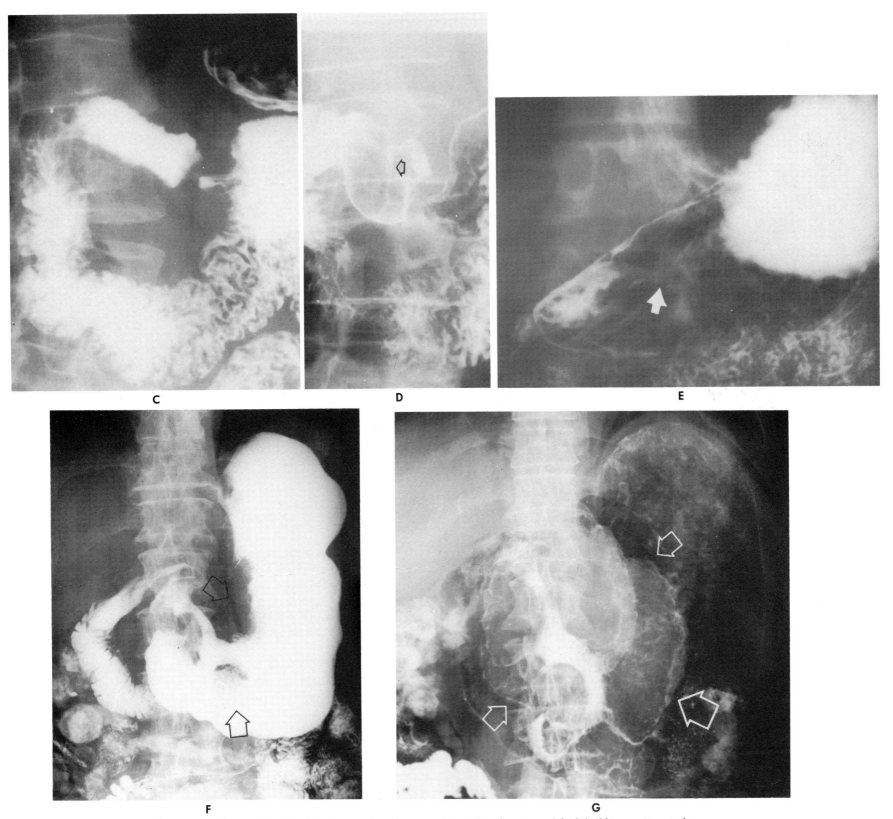

C

D

E

F

G

Figure 13–63 *Continued.* C and D. Once again a demonstration of the advantages of the left oblique supine study and double contrast demonstration of the ulcer on the posterior wall of the duodenum, not otherwise readily demonstrable. E. Double contrast barium-air representation of a healed gastric ulcer seen en face. The stellate radiation of the rugal pattern with a tendency to puckering of the mucosa with outright fleck formation is characteristic. F. Radiograph demonstrating large irregular carcinomatous filling defects of the stomach. G. Double contrast barium and air study of the stomach showing a large irregular polypoid carcinoma partly filling the stomach, in association with a markedly dilated stomach.

Figure 13–63 continued on the following page.

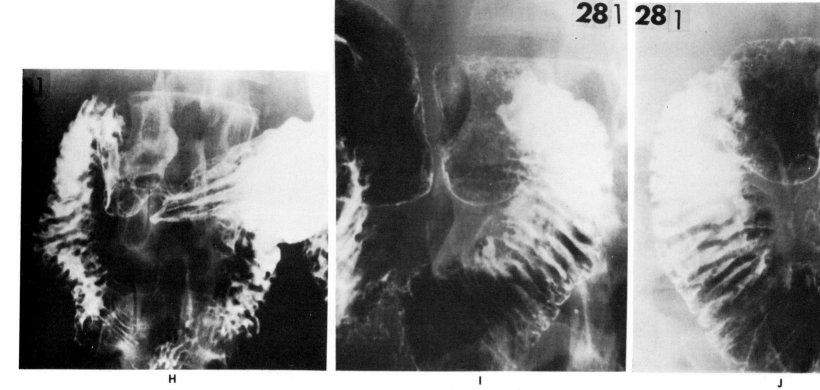

Figure 13–63 *Continued.*   Hypotonic duodenography. *H.* Routine film of the duodenum. *I* and *J.* Duodenum following hypotonic duodenography demonstrating the marked double contrast obtained in the duodenal bulb and duodenum.

For examination of the lower gastrointestinal tract, or in dehydrated patients, the use of these water soluble media is probably contraindicated since they are hyperosmotic and cause further water imbalance. They are also probably contraindicated in infants, in whom dehydration by the hyperosmotic medium may be disturbing unless intravenous fluids are administered simultaneously. However, in general, these agents (Hypaque or Gastrografin) may be used whenever barium mixtures can be used, with the proviso that small quantities be employed (Sidaway; Neuhauser).

Emergency Study of the Upper Gastrointestinal Tract for Bleeding.   When patients are unable to stand for any reason, we have modified our technique for fluoroscopy as follows:

1. The patient lies obliquely on his right side, prone, facing the examiner. He drinks one or two swallows of barium from a straw.

2. The swallowing function and esophagus are studied as the barium is swallowed and moves into the stomach.

3. The stomach is then studied with small and large quantities of barium, first in this position (right oblique, prone), then with the patient on his left side, and finally rotating the patient onto his back.

4. When the patient is supine, he is turned toward his left and lies obliquely on his left side, permitting a double contrast visualization of the antrum and duodenum.

5. Thick barium may be administered, particularly if esophageal varices are suspected. The patient may be asked to carry out, with caution, the Valsalva maneuver.

6. Spot films are taken as necessary throughout the procedure. There is a greater tendency in this examination to make "full spot" films of the entire stomach and duodenum rather than the smaller, more confined views.

7. Routine posteroanterior, right anterior oblique, right lateral, and left posterior oblique views are obtained. A left lateral decubitus view may also be obtained if desired.

This procedure is not intended to replace the routine gastrointestinal examination, which is repeated at a suitable interval after cessation of the emergency (Knowles et al.; Hampton).

Pharmacoradiology in Evaluation of Gastrointestinal Disease.   Smooth muscle stimulation by means of pharmacodynamic agents has long been recommended for evaluation of stomach and duodenum (Pancoast; Ritvo; Adler et al.; Bachrach; Rasmussen; Silbiger and Donner). Such agents as insulin, morphine, Dilaudid, atropine, Prostigmin, pethidine, Pro-banthine, opium derivatives, Mecholyl, physostigmine, Benzedrine, and Pantopon have found their proponents.

Morphine has been considered by some as the most reliable stimulant of gastric peristalsis (Silbiger and Donner). Eight milligrams of morphine were employed by the latter investigators. Within 2 to 10 minutes following intravenous administration, there was an increase in peristalsis which lasted 20 to 45 minutes. There was a second phase of prolonged depression of intestinal propulsion and diminution of tone. Neoplastic infiltrates of the gastric wall invariably resulted in disordered peristaltic patterns. Gastric ulcers, the postoperative stomach, and various infiltrating lesions may be studied to good advantage this way. Active intestinal bleeding and hypersensitivity to the drug are considered contraindications.

Parietography. In this examination, the gastric wall is isolated between two layers of air by gastric inflation and pneumoperitoneum. Body section radiography is also employed. This procedure permits definition of wall thickness of the suspected region and defines the extent of a tumor if present. Approximately 800 to 1200 ml. of air are introduced in the peritoneal cavity on the evening prior to the examination. The gas in the stomach is derived from tartaric acid which becomes mixed with a succeeding dose of sodium bicarbonate (250 to 300 ml. of gas estimated). Body section radiographs are obtained at 1 cm. intervals ordinarily, at 11 to 19 cm. from the posterior skin surface (Porcher and Buffard).

Celiac Angiography for Visualization of the Stomach, Duo-

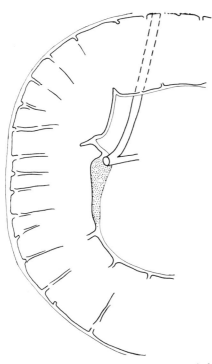

Figure 13–64. Anatomic diagram of normal features of duodenal hypotonic study. (From Ferrucci, J. T., Jr., Benedict, K. T., Page, D. C., Fleischli, D. J., and Eaton, S. B.: Radiology, 96:401–408, 1970.)

denum and Pancreas. See No. 11 in the following section on techniques of examination of the pancreas.

THE PANCREAS

Introduction. The radiologic diagnosis of pancreatic disease leaves much to be desired. The examination of the pancreas must be performed largely by indirect methods, such as careful study of the stomach and duodenum, as well as angiology. It is possible, however, that with greater expertise and refinement of technique our diagnostic accuracy will be considerably enhanced in the future.

Basic Anatomy. The pancreas is both an endocrine and an exocrine gland, its endocrine function being carried forward by the islets of Langerhans. The two hormones secreted are insulin and glucagon. These hormones help regulate glucose, lipid, and protein metabolism. The acini of the pancreas secrete digestive juices into the duodenum.

The pancreas is arbitrarily divided into four parts: *head, neck, body* and *tail*.

Head. The head of the pancreas lies within the curvature of the duodenum (Fig. 13–40 *B*). The prolongation of the left and caudal border of the head of the pancreas is called the "uncinate process" (Fig. 13–65). As shown in the posterior view of the pancreas and duodenum, the superior mesenteric artery and vein cross the uncinate process on its right aspect. The posterior surface of the pancreas is without peritoneum and is in contact with the aorta, inferior vena cava, common bile duct, renal veins, and right crus of the diaphragm (Fig. 13–51). The anterior surface is, in its lower part, below the level of the transverse colon, and is covered by peritoneum and separated from the transverse colon by areolar tissue.

The *neck* of the pancreas is that constricted portion just to the left of the head (Fig. 13–65). Superiorly it adjoins the pylorus. It is proximal to the origin of the portal vein and the gastroduodenal artery.

The *body* of the pancreas is separated anteriorly from the stomach by the omental bursa. The posterior surface of the body of the pancreas is closely related to the aorta, splenic vein, left kidney and its vessels, left suprarenal, the origin of the superior mesenteric artery, and the crura of the diaphragm. The inferior surface of the body is coated by peritoneum and is in close proximity to the duodenojejunal flexure, the coils of the jejunum, and the left flexure of the colon. Along its anterior aspect, the layers of the transverse mesocolon diverge. The superior border of the body of the pancreas is close to the celiac artery, with the hepatic artery to the right and the splenic artery to the left (Fig. 13–65).

The *tail* of the pancreas extends laterally toward the left to the surface of the spleen and is situated in the phrenicolienal ligament.

The exocrine secretions of the pancreas empty into the duo-

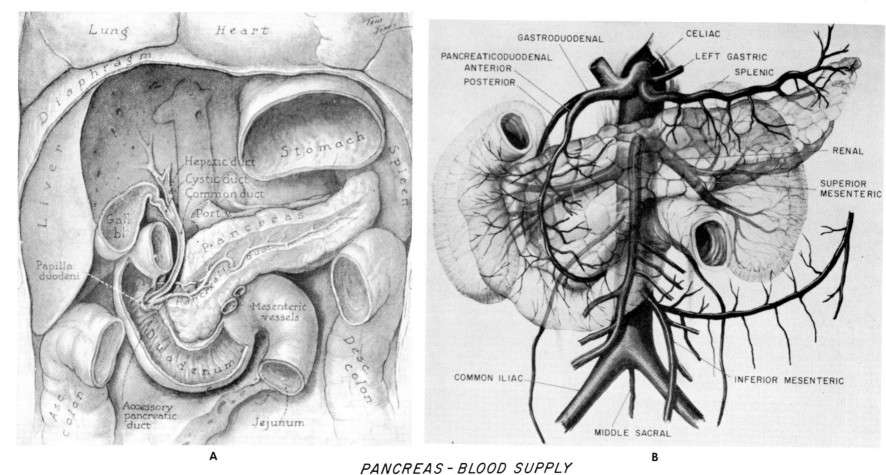

PANCREAS - BLOOD SUPPLY

Figure 13–65. A. The gross anatomy of the biliary system. (From Jones, T.: Anatomical Studies. Jackson, Michigan, S. H. Camp and Co., 1943.) B. Arterial circulation of the pancreas (isometric diagram). C. Pancreatic blood supply in simple diagram to demonstrate the anterior and posterior pancreaticoduodenal arcade in conjunction with the celiac axis and the superior mesenteric arteries and veins. The transverse pancreatic artery is also shown, in its relationship to the splenic artery and the pancreatica magna artery. (B and C from Bierman, H. R.: Selective Arterial Catheterization, 1969. Courtesy of Charles C Thomas, Publisher, Springfield, Illinois.)

denum through two ductal systems: first, a *major duct* (of Wirsung), which extends the full length of the pancreas toward the right, opening into the descending duodenum at a common orifice with the common bile duct, the *major papilla* (ampulla of Vater). Second, the *minor pancreatic duct* (of Santorini) drains

part of the head of the pancreas and enters the duodenum just above the duct of Wirsung by a separate opening in the duodenum.

The arterial blood supply of the pancreas (Fig. 13-66 *A*) is derived from *four* main sources: (1) numerous small branches

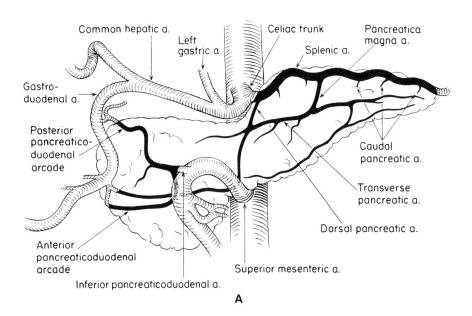

A

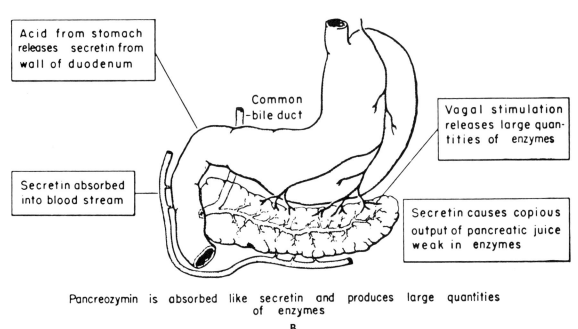

Pancreozymin is absorbed like secretin and produces large quantities of enzymes

B

Figure 13-66. *A.* Line drawing of arterial supply of the pancreas. The pancreatic branches are enlarged for emphasis. In this example, the dorsal pancreatic artery arises from the splenic artery and gives off the transverse pancreatic artery. It receives an anastomotic branch from the anterior pancreaticoduodenal arcade. The relationships of the pancreatic arteries are variable and must be evaluated in each patient. (From Reuter, S. R., and Redman, H. C.: Gastrointestinal Angiography. Philadelphia, W. B. Saunders Co., 1972.) *B.* Regulation of pancreatic secretion. (From Guyton, A. C.: Textbook of Medical Physiology, 4th ed. Philadelphia, W. B. Saunders Co., 1971.)

from the *splenic* artery; (2) the retroduodenal branch of the *gastroduodenal* artery; (3) the *superior pancreaticoduodenal* arising from the gastroduodenal artery; and (4) the *inferior pancreaticoduodenal* which arises from the superior mesenteric artery and anastomoses with the superior pancreaticoduodenal in the head of the pancreas.

A *dorsal pancreatic artery* may give rise from the celiac artery just distal to the origin of the splenic artery and opposite the point of origin of the left gastric. This supplies the body of the pancreas centrally with branches extending toward the head and tail. This artery, called by some the superior, instead of arising from the celiac trunk may originate from the superior mesenteric artery.

The *superior pancreaticoduodenal* artery may divide into two main segments, one anterior and one posterior, surrounding the head of the pancreas and its uncinate process. The arcade formed around the head of the pancreas also supplies the duodenum its ventral aspect.

The pancreas also receives branches directly from the *common hepatic artery*.

One of the branches from the splenic artery is often sufficiently large to be identified as a single branch called the *pancreatica magna artery*. It is distributed along the pancreatic duct.

The pancreatic veins drain directly into the portal vein by means of the *splenic and superior mesenteric veins*.

The *lymphatics* terminate in numerous lymph nodes near the root of the superior mesenteric artery, following the course of blood vessels and terminating in the pancreaticolienal, pancreaticoduodenal, and preaortic lymph nodes.

Pancreatic Exocrine Secretions. Pancreatic juice contains enzymes for digesting all three major types of food: proteins, carbohydrates, and fat. There are a number of proteolytic enzymes which, as synthesized in the pancreas, are inactive but become active after they are secreted into the intestinal tract by enzymes released from the intestinal mucosa whenever chyme comes in contact with the mucosa. If this were not the case, the pancreatic juice might digest the pancreas itself. There is additionally, however, another substance called trypsin inhibitor stored in the cells of the pancreas which prevents the activation of pancreatic proteolytic enzymes.

Pancreatic secretion, like gastric secretion, is regulated by both nervous and hormonal mechanisms. The most important hormone in this regard is *secretin*. A second hormone is *pancreozymin*. When chyme enters the intestine it causes the release and activation of secretin, which is absorbed into the blood and in turn causes the pancreas to secrete large quantities of fluid containing a high concentration of bicarbonate ion and a low concentration of chloride ion. Hydrochloric acid, particularly in the chyme, is capable of causing a great release of secretin, although almost any type of food will cause at least some release.

The secretin response is particularly important in the prevention of too great acidity in the small intestine, since the small intestine cannot withstand the intense digestive properties of gastric juice. Moreover, the tendency toward alkaline environment assists the action of the pancreatic enzymes per se.

Pancreozymin is largely responsible for secretion of the digestive enzymes from the pancreas and is somewhat similar to the effect of vagal stimulation. The type of secretion of the pancreas in response to secretin is called "hydrelatic" secretion and the secretion in response to pancreozymin is called "ecbolic" secretion (Fig. 13–66 *B*).

Technique of Examination of the Pancreas

1. **Plain Films of the Abdomen.** Anteroposterior and lateral views of the abdomen centered over the pancreas (with oblique views taken as necessary) are helpful from the standpoint of revealing (a) pancreatic calcification (Fig. 13–67); (b) an abnormal gas distribution, such as free air in the immediate vicinity of the pancreas or lesser omental bursa; or (c) displacement of adjoining organs such as the stomach, duodenum, kidney, or spleen.

2. **Air Contrast Studies of the Stomach and Duodenum.** Air contrast may be used in the stomach and duodenum to accentuate the pancreatic region, particularly when calcareous masses are noted therein. Air contrast ordinarily does not obscure the areas of calcification, whereas barium contrast introduced into the stomach and duodenum might do so. Body section radiography may be used in conjunction with the air contrast to enhance its efficacy.

3. **Endo- and Perigastric Gas with Selective Celiac Arteriography During the Phase of Maximal Secretion** (stimulation by pharmacologic agents) (Taylor, et al.). This combination of an angiographic identification of the pancreas, plus the visualization of the stomach and duodenum by gas intraluminally, permits the identification of the pancreas in conjunction with the gastric mucosa and thickness of the gastric wall.

Selective celiac arteriography in itself is very helpful in identifying certain lesions of the pancreas (Fig. 13–68). However, the interpretation of angiograms of the pancreas offers some difficulty and the efficacy of this technique for identification of carcinoma in the pancreas, for example, is somewhat controversial.

4. **Intubation of the Stomach and Duodenum with Opaque Tube.** The main purpose of this examination is to delineate the region of the pancreas for better visualization of any suspicious oblique or negative shadows in this area (Weens and Walker). A discussion of pancreatic calculi or calcified cysts of the pancreas is outside the scope of this text and the student is referred to special reports of these disorders for further information (Stein et al.; Poppel; Becker et al.; Meschan: *Analysis of Roentgen Signs,* Chapter 28).

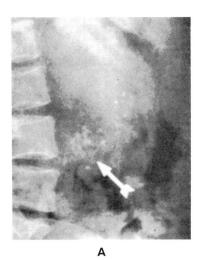 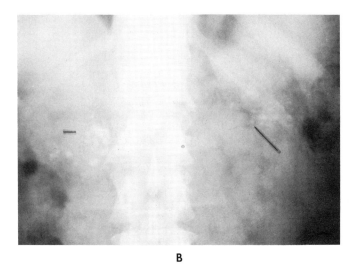

A   B

Figure 13–67. Pancreatic calculi. *A.* Lateral projection. The calcific shadows lie anteriorly to the second and third lumbar vertebrae. *B.* After the administration of an opaque meal. The calcific shadows are visualized within the loop of the duodenum (black marker). (From Ritvo, M., and Shauffer, I. A.: Gastrointestinal X-ray Diagnosis. Philadelphia, Lea & Febiger, 1952.)

5. **Opaque Meal in Stomach and Duodenum.** The close relationship of the pancreas to the stomach and duodenum has already been described. Impressions upon the stomach and alterations of the detailed mucosal pattern of the duodenum may be the only evidence of pancreatic abnormality. Cinefluorography and cineradiography are particularly useful for detailed analysis of areas of pliability or incipient rigidity in the second part of the duodenum (Salik). Greater variability in appearance, less rigidity and induration, and the absence of fixed corrugations favor a diagnosis of pancreatitis over carcinoma. Hypotonic duodenography is particularly helpful with opaque studies of the stomach and duodenum in revealing minute abnormalities related to the pancreas (Fig. 13–69).

6. **Barium Enema** (Chapter 14). The peritoneal reflection of the transverse mesocolon lies in very close proximity to the pancreas; and hence, lesions of the pancreas may extend to and involve the colon, especially its transverse portion. The barium enema may corroborate plain films of the abdomen that reveal inordinate shadows in the immediate vicinity of the transverse colon (Salik; Eyler et al.).

7. **Excretory Urogram** (Chapter 16). The tail of the pancreas may lie just anterior to the left kidney and extends to the hilum of the spleen. Abnormal enlargement of the pancreas, especially involving the lesser omental bursa, may displace or distort the left kidney, ureter, or spleen (Marshall et al.).

8. **Cholecystograms and Cholangiograms** (Chapter 15). Cholecystograms and cholangiograms may at times reveal evidence of an obstructed or a displaced common duct. The max-

imum diameter of the common duct in chronic pancreatitis for example, seldom if ever exceeds 25 mm. Obstruction of the common duct due to carcinoma may cause an enlargement of over 30 mm. Unfortunately, intravenous cholangiography fails in about one-third of the cases of acute inflammations of the pancreas (Schultz). Conspicuous dilatation of the pancreatic duct and its tributaries coupled with narrowness of the transduodenal portion of the common duct may also indicate inflammations of the pancreas (Sachs and Partington).

9. **Percutaneous Cholangiography** (Chapter 15). When complete obstruction of the common bile duct occurs at its site of entry into the pancreas, considerable dilatation of the more proximal regions in the biliary tree results. Direct percutaneous injection of a contrast agent through the liver into one of the dilated constituent branches will not only demonstrate severe dilatation, but also the more characteristic appearances of the common bile duct. At the site of obstruction, there may be a jagged, notched appearance and a reversal of the usual convexity of the common bile duct toward the left (Flemma et al.; Evans; Darke and Beal).

10. **Further Comments About Selective Pancreatic Angiography.** As indicated earlier, the arterial supply of the pancreas is somewhat variable, with the major supply coming from the splenic, celiac, gastroduodenal, and superior mesenteric arteries. Selective study of the pancreas is probably best accomplished by celiac or superior mesenteric angiograms. Inflation of the stomach in conjunction with this study is helpful (Lunderquist). Superselective catheterization of the hepatic, splenic, gastroduodenal, dorsal pancreatic, inferior pancreatic, or duodenal arteries

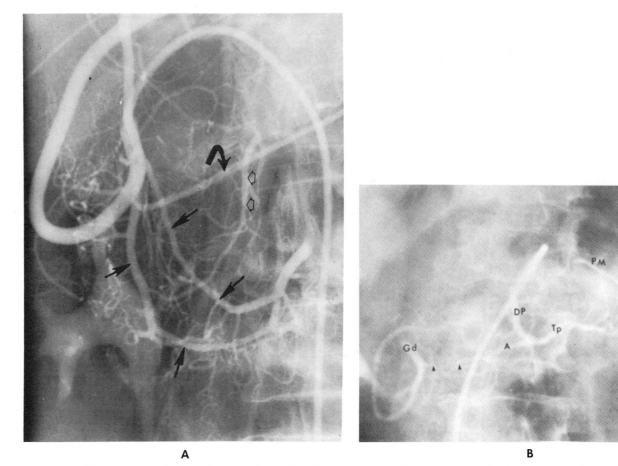

A   **B**

Figure 13–68. *A*. Normal pancreatic arcades. Direct serial magnification angiography during a gastroduodenal artery injection clearly demonstrates the pancreatic arcades (*straight arrows*), the transverse pancreatic artery (*curved arrow*) and the dorsal pancreatic artery (*open arrow*). (From Baum, S., and Athanasoulis, C. A.: Angiography. *In* Eaton, S. B., and Ferrucci, J. T. (ed.): Radiology of the Pancreas and Duodenum. Philadelphia, W. B. Saunders Co., 1973.) *B*. Selective dorsal pancreatic injection. Catheter passed via celiac artery. (*DP*). Dorsal pancreatic artery, (A and arrowheads), anastomotic branch from dorsal pancreatic artery to pancreaticoduodenal arcade, (*Gd*) gastroduodenal artery, (*Pm*) pancreatica magna, (*Tp*) transverse pancreatic. (From Ruzicka, F. F., Jr., and Rossi, P.: Radiol. Clin. N. Amer., 8:3–28, 1970.)

has been attempted, and it has been noted that injections must be made at least into both gastroduodenal and splenic arteries for adequate demonstration of the entire pancreas. It is probable that pharmacologic agents will serve to enhance these techniques (Bierman). (See also Fig. 13–68.)

11. **Splenoportography.** The splenic vein and tail of the pancreas are in close contiguity with one another. Splenic vein occlusion and distortion have been described in association with pancreatic tumors or large masses (pseudocysts) of the pancreas (Bookstein and Whitehouse; Rösch and Herfort; Varriale et al.).

12. **Retropneumoperitoneum with Body Section Radiography.** This method involves a combination of the retroperitoneal insufflation of a gas, gaseous distention of the stomach, and body section radiography in both the sagittal and coronal planes. Simultaneous pneumoperitoneum, introduction of con-

trast agent in the stomach, urinary tract, or biliary tree, and other expedients have also been utilized in conjunction with this method. These methods are still in the process of evaluation and it is questionable whether the discomfort and perhaps even the dangers of the procedure are justified when compared with other possible methods that might be employed in identical cases (Mosely).

13. **Direct Pancreatography.** This method involves direct insertion of a needle or catheter into the pancreatic duct at surgery (Doubilet et al., 1959). The original method involved transduodenal sphincterotomy and direct injection of a suitable contrast agent (from 2 to 5 ml. of 50 per cent sodium diatrizoate is recommended). This injection is made slowly during a 5 minute period, with the last 2 ml. introduced during the x-ray exposure. The tube may be left in place for drainage. Corrosion prepara-

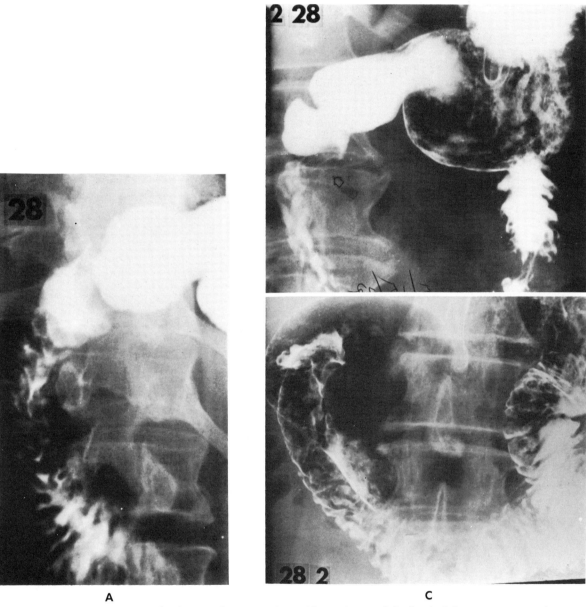

Figure 13-69. Hypotonic duodenography in a patient with carcinoma of the head of the pancreas. *A* and *B*. Prior to the hypotonic study. *C*. The hypotonic study. Although the rigid impression upon the duodenum is visible in *A* and *B*, it is better shown following the gaseous distention of the duodenal loop.

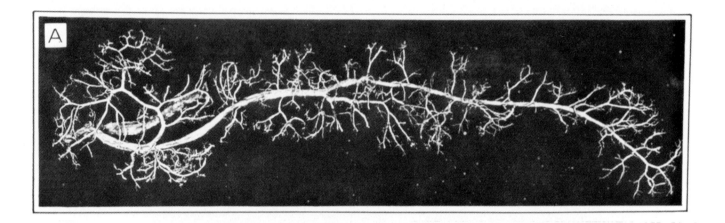

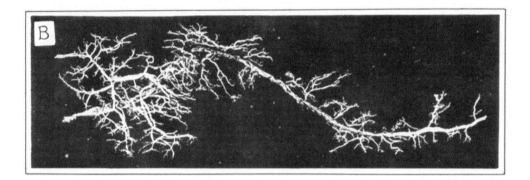

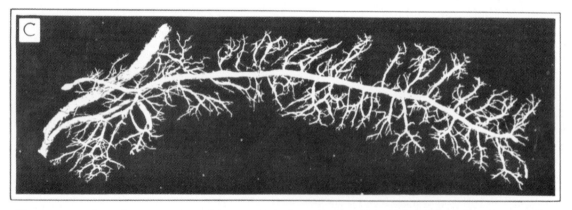

Figure 13–70. Corrosion preparations of the pancreatic ducts. *Dimensions:* total length 8.2 inches (average). The main duct begins 1 inch from the tail, and has a diameter of 0.5 mm., which gradually increases to 3.5 mm. in diameter in the head of the pancreas. (Reproduced by permission from J. C. B. Grant: An Atlas of Anatomy, 5th ed. Copyright © 1962, The Williams and Wilkins Company.)

tions of the pancreatic duct are shown in Figure 13–70. Normal pancreatograms reveal only the main ducts of the pancreas. With acute inflammation the radiopaque solution permeates the acinar tissue, showing not only the smaller ramifications as shown in Figure 13–70 but even some of the parenchymal tissue. Serial pancreatograms will depict resolution of such inflammation.

14. **Endoscopic Pancreatocholangiography** (peroral pancreaticobiliary ductography). Cannulation of the ampulla of Vater through a fiberoptic duodenoscope may be performed with the aid of x-ray television (Ogoshi et al.; Oi; Tagaki et al.; Gotton et al.; Kusagai et al.; Robbins et al.; Okuda et al.). The technique of the examination is described as follows: A fiberduodenoscope, Model JF-B of the Olympus Company, Tokyo, has been used. This instrument, 10 mm. in diameter and 1250 mm. long, is inserted perorally into the stomach and thereafter into the duodenum. Its tip is equipped with a rigid lens system that can be bent at will 120 degrees up and down, and 90 degrees right and left. It contains lenses and holes for illumination, fixed focus for visualization and photography, a small hole for injecting air and washing fluid, and a larger hole for passing a forceps and cannula. A Teflon cannula 1.7 mm. in external diameter is passed through the duodenoscope into the ampulla of Vater and sodium meglumine diatrizoate is then injected into the cannulated duct system. Usually only 2 to 3 cc. are required. The injection is terminated and left lateral and posteroanterior (sometimes left oblique) roentgenograms are taken. The cannula and scope are withdrawn and several more roentgenograms are taken in various projections, including the right oblique view and erect positions. The speed of disappearance or excretion of the contrast medium into the duodenum is checked on the television screen. If too great a volume of contrast agent is used, a pancreatitis may ensue and this should be avoided. After the procedure an antibiotic is used to prevent acute pancreatitis and infection.

After successful pancreatography the common duct may be visualized with a cannula withdrawn halfway and contrast medium reinjected (Fig. 13–71). The accessory pancreatic duct may be visualized as communicating with the duct of Wirsung. Usually, barium swallow study and hypotonic duodenography are carried out prior to the duodenoscopy. Representative ductograms are shown in Figure 13–71.

Okuda et al. note that the length of the normal pancreatic duct by this technique is usually 15.8 mm. on the average, and slightly longer in the presence of inflammation. The maximum duct diameter of the head of the normal pancreas is 3.9 mm., but this measurement is considerably larger in the presence of chronic pancreatitis. (There is no indication in this report of magnification in relation to these measurements.) Normally, the ductal system clears in an average of 4 minutes and 6 seconds, but considerably longer retention occurs in abnormal states.

15. **Measurement of the Retrogastric and Retroduodenal Spaces: an Index of Pancreatic or Lesser Omental Bursal In-** **volvement.** Various methods have been proposed for measurement of the retrogastric space (Poppel et al.; Scheinmel and Mednick; Meschan et al.; Poole). The normal range of distances in centimeters between the stomach and duodenum and the spine on left lateral roentgenograms of the abdomen according to body habitus has been proposed by a number of investigators. The limits of normal vary considerably according to the gross judgment of body habitus. Such great variations of normal make the validity of measurement difficult to interpret except in the presence of "extrinsic tumor impression on the visceral [which was] . . . the single most important statistical factor in evaluating the presence of a retroperitoneal mass" (Herbert and Margulis). Poole, in studying this issue, noted that "the only variable measurements in the midline cross-section at the level of the stomach are the thicknesses of the prepancreatic fat, and the width of the pancreatic neck, which is 1 to 1.5 cm. thick normally in the midline. Many other structures, however, are present such as the lesser sac, fat, aortic lymph nodes, and the aorta itself." Poole devised an anterior abdominal wall compression device which contained a nickel coin (measuring 2.1 cm. in diameter) on its flat surface. He used this device to press the midline stomach against the retroperitoneal structures. After the barium was swallowed, the fluoroscopic pressure cone was applied to the midline puddle of barium with sufficient force to splay the mucosal folds and flatten the column of barium. Adequate compression was noted by displacement of the central midbarium column to both sides of the midline. A lateral spot film was taken. The midline antrum-to-spine distance was measured from the posterior pressure defect to the anterior vertebral body. After the antrum-to-spine measurement, the patient was placed in the right lateral decubitus position to allow barium to enter the horizontal duodenum, and then he was brought upright and placed in the posteroanterior position. When the midline duodenum was identified in the posteroanterior projection, the patient was then turned laterally and a spot film taken without pressure (Fig. 13–72). The duodenum-to-spine distance was measured from the posterior aspect of the midline horizontal duodenum to the spine. The measurements obtained from spot films were corrected for magnification by the magnification of the coin marker on the compressor device. A nomogram is provided to correct for such magnification (Fig. 13–72). A direct linear correlation exists between the weight of the normal individual and his true antrum-to-spine measurement. For an average weight of 148 pounds the average corrected antrum-to-spine distance was 3.14 cm. The 95 per cent confidence limits are shown in the accompanying graph. The duodenum-to-spine normal measurement exhibited no relationship to body weight. The mean value was 1.3 cm., with a standard deviation of 5 mm. The upper limit of normal was 2.3 cm. (two standard deviations). This method obviates many of the variables previously noted by compressing the barium-containing midline viscus against the retroperitoneum, thus accurately defining its anterior margin.

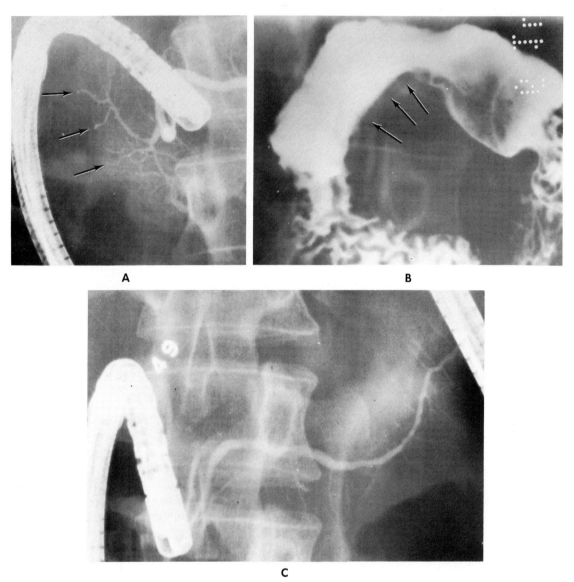

Figure 13–71. Detection of malignant disease by peroral retrograde pancreaticobiliary ductography. (From Robbins, A. H., et al.: Amer. J. Roentgenol., 117:432–436, 1973.)

A. Barium studies suggest pressure defect on second part of duodenum. B. Ductogram reveals normal tributary ducts in same region. C. Main pancreatic duct is normal and other branches are normal as well. (Patient had chronic pancreatitis.)

Figure 13–71 continued on the opposite page.

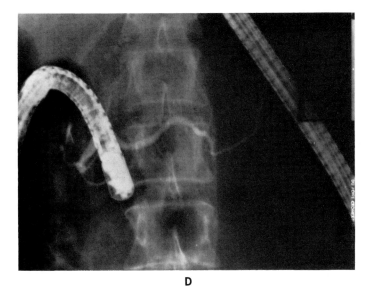

D

Figure **13–71** *Continued.* *D.* Another normal pancreatic ductogram. *E.* A normal cholangiogram.

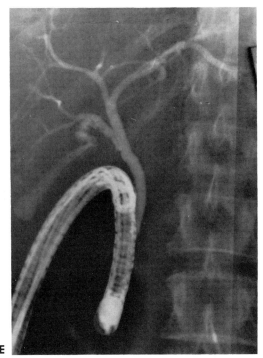

E

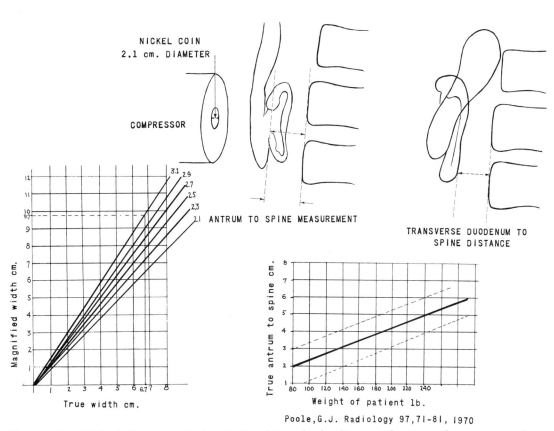

Figure **13–72.** Method of measuring "retroantral" and "retroduodenal" space. The coin on the compressor allows correction for magnification (graph, lower left). The normal standards for antrum to spine are shown in the graph, lower right. The transverse duodenum-to-spine distance plus 2 standard deviations was 2.3 cm. (From Poole, G. J.: Radiology *97:*71–81, 1970.)

GASTRIC AND DUODENAL ANGIOGRAPHY

Blood Supply of the Stomach

The Celiac Trunk. The celiac trunk or axis is the first unpaired branch of the abdominal aorta (Fig. 13–73). It arises from the ventral side, usually at about the upper margin of the first lumbar vertebra. It may vary in its origin, however, between the lower margin of T12 and the lower margin of L1. It is a very short branch and it lies ordinarily about an average of 1 cm. above the origin of the superior mesenteric artery, although this measurement may range between 1 and 2.2 cm. Usually the celiac artery terminates in three branches but occasionally in four. The three typical branches are the *left gastric, common hepatic,* and *splenic* (Fig. 13–73). Additional branches may occasionally go to the dorsal pancreatic, the left or right phrenic, and a middle or accessory middle colic.

The classical pattern of branching of the celiac artery is found in 93 per cent of cases (Ruzicka and Rossi) (Fig. 13–75). A representative simultaneous selective celiac and superior mesen-

teric artery angiogram of the type I pattern is shown in Figure 13–76.

The *left gastric artery* courses upward toward the cardiac end of the stomach and passes between the layers of the gastrohepatic ligament, following the lesser curvature of the stomach closely. After reaching the region of the cardia of the stomach it descends from left to right downward toward the pylorus, ultimately anastomosing with the right gastric artery (Fig. 13–74). It thus forms an arterial arch or arcade on the lesser curvature of the stomach with the right gastric artery. The main branches of the left gastric artery are the *esophageal* and the *hepatic.* One to three esophageal branches ascend along the right anterior and posterior surfaces of the esophagus, supplying the cardiac and distal portions of the esophagus. These branches anastomose with other esophageal arteries from the aorta, bronchial branches, posterior intercostal, and phrenic arteries as described in the section on the esophagus.

The hepatic branch of the left gastric artery occurs in about 25 per cent of individuals.

The *common hepatic artery* arises along the right aspect of the celiac trunk and to the right of the superior margin of the head of the pancreas (Fig. 13–73). In the region of the first part of the duodenum it gives off the *gastroduodenal artery,* and then turns forward into the hepatoduodenal ligament, where it continues toward the liver as the hepatic artery proper. In the hepatoduodenal ligament, the hepatic artery is situated on the ventral side of the portal vein to the left of the common bile duct. As it reaches the porta hepatis it divides into two main branches, a *right* and *left hepatic branches.* Some of the variations of normal branching of the hepatic arteries are shown in Figure 13–77.

The *right gastric artery* is ordinarily a branch of the hepatic artery proper. It usually arises distal to the origin of the gastroduodenal, but it may arise from other arteries, such as the left hepatic (40 per cent); right hepatic (5 per cent); middle hepatic (5 per cent); gastroduodenal (8 per cent); and common hepatic. The right gastric artery descends from its origin, giving off branches to the pylorus and stomach, and reaches the lesser curvature where it turns to the left and ascends along the lesser curvature, ultimately anastomosing with the left gastric artery in the arcade described previously.

The *right hepatic branch* of the hepatic artery passes between the portal vein and the common hepatic duct to enter the right lobe of the liver. It usually lies to the right of the right hepatic duct. Aberrant right hepatic arteries from other sources in the celiac trunk occur in about 18 per cent of individuals, usually as a branch of the superior mesenteric artery (Fig. 13–77). Outside the liver the right hepatic artery gives off the *cystic artery* to the gallbladder and it may also provide a *middle hepatic artery.* The intrahepatic distribution of the hepatic artery will be described subsequently in conjunction with the anatomy of the liver.

The *left hepatic artery* supplies the left lobe of the liver and is

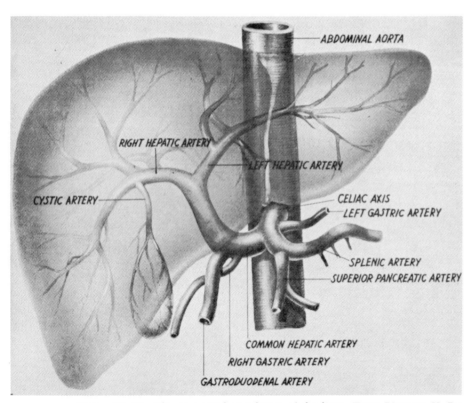

Figure 13–73. Classic arterial circulation of the liver. (From Bierman, H. R.: Selective Arterial Catheterization, 1969. Courtesy of Charles C Thomas, Publisher, Springfield, Illinois.)

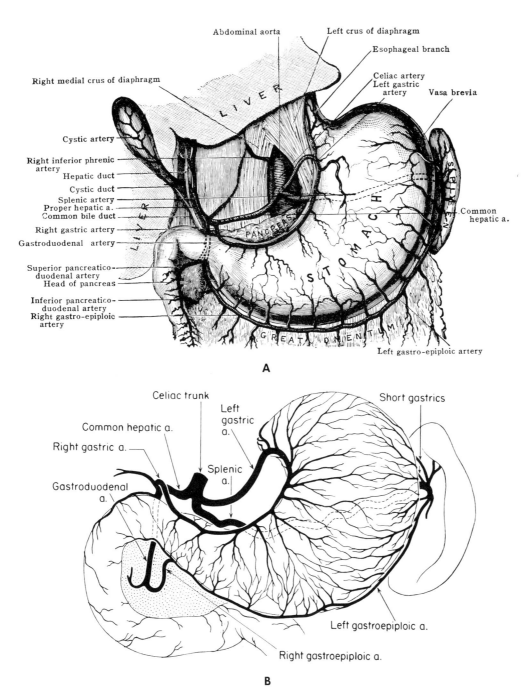

Figure 13–74. A. Celiac artery and its usual main branches. (From Anson, B. J. (ed.): Morris' Human Anatomy, 12th ed. Copyright © 1966 by McGraw-Hill, Inc. Used by permission of McGraw-Hill Book Company.) B. Line drawing of arterial supply of the stomach. The arteries to the stomach are enlarged for emphasis. The left gastro-epiploic and right gastric arteries are frequently not identified at angiography unless they are serving as a collateral pathway. (From Reuter, S. R., and Redman, H. C.: Gastrointestinal Angiography. Philadelphia, W. B. Saunders Co., 1972.)

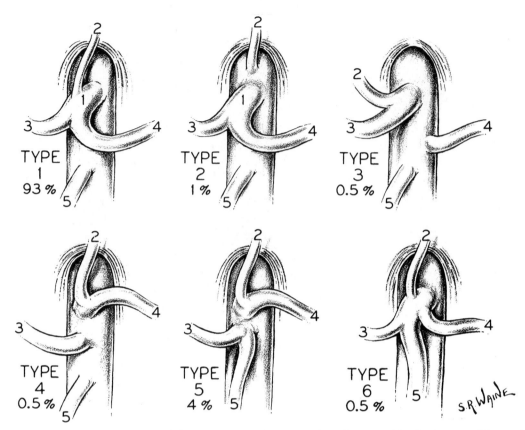

Figure 13–75. (1) Celiac trunk, (2) left gastric artery, (3) common hepatic artery, (4) splenic artery, (5) superior mesenteric artery, (6) right hepatic artery, (7) left hepatic artery, (8) gastroduodenal artery, (9) proper hepatic artery. (From Ruzicka, F. F., and Rossi, P.: N.Y. State J. Med., 23:3032–3033, 1968, reproduced with permission.)

usually considerably smaller than the right. An aberrant left hepatic artery occurs in about 25 per cent of individuals.

A *middle hepatic artery* supplies the quadrate lobe of the liver. It may arise from either the right or left hepatic artery and it gives off branches to the left side of the quadrate lobe and in some instances sends a branch to the left lobe. In rare instances, it gives rise to the cystic artery, to be described later.

The *gastroduodenal artery* descends dorsal to the first part of the duodenum to the lower margin of the pylorus, where it divides into a *right gastroepiploic artery* and an *anterior superior pancreaticoduodenal artery*. The gastroduodenal artery lies to the left of the common bile duct at its origin and terminally lies on the ventral aspect of the head of the pancreas, as described in the section on the pancreas. It has three main branches—*a posterior superior pancreaticoduodenal, an anterior superior pancreaticoduodenal,* and the *right gastroepiploic.* There may be other small duodenal branches. The pancreaticoduodenal branches form the arcade previously described in the section on the pancreas. The right

gastroepiploic artery courses along the greater curvature of the stomach, ultimately to anastomose with the left gastroepiploic artery, which arises from the splenic artery. The right gastroepiploic artery thereafter passes in the gastrocolic ligament or in the greater omentum. It is ordinarily larger than the left and passes much farther to the left than the midline. The right and left gastroepiploic arteries form an arcade supplying the anterior and superior surfaces of the stomach along its greater curvature.

The *splenic artery* is the largest branch arising from the celiac trunk and is generally the first branch of the celiac. It arises to the right of the midline and crosses the aorta to reach the spleen on the left, varying in length from 8 to 32 cm. It is often very tortuous, particularly in elderly persons. Its diameter varies from 4 to 11 mm. Generally, it embeds itself in the superior border of the pancreas and reaches the tail of the pancreas, where it divides into its *two main terminals* (Fig. 13–78), the *superior* and *inferior,* and occasionally, even a third branch called the *middle terminal.* Throughout its pancreatic course, it lies ceph-

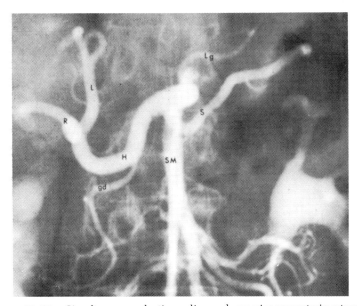

Figure 13–76. Simultaneous selective celiac and superior mesenteric artery injections show type I pattern (see Figs. 13–75 and 13–77 also). Anteroposterior view. (S) Splenic artery, (SM) superior mesenteric, (gd) gastroduodenal, (H) proper hepatic, (R) right hepatic, (L) left hepatic, (Lg) left gastric. (From Ruzicka, F. F., and Rossi, P.: Radiol. Clin. N. Amer., 8:3–29, 1970.)

alad to the splenic vein. Its most constant branches are the *pancreatic, left gastroepiploic, short gastric, superior and inferior terminal, and splenic branches.*

The pancreatic branches arising from the splenic artery are usually small, as previously indicated, but occasionally some may be very large. The largest of these is the *dorsal pancreatic*, which in turn forms the *inferior pancreatic artery* (supplying the inferior edge of the pancreas) and anastomoses with the caudal pancreatic branches of the *pancreatica magna*. The dorsal pancreatic may communicate with the superior mesenteric artery or its branches. The *pancreatica magna artery* is the largest pancreatic branch and enters the pancreas at the junction of its middle and left third. It represents the main blood supply of the tail of the pancreas. Caudal pancreatic branches arise from the splenic before its terminal division and penetrate the tail of the pancreas, anastomosing with the inferior pancreatic and pancreatica magna radicals.

The *left gastroepiploic artery* reaches the stomach below the fundus and descends along the left side of the greater curvature in the anterior layer of the greater omentum. As previously mentioned, it anastomoses with the right gastroepiploic artery and provides an arcade on the greater curvature of the stomach. It

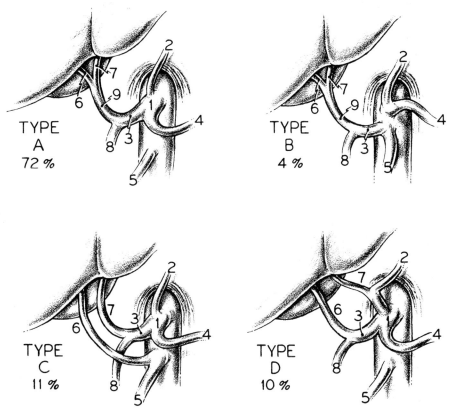

Figure 13–77. (1) Celiac trunk, (2) left gastric artery, (3) common hepatic artery, (4) splenic artery, (5) superior mesenteric artery, (6) right hepatic artery, (7) left hepatic artery, (8) gastroduodenal artery, (9) proper hepatic artery. (From Ruzicka, F. F., and Rossi, P.: N.Y. State J. Med., 23:3032–3033, 1968, reproduced with permission.)

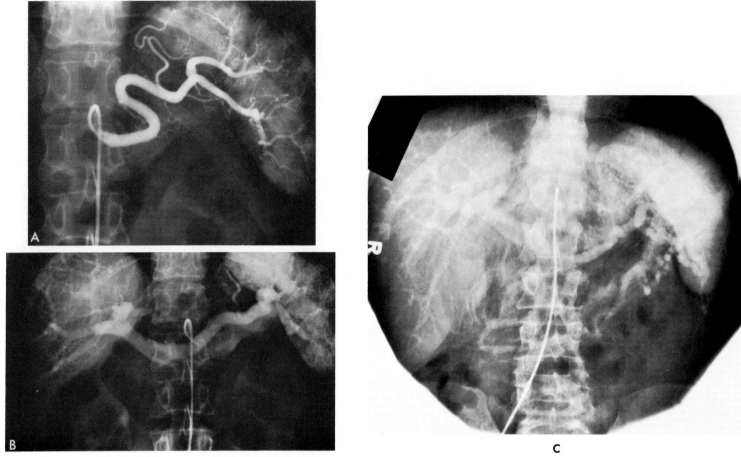

Figure 13-78. Normal splenic arteriogram in the evaluation of the pancreatic body and tail.

A. Arterial phase of a selective splenic arteriogram demonstrates the pancreatica magna and short pancreatic arteries supplying the body and tail of the pancreas.

B. During the venous phase of the same injection, the splenic vein and portal vein are optimally visualized. The close association of the splenic vein with the opacified normal pancreatic body and tail is apparent. (From Eaton, S. B. and Ferrucci, J. T., Jr., Radiology of the Pancreas and Duodenum, W. B. Saunders Co., 1973.)

C. Portal or splenoportal venogram following celiac arteriogram.

Figure 13-78 continued on the opposite page.

gives off various gastric, pancreatic, and splenic arterial branches. The *short gastric arteries* are small branches from the splenic artery which pass to the greater curvature of the stomach in its cardiac or fundic region.

The *terminal arteries* of the splenic send from two to twelve small splenic branches into the substance of the spleen.

Venous Drainage. The *veins of the stomach* drain directly or indirectly into the portal vein which will be described in more detail in Chapter 14. However, short gastric veins from the greater curvatures and fundus may drain into the splenic vein (Fig. 13-78 *C, D*), and the left gastroepiploic vein also drains into the splenic from the greater curvature of the stomach. The right

gastroepiploic from the right end of the greater curvature drains into the superior mesenteric vein. *A coronary vein* runs the length of the lesser curvature from the cardia to the portal vein in the same distribution as the left and right gastric arteries. There are additional pyloric veins along the pyloric part of the lesser curvature which join directly into the portal vein.

Lymphatic Drainage. The *lymphatic drainage of the stomach* and its zones of flow are illustrated in Figure 13-79. The visceral nodes consist of gastric, hepatic, and pancreaticolienal. The gastric nodes are situated along the left gastric artery and the right half of the greater curvature. The hepatic nodes are situated along the hepatic artery, near the neck of the gallbladder and in

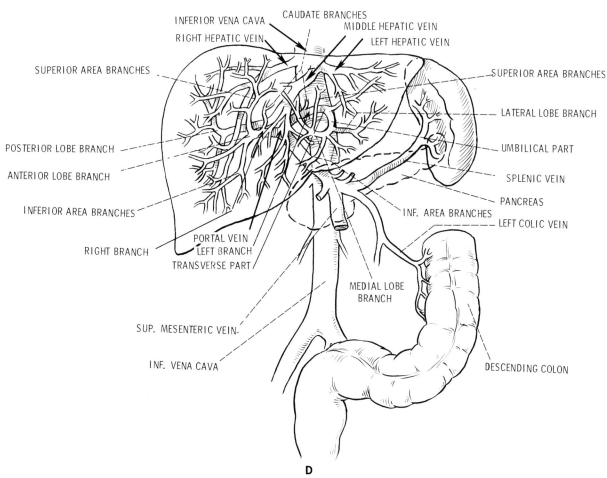

Figure 13-78 *Continued.* D. Scheme of portal system of veins and its connections with systemic veins. It must be remembered that the systemic blood carried by the hepatic artery also enters the capillaries of the liver, and the hepatic veins contain, therefore, both portal and systemic blood.

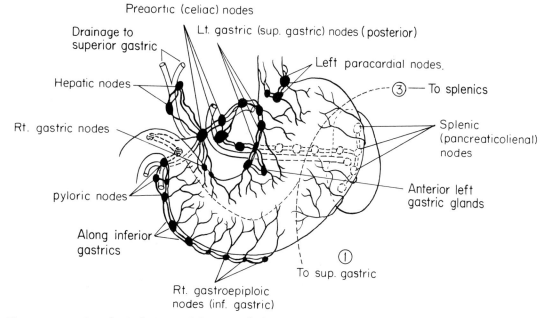

Figure 13-79. Lymphatic drainage of the stomach showing major lymph nodes, zones and flow of lymphatics.

the angle between the superior and descending duodenum. The pancreaticolienal nodes lie along the splenic artery. The lymphatic channels course along the following paths: along the left gastric artery to the superior gastric nodes; from the fundus and body to the left of the esophagus along the left gastroepiploic artery to the pancreaticolienal nodes; from the right part of the greater curvature to the inferior gastric and hepatic nodes; and from the pyloric region to the hepatic and superior gastric nodes (Pansky and House).

The Technique of Selective Celiac and Superior Mesenteric Arteriography

A Kifa x-ray opaque catheter with an outer diameter of 2.85 mm., an internal diameter of 1.5 mm., and a length of 45 to 50 cm. is usually employed. A Seldinger technique (see Chapter 11) is utilized. A C-shaped curve is imparted to the tip of the catheter by immersion in hot water to permit easier entry of the tip of the catheter into the celiac trunk. Precise localization is accomplished under fluoroscopic control. A few milliliters of heparinized saline are used to flush the catheter to ascertain that the tip is not obstructed. A few milliliters of 50 per cent sodium diatrizoate or meglumine diatrizoate are then instilled for visualization of the catheter in the vascular trunk. Finally, as a test, 10 to 15 ml. of heparinized saline are forcibly injected as rapidly as possible with the catheter tip under visual control. This will deter-

mine whether the catheter tip is in a secure position. If the catheter recoils or is dislodged, repositioning is necessary.

Twenty to 25 ml. of 75 per cent sodium diatrizoate (or meglumine diatrizoate) are used for demonstration of the celiac axis and its branches.

Mechanical injection apparatus may be utilized, with flow rates of 10 to 15 ml. per second.

Sequential films are obtained rapidly, two to three per second, so that arterial, capillary, and venous phases are all visualized. At times, a 2 to 4 second delay may be interposed following a 4 second interval at the end of the arterial phase. Very often filming must be planned to cover a total interval of between 17 and 25 seconds to visualize the venous phase adequately. Time delays in programming and special space loading of the film (if cut film is employed) are used to accomplish this format.

For visualization of the pancreas, a two catheter technique is virtually essential since the major blood supply of the pancreas is derived from the celiac and superior mesenteric trunks.

The celiac and superior mesenteric arteries may also be visualized by a translumbar approach. For this purpose a 15 cm., 16 gauge needle with stylet is employed. The needle is inserted approximately 4 cm. from the midline at the lower edge of the left twelfth rib and directed upward and medially, where it is gently advanced toward the eleventh thoracic vertebra. Once properly placed in the aorta, 40 to 50 ml. of contrast agent are rapidly injected by hand. A single film technique or serialography may be employed. A better visualization of the stomach and its blood supply is obtained if approximately 1000 to 1500 cc. of air are injected into the stomach just before the arterial and venous visualization. This may be done by nasogastric tube.

REFERENCES

Adler, D. C., Jacobson, G., Heitmann, K. A., and Watson, D. D.: Insulin-induced hypermotility in the roentgen examination of the stomach and duodenum. Radiology, 65:530–537, 1955.

Adler, R. H.: What is the cardia? J.A.M.A., 182:1045–1047, 1962.

Anson, B. J.: An Atlas of Human Anatomy. Philadelphia, W. B. Saunders Co., 1963.

Anson, B. J. (ed.): Morris' Human Anatomy. 12th edition. New York, McGraw Hill, 1966.

Bachrach, W. H.: Action of insulin hypoglyssemia on motor and secretory function of the digestive tract. Physiolog. Rev., 38:566–592, 1953.

Becker, W. F., Welsh, R. A., and Pratt, H. S.: Cystadenoma and cystadenocarcinoma of the pancreas. Ann. Surg., 161:845–863, 1965.

Berridge, F. R.: Mechanism of cardia. Symposium: three radiologic aspects. Brit. J. Radiol., 34:487–498, 1961.

Berridge, F. R., Friedland, G. W., and Tagart, R. E. B.: Radiological landmarks at esophagogastric junction. Thorax, 21:499–510, 1966.

Bierman, H. R.: Selective Arterial Catheterization. Springfield, Illinois, Charles C Thomas, 1969.

Bookstein, J. J., and Whitehouse, W. M.: Splenoportography. Radiol. Clin. N. Amer., 2:447–460, 1964.

Burhenne, H. J.: Technique of examination of the stomach and duodenum, In Margulis, A. R., and Burhenne, H. J. (eds.): Alimentary Tract Roentgenology. St. Louis, C. V. Mosby Co., 1973.

Chisholm, D. M., Blair, G. S., Low, P. S., and Whaley, K.: Hydrostatic sialography as an index of salivary gland disease in Sjögren's syndrome. Acta Radiol. (Diag.), 11:577–585, 1971.

Cunningham, D. J.: Manual of Practical Anatomy. 12th edition. London, Oxford University Press, 1958.

Darke, C. T., and Beal, J. M.: Percutaneous cholangiography. Arch. Surg., 91:558–563, 1965.

Doubilet, H., Poppel, M. H., and Mulholland, J. H.: Pancreatography. Ann. N.Y. Acad. Sci., 78:829–851, 1959.

Doubilet, H., Poppel, M. H., and Mulholland, J. H.: Pancreatography. Radiology, 64:325–339, 1955.

Evans, J. A.: Specialized roentgen diagnostic techniques in the investigation of abdominal disease. Radiology, 82:579–594, 1964.

Eyler, W. R., Clark, M. D., and Rian, R. L.: An evaluation of roentgen signs of pancreatic enlargement. J.A.M.A., 181:967–971, 1962.

Ferrucci, J. T., Jr., Benedict, K. T., Jr., Page, D. L., Fleischli, D. J., and Eaton, S. B.: Radiographic features of normal hypotonic duodenogram. Radiology, 96:401–408, 1970.

Flemma, R. J., Schauble, J. F., Gardner, C. E., Anlyan, W. G., and Capp, M. P.: Percutaneous transhepatic cholangiography in the differential diagnosis of jaundice. Surg. Gynec. Obstet., 116:559–568, 1963.

Gotton, P. B., Salmon, P. R., and Blumgart, L. H.: Cannulation of papilla of Vater via fiber duodenoscope: assessment of retrograde cholangiopancreatography in 60 patients. Lancet, 1:53–58, 1972.

Grant, J. C. B.: Atlas of Anatomy. Fifth edition. Baltimore, Williams and Wilkins Co., 1962.

Guyton, A. C.: Textbook of Medical Physiology. Fourth edition. Philadelphia, W. B. Saunders Co., 1971.

Hampton, A. O.: A safe method for the roentgen demonstration of bleeding ulcers. Amer. J. Roentgenol., 38:565–570, 1937.

Herbert, W. W., and Margulis, A. R.: Diagnosis of retroperitoneal masses by gastrointestinal roentgenographic measurements: a computer study. Radiology, 84:52–57, 1965.

Jacobson, G., Berne, C. J., Meyers, H. I., and Rosoff, L.: The examination of patients with suspected perforated ulcer using a water soluble contrast medium. Amer. J. Roentgenol., 86:37–49, 1961.

Johnstone, A. S.: Observations on the radiological anatomy of the esophagogastric junction. Radiology, 73:501–510, 1959.

Knowles, H. C., Felson, B., Shapiro, N., and Schiff, L.: Emergency diagnosis of upper digestive tract bleeding by roentgen examination without palpation. ("Hampton" technique.) Radiology, 58:536–541, 1952.

Kusagai, T., Kuno, N., and Aoki, I.: Fibroduodenoscopy: analysis of 353 examinations. Gastrointestinal Endoscopy, 18:9–16, 1971.

Lerche, W.: The esophagus and pharynx in action: a study of structure in relation to function. Springfield, Illinois, Charles C Thomas, 1950.

Lowman, R. M.: Retroperitoneal tumors: a survey and assessment of roentgen techniques. Radiol. Clin. N. Amer., 3:543–566, 1965.

Lunderquist, A.: Angiography in carcinoma of the pancreas. Acta Radiol. (Diag.), Suppl. 235:1, 1965.

Marshall, S., Lapp, M., and Schulte, J. W.: Lesions of the pancreas mimicking renal disease. J. Urol., 93:41–45, 1965.

Morcttin, L. B.: Normal and abnormal sialograms of the parotid gland. Personal communication.

Meschan, I., Landsman, H., Regnier, G., et al.: The normal radiographic adult stomach and duodenum. A study of their contour and size and their critical relationships to spine in both symptomatic and asymptomatic individuals. South Med. J., 46:878–887, 1953.

Mosely, R. D., Jr.: Roentgen diagnosis of pancreatic disease. Arch. Intern. Med., 107:31–36, 1961.

Neuhauser, E. D. B.: quoted in Sidaway, M. E.: The use of water soluble contrast medium in pediatric radiology. Clin. Radiol., 15:132–138, 1964.

Ogoshi, K., Tobita, Y., and Hara, Y.: Endoscopic observation of duodenum and pancreatocholedochography using duodenal fibroscope under direct vision. Gastroenterology, 12:83–96, 1970.

Oi, I.: Fibroduodenoscopy and endoscopic pancreato-cholangiography. Gastrointestinal Endoscopy, 17:59–62, 1970.

Okuda, K., Someya, N., Goto, A., Tadahiko, K., Emura, T., Yasumoto, M., and Shimokawa, Y.: Endoscopic pancreato-cholangiography. Amer. J. Roentgenol., 117:437–445, 1973.

Pancoast, H. K.: Possible effects of morphine on intestinal motility. Amer. J. Roentgenol., 2:549–551, 1914.

Pansky, B., and House, E. L.: Review of Gross Anatomy. New York, MacMillan Co., 1964.

Park, W. M., and Mason, D. K.: Hydrostatic sialography. Radiology, 86:116, 1966.

Pernkopf, E.: Atlas of Topographical and Applied Human Anatomy. Volumes 1 and 2. Philadelphia, W. B. Saunders Co., 1963.

Poole, G. J.: A new roentgenographic method of measuring the retrogastric and retroduodenal spaces: statistical evaluation of reliability and diagnostic utility. Radiology, 97:71–81, 1970.

Poppel, M. H.: Roentgen Manifestations of Pancreatic Disease. Springfield, Illinois, Charles C Thomas, 1951.

Poppel, M. H., Sheinmel, A., and Mednick, E.: The procurement and critical appraisal of the width diameter of the midline retrogastric soft tissues. Amer. J. Roentgenol., *61*:56–60, 1949.

Porcher, P., and Buffard, P.: Malignancy of the stomach. *In* Margulis, A. R., and Burhenne, H. J. (eds.): Alimentary Tract Roentgenology. St. Louis, C. V. Mosby Co., 1967.

Porrath, S.: Roentgenologic considerations of the hyoid apparatus. Amer. J. Roentgenol., *105*:63–73, 1969.

Quigley, J. P., and Louckes, H. S.: Gastric emptying. Amer. J. Digest. Dis., 7:672–676, 1962.

Quigley, J. P., and Meschan, I.: The gastric evacuation of fat with special reference to pyloric sphincter activity. Gastroenterol., *4*:272–275, 1937.

Rasmussen, T.: Pharmacoradiography of the stomach. Nord. Med., *44*:1563–1566, 1950.

Rea, C. E.: Conservative versus operative treatment of perforated peptic ulcer. Surgery, *32*:654–657, 1952.

Ritvo, M.: Drugs as an aid in roentgen examination of the gastrointestinal tract: the use of Mecholyl, physostigmine, and Benzedrine in overcoming atonicity, sluggishness of peristalsis, and spasm. Amer. J. Roentgenol., *36*:868–874, 1936.

Robbins, A. H., Paul, R. E., Jr., Norton, R. A., Schimmel, E. M., Tomas, J. G., and Sugarman, H. J.: Detection of malignant disease by peroral retrograde pancreatico-biliary ductography. Amer. J. Roentgenol., *117*:432–436, 1973.

Rösch, J.: Roentgenology of the Spleen and Pancreas. Springfield, Illinois, Charles C Thomas, 1967.

Rösch, J., and Herfort, K.: Contribution of splenoportography to the diagnosis of diseases of the pancreas. Acta Med. Scand., *171*:263–272, 1962.

Ruzicka, F. F., and Rossi, P.: Normal vascular anatomy of the abdominal viscera. Radiol. Clin. N. Amer., *8*:3–29, 1970.

Sachs, M. D., and Partington, P. F.: Cholangiographic diagnosis of pancreatitis. Amer. J. Roentgenol., *76*:32–38, 1956.

Salik, J. O.: Pancreatic carcinoma and its early roentgenologic recognition. Amer. J. Roentgenol., *86*:1–28, 1961.

Schultz, E. H.: Aid to diagnosis of acute pancreatitis by roentgenologic study. Amer. J. Roentgenol., *89*:825–836, 1963.

Schultz, E. H.: Cervical disk disease simulating intramedullary neoplasms by myelography. Radiology, *84*:389, 1965.

Sheinmel, A., and Mednick, E. A.: The roentgen diagnosis of upper abdominal retroperitoneal space-occupying lesions. Amer. J. Roentgenol., *65*:77–92, 1951.

Sidaway, M. E.: The use of water soluble contrast medium in pediatric radiology. Clin. Radiol., *15*:132–138, 1964.

Siebert, T. L., Stein, J., and Poppel, M. H.: Variations in the roentgen appearance of the "esophageal lip." Amer. J. Roentgenol., *81*:570–575, 1959.

Silbiger, M. L., and Donner, M. W.: Morphine in the evaluation of gastrointestinal disease: a cineradiographic study. Radiology, *90*:1090–1096, 1968.

Stein, G. N., Kalser, M. H., Sarian, N. N., and Finkelstein, A.: An evaluation of the roentgen changes in acute pancreatitis: correlation with clinical findings. Gastroenterology, *36*:354–361, 1959.

Tagaki, K., Ikeda, S., and Nakagawa, Y.: Retrograde pancreatography and cholangiography by fibroduodenoscope. Gastroenterology, *59*:445–452, 1970.

Taylor, D. A., Macken, K. L., Fiore, A. S., Colcher, H., Bachman, A. L., and Seaman, W. B.: New method of visualizing gastric wall. Further studies. Radiology, *86*:711–717, 1966.

Varriale, P., Bonanno, C. A., and Grace, W. J.: Portal hypertension secondary to pancreatic pseudocysts. Arch. Intern. Med. (Chicago), *112*:191–198, 1963.

Weens, H. S., and Walker, L. A.: Radiologic diagnosis of acute cholecystitis and pancreatitis. Radiol. Clin. N. Amer., *2*:89–106, 1964.

Wolf, B. S.: Roentgen features of normal and herniated esophagogastric region. Amer. J. Digest. Dis., *5*:751–769, 1960.

Wolf, B. S.: Roentgen features of the normal and herniated esophagogastric region; clinical correlations. *In* Glass, G. B. J. (ed.): Progress in Gastroenterology. Vol. 2, New York, Grune and Stratton, 1970, pp. 288–315.

Wolf, B. S.: Sliding hiatal hernia: the need for re-definition. Amer. J. Roentgenol., *117*:231–247, 1973.

Small Intestine, Colon, and Biliary Tract

THE SMALL INTESTINE

Gross Anatomy. The small intestine during life varies considerably in length. It is well known, for example, that the entire small intestine can be traversed by a Miller-Abbott tube several feet in length, whereas its length at autopsy is usually 20 to 22 feet; probably with good muscle tone during life it varies between 15 and 17 feet. In formalin-hardened bodies, it rarely measures longer than 12 or 13 feet in length. There is a gradual diminution in diameter from the pylorus to the ileocecal valve (valvula coli).

The jejunum and ileum are completely covered with peritoneum and therefore vary considerably in position, except at the two ends where relative fixation occurs. However, the small intestine is usually distributed in the abdomen according to a fairly regular pattern (Fig. 14-1). Thus, the proximal jejunum usually lies in the left half of the abdomen between the level of the pancreas and the intercrestal line. The distal ileum usually lies deep in the pelvis posteriorly, with the terminal ileum arising out of the pelvis to meet the cecum in the right lower quadrant anteriorly. The distal jejunum and proximal ileum are distributed in the right half of the abdomen for the most part.

The root of the mesentery, about 15 cm. long, is attached to the posterior abdominal wall along a line running obliquely from the left side of the body of the L2 vertebra to the right sacroiliac joint, crossing the third part of the duodenum, the aorta, the inferior vena cava, the right gonadal vessels, the right ureter, and the right psoas muscle (Fig. 14-2). It is approximately 20 cm. broad, on the average, tending to become narrower as it reaches the lower end of the ileum. The mesentery contains blood vessels, lymphatics, lymph nodes, and nerves of the small intestine, as well as fat.

The mucous membrane of the small intestine is enormously increased in surface area by the formation of circular folds (valvulae conniventes), upon which are mounted intestinal villi (Figs. 14-3 and 14-4). The circular folds give a characteristic coiled-spring appearance to the inner aspect of the small intestine. These folds reach their maximum development in the distal half of the duodenum and proximal part of the jejunum, where

they may be as much as 8 mm. in height and extend around two-thirds of the circumference of the bowel, branching in the course of their extension. Thereafter they gradually become smaller and less numerous so that they are virtually absent in the lower ileum (Fig. 14-3). Although they extend through the wall of the bowel and involve the whole thickness of the mucous membrane and a core of submucosa, they do not involve the serosa, unlike the valvulae semilunares of the colon.

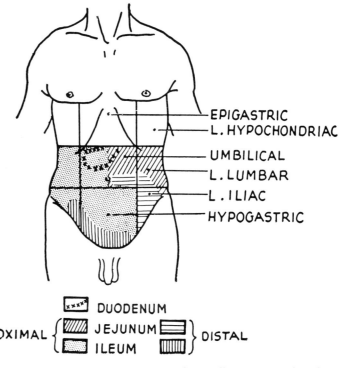

SCHEME OF NORMAL POSITION OF SMALL INTESTINE

PROXIMAL / DISTAL

DUODENUM

JEJUNUM

ILEUM

EPIGASTRIC
L. HYPOCHONDRIAC
UMBILICAL
L. LUMBAR
L. ILIAC
HYPOGASTRIC

Figure 14-1. Approximate distribution of the small intestine within the abdomen.

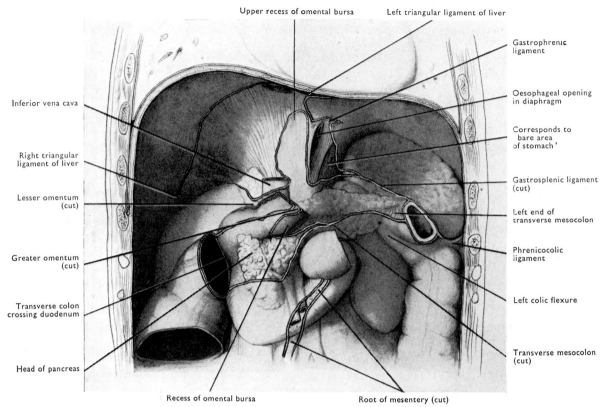

Figure 14–2.   Peritoneal relations of duodenum, pancreas, spleen, kidneys, etc. From a body hardened by injection of formalin. When the liver, stomach, and intestines were removed the lines of the peritoneal reflections were carefully preserved. (From Cunningham's Textbook of Anatomy, 10th ed. London, Oxford University Press, 1964.)

The intestinal villi are mounted on these folds and measure less than half a millimeter in height. They begin at the pyloric orifice where they are broad and short, becoming longer and narrower as they approach the ileocecal valve. These villi are actu-

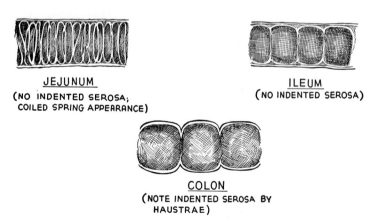

Figure 14–3.   Differences in roentgen appearance of distended small and large intestines.

ally present on and between the circular folds but never over solitary lymph nodules. In the center of each villus there is a lymph channel — a central lacteal — which joins the submucous lymph plexuses and a vascular capillary network that drains into a vein at the base of the villus.

Major Differences Between Jejunum and Ileum.   The main differences between the jejunum and ileum from the radiographic standpoint can be summarized as follows:

1. There is a gradual diminution in diameter as the cecum is approached, and thus the lumen of the ileum is smaller than that of the jejunum. The average diameter of the jejunum measures 3 to 3.5 cm.; that of the ileum, 2.5 cm. or less.

2. The plicae circulares commence in the second part of the duodenum (see the description in the preceding chapter). The maximum number and size of plicae circulares are found in the midjejunum, and they diminish toward the ileum, practically ceasing a little below the middle of this portion. This fact is important because the mucosal pattern of the ileum differs from that of the proximal jejunum by being considerably smoother and less feathery (Fig. 14–5). Barium tends to have a more clumped appearance in the ileum than in the jejunum as a result of this fundamental difference. In the ileocecal region, the rugae tend to be

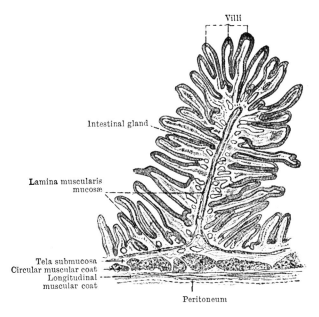

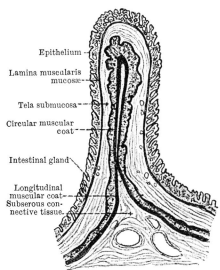

Figure 14–4. Diagrammatic presentation of the differences in transverse section between the plicae circulares of the small intestine and plicae semilunares of the large intestine. (From Cunningham's Textbook of Anatomy, 6th ed. London, Oxford University Press, 1931.)

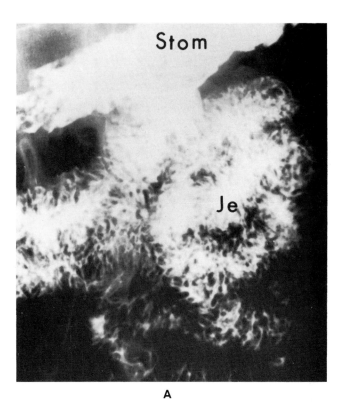

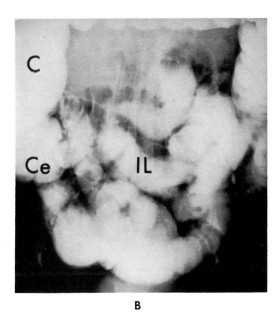

Figure 14–5. *A.* Radiograph of jejunal mucosal pattern. *B.* Radiograph of ileal mucosal pattern.

parallel in type approaching the appearance of the rugae in the pylorus.

3. The aggregate lymphatic nodules, or Peyer's patches, are most numerous in the ileum and considerably fewer in number in the jejunum. They are more prominent in young people and tend to atrophy as age advances. They are not ordinarily distinguishable radiographically and normally do not play a significant role in radiographic diagnosis.

4. In the adult, because the mesentery of the ileum contains

considerably more fatty tissue than that of the jejunum, it appears to be considerably thicker than the latter structure.

Intestinal Glands. The crypts between the villi contain one or two tubular structures connected with intestinal glands or "crypts of Lieberkühn." The villi are otherwise covered by a single layer of cylindrical epithelial cells with glandular cells of three types occasionally interspersed: (1) goblet cells, (2) oxyphilic granular cells of Paneth, and (3) argentaffine cells.

The goblet cells secrete mucous fluid. Generally, they are found low in the crypts along the lower part of the villi, but occasionally they are located in the upper regions of the villi as well. The oxyphilic granular cells of Paneth are characteristically situated in the floor of the crypts; they participate in enzyme production. Argentaffine or yellow cells have a high affinity for silver and chromium, and their characteristic site is in the fundi of the crypts of Lieberkühn. They are associated with the production of serotonin, and they are found with particular frequency in the duodenum and the appendix.

The secretions from these glands are rapidly reabsorbed by the villi so that there is a constant circulation of fluid from the crypts to the villi, thus supplying a watery vehicle for absorption of food substances from the small intestine. The epithelial cells of the mucosa of the small intestine contain large quantities of digestive enzymes, enabling them presumably to digest food substances during absorption through the epithelium (Guyton).

There is a constant reproductive cycle of these epithelial cells from deep within the crypts of Lieberkühn toward the surface of the mucosa. The life cycle of an intestinal epithelial cell is approximately 48 hours. Thus, excoriation of the small intestine is rapidly repaired. One of the chief effects of radiation on the small intestine, however, is significant impairment of the reproductive capacity of the crypts of Lieberkühn.

Motility Study of the Small Intestine. It has been well established that many systemic diseases (such as vitamin deficiency, protein deficiency, certain anemias, allergic states, and so on) are capable of producing considerable changes in the motility pattern of the small intestine, and for that reason, a close study of the normal small intestinal motility is imperative.

Cannon was one of the first investigators to demonstrate intestinal motility, both by direct inspection of the exposed intestine in anesthetized animals and also by radiographic studies in the intact animal. He described *rhythmic segmentation, pendulum movements* and *peristaltic waves.*

The movements of rhythmic segmentation occur at a rate of 8 to 9 per minute in the duodenum, becoming progressively slower farther down the small intestine. These contractions appear to divide the small intestine into segments, imparting to it the appearance of a "chain of sausages." Such chopping movements of the intestinal chyme tend to mix the chyme with intestinal secretions and promote absorption.

The pendular movements consist of small constrictive waves that sweep forward and then backward, up and down a few centimeters of the gut. By moving the contents back and forth within the intestinal lumen these movements further keep the intestinal contents thoroughly mixed.

Peristaltic waves propel the intestinal contents toward the anus at a velocity of approximately 1 to 2 cm. per second. Usually, the contents travel visibly only a few centimeters at a time. Peristaltic activity generally increases immediately after a meal and is produced by the so-called "gastroenteric reflex." Intense irritation of the intestinal mucosa may produce a rapid peristaltic movement, the so-called "peristaltic rush," which may pass over large lengths of intestine in a few minutes, sweeping the contents into the colon.

A significant delay of the intestinal contents may occur in the region of the ileocecal valve, often relieved by a gastroileal or gastroenteric reflex at the time of another meal.

Actually, our present-day concept is not quite so clear-cut as Cannon's description might indicate. Barium usually passes quite rapidly into the jejunum for approximately 30 or 40 cm., and thereafter the movement of the barium column proceeds quite slowly. The lumen of the jejunum is usually sufficiently collapsed to permit a ready and accurate visualization of the rugal pattern. Peristaltic waves are the most common type of motility, but occasionally an overall circular movement of a whole segment of small bowel is superimposed. The barium column gradually moves on into the ileum, where there is a smoother and less fluffy pattern, and where the barium tends to remain longer in continuous cylinders. Ordinarily, the barium remains clumped in the distal ileum for a considerable period of time, and periodically a peristaltic wave will be seen to carry a small portion of the barium into the terminal ileum, which rises out of the pelvis to meet the cecum. Peristaltic waves are intermittent over the terminal ileum. In the distal ileum, there is virtually no rugal pattern visible, and all movement is difficult to observe fluoroscopically, since the ileal loops are conglomerated and difficult to palpate in view of their posterior position.

The average time for the head of the barium column to reach the ileocecal region is $1\frac{1}{2}$ to 2 hours, but it is not unusual for a period of 4 hours to elapse before barium appears in the cecum. Abnormality, either primary or secondary, in the emptying of the stomach will of course affect the emptying time of the small intestine, and any abnormality of the terminal ileum may be reflected in a delayed emptying of the stomach.

Special Anatomy of the Ileocecal Valve (Valvula Coli). The terminal ileum projects into the cecum at its termination, producing folds or a papillary protrusion that function as a sphincter. The serosa of the ileum does not participate in this protrusion and helps to prevent abnormal invagination of the terminal ileum into the ascending colon (called "intussusception"). The filling defect produced by this anatomic structure is readily visualized radiographically (Figs. 14–6, 14–7).

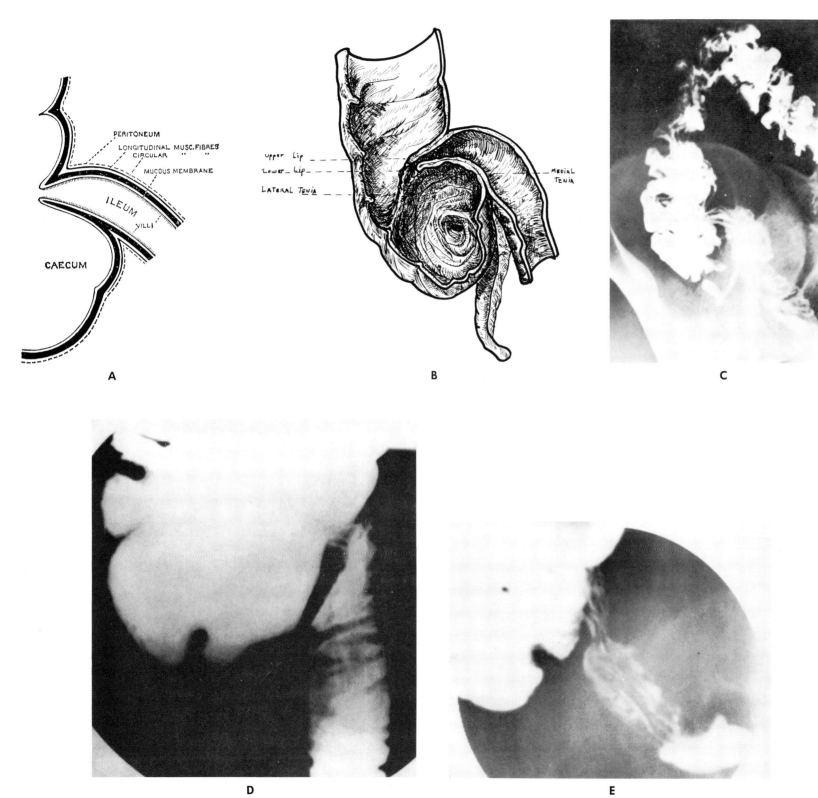

Figure 14–6. Ileocecal junction. *A.* Diagrammatic section. (From Cunningham's Textbook of Anatomy, 6th ed. London, Oxford University Press, 1931.) *B.* Line drawing of the ileocecal valve. (From Rubin, S., Dann, D. S., Ezekial, C., and Vincent, J.: Amer. J. Roentgenol., *87*:708, 1962). *C, D, E.* Ileocecal junction; spot film studies.

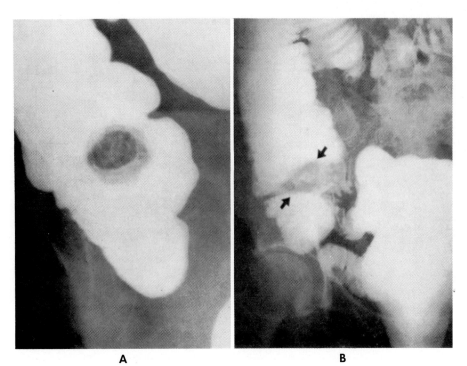

A   B

Figure 14–7. Difference between prolapse (A) and prominent ileocecal valves (B). In the former the central slitlike valve orifice is not filled with barium, whereas in the latter it stands out clearly. This is a posteriorly situated valve. (From Hinkel, C. L.: Amer. J. Roentgenol., 68, 1952.)

The function of this valve is sphincteric—much like that of the pyloric valve—but it is unknown if its main function is to prevent regurgitation as is the case with the pyloric sphincter. In performing barium enema examinations, it is possible to force barium from the colon into the terminal ileum in at least half of the cases, and this incompetency is probably of no pathologic significance. Ordinarily, however, in gaseous distention of the colon from any mechanical obstructive cause at a lower level in the colon, the ileocecal valve will prevent passage of the gas back up into the small intestine for a considerable period of time.

THE LARGE INTESTINE

Gross Anatomy. The large intestine is approximately 5 to 5½ feet in length and varies in diameter from 1½ to 3 inches. Commencing at the cecum, it is further subdivided into ascending colon, transverse colon, descending and iliac colon, sigmoid or pelvic colon, and rectum.

The cecum is found in the right lower quadrant of the abdomen ordinarily, but its position is most variable. It is usually situated anteriorly, with only the omentum and abdominal wall lying over it. The terminal ileum joins the cecum usually on its medial or posterior aspect, and the vermiform appendix springs from the cecum on the same side as the ileocecal junction. The upper end of the cecum is continuous with the ascending colon. There is considerable variation, however, in the position of the cecum, both in respect to its posterior peritoneal attachment and to its relationship to the pelvic rim or the abdomen. Some variations in attachment of the posterior peritoneum to the cecum are shown in Figure 14–8. Variations in the contour of the cecum, terminal ileum, and appendix, when on the right side of the abdomen, are shown in Figure 14–9. Variations in position of the appendix and cecum are shown in Figure 14–10.

The vermiform appendix is part of the cecum. It arises from the point where the three taeniae of the large intestine merge into one uniform coat of longitudinal muscle. It varies considerably in length from 2.5 to 25 cm., averaging 6 to 9 cm. Unless inflamed, it varies in position freely in the same individual in relation to its attachment to the cecum. Its movement depends considerably on the length and width of the peritoneal fold that represents its mesentery. At times it points upward toward the liver and sometimes it is "retrocolic" rather than retrocecal, lying behind or to the right of the ascending colon. It contains masses of

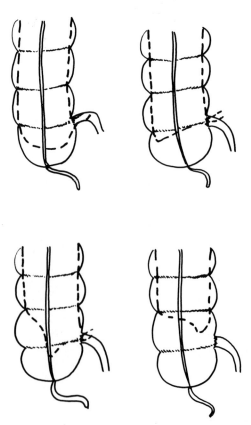

Figure 14–8. Diagram showing variations in position of the posterior peritoneal attachment of the cecum.

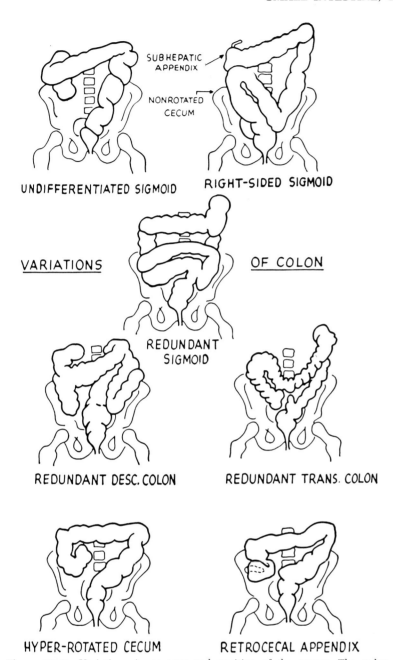

UNDIFFERENTIATED SIGMOID   RIGHT-SIDED SIGMOID

SUBHEPATIC APPENDIX

NONROTATED CECUM

VARIATIONS   OF COLON

REDUNDANT SIGMOID

REDUNDANT DESC. COLON   REDUNDANT TRANS. COLON

HYPER-ROTATED CECUM   RETROCECAL APPENDIX

Figure 14–9. Variations in contour and position of the cecum. The redundancy of various parts of the colon is also illustrated.

The lower portion of the ascending colon may be on a partial mesentery, and, like the cecum, rather anterior in position, but very soon it proceeds posteriorly in most instances, assuming a partially covered retroperitoneal position. When it reaches the inferior surface of the liver, it turns forward and to the left (forming the hepatic flexure). It lies between the quadratus lumborum laterally, and the psoas major muscle medially. Its posterior surface is ordinarily not peritonealized, thus giving it a relatively fixed position, but it is surprisingly mobile radiographically despite these anatomic limitations.

The hepatic flexure is ordinarily situated lateral and anterior to the descending portion of the duodenum, and posterior to the thin anterior margin of the liver. Its peritoneal relations are similar to those of the ascending colon.

The transverse colon has a long mesentery, and as a result is subject to wide variation in length and position. It usually hangs down in front of the small intestine, at a considerable distance from the posterior abdominal wall, with only the greater omentum and anterior abdominal wall lying over it. *Along its first few centimeters, however, it is usually firmly attached to the anterior surface of the second part of the duodenum and the head of the pancreas* — a factor of considerable importance when these structures are distended by a space-occupying lesion, since there is in such cases a secondary displacement of this portion of the colon. Toward the left, the mesentery shortens, bringing this segment close to the tail of the pancreas, with the stomach lying anterior and to the right. At the inferior surface of the spleen, it passes into the splenic flexure, which is again retroperitoneal *but at a higher level than the hepatic flexure.*

The posterior surface of the greater omentum adheres to the upper surface of the transverse mesocolon and to the serosal coating on the anterior side of the transverse colon. The omentum droops down from the greater curvature of the stomach, forming a double fold over the middle part of the transverse colon.

The splenic flexure is perhaps the most constant part of the colon, being held in position by the phrenicocolic ligament, which is attached laterally to the diaphragm opposite the ninth to the eleventh rib posteriorly.

The descending and iliac portions of the colon are the narrowest parts. The descending colon first lies in contact with the lateral margin of the left kidney, and then in a comparable position with the ascending colon on the right. The posterior surface is not peritonealized and the descending colon is less mobile ordinarily than the ascending.

The iliac colon lies in the iliac fossa and, like the descending colon, is not peritonealized on its posterior surface.

The pelvic or sigmoid colon has a mesentery of its own, which accounts for the mobility of this portion of the colon, and is somewhat variable in width. It usually lies for the most part in the pelvis minor, but occasionally with marked redundancy it may escape above into the abdominal cavity. In the child at birth,

lymphoepithelial tissue and some glandular elements such as argentaffine cells, the latter of which give rise to carcinoid tumors, the appendix being a frequent site of these neoplasms. Since the lumen of the vermiform appendix is often patent, it may be visualized radiographically at the time of a barium enema or following the ingestion of oral barium.

THE COLON

ANOMALIES OF THE CECUM, ABNORMALITIES OF POSITION

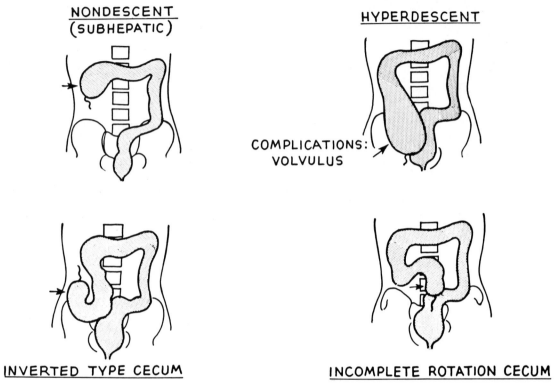

NONDESCENT (SUBHEPATIC)

HYPERDESCENT

COMPLICATIONS: VOLVULUS

INVERTED TYPE CECUM

INCOMPLETE ROTATION CECUM

Figure 14–10. Variations of the contour of the ascending colon in particular, demonstrating abnormalities of contour as well as position of the cecum.

owing to the small size of the pelvis minor, only the terminal part of the pelvic colon lies in this area. In the child, the pelvic colon usually arches over to the right side, and lies in great part in the right iliac fossa. At the termination of the pelvic colon, it arches backward and downward to form the rectosigmoid junction.

The rectosigmoid junction is usually the narrowest point in the colon, and this narrowness may extend for 1 to 1.5 cm. *This narrowness sometimes is difficult to distinguish from an abnormal constriction,* and the radiologist must be thoroughly familiar with the normal variations of this region (Fig. 14–20D). Ordinarily, the rectosigmoid junction is found at the level of the third sacral vertebra. The peritoneal coat continues down from the sigmoid but only over the anterior and lateral rectal walls for about 1 to 2 cm.

The rectum is a true retroperitoneal organ. The peritoneal reflection between the rectum and the bladder in the male, or between the rectum and the uterus in the female forms the *rectovesical* or *rectouterine recess or pouch.*

Rectum and Anal Canal. *The rectum and anal canal are more accurately examined by the proctoscope and sigmoidoscope and by digital palpation than by radiographic methods,* and for that reason less radiographic emphasis is placed upon these regions. The rectum has only a partial covering of peritoneum, and no sacculations; it is very distensible, particularly in its midportion, and this area is therefore called the rectal ampulla. The rectum first follows the hollow of the sacrum and coccyx, and then turns gently forward and finally abruptly downward to join the anal canal. There are three (and sometimes as many as five) crescentic folds, called the plicae transversales (plicae of Houston), which project into the lumen of the rectum. These pass around two-thirds of the rectal circumference and produce indentations on the radiograph of the rectum. They are variable in position and occasionally are poorly developed or virtually absent. It is probable that these are similar in origin to the plicae semilunares of the rest of the colon, but in the absence of the taeniae coli they take on a somewhat different appearance. There are creases in addition, however, that involve the entire wall of the rectum in their structure.

Some of the distinguishing features of the anal canal and rectum in relation to the sigmoid are shown in Figure 14–11. The superior and inferior plicae of Houston or rectal valves (also called the plica transversalis of Kohlrausch) are located on the left side, between 2 and 4 cm. from the rectosigmoid junction. The middle rectal valve lies just inferior to the peritoneal cul-de-sac, usually on the right side at or slightly above the level of the peritoneal reflection, approximately the distance that a probing finger can reach in rectal digital examination. This is usually the largest of the three valves, but their size varies individually, as does their number. These rectal valves occupy one-third to one-half the circumference of the rectum. The superior rectal valve is below the level of the rectosigmoid junction, which has also been called the

"third sphincter" (Cohen). Although there is considerable variability in the rectal valves, some identification of them is possible roentgenographically (in 83 per cent of cases in the lateral projection, according to Cohen).

The sphincteric portion of the rectum is actually the upper third of the surgical anal canal, usually about 4 to 6 cm. above the anal verge.

The lower two-thirds of the surgical anal canal is identical with the *anatomic anal canal*, and extends to the margin where the anal tube opens outward, approximately where hair stops growing in the margin of the anal skin.

The axis of the anal canal is, in adults, directed anteriorly toward the umbilicus, in contrast to that of the rectum, which is directed posteriorly along the margin of the sacrum. *However, in infants, both the rectal and anal axes take the same direction because the child still lacks the adult rectal curves. This may predispose to anal and rectal prolapse in childhood.*

The average width of the prominent rectal fold is 4.3 mm. ± 1.1 mm., with a range of 2 to 7 mm. The 95 per cent limit is therefore approximately 6.5 mm.

The fascia of Waldeyer is a thin layer of fatty areolar tissue which lies anterior to the sacrum between it and the rectal wall. This layer is continuous with the extraperitoneal layer of areolar tissue. When the rectum is filled with barium, it balloons out to fill the hollow of the sacrum so that the presacral space normally becomes very small. Examples of normal and abnormal appearances are shown in Figure 14–12. When the rectum is empty the space is rather large because the rectum falls away from the sacral concavity. The retrosacral distance in randomly selected normal patients is usually less than 1 cm. in width, with a mean value of 0.7 cm. and a range of 0.2 to 1.6 cm. It is thought that any measurement above 2 cm. can be interpreted as abnormal (Chrispin and Fry). Others have measured this distance more conservatively (Edling and Eklof), but in our experience the measurements of Chrispin and Fry apparently are more applicable. When this space was measured in a large series of children without signs of inflammatory large bowel disease, it was found to range between 1 and 5 mm., with over half of the measurements falling at 3 mm. (Eklof and Gierup). These measurements are 2 mm. below those given by Rudhe.

Normal Anatomic Relationships and Variations of Position in the Colon

1. Although in most patients the ascending colon is "retroperitoneal," usually to the point where it passes over the inferior portion of the right kidney, there is a mesentery, albeit short, of the ascending colon in 26 per cent of persons (Treves).

2. It will be recalled that the transverse mesocolon is attached to the midportion of the head of the pancreas and to the inferior surface of the body and tail of the pancreas. It passes above the duodenojejunal junction and over the upper portion of the an-

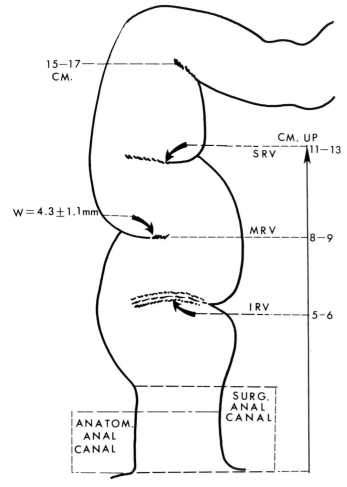

Figure 14–11. Diagram illustrating the rectum, the valves of Houston, and the position of the rectosigmoid junction. (W) Width, (SRV) superior rectal valve, (MRV) middle rectal valve, (IRV) inferior rectal valve.

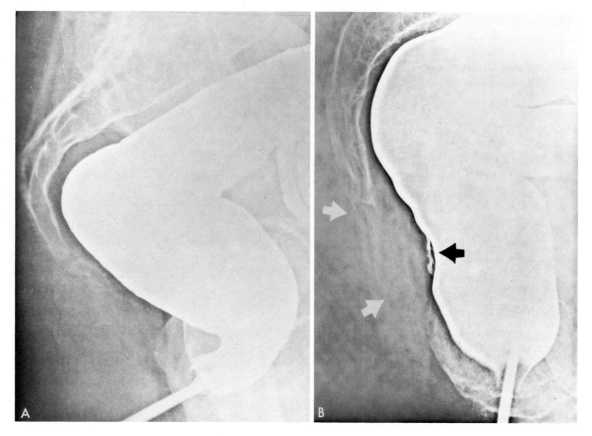

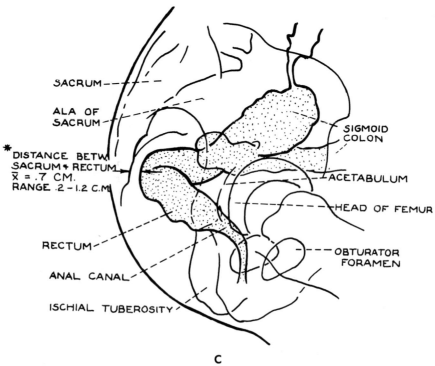

Figure 14–12. Lateral view of sacrum, coccyx, and barium-filled rectum, demonstrating (A) normal close application of rectum to sacrum and coccyx even with sharp angulation of the sacrum, and (B) displacement of barium-filled rectum by a chordoma which has partially destroyed the tip of the sacrum and adjoining coccyx. C. Diagram showing rectosacral distance and its measurement.

terior surface of the left kidney, and then descends abruptly. It is fixed at this level by the phrenicocolic ligament.

3. The colon in this region is related closely to the inferior and posterior portions of the tip of the spleen—this relationship is illustrated in Figure 14–13. This ligament is a strong peritoneal fold, extending from the splenic flexure of the colon to the parietal peritoneum overlying the posterolateral aspect of the diaphragm at the level of the eleventh rib. This is the most posterior portion in position of the entire colon. The splenic angle, radiographically visualized because of contrast afforded by extraperitoneal fat (see Chapter 15), marks the site of the phrenicocolic ligament on a plain radiograph. At this site the colon becomes retroperitoneal and starts to descend. This ligament also bridges the limit of the left paracolonic gutter and is related to some of the roentgen signs of abnormality, thus assuming considerable significance at times (Meyers) (for more detail on the colon "cutoff sign" see *Analysis of Roentgen Signs*).

4. The descending segment of the colon is without a mesen-

tery in 64 per cent of the cases, while 36 per cent do have a mesocolon (Treves).

5. The relationship of frontal and lateral perspectives of the colon has been very carefully documented by Whalen and Riemenschneider, and is shown in Figure 14–14. In this correlation they point out that the splenic flexure as visualized roentgenographically may not actually represent the point of anatomic splenic flexure. Thus, in their diagram, all of the area from points 4 to 5 (Fig. 14–14) is mesenteric, since although point 4 is that portion of the colon which has been called the splenic flexure roentgenographically, it is point 5 that is actually fixed retroperitoneally, is in constant relation to the inferior tip of the spleen, and hence, is the point of attachment of the phrenicocolic ligament. The area of attachment of the phrenicocolic ligament is indeed a constant one to look for.

6. Such close analysis of the relationship of the colon to contiguous organs is important in predicting causes of displacement of the colon, such as: (a) enlargement of the liver will depress

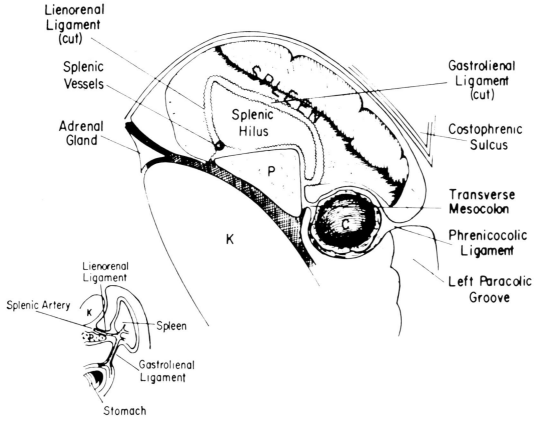

Figure 14–13. The phrenicocolic ligament is continuous with the transverse mesocolon and the gastrolienal ligament and indirectly with the lienorenal and gastrocolic ligaments. Posteriorly and laterally, it reflects to the parietal peritoneum. The small horizontal diagram shows the tail of the pancreas ensheathed intraperitoneally by the leaves of the lienorenal ligament. (From Meyers, M. A.: Radiology, 95:539–545, 1970.)

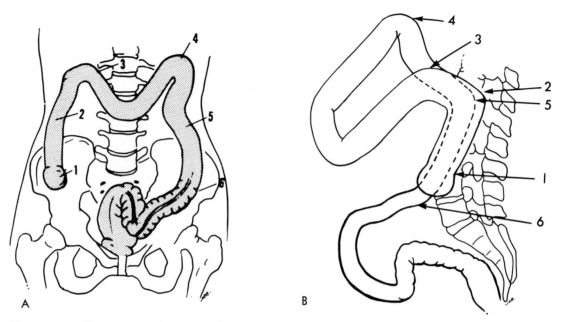

Figure 14–14. Diagrammatic drawings of the entire colon in frontal (*A*) and lateral (*B*) projections. The known anatomic portions of the colon are labeled from 1 to 6. (1) Ileocecal area; (2) the most distal portion of the fixed retroperitoneal right colon, the most posterior portion of the right flexure; (3) the area of the colon as it passes over the second portion of the duodenum, where the mesentery begins to lengthen; (4) the roentgenographic splenic flexure; (5) the anatomic splenic flexure; (6) that portion of colon which again becomes mesenteric, the beginning of the sigmoid colon. (From Whalen, J. P., and Riemenschneider, P. A.: Amer. J. Roentgenol., 99:55–61, 1967.)

point 2 of the colon (Fig. 14–14) and push to the left the area between points 2 and 3; (b) enlargement of the gallbladder will depress point 3, but will not affect the area from points 2 to 3; (c) right kidney masses will displace anteriorly the area from points 2 to 3 and will depress this segment (with the exception of lesions of the inferior pole of the right kidney which lie beneath the mesocolon, and which would thus elevate the segment from points 2 to 3); (d) right adrenal masses will displace the colon in the same way as would masses affecting the upper pole of the right kidney.

(e) Lesions of the pancreas will depress the area of the colon between points 3 and 4, at the point of insertion of the mesocolon.

(f) Lesions of the left kidney will ele ate the distal portion of the segment from point 3 to point 4, an .1l laterally displace the portion of the colon from point 4 to point 5. Most of the kidney tissue on the left side is below the insertion of the mesocolon, and the fixed portions of the left colon are lateral to the kidney (exception: a mass arising in the superior pole of the left kidney).

(g) Left adrenal masses will displace the colon in the same way as a mass situated in the superior portion of the left kidney, depressing the segment between points 4 and 5.

(h) Enlargement of the spleen will depress point 5 of the colon and displace to the right and anteriorly the portion from point 4 to point 5. An enlargement in the region of the tail of the

pancreas could displace the colon in the same way as masses in or enlargements of the spleen.

(i) Retroperitoneal tumors will displace the colon anteriorly from points 1 to 3 and points 5 to 6.

Distinguishing Features between the Large and Small Intestines. Those features which distinguish the large from the small intestine are: (1) the *taeniae coli*, which are longitudinal bands of muscle running along the outer surface of the large intestine and symmetrically placed around its circumference; (2) the *appendices epiploicae*, which are small peritoneal processes projecting from the serous coat of the large intestine; and (3) the *haustral sacculations* of the large intestine (Fig. 14–15).

The taeniae coli are the three longitudinal muscle bands into which the longitudinal musculature of the large intestine is principally concentrated; they pass from the cecum to the rectum, where they disappear in a fan-shaped process to form a more continuous layer of muscle around the rectum.

The appendices epiploicae usually contain fat and project from the serous coat of the entire large intestine, with the exception of the rectum. Their importance radiologically lies in the fact that occasionally they undergo calcification.

The haustral sacculations are produced by crescentic folds of the entire wall of the large bowel that result in a segmented appearance, each haustral segment measuring 3 to 5 cm. in length.

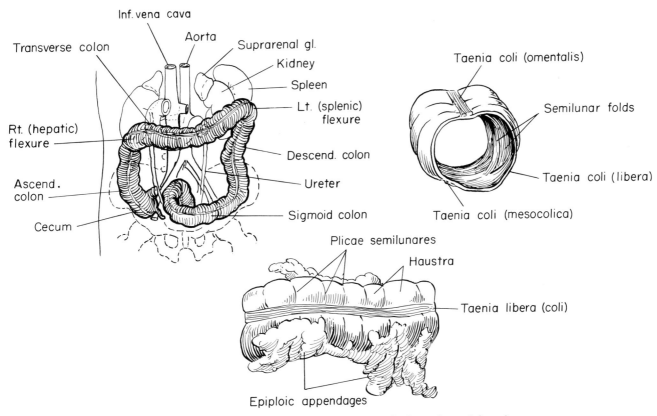

Figure 14–15.   Distinguishing anatomic features and relationships of the colon.

There are creases or folds on the interior of the large intestine that correspond with the external folds, which are called the plicae semilunares of the colon. These plicae differ from those of the small intestine in that: (1) they contain not only the mucosal fold, but the submucosal layer and also a portion of the muscular layer as well; and (2) they are much more widely separated — each of these folds extends around one-third the circumference of the wall of the large intestine between two taeniae coli.

The radiographic representation of these differences (Fig. 14–3 and 4) between the plicae circulares of the small intestine and the plicae semilunares of the colon is of considerable practical significance in attempting to differentiate the gas-distended small and large intestine. The plicae circulares are very closely placed with respect to one another, and are most conspicuous in the jejunum and least conspicuous in the ileum. Occasionally, they are completely effaced in the ileum. They form a sharp margin with the outer wall of the small bowel, since they are purely mucosal folds, and have no contribution from the outer layers of the wall of the small bowel. The plicae semilunares of the colon, on the other hand, are usually 3 to 5 cm. apart, are most conspicuous in the transverse colon, and have rounded margins, in which there is a contribution from the entire wall of the large intestine.

The widest parts of the colon are the cecum and the full rectum. There is a gradual diminution in the caliber of the colon from the cecum to the rectosigmoid junction.

Mucosal Pattern of the Large Intestine.   When the colon is full (Fig. 14–16) only the normal haustral pattern of the colon is visible. This is slightly more irregular in the ascending colon than in the transverse, and *may be virtually absent in the descending colon and sigmoid* when the latter portions of the colon are examined radiographically. The haustral appearance of the descending and pelvic colons is therefore variable.

When the colon is empty (Fig. 14–17), its mucosa is thrown into numerous irregular folds. These folds, however, are coarser than those of the small intestine because of the lack of the plicae circulares and villi. The pattern, however, is an irregular mosaic throughout the colon, except in the iliac and pelvic colons where these folds assume a more regular and parallel appearance. The pattern of the cecum (Fig. 14–18) differs also slightly from that of the rest of the colon, in that there is a greater tendency toward a spiral arrangement of the rugal pattern.

An examination of the rugal pattern of the colon is a very important part of the colonic examination, and for that reason a film after evacuation of a barium enema is never omitted.

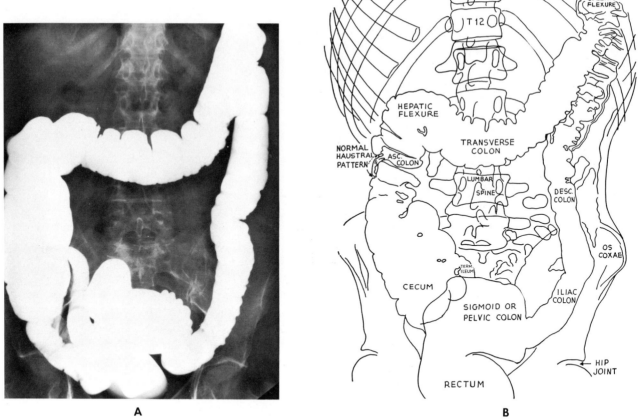

Figure 14–16.   Colon distended with barium. *A.* Radiograph. *B.* Tracing.

Special Anatomy of the Vermiform Appendix.   The appendix usually arises from the cecum on its medial or posterior aspects, about 2.5 to 4 cm. from the ileocecal valve. It is extremely variable in size and position (Figs. 14–9; 14–10). There is a "valve" at its orifice in the cecum that probably does not function in life, although occasionally the appendix even with a patent lumen will not fill immediately at the time of a barium enema and will be seen to contain barium 24 or more hours later.

At postmortem examination total occlusion of the lumen of the appendix is found in 3 or 4 per cent of cases, whereas almost total or partial obliteration of the lumen is found in an additional 25 per cent (Cunningham). In persons past the age of 60, the lumen is obliterated in more than 50 per cent of the cases, and may represent a retrogressive normal change with age.

In disease of the appendix, its lumen is obliterated in practically all (but not all) instances, but since obliteration of the appendix in the adult is such a frequent finding without definite disease, the mere lack of visualization of the appendix radiographically is not indicative of abnormality. However, when the appendix is visualized, it can be taken as good evidence, though not conclusive, of a normal appendix.

Fecal concretions and calculi (called "coproliths") are found in the appendix under many circumstances, and may permit a partial visualization of this structure, despite their presence. In infants and children a coprolith of the appendix usually is indicative of associated appendicitis.

Variation in Size and Position of the Subdivisions of the Colon.   The dividing line between anatomic variations and congenital malformations is not a sharp one. Marked redundancies of the sigmoid colon and transverse colon are found so frequently that they can be considered anatomic variants. These various types of redundancies are illustrated in Figure 14–19.

Failures of rotation, however, are congenital aberrations which have considerable practical significance. These are outside the scope of the present text, but the most frequent of these are illustrated (Fig. 14–19). In nonrotation of the cecum, the cecum lies lateral to the ascending colon, and the appendix ascends toward the liver, giving rise to the so-called subhepatic appendix (Fig. 14–9). In hyper-rotation of the colon, the cecum appears to acquire an extra twist which places it medial to the ascending colon, pointing medially or upward (Figs. 14–9, 14–19). The appendix is in a variable position in these cases, but is not found

half of the colon. The hindgut consists of the distal half of the colon beyond the midtransverse colon to the rectum. These areas correspond closely to major blood supply.

Anomalies of intestinal rotation are principally limited to

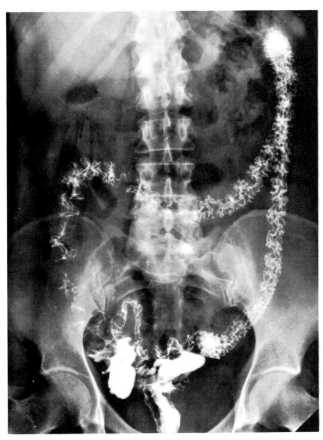

Figure 14–17. Radiograph of colon after evacuation of barium.

in its usual location. A schematic representation of the normal fetal rotation of the midgut in successive stages is shown in Figure 14–19 C. The foregut consists of the stomach and superior portion of the duodenum down to approximately the major papilla of the duodenum. The midgut consists of the remaining portion of the duodenum, the whole of the small intestine, and the proximal

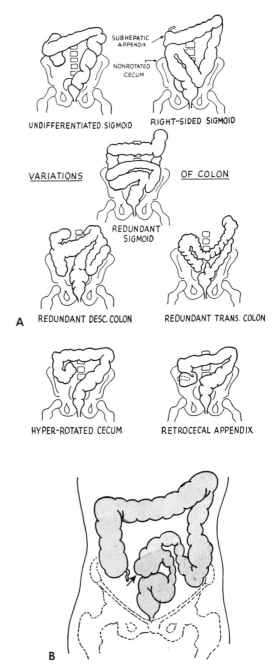

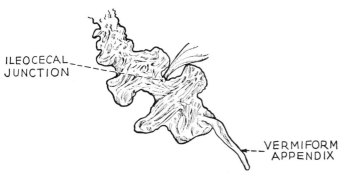

Figure 14–18. Representative mucosal pattern of cecum.

Figure 14–19. *A.* Variations in contour of the normal colon. *B.* Tracing of a colon with marked redundancy of the sigmoid region.

Figure 14–19 continued on the following page.

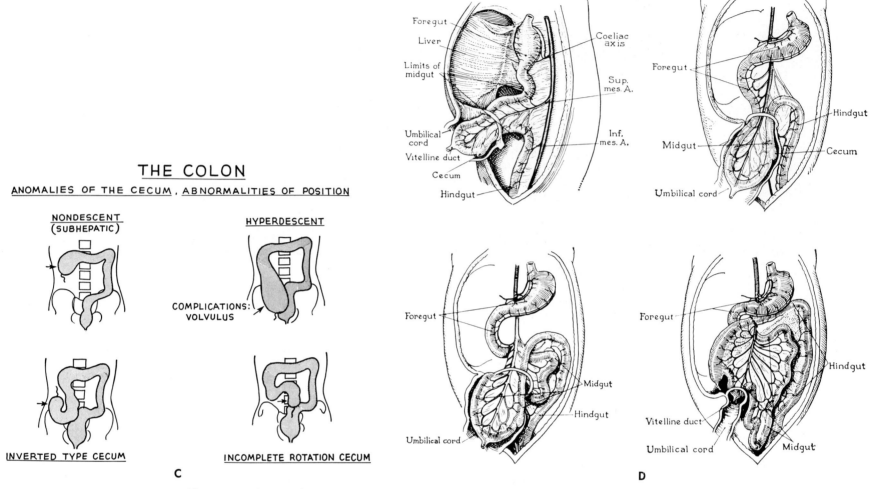

Figure 14–19 *Continued.* C. Variations of the contour of the ascending colon in particular, demonstrating abnormalities of contour as well as position of the cecum. *D.* Schematic representation of normal fetal rotation of the midgut in successive stages. *Upper left,* Lateral view at the fifth fetal week. The foregut, hindgut, and midgut are suspended from the posterior wall in the common dorsal mesentery. Part of the midgut and superior mesenteric artery protrudes out into the umbilical cord and forms a physiologic umbilical hernia. The foregut derives its blood supply from the celiac axis, the midgut from the superior mesenteric artery, and the hindgut from the inferior mesenteric artery. *Upper right,* Frontal view at the eighth fetal week. The midgut has rotated 90 degrees counterclockwise so that the prearterial segment now lies on the right and the postarterial segment on the left. External rotation is complete. *Lower left,* Frontal view at the tenth fetal week. The midgut is returning to the abdominal cavity and is undergoing internal rotation. *It is noteworthy that the proximal end of the midgut returns first and that it passes to the right and behind the superior mesenteric artery.* Succeeding loops are then packed into the left upper abdominal quadrant and later in the right side and lower portions of the abdomen. *Lower right,* At approximately the eleventh fetal week all of the midgut has returned to the abdominal cavity and has rotated an additional 180 degrees counterclockwise from its position as shown at upper right and a total of 270 degrees from its original position as shown at upper left. The process of rotation is now complete and the mesenteries are then fixed onto the posterior wall of the abdomen in the areas which are indicated in stipple.

In the case of failure of rotation or incomplete rotation the cecum and small intestine remain in their early fetal patterns and, more important, the stage of fixation is missed. Without its anchorage to the posterior abdominal wall, the malplaced midgut is prone to twist around the superior mesenteric artery on a narrow mesenteric pedicle to form a volvulus. The volvulus usually impinges on the third portion of the duodenum and causes complete or incomplete obstruction at this level. (Modified from Golden, Radiologic Examination of the Small Intestine, *in* Caffey, J.: Pediatric X-Ray Diagnosis, 4th ed. Chicago, Year Book Medical Publishers, 1961.)

Figure 14–19 continued on the opposite page.

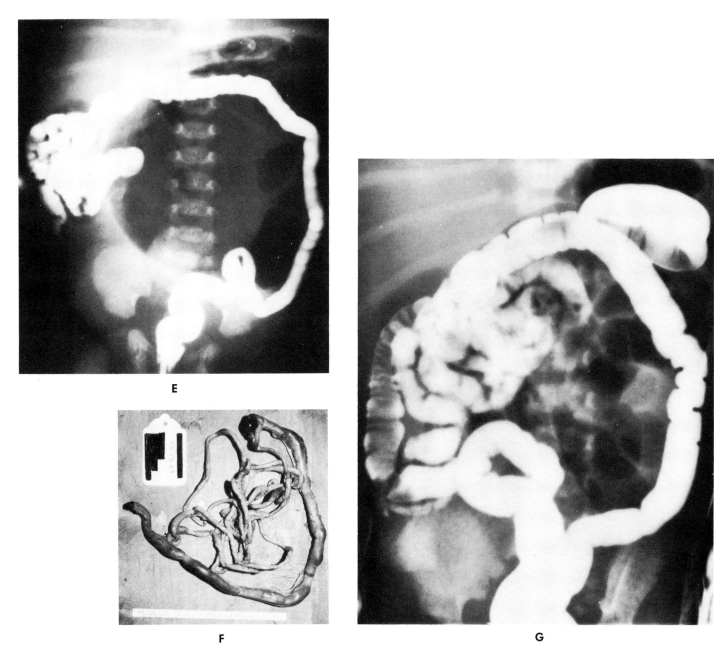

E

F   G

Figure 14-19 *Continued.* *E.* Barium enema in an "unused colon" in a neonate with a large peritoneal abscess. *F.* Photograph of a neonatal "unused colon." *G.* Barium enema in a neonate with jejunal atresia, but with meconium in the colon.

the midgut. The most common problem is incomplete rotation—the cecum fails to migrate completely from the left lower quadrant to its normal position in the right lower quadrant. The midgut hangs on the superior mesenteric artery. The cecum and terminal ileum are either free or attached in the subhepatic region by peritoneal bands. If the entire midgut is unattached, a

twisting (volvulus) may occur, usually in a clockwise direction. This not only occludes the blood supply to the midgut but also increases the pressure on the duodenum.

Variations in Appearance of the Normal Colon. Apart from the marked redundancy of the descending colon or sigmoid, or increased mobility of the cecum on its long mesentery with

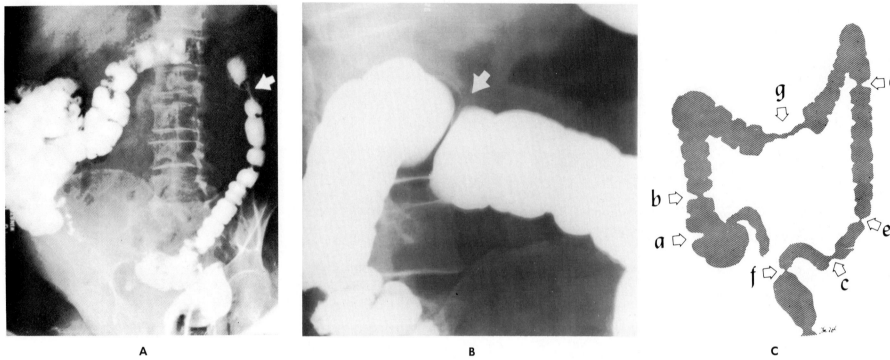

Figure 14–20. *A.* Annular constriction in the distal portion of the splenic flexure representing a segmental contraction simulating an area of abnormal narrowness. This is the so-called Payr-Strauss focal contraction. *B.* Radiograph demonstrating an area of segmental contraction in the transverse colon just beyond the hepatic flexure at Cannon's ring point. *C.* The approximate locations of inconstant segmental contractions which may simulate disease in the barium-filled colon. They are designated by the names of their describers; *a*, Busi; *b*, Hirsch; *c*, Moultier; *d*, Payr-Strauss; *e*, Balli; *f*, Rossi; *g*, Cannon's ring. (Part *C* after Templeton, *in* Bockus, H. L.: Gastroenterology. Vol. 2, 2nd ed. Philadelphia, W. B. Saunders Co., 1964.)

Figure 14–20 continued on the opposite page.

various rotational abnormalities, there are other variations of normal as follows:

1. *Variations in the Appearance of the Haustral Pattern.* There are seven areas of normal narrowness or focal contraction of the colon that are inconstantly seen radiographically and that are not found at autopsy. These must be carefully differentiated from organic or neoplastic defects. The most common of these is Cannon's ring, which is located approximately in the middle of the transverse colon and represents the junction of the primitive midgut and hindgut. The other areas of narrowness producing somewhat similar appearances are shown in Figure 14–20 *A, B, C,* and *D.*

2. *Innocuous Filling of Intestinal Glands or Innominate Grooves* (Williams; Sasson; Dassel). The major secretion obtained from the colon is mucus from small cryptlike glands—the glands of Lieberkühn. Ordinarily, mucus is not grossly discernible in the feces unless excretion is excessive. When barium sulfate enters the colonic glands or small innominate grooves, particularly in the sigmoid colon, a spiculated appearance is produced along the margins of the colon that simulates small mucosal ulcers and sawtoothing (Fig. 14–21 *A, B*). The glands of

Lieberkühn are straight tubular glands with central crypts 0.5 to 0.7 mm. long. These are ordinarily perpendicular to the surface and are regularly and profusely distributed over the mucosa of the colon. The individual spicules may be scattered 3 to 5 mm. apart, and they may be limited to a single segment or distributed throughout the entire colon. Patients in whom this appearance was seen have ranged in age from 2 ½ to 49 years. This should be regarded as a transient, normal observation when the colon is otherwise normal in length, caliber, and haustral pattern.

3. *The "Unused" Colon of a Neonate.* The gastrointestinal tract in the healthy newborn infant has received considerable study, but generally results are so variable that conclusions are difficult (Henderson; Smith, 1959). The intestinal tract at birth is longer in proportion to the length of the body than is the case in adult life, and this disproportion is even more marked during the second year of infancy. Apparently, all the glandular elements found in the normal gastrointestinal mucosa of adults are present at birth, although glandular structures are more shallow, especially at premature birth. In the newborn, the colon is redundant, its haustrations are relatively shallow, and its musculature is relatively active. Its capacity would appear to be between 6 and

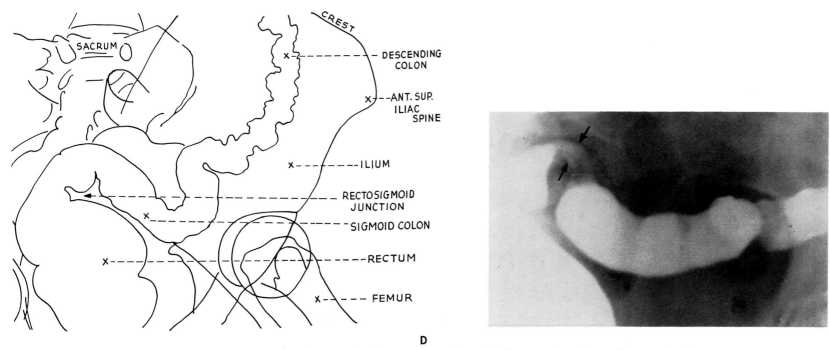

D

Figure 14–20 *Continued.* *D.* Oblique study of the rectosigmoid junction demonstrating a frequently encountered normal narrowness. A labeled tracing from another normal patient is shown for comparison.

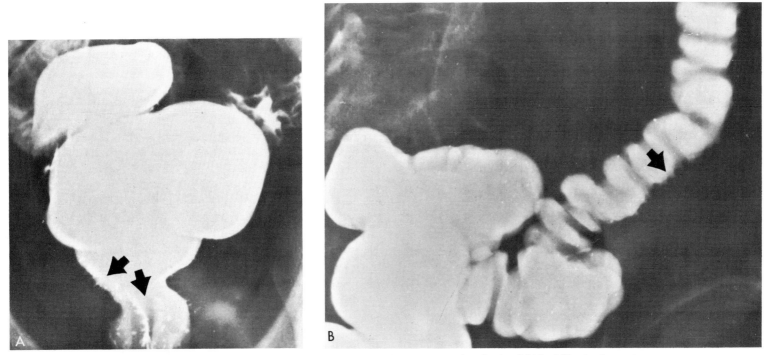

Figure 14–21. *A.* Radiograph demonstrating barium sulfate entering the glands of Lieberkühn in the rectum. When perpendicular to the surface, these present a dotlike pattern. *B.* Similar granular crypts demonstrated in profile in the region of the sigmoid simulating diverticulosis.

75 ml. of an opaque mixture. The neonatal intestine shows a relatively greater thickness of mucosa as compared to the muscle coats. Thus, the ratio of mucosa to muscle in the newborn subject is 23 to 26, whereas in the adult it is 27 to 41. The wall of the colon is relatively better developed than that of the small bowel.

There is no uniformity in the appearance of the colon; dogmatic descriptions are unwarranted and anatomic classification is highly variable. Generally, motility, especially of the stomach, is much more variable than it is in adults, and the stomach empties more slowly in the newborn period than at any other time of life. It is probable that the composition of the substance ingested is important since human milk leaves the stomach and reaches the large intestine more rapidly than does cow's milk in particular formulas. The jejunum in the newborn lacks sufficient muscle to throw the outline of its contents into the mucosal folds as is commonly observed in older subjects. Segmentation into isolated masses is therefore the most frequent observation, and "puddling" is the most frequent description of the ileum. Food eaten by a newborn infant requires from 3 to 6 hours at least before it begins to arrive at the cecum, and it appears in the stool in only a little more than 8 hours.

Meconium is first demonstrable in the bowel of the human fetus at 4 or 5 months gestation. The meconium tends to become increasingly firm, solid, and dark as gestational life progresses. At birth its amount is estimated to be from 60 to 200 grams, and it is described as "viscid, sticky, dark greenish-brown to black." In meconium ileus, the meconium is extremely viscid and it tends not to be propelled satisfactorily in the gastrointestinal tract. Hence, it is felt that pancreatic enzymes, which are lacking in meconium ileus, are responsible for the normally semifluid state of meconium. Usually, the normal infant passes some meconium within the first 10 hours of life, although failure to pass meconium in the presence of a normal alimentary tract may occur for over 24 hours after birth. Ninety per cent of normal infants will, however, pass meconium during the first 24 hours. The meconial characteristics disappear from the fecal mass by about the fourth day.

In a series of studies on the gastrointestinal tract from the small intestine to the colon in the newborn, it was noted that the caliber of the ileum and the colon after an opaque meal were so nearly the same that this measurement alone gave no clue to the location of the barium (Henderson). Often it was only when the barium was seen in the rectosigmoid colon that the examiner was certain that he had been observing barium-filled segments of the colon and not ileum. In antegrade studies in the newborn it is very difficult to outline the cecum, but by means of a barium enema the cecum begins to resemble its adult shape, although smaller.

The cecum at times appears to be separated from the ascending colon by a valvelike constriction at the ileocecal level. Although the appendix is not infrequently demonstrated by barium

enema, it does not usually appear when the barium mixture has been orally administered.

When antegrade study of the colon is performed, the barium tends to be clumped as it is in the ileum, and it is not until 7 or 8 hours after a barium meal that one sees a continuously filled portion of colon; this usually appears in the descending and sigmoid area. Motility in the colon is generally more rapid in the infant than in the adult. In antegrade studies at the end of 24 hours, most of the barium meal has left the intestinal tract.

In studies utilizing a barium enema there is considerable variation in the total length and regional topography of an infant's colon compared with that seen in an adult. It is indeed difficult to fill the colon around to the cecum in the newborn infant. Colonic spasm occurs frequently. Marked variation in total length of the colon is seen; some are slightly redundant while in others there is a great deal of reduplication, sometimes to such an extent that it is difficult to follow the course of the bowel. The contour of the colon in the newborn is almost invariably smooth and its contents are "mushy." At times, meconium, adherent to the wall, imparts a ragged contour to the mucosa. Approximately four-fifths of infants studied will have some indication of a haustral pattern, although in most this pattern will be shallow. Haustrations are more evident after evacuation of the barium.

Although initially the "unused" or relatively unused colon may be of very small caliber and not redundant, it is apparent as additional barium flows into the colon that the sigmoid particularly is capable of much dilatation and apparent elongation; hence, the visible redundancy is dependent on the amount of mixture used. This is particularly true if the ileocecal valve is not relaxed.

A right-sided sigmoid is visible more often than one in the left abdomen, and in most cases the sigmoid is in the midline. The lumen size can be controlled by the amount of mixture used. The appearance of reduplication of the descending colon may be obtained in approximately a third of the cases, and the incidence of redundancy in the splenic flexure and in the transverse colon is about the same as it is in the descending portion (Henderson and Bryant).

The site of the ileocecal valve is much more clearly demarcated in the colon of the newborn infant than in the adult, and a definite separation is seen in the majority of infants. The fetal type of cecum can be anatomically described as conical, with the appendix arising from the apex of the cone and forming a continuation of the long axis of the colon. This is found quite frequently. It is probable that descent of the cecum is completed by the eighth month of fetal life (MacLean and Hertwig, quoted from Henderson and Bryant).

The accompanying illustrations (Fig. 14–19 D, E, F) show a barium enema in an "unused" colon in a neonate with a large peritoneal abscess, a photograph of a neonatal "unused" colon, and a barium enema in a neonate with jejunal atresia, but with meconium in the colon suggesting that complete obstruction by the jejunal atresia did not occur until at least some of the meconium content of the small bowel had passed into the colon. This conclusion, however, is not absolute, particularly since autopsy in stillborn infants reveals tenacious meconium adherent to the walls of the colon (Henderson and Bryant).

MOTILITY STUDY OF THE LARGE INTESTINE

The passage of a barium mixture in the adult as viewed fluoroscopically through the large intestine is usually slow and almost imperceptible. While the contents are still fluid, peristaltic activity and a constant head of pressure from the ileum force the barium column onward. When the barium mixture becomes semisolid or solid, it is a mass movement that forces the passage of the colonic contents. In a matter of seconds, the normal haustral pattern of the colon disappears, and an entire long segment of the large bowel appears to close down into a ribbonlike structure. This mass movement then gradually passes over the bowel distal to its site of origin and forces the bowel contents toward the rectum. It may reach the rectum in a matter of 15 or 20 seconds, and shortly thereafter, the original haustral markings once again make their appearance.

Normally, these mass movements do not occur many times during the day, but during a barium enema examination, especially in an irritable colon, they may be seen repeatedly, eventually forcing the evacuation of the colonic contents.

Some investigators, such as Wright, Cole and others, have described a haustral churning motion in which the haustra remain in evidence but change their size. This is a very slow movement, and can be detected ordinarily only in serial radiographic studies. This churning or mixing movement is the same as the segmentation movement previously described in the small intestine. About 2.5 cm. of the circular muscle contracts, sometimes constricting the lumen of the colon to almost complete occlusion. At the same time, the taeniae coli contract longitudinally. These latter haustral contractions reach a peak in about 30 seconds and then disappear during the next 60 seconds, and they may at times move slowly toward the anus during the period of contraction.

The rate of movement through the large intestine is very variable, but under ordinary circumstances the cecum is visualized in 1½ to 4 hours after the oral administration of barium. The head of the barium column will reach the hepatic flexure in 3 to 6 hours, and the splenic flexure in 6 to 12 hours. By 24 hours, usually about one-half of the barium has been evacuated and the remainder scattered in the colon. Ordinarily, the colon is virtually empty of barium in 48 hours, except for a few scattered foci. Variations from this sequence are very frequent, and caution must be exercised in the interpretation of abnormal motility of the large intestine.

Fluid is progressively absorbed from the colon until only about 80 ml. of the 450 ml. daily load of chyme is lost in the feces (Guyton). The content of the colon tends to be fluid in the ascending colon normally, semifluid as it approaches the hepatic flexure, mushy in the transverse colon, and solid in the lower descending colon. Excess motility causes less absorption and diarrhea or loose feces.

Secretions of the Large Intestine.   The surface epithelium of the large intestine contains a large number of goblet or mucus-secreting cells dispersed among the upper epithelial cells; the only significant secretion in the large intestine is mucus. When a segment of the large intestine becomes irritated, however, the mucosa then secretes large quantities of water and electrolytes in addition to the mucus, and this acts to dilute the irritating factors and causes rapid movement of the feces toward the anus. *The lost electrolytes, under these circumstances, contain an especially large amount of potassium (Guyton).*

TECHNIQUE OF RADIOLOGIC EXAMINATION OF THE SMALL INTESTINE (EXCEPT ANGIOGRAPHY)

Barium Meal.   Many different types of barium meals have been tested and many different adjuvant agents have been employed. Generally, nonflocculating barium mixed with 50 per cent water is considered most satisfactory (Zimmer; Ardran et al.; Miller; Nelson et al., 1965b; Stacy and Loop).

Different volumes have been recommended — some have used 8 ounces, others, 19 ounces (Schlaeger); Marshak has recommended at least 16 ounces and at times 20 ounces (this has been corroborated by Caldwell and Flock).

Our own experience has favored the utilization of 8 ounces initially under fluoroscopic control. During this time the esophagus, stomach, and duodenum are examined, thereafter an additional 8 ounces are administered prior to the routine film studies. At predetermined intervals (30 to 60 minutes) each film is viewed before the next, and spot filming is done as necessary.

Acceleration of the Barium Meal.   From time to time different drugs have been advocated to enhance motility and shorten the time of the small bowel examination. Marshak and Lindner recommend a subcutaneous or intramuscular injection of 0.5 mg. neostigmine. They do not, however, recommend the use of this drug in the elderly or in patients with heart disease, asthma, or mechanical intestinal or urinary tract obstruction. Atropine should be readily available in case a reaction should occur. Sovenyi and Varro have recommended the addition of 30 grams of sorbitol to a barium meal consisting of 400 cc. of water and 125 to 130 grams of nonflocculent barium for study of the small intestine. The small intestinal transit time is thereby shortened to approximately 40 to 60 minutes, and they claim that there is no apparent interference with accuracy of study.

Goldstein et al. compared various methods for acceleration of the small intestinal radiographic examination such as 0.5 mg. neostigmine methylsulfate, the right lateral decubitus position except during roentgenography, and the addition of Gastrografin to the barium mixture. They concluded that adding 10 ml. of Gastrografin to the barium mixture was the most effective method.

Other drugs have also been utilized but may tend to alter the size of the small intestine or its motility—hence, serious doubt is cast on the use of any medication to alter the procedure (Lumsden and Truelove; Holt et al.).

Cold isotonic saline has also been shown to hasten both motility of the small intestine and gastric evacuation (Weintraub and Williams). After the administration of barium sulfate in examination of the stomach and duodenum, the patient is given a glass of cold isotonic saline to drink. One half hour later he is given another glass of the saline. Under these circumstances the ileocecal region is reached in a half hour or an hour instead of the usual longer interval. In a variance of this basic technique, the second glass of isotonic saline is mixed with approximately 100 grams of barium which may enhance the contrast within the small intestine.

Conventional Small Intestinal Series. It is always desirable to have a film of the abdomen without contrast prior to the introduction of any contrast agent.

The patient is allowed no food or drink following the evening meal on the night before the examination.

A routine examination of the esophagus, stomach, and duodenum is carried out as previously described (Chapter 13). The barium column is watched as it passes into the jejunum. When it appears relatively stationary, it has been our practice to administer another 8 ounces of nonflocculent barium mixture as described above and then to obtain a film of the abdomen. Fifteen to thirty minutes later another film of the abdomen is obtained. This film is inspected, and time intervals are designated for the further examination of the passage of the barium in the small bowel. Usually these intervals are approximately 30 to 60 minutes. When the barium has reached the ileocecal region, the patient is examined fluoroscopically once again and spot-film compression studies of the ileocecal region are obtained.

If any abnormalities are seen in the course of the small intestinal series, the patient is restudied by fluoroscopy and the area in question is carefully compressed, palpated, and refilmed by spot-film compression techniques.

A representative routine series is shown in Figure 14–22.

If small bowel or large intestinal obstruction is suspected, a routine series of films for investigation of the abdomen without additional contrast is used prior to the small bowel series. These include chest film, supine anteroposterior view of the abdomen, and upright film of the abdomen or a lateral decubitus if the patient is unable to stand (see Chapter 15). If obstruction is suspected in the large intestine, we have preferred to administer a barium enema first to make certain of the site of the obstruction.

An obstruction in the small intestine is not considered a contraindication to examination with oral barium (Frimann-Dahl; Nelson et al., 1965b).

Small Intestinal Enema. Following the passage of a tube into the duodenum, 500 to 1000 cc. of thin barium solution may be given in a continuous stream by gravity. Thereafter, the entire small bowel is studied as this continuous stream of barium passes through it. Schatzki has indicated that barium reaches the cecum in about 15 minutes under these circumstances.

Modification of Technique with the Postoperative Partially Resected Stomach. The basic modification required for examination of a patient with a partially resected stomach is the study of the small intestine at more frequent intervals, particularly shortly after the administration of the oral barium. Motility through the proximal small intestine is more rapid than normal, but as the barium column reaches the ileum and beyond, motility occurs at normal time intervals.

Intubation Techniques for Study of Small Foci of Involvement. A Miller-Abbott or Cantor tube may be passed and allowed to move down the small intestine until it meets a point of delay or obstruction. The barium mixture is injected through the tube at this point, and the intestine at the site of obstruction is carefully studied without interference of adjoining loops. This technique is particularly useful for studying an area of obstruction, either partial or complete. A length of 6 to 8 feet of tubing is sufficient to extend from the pylorus to the cecum ordinarily. Approximately 3 hours are required for passage. The tube is withdrawn when it has reached the cecum if an obstruction is not present. The instillation of 4 to 8 cc. of liquid metallic mercury into the rubber balloon of the tube facilitates the passage of the tube through the pylorus and increases the rapidity with which the tube passes down the small intestine.

Radiologic Study of the Small Intestine with Water Soluble Iodinated Contrast Media. Various mixtures of water soluble iodide have been utilized for examination of the gastrointestinal tract both orally and rectally.

1. Forty per cent sodium diatrizoate solution (Hypaque) (Shehadi).

2. Forty per cent sodium diatrizoate with oxyphenisatin.

3. Twenty-five per cent diatrizoate solution plus an equal volume of barium sulfate suspension.

4. Forty per cent sodium diatrizoate or methylglucamine diatrizoate (Gastrografin).

5. Fifty grams of sodium diatrizoate dissolved in 75 cc. of sterile water to which 10 drops of a wetting agent such as Tween-80 have been added, to aid in the coating of the mucosa (Jacobson et al.). A flavoring agent must be added if this is used orally.

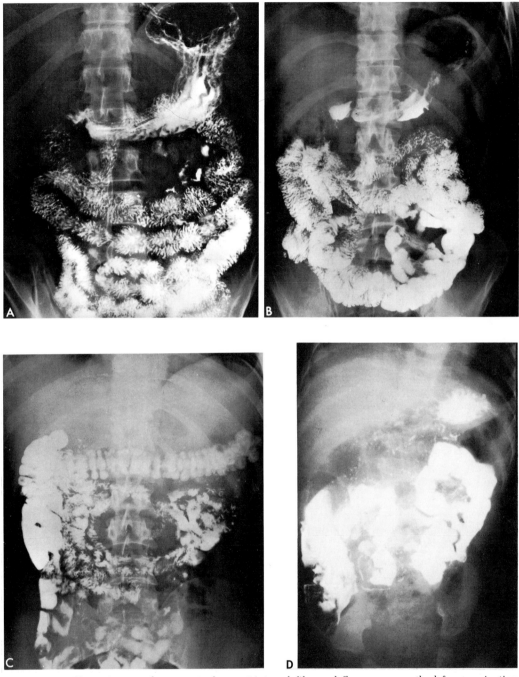

Figure 14–22. Illustrations to demonstrate frequent-interval film and fluoroscopy method for examination of small intestine: *A.* At 1 hour following administration of the barium; *B.* at 2 hours; *C.* at 3 hours. *D.* Representative small intestinal pattern of a normal infant on a predominantly milk diet. Note that the clumping and scattering are relatively normal for infants at this stage of development.

Because of the high tonicity of these water soluble agents, they have not been recommended, especially in children (Neuhauser; Nelson et al., 1965a). The high tonicity of these contrast agents has another result – they are diluted in the small intestine and become less radiopaque in the jejunum and ileum. However, in the colon water is reabsorbed and the contrast improves. The transit time is more rapid than with barium (30 to 90 minutes unless obstruction is encountered).

These water soluble contrast media may be particularly preferred in severely debilitated patients just prior to surgery, in the presence of suspected mesenteric occlusion, and in patients with known diverticulitis when there is a danger of impending perforation or the possibility of leakage of barium into the peritoneal space (Ostrum and Heinz). In general, however, it has been our preference to use the nonflocculent barium mixture described above.

Differences in Infants and Children. Small barium feedings of 1 to 3 ounces are utilized for infants and children. The transit time may be long in the very young (Lonnerblad). Fluoroscopy should be limited to the smallest possible field.

In the first weeks and months of life the normal feathery pattern of the small intestine does not appear. Distinct jejunal markings, however, are usually visible after the fifth month. Segmentation persists much longer (Fig. 14–22 *D*).

During the first year and until the infant assumes the erect posture, the small intestine lies almost entirely above the pelvis.

Large amounts of gas may be found in the jejunum and ileum during the first two or three years of life.

In general, clumping and segmentation of the barium column are so relatively common in the child (both healthy and sick) that this adult criterion of abnormality cannot be applied (Fig. 14–22 *D*). Also, the mucosal contours in the terminal segment of the ileum that are usually longitudinal and linear in the adult may normally have a cobblestone pattern in the child. They are probably caused by the greater abundance in the child of solitary and conglomerate lymph follicles, and are largest in the terminal ileum during preadolescence and adolescence.

Intestinal Biopsy Techniques (Wood et al.; Tomenius). In general, these instruments consist of flexible tubes at the lower end of which is a small metal cylinder provided with a circular lateral hole about 2 to 3 mm. in diameter. The capsule contains a circular knife blade. Suction applied with a vacuum pump or a large syringe aspirates a fragment of the mucosa through the opening of the capsule. The knife blade is released, cutting the mucosa fragment, which is then contained within the capsule. In the Crosby capsule the hole is somewhat enlarged, minimizing the occurrence of hemorrhagic artefacts. The capsule is removed as quickly as possible from the gastrointestinal tract, the terminal cylinder is unscrewed, and the mucosal fragments are collected and oriented on a small piece of wet lens paper with the cut surface downward. They are promptly immersed in 10 per cent formalin or a modified Bouin's solution and embedded in paraffin. They are thereafter stained with hematoxylin-eosin or by special staining techniques.

String Test for Bleeding in Upper Gastrointestinal Tract (Fig. 14–23). The original Einhorn string test of 1909 has been modified in two important ways: (1) the application of guaiac stains to the string, and (2) the administration of sodium fluorescein (20 ml., 5 per cent solution) intravenously and the withdrawal of the

string 4 minutes thereafter. The string is then examined for fluorescence with a Wood's lamp. The string is a common type with a mercury bag tied to its end. There are small radiopaque gauze markers tied to the string at designated intervals. Approximately the first 40 cm. on the string lie in the esophageal area, 40 to 55 cm. in the gastric area, and beyond 55 to 60 cm. in the duodenal and jejunal areas. The total string length is approximately 150 cm. (Traphagen and Karlan; Smith; Haynes and Pittman).

According to Smith, the incidence of false negative tests is 1.2 per cent. False positive tests can be attributed to eating of meats, beets, tomatoes, gelatin, cherries (red), or chocolate, or to trauma in passing the string. The string must be withdrawn 4 minutes after the intravenous administration of the fluorescein, since fluorescein would be excreted by the major papilla (of Vater) if the procedure is prolonged.

ROENTGENOLOGIC VARIATIONS OF NORMAL

Variations With Age. During the first 3 or 4 months of life, while the infant is still on a milk diet, there is a tendency toward segmentation and lack of continuity of the barium column and delay of transit time. The stomach-to-colon time may be as long as 9 hours in the newborn (Fig. 14–22).

Gas in the small bowel is abnormal except in the very young and the very old (when not excessive). In the young it is due to air swallowing and in the old to a relative hypotonicity of the small intestine. Such changes begin to be particularly manifest beyond the age of 60 years.

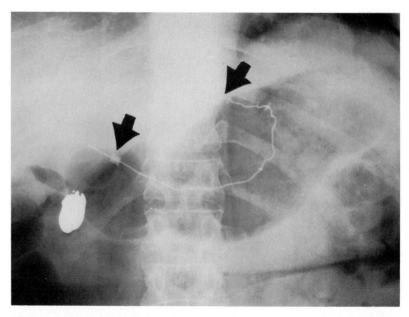

Figure 14–23. Radiograph demonstrating string test for gastrointestinal bleeding.

A persistent deficiency of gas in the small intestine of the newborn infant beyond the first day may be a cardinal sign of intestinal obstruction. However, there are other entities which may be responsible for this appearance, such as adrenal insufficiency, dehydration, diarrhea, and other interference with the normal transport mechanisms.

TECHNIQUE OF RADIOLOGIC EXAMINATION OF THE COLON (EXCEPT ANGIOGRAPHY)

The methods of examination are: (1) the plain radiograph of the abdomen; (2) the barium enema, under fluoroscopic visualization, and accompanied by spot-film compression radiography, in addition to certain routine film studies; (3) the barium meal, followed through until the colon is visualized, and thereafter at 6 hours, 24 hours, and further intervals if desired; and (4) the barium-air double contrast enema (see Fig. 14–24).

Preliminary Plain Radiograph of the Abdomen. If a film of the abdomen has not been obtained in the course of other studies prior to the barium enema, it is well to obtain a posteroanterior film of the abdomen prior to the introduction of any contrast agent. The routine base line film of the abdomen is not only useful from the standpoint of later evaluation after contrast is introduced, but in itself it may reveal significant abnormality (Rosenbaum et al.). Moreover, the appearance of dense inspissated fecal material may indicate the presence of a bowel obstruction. This appearance must also be differentiated at times from extraluminal gas which may produce a somewhat similar appearance.

The Routine Barium Enema

Preparation of the Patient. Thorough cleansing of the colon prior to the barium enema is essential, since any fecal material will obscure the normal anatomy and give rise to false filling defects and mucosal aberrations. This is best accomplished, in our experience, by the following routine:

1. Clear liquid diet for at least 24 hours prior to the examination forcing liquids.

2. One and one-half ounces of X-Prep liquid or its equivalent for catharsis, at 6 P.M. on the evening prior to the examination. As an alternative, a 10 ounce dose of liquid magnesium citrate (U.S.P.) may be administered at 8:00 P.M., followed by 4 Dulcolax tablets (5 mg. bisacodyl each) at 10:00 P.M. (Barnes). If magnesium citrate is used, the patient must drink about 6 glasses of water additionally before midnight.

3. Cleansing enemas prior to the barium enema examination until the returning fluid is clear, unless thorough cleansing of the colon has otherwise been accomplished following the catharsis. A Dulcolax suppository (10 mg.) in the rectum at 7:00 A.M. may be used.

Ordinarily the patient is examined without breakfast, as the breakfast meal will introduce gas in the stomach and occasionally in the colon.

Flocculent barium sulfate suspension is used (Barotrast or its equivalent) and is made by mixing the compounds in a 1 to 4 or up to 1 to 6 mixture, depending upon preference.

TANNIC ACID. Up until March, 1964 we had found it advantageous to introduce ½ to 1 tablespoon of tannic acid per quart of nonflocculating barium suspension in the mixture used for the barium enema. On March 17, 1964 the Commission of Food and Drugs indicated that the medical literature reported "a number of deaths associated with the addition of tannic acid to barium enemas." It indicated that tannic acid "is capable of causing diminished liver function and severe liver necrosis when absorbed in sufficient amounts." In view of these hazards, the Commission of Food and Drugs declared that "tannic acid for rectal use to enhance x-ray visualization is regarded as a new drug," and was not to be used in enemas until complete and further testing had established its safety (Federal Register, March 21, 1964; McAlister et al.). Various substitutes for tannic acid have been recommended, but none to our satisfaction has thus far been found (Reboul et al.). It is probable that adequate colon cleansing, a preparatory clear liquid diet, and the use of well-suspended barium preparations go far toward obtaining satisfactory studies.

At this time, the only tannic acid preparation that may be used as a colonic evacuant is Clysodrast (bisacodyl tannex).* This preparation must be used in accordance with directions. The dosage and administration according to the manufacturer's directions are as follows:

"It is important that the entire medical history and condition of the patient be considered in deciding the dosage regimen. Traumatizing procedures, such as repetition of enemas (with or without Clysodrast) should be kept at the minimum necessary to achieve the desired result.

"*Cleansing enema:* Prepare the cleansing enema by dissolving the contents of one packet (2.5 gm.) of Clysodrast in one liter of lukewarm water and administer.

"*Barium enema:* Prepare the barium enema by dissolving the contents of one or not more than two packets (2.5 gm. or 5.0 gm.) of Clysodrast in one liter of barium suspension. If more than one liter of barium suspension is prepared, it is important that the concentration of Clysodrast (bisacodyl tannex) never exceed 0.5 per cent (two packets per liter). The total dosage of Clysodrast for any one complete colonic examination, including the cleansing enema, should not exceed 7.5 gm. (three packets). No more than 10 gm. (four packets) of Clysodrast should be administered to any individual within a 72 hour period."

A cooperative efficacy study of Clysodrast suggests that in a 0.25 per cent concentration it probably plays an insignificant role

---

*Barnes-Hind Diagnostics, Inc.

in the cleansing of the colon when administered as a preparatory enema (Lasser et al.). It is likely that the completeness of filling of the colon outweighs any other consideration including the ingredients of the agent, in determining the adequacy of a preparatory enema. However, there is good evidence that the Clysodrast in the concentration utilized promoted a more complete contraction of the colon than did any placebo and that the evaluation of mucosal detail of the empty colon was enhanced by the Clysodrast. It has been our impression that this is indeed the main efficacy of the 0.25 per cent tannic acid–barium enema. It should, however, be utilized exactly as directed above. The chemistry of tannic acid, its analysis and toxicology have been reviewed by Krezanoski and the student is referred to this article for greater detail.

For *double contrast enemas* only barium sulfate specially processed for this purpose should be used. The Clysodrast may be added to this barium enema examination as described earlier, but (to repeat) *no more than four packets (10 gm.) of Clysodrast should be administered to any individual within a 72 hour period.* In this instance air without barium may be used following evacuation of the barium enema containing Clysodrast in order to obtain the double contrast.

The manufacturer further states that "Clysodrast is contraindicated in patients under the age of 10 and safe usage in pregnancy of Clysodrast has not been established with respect to the adverse effects upon fetal development. Therefore, it should not be used in women of child-bearing potential, particularly during early pregnancy, except where, in the judgment of the physician, the potential benefits outweigh the possible hazards."

In general, preparation of the patient begins with a residue-free diet the day before the examination. One to two ounces of castor oil (or its equivalent) is administered approximately 16 hours before the examination. On the day of the examination the Clysodrast cleansing enema is given and expelled as described above; it may be repeated if necessary. The patient is then given a barium enema and Clysodrast may be incorporated into the barium sulfate mixture as described above.

Order of the Barium Enema Examination. It has been our preference to perform the barium enema examination *prior* to the study of the upper gastrointestinal tract to avoid any possibility of barium lodging above an unsuspected obstruction in the colon.

We prefer also to examine the urinary tract and biliary system *prior* to the administration of barium orally or by rectum. Telepaque will, of course, introduce opaque material into the colon, and for the best results, the examination of the colon cannot be carried forward on the same day as oral cholecystograms (with Telepaque). In the *massively* bleeding patient, angiograms should be performed before the introduction of any opaque material in the abdomen.

Administration of the Enema. A plastic disposable enema tip and tube are strongly recommended, combined if possible with an enema reservoir. The enema reservoir may also be disposable, or a suitable cap provided between the enema tip and the reservoir to prevent contamination. The reservoir is elevated 3 feet above the table top in adults (or 18 inches in the newborn). For adults the enema reservoir usually contains 2 quarts of the mixture, which is usually adequate for most patients. Occasionally, additional barium must be used. In the newborn infant, 90 ml. of the barium mixture should be more than adequate since the average volume required is 70 mm. Volumes between these two extremes are utilized in the reservoir for different age groups.

The barium is introduced slowly and the examiner should allow the patient to accommodate small increments of the barium as it is introduced. Such slow introduction also allows the examiner to keep "ahead of the barium column" and thus to detect patterns of flow, blockage, filling defects, and mucosal pattern to best advantage. The routine of introduction of the barium and positioning of the patient as well as spot filming is shown in Figure 14–24.

Debilitated patients and those with a relaxed anal sphincter may require an enema tip with a retaining balloon. Great caution must be exercised in the insertion and inflation of such a balloon, since injury to the rectum may result. It is best for the examiner to perform a rectal examination prior to insertion of the balloon, to inflate the balloon very carefully, and to study its position and size fluoroscopically immediately following its insertion. In the presence of a low rectal carcinoma or ulcerative colitis, a balloon is definitely contraindicated. In any case, the use of the balloon should rarely be necessary, since most patients, when properly prepared, experience no difficulty in retaining the enema.

The Fluoroscopic-Radiographic Equipment. The radiographic equipment should be capable of high kilovoltage and high milliamperage with short exposure times. The kilovoltage should be at least 120 Kv. to permit overpenetration of the barium. Photo-timing for spot films is desirable. Image amplifier fluoroscopy is also preferred.

It is our preference to use one hand (left) for manipulation of the exposures and the fluoroscopic screen; the right hand, protected by a heavy lead glove, and kept over the heavy column of barium or outside the direct beam, is used to palpate the patient's abdomen.

Routine for Fluoroscopy. The routine for fluoroscopy is as follows:

1. The patient's abdomen and chest are initially surveyed.

2. Following this survey, the examination is carried out as detailed in Figure 14–24 *A.* The patient first lies on his left side, at an angle of about 60 degrees to the table. The barium mixture is allowed to flow slowly into the rectum to permit the patient to adjust to the liquid mixture being introduced. It should have been warmed to body temperature prior to introduction.

A spot film of the rectosigmoid junction is obtained when this

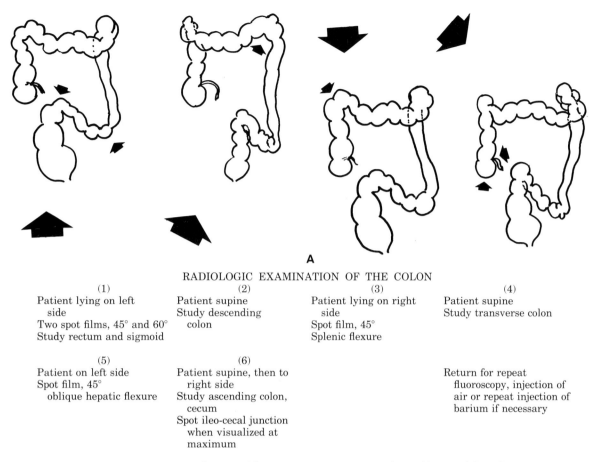

A

RADIOLOGIC EXAMINATION OF THE COLON

(1)
Patient lying on left
   side
Two spot films, 45° and 60°
Study rectum and sigmoid

(2)
Patient supine
Study descending
   colon

(3)
Patient lying on right
   side
Spot film, 45°
Splenic flexure

(4)
Patient supine
Study transverse colon

(5)
Patient on left side
Spot film, 45°
   oblique hepatic flexure

(6)
Patient supine, then to
   right side
Study ascending colon,
   cecum
Spot ileo-cecal junction
   when visualized at
   maximum

Return for repeat
   fluoroscopy, injection of
   air or repeat injection of
   barium if necessary

Figure 14–24. A. Technique of fluoroscopic examination and spot filming of the colon.

Figure 14–24 continued on the following page.

junction is observed to fill and the barium flow momentarily stops (Fig. 14–24 B).

The patient is then lowered slightly to a 45 degree angle and a small amount of barium is introduced so that the entire sigmoid and lower descending colon are filled. Once again there is a cessation of the barium flow and a second spot film is obtained to demonstrate the entire sigmoid and junction with the descending colon (Fig. 14–24 C).

The patient then is turned on his back, fully supine, and the barium mixture is again allowed to flow until the descending colon to the level of the splenic flexure can be carefully examined.

The patient is then slowly turned to his right side as the barium mixture is allowed to flow around the splenic flexure, and again the flow ceases while a spot film is obtained of the splenic flexure (Fig. 14–24 D).

With the patient supine once more the barium is allowed to flow to fill the transverse colon and the beginning of the ascending colon around the hepatic flexure. The patient is then turned on his left side at an angle of approximately 45 degrees so that the

hepatic flexure is completely unwound, and another spot film is obtained (Fig. 14–24 E).

With the patient once again supine, the barium flow continues until the entire cecum is identified and reflux into the ileum through the ileocecal junction is obtained if possible. The patient is turned so that the ileocecal junction is seen to best advantage without interference from adjoining loops of bowel. A spot film is obtained (Fig. 14–24 F).

Usually the patient will experience moderate discomfort once the barium column has passed the hepatic flexure into the ascending colon, and the examination must be carried forward expeditiously at this point. Routine films are immediately obtained after the filling and reflux into the distal ileum.

Each of the films must be carefully inspected before the patient is allowed to leave. A repeat study may be undertaken if any questionable areas are seen during the film review. Air may also be injected at this time if necessary, although the ideal double contrast barium enema is a separate examination, as pointed out later.

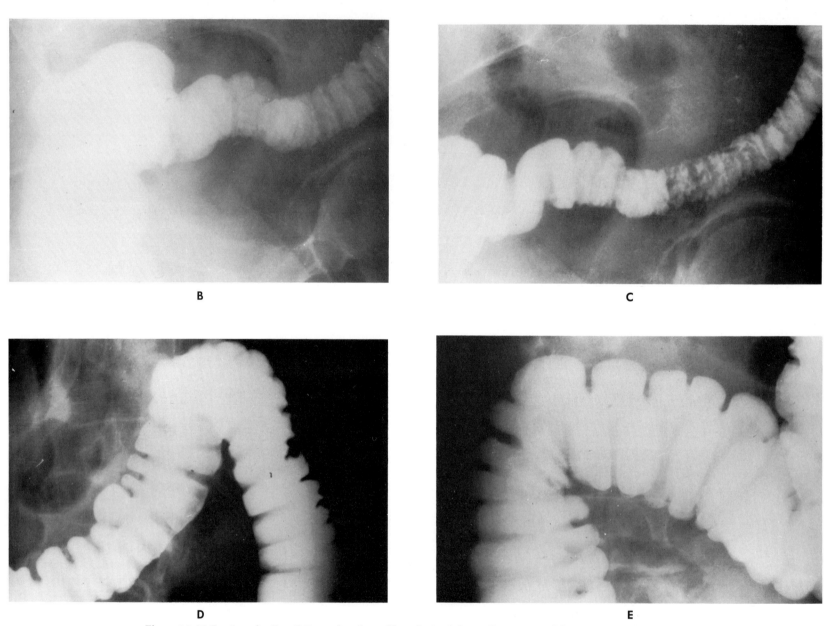

Figure 14–24 *Continued.*   *B* to *F*. Examples of spot films obtained during fluoroscopy of the rectosigmoid, sigmoid, splenic flexure, hepatic flexure, and ileocecal junction.

Figure 14–24 continued on the opposite page.

Routine films following fluoroscopy and spot filming are taken as follows: (1) a high kilovoltage posteroanterior view of the entire colon (Fig. 14–25), (2) a right or left lateral film of the colon centered at the rectosigmoid (Fig. 14–26 *A, B, C*). Oblique films are ordered as required. The spot films may be adequate for this purpose (Fig. 14–27).

Special studies of the rectosigmoid, such as the Chassard-Lapiné view of the rectum and sigmoid may be employed to "unravel" a tortuous and redundant sigmoid (Fig. 14–28). An alternate oblique study of the rectosigmoid and sigmoid colon may be obtained as shown in Figure 14–29 *A* and *B*. Here, the patient lies prone and the central x-ray beam, centered at the level of the anal canal, is directed approximately 35 degrees cephalad. A view very similar to the Chassard-Lapiné view is thereby obtained.

Following colonic evacuation, another posteroanterior prone film of the empty colon is obtained. If the evacuation has not been sufficient, the patient is asked to return after further evacuation for more film studies of the empty colon (Fig. 14–17).

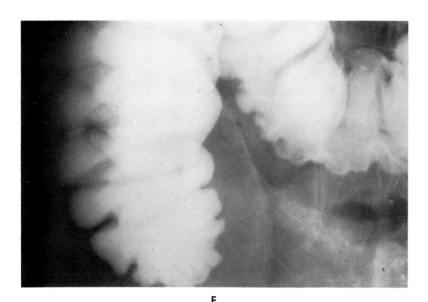

F

Figure 14–24 *Continued. F. See opposite page for legend.*

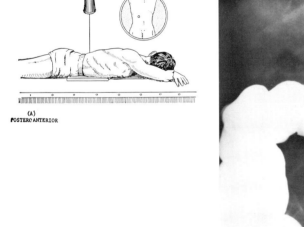

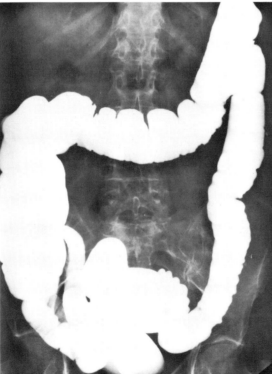

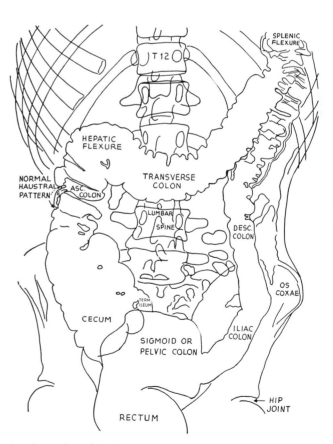

Figure 14–25. Colon distended with barium: positioning of patient, radiograph, and tracing.

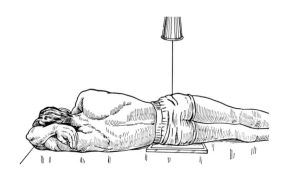

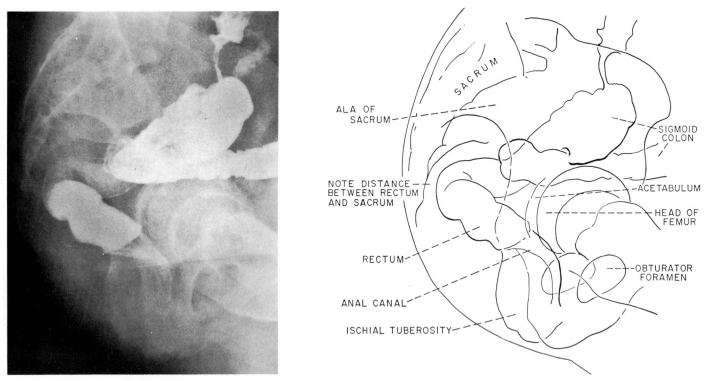

Figure 14–26.   Lateral view of the rectosigmoid: positioning of patient, radiograph, and tracing.

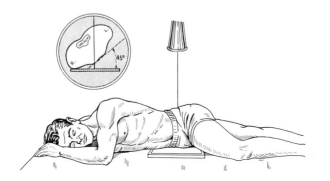

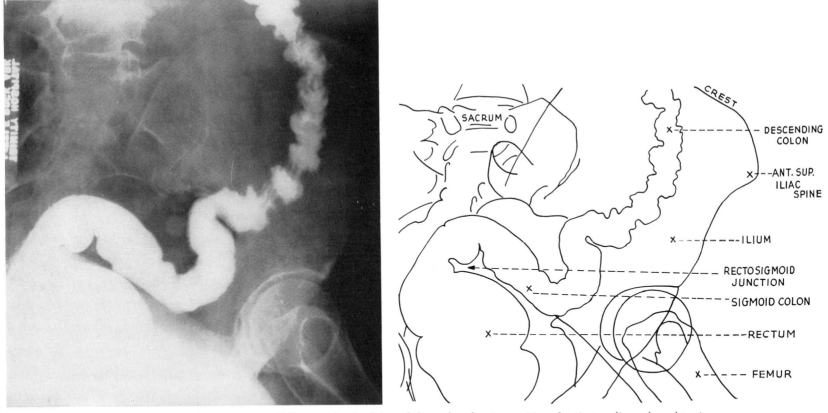

Figure 14–27. Oblique study of pelvic and iliac colon showing position of patient, radiograph, and tracing.

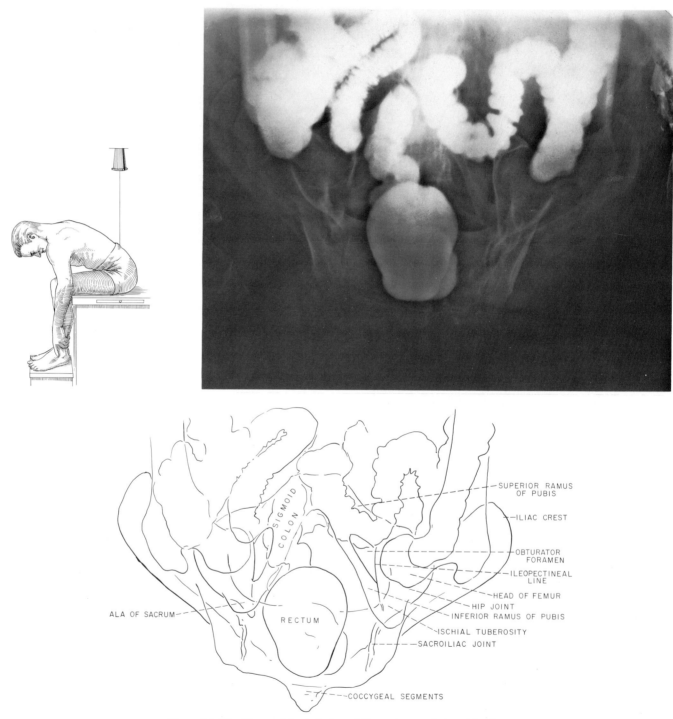

Figure 14–28.   Chassard-Lapiné view of the rectum and sigmoid colon.

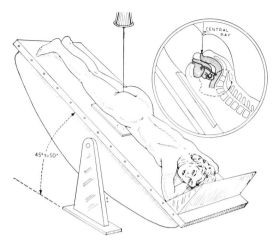

A

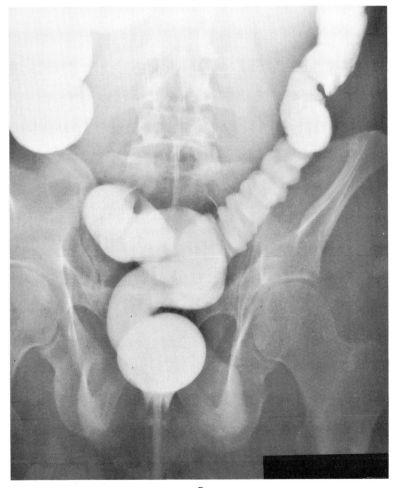

B

Figure 14–29. Distorted view of sigmoid colon. *A.* Position of patient in relation to central x-ray beam. *B.* Radiograph so obtained.

If indicated, air may be introduced at this juncture for optimal visualization of questionable polypoid defects. *This adjunct is not necessarily a substitute for a properly performed barium-air double contrast enema which will be described later.*

Limitations of the Routine Barium Enema. The barium enema examination should not be considered a substitute for the digital or sigmoidoscopic examination of the rectum. The rectum is often obscured by its voluminous barium content, or by a balloon, if such was employed, and in the postevacuation study the sigmoid and rectal loops may fold over one another in such a way as to mask a lesion.

Redundancy and overlapping of portions of the colon may obscure one of the anatomic parts—hence, a complete examination of all flexures in the fluoroscopic visualization is essential. Occasionally, such complete examination is virtually impossible and careful notation of this inadequacy should be made.

Haustral points of narrowness and the rectosigmoid junction may give the impression of abnormal areas of narrowness unless the examiner is thoroughly conversant with the wide variation in the normal appearance of the colon.

Unless the terminal ileum or appendix has been visualized, it is difficult to be completely certain that the cecum has been seen, and for that reason caution must be exercised in assuming that the colon has been completely filled when the terminal ileum and appendix have not been visualized. Unfortunately, it is sometimes impossible to fill the terminal ileum and appendix, so experience must dictate when the colon has been entirely distended with barium.

Fluoroscopy is not as accurate as film studies for revealing minute mucosal changes such as those seen in the earliest aberrations of mucosal structure. It is important to become familiar with the normal appearance of both the full and empty colon in this regard, so that minimal abnormalities may be recognized on the film.

When patients are unable to retain the enema and evacuation is forced before complete filling of the colon and cecum, it must not be assumed that an obstructive abnormality of an organic type necessarily exists in the colon. A repeat examination, especially with the aid of a carefully inserted rectal balloon, may be necessary.

The diagnosis of small polyps is fraught with difficulty. Moreton et al. have pointed out some of these difficulties. They found that in 267 colons studied by the double contrast method 63, or 23.5 per cent, showed fictitious polyps.

The importance of proctosigmoidoscopy is shown by the fact that this adjunctive study may permit observation of: thromboulcerative colitis; ulcerations occurring in amebic, bacillary, and tuberculous colitis; 90 per cent of the organic pathology occurring in the colon; 70 per cent of the nonmalignant tumors; 75 per cent of the malignant tumors originating in the colon; factitial prostatitis and lymphogranuloma venereum; foreign bodies; rectovesical and rectourethral fistulas; and perforation of the rectum or sigmoid by foreign bodies.

Complications of a Barium Enema

Perforation or rupture of the colon, which may be either *intra- or extraperitoneal.*

Perforation of the colon into the venous system (Rosenberg and Fine; Zatzkin and Irwin).

Water intoxication, especially in children (Steinbach et al.).

Colonic intramural barium (Seaman and Bragg). This complication results from mucosal rupture, which permits the barium to dissect into the colonic wall. The outstanding roentgen feature is a transverse striated pattern that is probably produced by the inner layer of circular muscle fibers.

Examination of the Colon Through a Colostomy. In preparation of the patient, a low residue diet for 24 to 48 hours and thorough cleansing of the colon through the colostomy is ordinarily sufficient.

If a Foley catheter is employed as the enema tip in order to prevent spillage of the barium out of the colostomy, the inflation of the Foley bag must be carried out with great caution and under careful fluoroscopic control. Perforation of the bowel may result (Seaman and Wells). Some have urged that a Foley catheter with a long tubular section ahead of the balloon be employed, the balloon being applied with pressure on the outside of the colostomy to prevent spillage (Margulis). Various other techniques for preventing spillage have been advocated.

The introduction of the barium and the rolling of the patient from one side to the other is very much the same as previously described for the routine barium enema. Spot films are taken as necessary. Likewise, the routine filming following the enema through the colostomy is very similar, care being exercised once again to obtain the films as quickly as possible after the filling to prevent spillage.

Barium-Air Double Contrast Enema. There are two types of double contrast barium-air enemas. After a conventional barium enema with a nonflocculating Barotrast-type mixture and after evacuation of the conventional barium enema, air may be insufflated. Results from this type of enema are not usually as good as those from a double contrast enema performed as a separate examination as follows.

The preparation of the patient must be especially carefully done under these circumstances. We have preferred placing the patient on a low residue diet for a period of 2 days, and on 2 successive nights prior to the morning of the examination we have recommended the administration of 1½ ounces of X-Prep liquid. *If 2 ounces of castor oil are used, they should be given on only one occasion, the evening before the examination as in the routine barium enema examination.*

Breakfast is omitted on the morning of the examination and *further cleansing enemas may be given if it is thought necessary.* It has been our usual experience that after 2 such consecutive days of preparation (sometimes 3), the colon is thoroughly cleansed and no further cleansing enemas are necessary.

The colloidal barium mixture (Barotrast may be utilized) is introduced to the mid-descending colon or lower descending colon, and this is followed immediately by forceful insufflation of air, with rotation of the patient first to the left prone position and then to the right prone to accomplish proper dispersion of the heavy barium mixture.

Another variant of this technique requires that the colloidal barium mixture be introduced into the splenic flexure or the middle of the transverse colon and aspirated into a special bag, after which air is injected.

There are various colloidal barium sulfate preparations available, each with specific directions for mixing. Some of these are Baroloid, which is easy to mix, Barotrast, Baridol, and Stabarium. Since the colloidal barium mixture is viscous, pressure is required to force it through the enema tubing. This may be done by elevation of the barium reservoir, by "milking" the tube, by piston-type syringes, or by pumping devices.

When suction and control drainage are required, various devices are available—the three-way valve box (designed by Templeton and Addington) which is attached to a sink and works on a Venturi siphon principle, or simple Y-tube and clamp devices which permit drainage through one branch of the Y and injections through the other.

The films we have obtained routinely are both oblique views, prone and supine films, and both horizontal, lateral, and decubitus films (Fig. 14–30). Chassard-Lapiné views and other special views of the rectosigmoid may be obtained as necessary.

It is our preference to utilize this special method of double contrast visualization of the colon only if the routine examination of the colon does not yield all information necessary.

It is unfortunate that both the routine barium enema examination and this special double contrast type cannot be done on the same day to best advantage. They are best done 1 or 2 days apart as indicated by the clinical history.

The Importance of the Lateral View of the Rectum and Sigmoid Colon. The direct lateral view of the rectosigmoid (Fig. 14–26 *A*) is important for the study of the soft tissue space between the rectum and sacrum; and in the infant, to determine the lowest point of obstruction, particularly in patients with Hirschsprung's disease. The retrorectal soft tissue space ordinarily measures between 0.2 and 1.6 cm. (mean, 0.7 cm.) and ordinarily does not exceed 2 cm. It may on occasion, however, even in a normal patient, exceed this measurement and still be of no pathologic significance.

Apart from detection of infiltration of the retrorectal space in patients with ulcerative colitis, this view is especially useful for visualization of retrorectal masses and sacral tumors.

Examination of the Colon After a Barium Meal. The barium

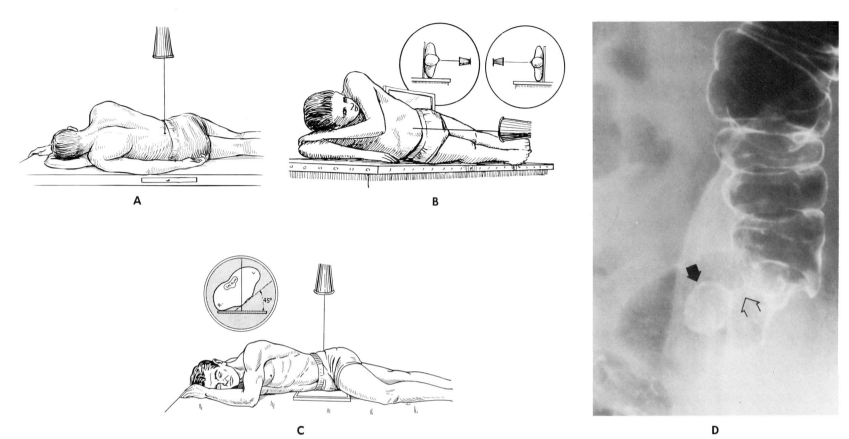

Figure 14–30. *A, B, C.* Positioning of patient for film studies with a double-contrast enema. In addition to the two oblique and the two horizontal beam views shown, straight posteroanterior and left lateral views are also obtained. *D.* Polyp in the colon as seen by double contrast. The closed arrow demonstrates the polyp; the open arrow shows the stalk.

meal method for examination of the colon is employed only if a barium enema is not feasible. It should never be employed unless it is certain that no colonic obstruction exists. When the barium reaches the distal portions of the colon, it is usually dehydrated and caked, giving rise to inaccurate analysis of the colonic structures.

It is possible that a more accurate concept regarding the irritable or spastic colon is obtained by this method.

When oral barium is used, films of the abdomen are taken at 2 and 6 hours, and at 12 and 24 hours if full visualization of the colon has not been obtained by the 6 hour interval. Usually a 24 hour study is necessary.

Silicone Foam in the Diagnosis of Lesions of the Rectum and Sigmoid. Cook and Margulis have employed a radiopaque silicone elastomer introduced into the rectum and sigmoid under fluoroscopic control for study of the rectum and sigmoid. The mixture utilized is spongy and capable of expanding into small crevices. Approximately 50 cm. of the distal colon is filled; 5 minutes later the foam sets and radiographs of the lower colon are ob-

tained. Neostigmine (0.5 ml.) is then given subcutaneously (unless clinically contraindicated), and the patient expels the mold within a few minutes. Generally a balloon is used to fill the rectal ampulla, permitting a painless spontaneous expulsion of the foam mold. The addition of uniformly distributed barium sulfate or Hypaque powder to the silicone mixture before it is introduced into the colon results in radiopacity and allows fluoroscopic control of the filling of the rectum and sigmoid. The method should not be utilized in the presence of a tight or fibrotic anal sphincter, or if there is suspected perforation of the colon. Likewise, patients who have suffered from chronic constipation should not be so examined.

The Water Enema Examination for Lipoma. The water enema examination for identification of lipomas (Margulis and Jovanovich) is based upon the concept of a difference of absorption coefficients of water and fat in roentgenograms obtained in a lower kilovoltage range. This examination is performed only after a routine study has revealed a lesion suspected of being a lipoma.

ANGIOGRAPHY OF THE SMALL AND LARGE INTESTINES

Basic Arterial Anatomy

The *superior mesenteric artery* is the second unpaired branch of the abdominal aorta (Fig. 14–31). It arises from the front of the abdominal aorta from 1 to 23 mm. below the celiac trunk (preponderantly 1 to 6 mm.), usually opposite the lower third or middle of the first lumbar vertebra. It may arise anywhere from the lower border of the twelfth thoracic to the disk between the second and third lumbar vertebrae. It may arise as a common trunk with the celiac artery; indeed, it may give rise to the splenic or to both the splenic and hepatic arteries, or to the right gastroepiploic. For example, the right hepatic artery is a branch of the superior mesenteric in about 14 per cent of cases.

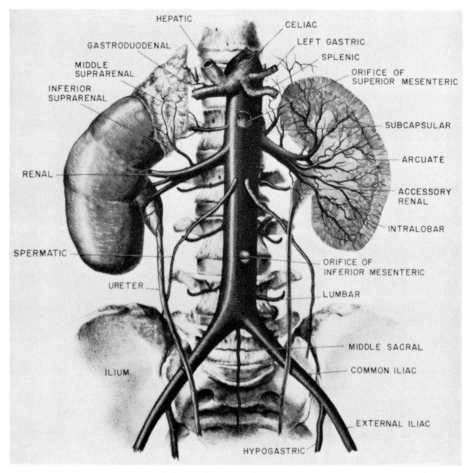

Figure 14–31. Abdominal aorta and its branches. (From Bierman, H. C.: Selective Arterial Catheterization. 1969. Courtesy of Charles C Thomas, Springfield, Illinois.)

The superior mesenteric artery crosses the duodenum and enters the mesentery following the route of the mesentery, and crossing the aorta, inferior vena cava, right ureter, and psoas major muscle. Its branches are: the *inferior pancreaticoduodenal,* feeding the duodenum and head of the pancreas; *intestinal; middle colic; right colic;* and *ileocolic.* It has a number of inconstant important branches to the pancreas (such as the *dorsal* or *transverse pancreatic artery*) in perhaps 14 to 20 per cent of cases, and a *right hepatic branch* in about 14 per cent of cases (Fig. 14–32). Other variations may occur.

The inferior pancreaticoduodenal arteries help form an arcade along the head of the pancreas and third part of the duodenum (see Chapter 13).

The *intestinal arteries*—branches of the superior mesenteric—arise from the left convex side of the superior mesenteric artery and number anywhere from 12 to 20, radiating into the mesentery. There are three to seven purely jejunal branches and eight to seven below the origin of the ileocolic artery that supply the jejunum, ileum, and proximal half of the colon. They form arcades by uniting and anastomosing in and around these organs. The arcades for the jejunum tend to be less tiered and multiplex when compared with those for the ileum. The *straight terminal arteries* alternate to one side or the other of the small intestine; their number increases as one proceeds distally along the intestine (Fig. 14–32 *A*).

The first intestinal artery anastomoses with the inferior pancreaticoduodenal artery (Fig. 14–32 *B*) may originate this artery. The terminal branches of the first intestinal artery also anastomose with the ileal branch of the ileocolic.

The *middle colic artery* arises somewhat variably from the superior mesenteric distal to the origin of the inferior pancreaticoduodenal artery and below the pancreas, but proximal to the jejunal or ileocolic branches (Fig. 14–32). It divides into right and left branches coursing along the margin of the colon. The *right branch* forms an anastomosis with the ascending branch of the right colic, and the *left branch* an anastomosis with the ascending branch of the left colic artery. The left colic is a branch of the inferior mesenteric.

Considerable variation exists in respect to the middle colic artery. It may be single; it may arise from a common stem with the right colic; or accessory middle colics may arise from any part of the superior mesenteric branching system (Netter).

The *right colic artery* crosses the ureter and gonadal vessels and divides into ascending and descending branches near the ascending colon. The *ascending branch* forms an anastomosis with the right branch of the middle colic; the *descending branch* forms an anastomosis with either the ascending or the colic branch of the ileocolic artery. Again, considerable variation exists in its relationship to the superior mesenteric or adjoining branches. The right colic artery is absent in 13 per cent of individuals.

The *ileocolic artery* arises in the root of the mesentery on the

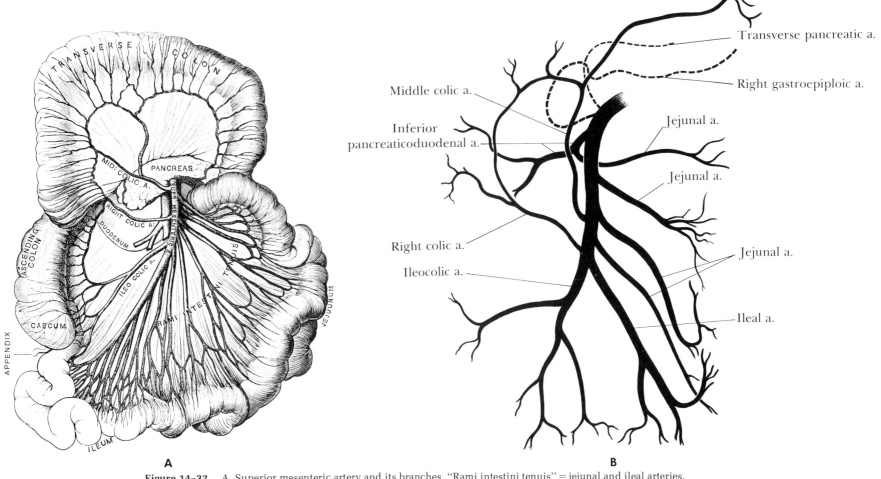

A

B

Figure 14–32. *A.* Superior mesenteric artery and its branches. "Rami intestini tenuis" = jejunal and ileal arteries. (From Cunningham's Manual of Practical Anatomy, 12th ed. Vol. 2. London, Oxford University Press, 1958.) *B.* Superior mesenteric artery and its branches. Constant branches are shown in solid lines, inconstant branches in interrupted lines. (From Ruzicka, F. F., and Rossi, P.: Radiol. Clin. N. Amer., 8:3–29, 1970.)

concave side of the superior mesenteric and its course crosses the psoas major muscle, gonadal vessels, and ureter. It may even cross the third part of the duodenum if it arises sufficiently high. It may arise independently from the superior mesenteric. When it reaches the cecum, the artery divides into approximately five branches supplying their corresponding regions: the *ileal, ascending colic, anterior cecal, posterior cecal,* and an *appendicular artery* (Fig. 14–33).

Figure 14–33. Blood supply of caecum and vermiform appendix (modified from Jonnesco, 1895.) The illustration on the left is from the front, the right from behind. In the latter the appendicular artery and the three taeniae coli springing from the root of the appendix should be specially noted. (From Cunningham's Textbook of Anatomy, 10th ed. London, Oxford University Press, 1964.)

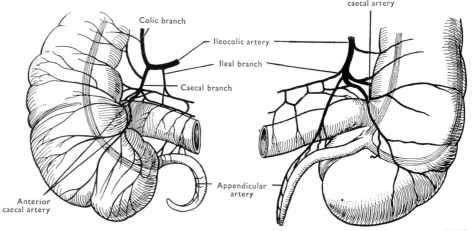

The *inferior mesenteric artery* is the third unpaired branch in the abdominal aorta, arising opposite the lower third of L3 vertebra (Fig. 14–31). This is usually about 4 cm. above the aortic bifurcation. It runs obliquely downward to the left behind the peritoneum and crosses the lower part of the abdominal aorta, the left psoas muscle, and the left common iliac artery. It descends into the pelvis in the sigmoid mesacolon and terminates on the rectum as the *superior rectal artery* (Figs. 14–34 *A, B;* 14–35).

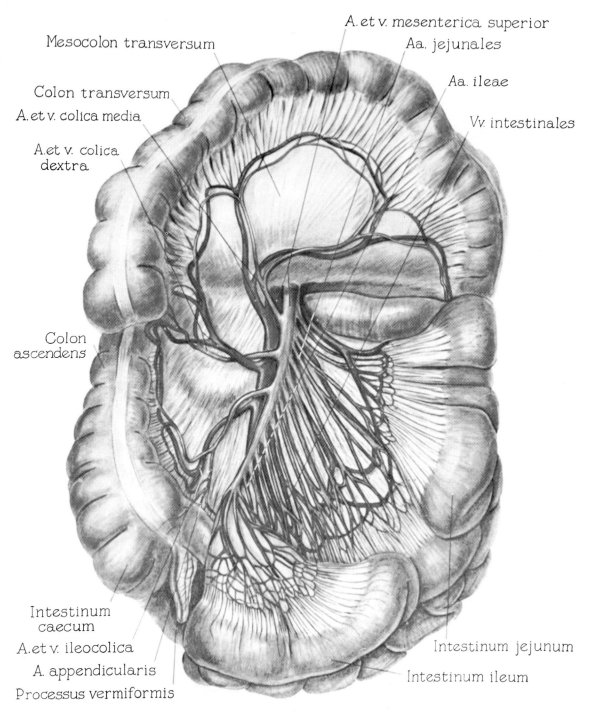

Mesocolon transversum

Colon transversum
A. et v. colica media

A. et v. colica dextra

Colon ascendens

Intestinum caecum

A. et v. ileocolica

A. appendicularis

Processus vermiformis

A. et v. mesenterica superior
Aa. jejunales

Aa. ileae

Vv. intestinales

Intestinum jejunum

Intestinum ileum

A

Figure 14–34.   A. Blood supply of the intestines. The transverse colon is lifted to show the patterns of distribution of the intestinal and colic branches of the superior mesenteric artery, and the accompanying venous tributaries to the portal vein. (From Warren, Handbook of Anatomy, Harvard University Press.)

Figure 14–34 continued on the opposite page.

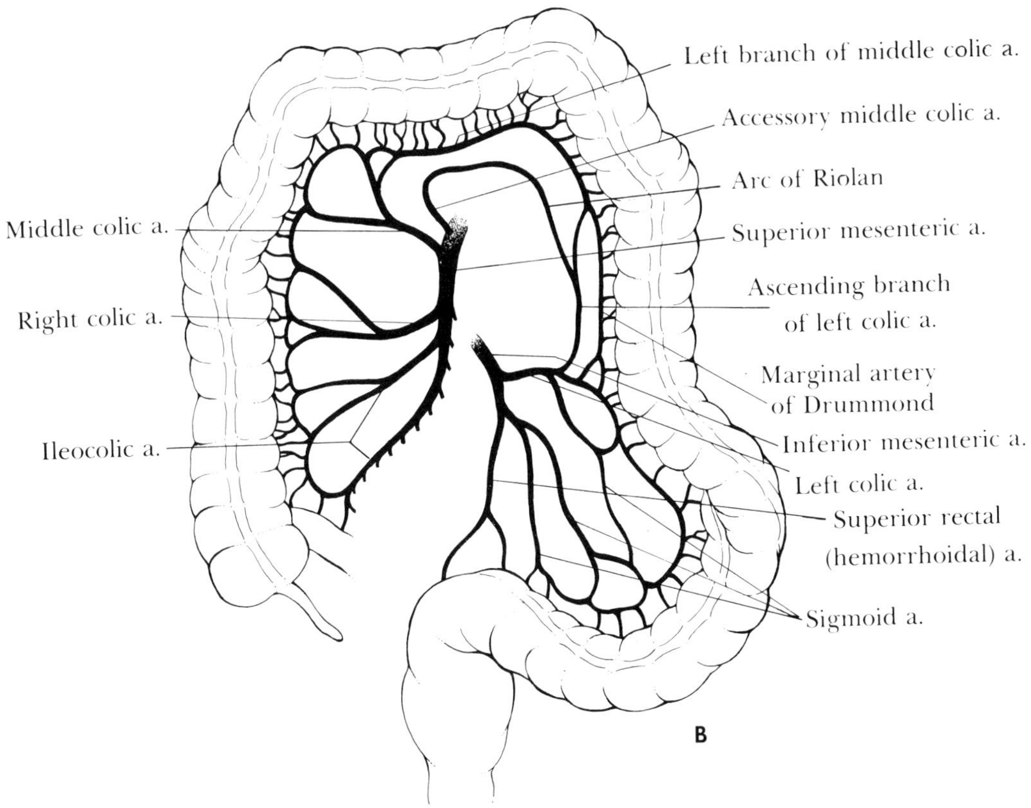

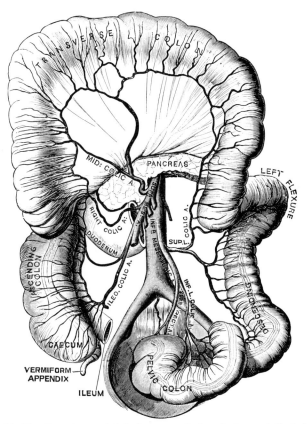

Figure 14–34 *Continued. B.* Superior and inferior mesenteric arterial systems, showing the arc of Riolan and the marginal artery of Drummond. The arc of Riolan is made up of the accessory middle colic artery, the ascending branch of the left colic artery, and an anastomotic branch between the two. The marginal artery of Drummond is shown here as a continuous vessel from sigmoid to cecum. In actuality, it is often interrupted, especially in the right colon. (From Ruzicka, F. F., and Rossi, P.: Radiol. Clin. N. Amer., 8:3–29, 1970.)

Labels in figure B:
- Left branch of middle colic a.
- Accessory middle colic a.
- Arc of Riolan
- Superior mesenteric a.
- Ascending branch of left colic a.
- Marginal artery of Drummond
- Inferior mesenteric a.
- Left colic a.
- Superior rectal (hemorrhoidal) a.
- Sigmoid a.
- Middle colic a.
- Right colic a.
- Ileocolic a.

The branches of the inferior mesenteric artery are: the *left colic*, which ascends to anastomose with a branch of the accessory middle colic artery and forms another tier which in turn anastomoses with a branch of the middle colic artery itself, the *sigmoid*, and the *superior rectal*. These are indicated in diagram in Figure 14–34 *B.* They supply the corresponding portions of the rectum and colon. In about 27 per cent of persons the ascending branch of the left colic artery extends to the descending colon. In the remainder the ascending branch is directed toward the splenic flexure. There are numerous anastomoses between the left colic and sigmoid arteries in various arcades.

The *superior rectal artery* is actually the continued trunk of the inferior mesenteric artery (Fig. 14–35), and as it bifurcates it forms an arcade around the rectum continuous with similar arcades around the sigmoid.

Along their course, the branches of the superior rectal artery anastomose with branches of the middle and inferior rectal and middle sacral arteries which participate in supply of the two lowest segments of the intestinal tract, the rectum and anus, and thereby communicate with branches of the abdominal aorta more inferiorly.

The *middle rectal arteries* have a varied origin but most commonly arise from the anterior division of the hypogastric or internal iliac arteries.

The *middle sacral artery* is a single vessel originating from the posterior surface of the aorta, a little more than 1 cm. above the aortic bifurcation, and extending to the tip of the coccyx.

Figure 14–35. Superior and inferior mesenteric arteries and their branches. Usually, there is more than one inferior left colic (sigmoid) artery. (From Cunningham's Manual of Practical Anatomy, 12th ed. Vol. 2. London, Oxford University Press, 1958.)

881

Marginal Artery of Drummond.   One of the significant arcades is formed by a continuous channel, the *marginal artery of Drummond* (Fig. 14–34 B), which links the blood stream of all the vessels sustaining the various portions of the colon, including the rectum. It acts as a terminal arcade from which smaller vessels permeate the colon perpendicularly. It begins with the terminal portion of the colic branch of the ileocolic artery and ends in the region of the upper sigmoid. Unfortunately, the *arteriae rectae* (perpendicular branches from the marginal artery) constitute an element of danger in so far as gangrene is concerned because these arteries are widely spaced and gangrene may result when two or more of them are severed.

Venous Drainage of the Small and Large Intestines

Generally, the veins involved in the drainage of the small and large intestines follow a design similar to that of the arteries. The exception to this rule is the right gastroepiploic vein, which drains directly into the superior mesenteric just before the latter enters the portal vein. However, the other tributaries of the superior mesenteric vein such as the *inferior pancreaticoduodenal, dorsal pancreatic, transverse pancreatic, jejunal, ileal, ileocolic,* and the *right and middle colic veins* follow a course almost identical with that of the arteries.

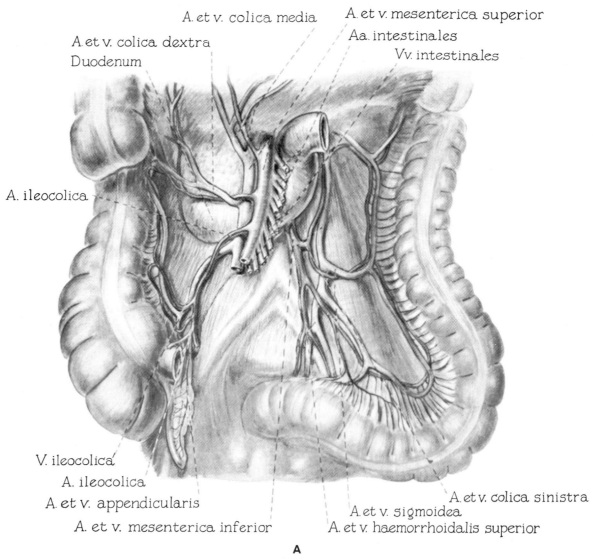

A. et v. colica media
A. et v. colica dextra
Duodenum
A. et v. mesenterica superior
Aa. intestinales
Vv. intestinales
A. ileocolica
V. ileocolica
A. ileocolica
A. et v. appendicularis
A. et v. mesenterica inferior
A. et v. colica sinistra
A. et v. sigmoidea
A. et v. haemorrhoidalis superior

A

Figure 14–36.   A. Blood supply to the large intestine. The jejunal and ileal divisions of the small intestine have been removed in order to expose the arterial branches of the inferior mesenteric and the corresponding veins of colic drainage. (From Warren: Handbook of Anatomy, Harvard University Press.)

Figure 14–36 continued on the opposite page.

The *pancreaticoduodenal arcades* are similar in respect to arteries and veins (see Chapter 13). Starting in the terminal ileum and taking in the root of the mesentery, the *superior mesenteric vein* lies to the right and somewhat in front of the corresponding artery. Both vessels are convex toward the left, and both cross in front of the third portion of the duodenum. The *inferior mesenteric vein* is similarly arranged, with the tributaries following closely corresponding arteries mostly to their left. *However, when the left colic and the upper sigmoid arteries take their origin from the inferior mesenteric artery, the corresponding vein follows a separate course.* The vein moves directly upward, ascending behind the peritoneum over the psoas muscles and to the left of the fourth part of the duodenum. It drains into the splenic vein behind the body of the pancreas. The course of the inferior mesenteric vein varies considerably, however, and it occasionally enters the superior mesenteric, in some individuals joining both the superior mesenteric and splenic veins (Fig. 14–36 *A, B*).

The *splenic vein* is formed by large veins from the hilus of the spleen, and it traverses the superior border of the pancreas ventral to the aorta, caudal to the celiac trunk, joining the superior mesenteric vein behind the head of the pancreas — the portal vein proper. It receives such tributaries as the *short gastric, left gas-*troepiploic, and *pancreatic veins*. In about 60 per cent of cases the inferior mesenteric vein may join the splenic vein.

The *portal vein* is a thick trunk, 7 or 8 cm. long, originating just dorsal to the pancreas and opposite the right aspect of L2 vertebra. It passes between the layers of a hepatoduodenal ligament and dorsal to the hepatic artery and common bile duct proper. It enters the porta hepatis and divides into right and left branches.

The portal vein receives a *prepyloric vein, right and left gastric veins,* and the *posterior superior pancreaticoduodenal vein.* There may be other tributaries. In the liver, it corresponds in course and distribution to the hepatic artery and biliary duct. There are usually three portal branches to the caudal lobe.

The three structures — hepatic artery, portal vein, and biliary duct — are enclosed within the liver in a connective tissue sheath called the *perivascular fibrous capsule.*

The *hepatic veins* are quite large in diameter but have a short intra-abdominal length. Three hepatic veins begin within the liver and converge toward the inferior vena cava. Although they are relatively constant, *they do not parallel the intrahepatic course of the portal vein, hepatic artery, and bile duct,* but rather lie in intersegmental planes draining adjacent segments. *In the event of obstruction of the intrahepatic portal system, there are im-*

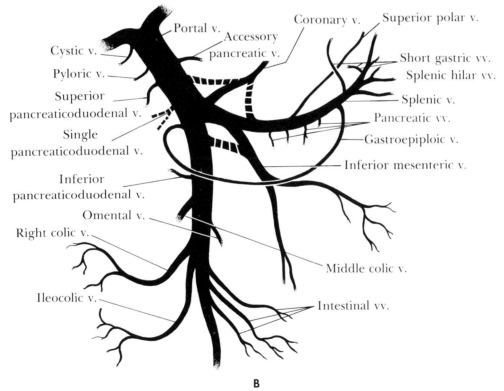

B

Figure 14–36 *Continued.* B. Portal venous system. Solid line drawing represents the most frequent pattern. Interrupted lines show variations of coronary, inferior mesenteric, and pancreaticoduodenal veins. When the pancreaticoduodenal vein is single, it empties into the right wall of the portal vein just above the confluence of the splenic and superior mesenteric veins. (From Ruzicka, F. F., Jr., and Rossi, P.: Radiol. Clin. N. Amer., 8:3–29, 1970. Modified from Douglass, B. E., Baggenstoss, A. H., and Hollinshead, W. H.: Surg., Gynec., Obstet., 91:562–576, 1950, by permission of Surgery, Gynecology, and Obstetrics.)

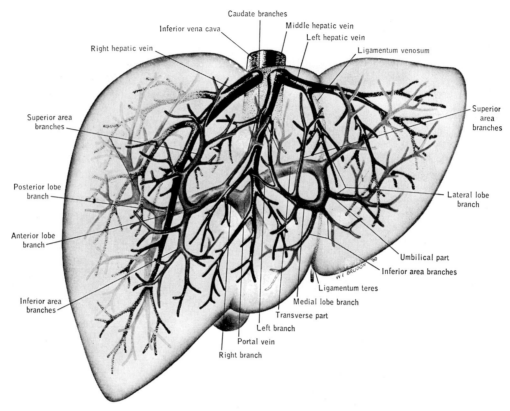

Figure 14–37. Intrahepatic distribution of the hepatic and portal veins. (From Anson, B. J. (ed.): Morris' Human Anatomy, 12th ed. Copyright © 1966 by McGraw-Hill, Inc. Used by permission of McGraw-Hill Book Company.)

portant bypass tributaries such as: (1) those between esophageal veins that are tributaries to the azygos and to the left gastric vein; (2) those between superior rectal veins that are tributary to the inferior mesenteric, and between middle and inferior rectal veins that are tributary to the internal iliac veins; (3) those between retroperitoneal, posterior, abdominal wall veins (such as those around the kidney, the inferior phrenic, and the azygos system) and the veins of the pancreas, duodenum, and liver; and (4) those between the epigastric anastomosis around the umbilicus, and the left branch of the portal vein by means of its periumbilical tributary.

When these collateral channels are used because of portal obstruction, varicosities and tortuous enlargements are produced which on occasion may bleed.

Illustrative angiograms of the celiac trunk, superior mesenteric artery, inferior mesenteric artery, and portal venous system are provided in Figures 14–38 to 14–41.

Some Variations of Arterial Patterns

The Celiac, Superior, and Inferior Mesenteric Trunks. Extensive studies have been made after dissection of the hepatic,

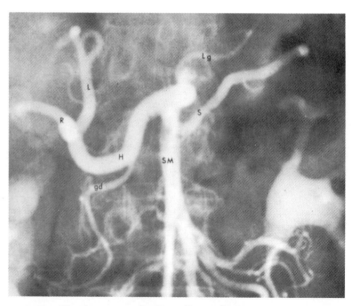

Figure 14–38. Simultaneous selective celiac and superior mesenteric artery injections show type I pattern (see Figs. 14–42 and 14–43 and text). Anteroposterior view. (S) Splenic artery, (SM) superior mesenteric, (gd) gastroduodenal, (H) proper hepatic, (R) right hepatic, (L) left hepatic, (Lg) left gastric. (From Ruzicka, F. F., Jr., and Rossi, P.: Radiol. Clin. N. Amer., 8:3–29, 1970.)

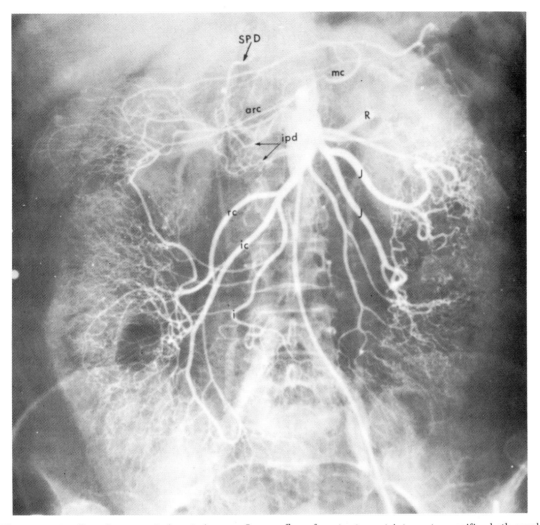

Figure 14–39. Superior mesenteric arteriogram. Some reflux of contrast agent into aorta opacifies both renal arteries. Note filling of pancreaticoduodenal arcades and superior pancreaticoduodenal artery from inferior pancreaticoduodenal arteries. *(R)* Renal, *(J)* jejunal artery, *(i)* ileal artery, *(ic)* ileocolic artery, *(rc)* right colic, *(mc)* middle colic, *(arc)* accessory right colic, *(ipd)* inferior pancreaticoduodenal, *(SPD)* superior pancreaticoduodenal artery. (From Ruzicka, F. F., Jr., and Rossi, P.: Radiol. Clin. N. Amer., 8:3–29, 1970.)

celiac, superior mesenteric, and inferior mesenteric arteries, and these variations do have practical significance in the interpretation of angiograms (Odnoralov).

As pointed out by Ruzicka and Rossi, if the main celiac trunk and the superior mesenteric artery are considered together, *six different basic types* can be proposed that include most of the variations encountered (Fig. 14–42). The classical pattern, illustrated here, occurs in approximately 93 per cent of cases. In a few instances, as shown, there is a separate origin for (1) the left gastric artery, (2) the splenic artery, and (3) the common hepatic artery. In another pattern, the left gastric and the splenic arise from the celiac artery, and the common hepatic arises from the superior

mesenteric. In this instance there is a single common trunk for both the celiac and superior mesenteric branches. There are minor variations of each of these patterns.

Hepatic Artery. A number of hepatic artery variations occur also. For example, the most common type is Type 1, illustrated in Figure 14–42. In this instance the common hepatic artery arises from the celiac artery and the gastroduodenal artery in turn arises from it.

One variation of the hepatic artery is Type 5, shown in Figure 14–42, where the entire arterial blood supply of the liver arises from the superior mesenteric artery. As a further variation, the left hepatic may arise from the common hepatic, which

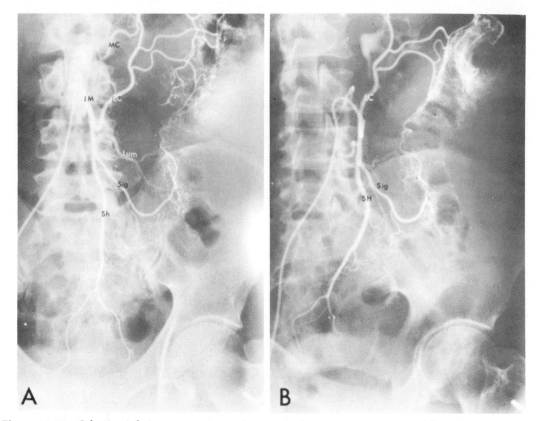

Figure 14–40. Selective inferior mesenteric arteriogram. *A.* Anteroposterior view. Middle colic artery fills via communications (not shown) with left colic branches. A small amount of reflux defines adjacent aorta, and lumbar artery is also opacified because of this reflux. (*MC*) Middle colic, (*LC*) left colic, (*Lum*) lumbar artery, (*Sig*) sigmoid, (*Sh*) superior hemorrhoidal, (*IM*) inferior mesenteric artery. *B.* Left posterior oblique view. (From Ruzicka, F. F., Jr., and Rossi, P.: Radiol. Clin. N. Amer., 8:3–29, 1970.)

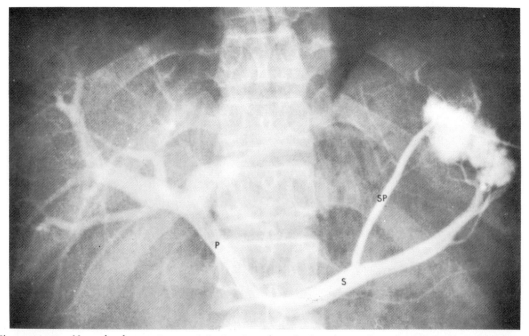

Figure 14–41. Normal splenoportogram. Injection into the splenic pulp results in visualization of splenoportal axis. Superior polar vein (*SP*) is part of splenoportal axis. Tributaries are not visualized normally by this technique. However, capsular veins of spleen and adjacent small vessels may fill during splenic injection in the normal patient. (*S*) Splenic vein, (*P*) portal vein. (From Ruzicka, F. F., Jr., and Rossi, P.: Radiol. Clin. N. Amer., 8:3–29, 1970.)

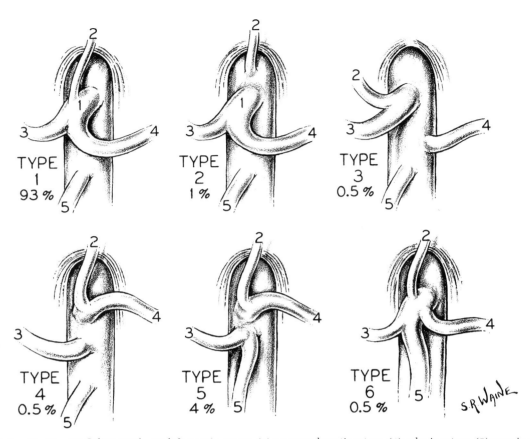

Figure 14-42. *(1)* Celiac trunk, *(2)* left gastric artery, *(3)* common hepatic artery, *(4)* splenic artery, *(5)* superior mesenteric artery, *(6)* right hepatic artery, *(7)* left hepatic artery, *(8)* gastroduodenal artery, *(9)* proper hepatic artery. (From Ruzicka, F. F., and Rossi, P.: N.Y. State J. Med., 23:3032–3033, 1968, reproduced with permission.)

in turn arises from the celiac artery. Probably the fourth most frequent variation is one in which the right hepatic arises from the common hepatic but the left hepatic arises from a left gastric. Four of the most frequent variations in patterns of arterial blood supply to the liver are shown in Figure 14–43.

Splenic Artery. There are also numerous variations of the splenic artery and its branches (Michels). Apart from the splenic artery's pancreatic branches, which will be separately considered, the terminal branches of this artery need further comment. The superior polar artery, one of the terminal branches, may be short or long – 12 cm. or more. It may arise separately from the celiac axis and appear as a second splenic artery. There are also many short gastric arteries that may arise from either the splenic or any of its branches, and these help supply the posterior and anterior aspects of the cardia and fundus of the stomach.

PANCREATIC ARTERIAL DISTRIBUTION

The classical pattern of pancreatic arterial distribution has been described in Chapter 13. It will be recalled that the main ar-

terial blood supply for the pancreas is derived from: (1) the splenic artery, (2) the retroduodenal branch of the gastroduodenal artery, (3) the superior pancreaticoduodenal from the gastroduodenal artery, and (4) the inferior pancreaticoduodenal artery – a branch of the superior mesenteric.

The *dorsal pancreatic artery,* a branch of the splenic, is probably the principal nutrient vessel of the pancreas. The *transverse pancreatic artery,* at the inferior margin of the pancreas, is usually a branch of the dorsal. Branches of the great pancreatic artery (from the splenic artery) and the caudal artery anastomose with the transverse (Fig. 14–44). The *pancreatica magna* or large artery of the pancreas is indeed often smaller than the dorsal pancreatic artery, but it does constitute the principal blood supply to the tail of the pancreas. The dorsal pancreatic artery may, in turn, act as a collateral route between celiac and superior mesenteric arteries (Fig. 14–44 *C*).

Although the transverse pancreatic artery is in 90 per cent of the cases a branch of the dorsal pancreatic, it may take origin from the gastroduodenal, the right gastroepiploic, or the superior

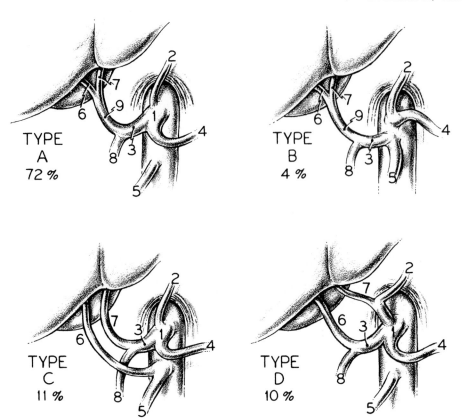

Figure 14–43. (1) Celiac trunk, (2) left gastric artery, (3) common hepatic artery, (4) splenic artery, (5) superior mesenteric artery, (6) right hepatic artery, (7) left hepatic artery, (8) gastroduodenal artery, (9) proper hepatic artery. (From Ruzicka, F. F., and Rossi, P.: N.Y. State J. Med., 23:3032–3033, 1968, reproduced with permission.)

pancreaticoduodenal (Michels). Indeed, at times there may be two transverse pancreatic arteries.

One of the most important variant branches of the superior mesenteric artery is an aberrant hepatic artery (Type C, Fig. 14–43). Other normal variations already mentioned are the dorsal pancreatic and transverse pancreatic arteries originating from the superior mesenteric instead of the splenic.

Occasionally, the right gastroepiploic arises from the superior mesenteric artery directly or from one of the branches.

Other variations of normal are seen around the origin of the middle colic and acessory middle colic arteries. The reader is referred to an excellent succinct review of the major anastomotic patterns of these vessels of the abdominal viscera by Ruzicka and Rossi; see also Michels.

Neonatal Umbilical Catheterization and Angiography

Basic Anatomy. The *umbilical vein* ascends to reach the liver by way of the falciform ligament, entering the *left portal vein* opposite the ductus venosus. If the latter is patent, a catheter may pass directly to the inferior vena cava, right atrium, and ultimately through the septum into the left atrium.

The paired umbilical arteries in the fetus are the main channels from the aorta to the placenta by way of the umbilical cord. The proximal parts of this main channel are the common iliac and internal iliac arteries. Atrophy of the umbilical artery leading to the internal iliac artery is incomplete, and a superior vesical artery arises as a result. A schematic drawing of the umbilical vein and umbilical arteries is shown in Figure 14–45. A catheter in the umbilical vein rises directly beneath the anterior abdominal wall toward the liver, joining the portal vein in the ductus venosus (Fig. 14–46 A). A catheter in the umbilical artery, however, descends to the pelvis minor and enters the aorta via either the common iliac or internal iliac artery (Fig. 14–46 B).

Injections of contrast media may be made into the catheter in the umbilical vein for visualization of the liver (transumbilical portography).

Selective catheterization of the abdominal branches of the newborn is possible through the umbilical artery. This method is often used to study vascular masses in the liver or kidney of the newborn. Failure to visualize renal arteries by this route is often confirmatory evidence of renal agenesis—another application of this kind of angiography.

Prolonged neonatal therapeutic canalization of umbilical vessels may lead to an acquired arteriovenous connection, which must be avoided. Short-term catheterization of these vessels presents no serious problems. Unfortunately, however, catheterization of the umbilicus is attended by thrombosis and intravascular clotting. Introduction of a catheter into the portal vein may lead to portal thrombosis with later portal hypertension and esophageal varices. Hence, this technique is reserved for cases in which special information or important therapeutic canalization is required (Kessler et al.; Salerna et al.; Emmanoulides et al.).

THE BILIARY TRACT

The radiographic examination of the gallbladder is at the same time a means of visualization of the anatomic structures of the gallbladder and cystic duct, and a test of hepatobiliary function. One can hardly be considered without the other, and a detailed knowledge of both is essential if we are to carry out the examination with accuracy.

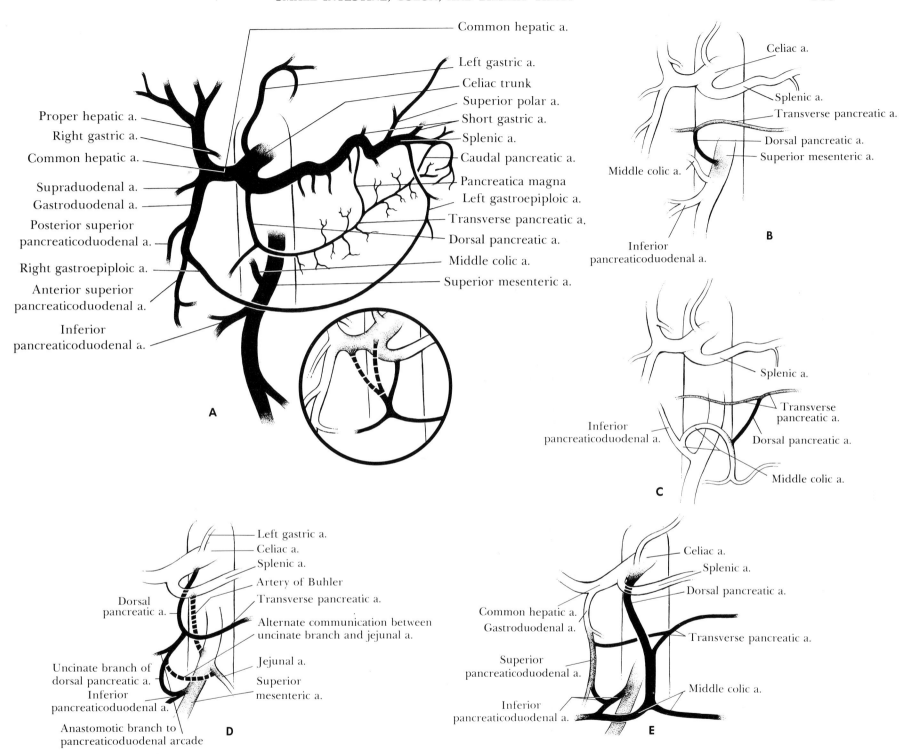

Figure 14–44. Pancreatic artery variations. The classical pattern of pancreatic arteries, as well as the major branches of the celiac system, are shown in A. Inset demonstrates the more usual variations of the dorsal pancreatic artery. Vessels portrayed by interrupted lines are alternate routes. Unusual sites of origin of the dorsal pancreatic artery are shown in B and C. D and E. The dorsal pancreatic artery as a major anastomotic channel. Two variations of this role are shown. The artery of Buhler, which is distinct from the dorsal pancreatic artery, similarly joins the celiac and superior mesenteric systems. (From Ruzicka, F. F., Jr., and Rossi, P.: Radiol. Clin. N. Amer., 8:3–29, 1970.)

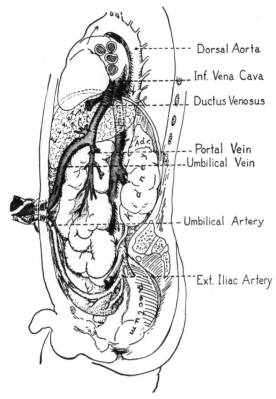

Figure 14-45. Semischematic drawings to show the vestiges in the adult of the umbilical vessels of the fetus. (From Cullen, The Umbilicus and Its Diseases, *in* Anson, B. J. (ed.): Morris' Human Anatomy, 12th ed. Copyright © 1966 by McGraw-Hill, Inc. Used by permission of McGraw-Hill Book Company.)

The Microscopic and Gross Anatomy of the Biliary Tract (Figs. 14–47, 14–48).   The liver is composed of many hundreds of units called lobules, and each lobule is composed of radial columns of parenchymal cells. Between these columns of cells lie the bile capillaries, the walls of which are the liver cells themselves. On the opposite side of these cells are the stellate cells of the lymph channels and reticulodenothelial system, and the endothelium of the venules leading into the central vein. The bile capillaries empty into interlobular bile ducts, which enter in their turn into larger bile ducts, until finally two chief branches are obtained: a large branch from the right, and a small branch from the left lobe of the liver, called the right and left hepatic ducts respectively (Fig. 14–48). These ultimately unite to form the common hepatic duct.

The common hepatic duct passes downward, and just beyond the porta hepatis, it is joined by the cystic duct from the gallbladder (a pear-shaped enlargement lying distal to the cystic duct) to form the common bile duct. The common hepatic duct is about 25 to 30 mm. in length, and about 6 mm. in diameter.

The cystic duct is about half the diameter of the hepatic duct but somewhat longer—about 30 to 37 mm. in length. It pursues a course backward and medially to join the hepatic duct.

The spiral constriction at the neck of the gallbladder (to be described below) is continued into the proximal portion, called the valvular portion of the cystic duct, in contrast to the nonvalvular portion, or pars glabra.

The common bile duct is about 7.5 cm. in length and about the same diameter as the hepatic duct. It passes downward between the two layers of the hepatoduodenal ligament, with the portal vein behind and the hepatic artery to its left. It then passes behind the superior part of the duodenum and runs in a groove between the duodenum and head of the pancreas. Joining the pancreatic duct (still maintaining a separate lumen), it pierces the descending part of the duodenum in its midportion, to open

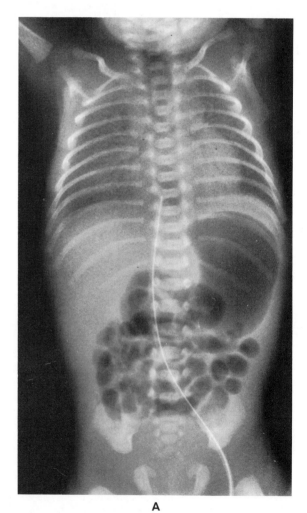

A

Figure 14-46.   A. Anteroposterior view of newborn whose umbilical vein has been catheterized.

Figure 14–46 continued on the opposite page.

obliquely into the lumen at the duodenal papilla. Two common variations at the juncture with the duodenum are indicated in Figure 14–50.

The gallbladder is arbitrarily divided into four parts (Fig. 14–49): the distal end or *fundus* usually reaches the anterior border of the liver; the *body* runs backward, upward, and to the left; the *infundibulum* is situated between the body and neck, and consists of that portion tapering toward the neck; the *neck* is curved medially toward the porta hepatis and contains spiral crescentic folds around the interior of its lumen, forming the spiral valve of Heister. The neck of the gallbladder usually curves sharply like the letter "S." This continues into the valvular portion of the cystic duct as previously described. Smooth muscle fibers are found in the fundus and infundibulum but are almost completely absent in the body; conversely, there is much elastic

tissue in the body and very little in the fundus and infundibulum. The muscle fibers are longitudinal and oblique in the fundus but circular in the infundibulum, and this circular conformation is continued into the spiral valves.

The gallbladder, when measured angiographically, is 2 to 3 mm. thick, less than 35 sq. cm. in area, and 5 cm. or less in width (Rösch et al.; Deutsch; Redman and Reuter). The gallbladder may often appear larger than this in oral cholecystograms when distended and magnified, but a gallbladder that is somewhat enlarged and concentrates well is difficult to interpret.

Usually the gallbladder is not covered with peritoneum on its hepatic side, but occasionally it is suspended from the liver by a short peritoneal ligament. The gallbladder usually rests on the transverse colon in front, and its neck is usually in close proximity with the duodenum.

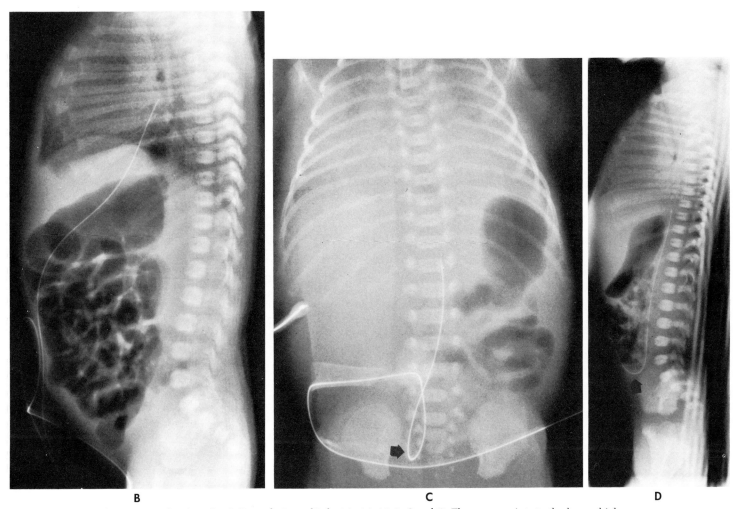

B   C   D

Figure 14–46 *Continued.* *B.* Lateral view of infant in 14–46 *A. C* and *D.* The arrow points to the loop which extends down to the hypogastric artery, which in frontal perspective establishes the arterial position of the catheter.

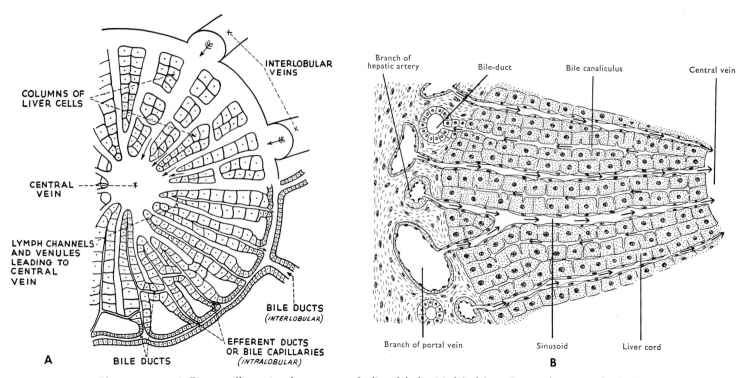

Figure 14–47. A. Diagram illustrating the structure of a liver lobule. (Modified from Cunningham's Textbook of Anatomy, 10th ed. London, Oxford University Press, 1964.) B. The structure of the liver lobule (human). (From Cunningham's Textbook of Anatomy, 10th ed. London, Oxford University Press, 1964.)

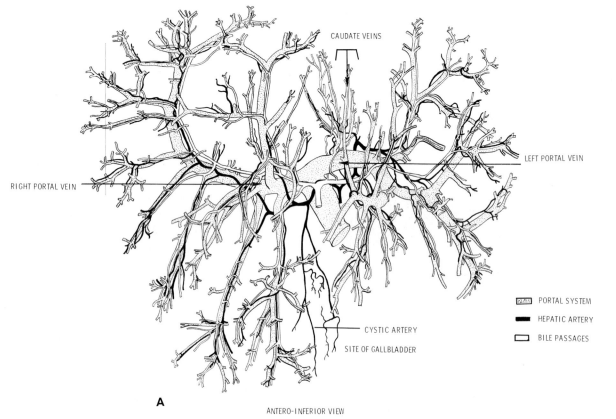

Figure 14–48. A. Venous drainage of the liver into the caval system as compared with the portal venous system.

892

Figure 14–48 continued on the opposite page.

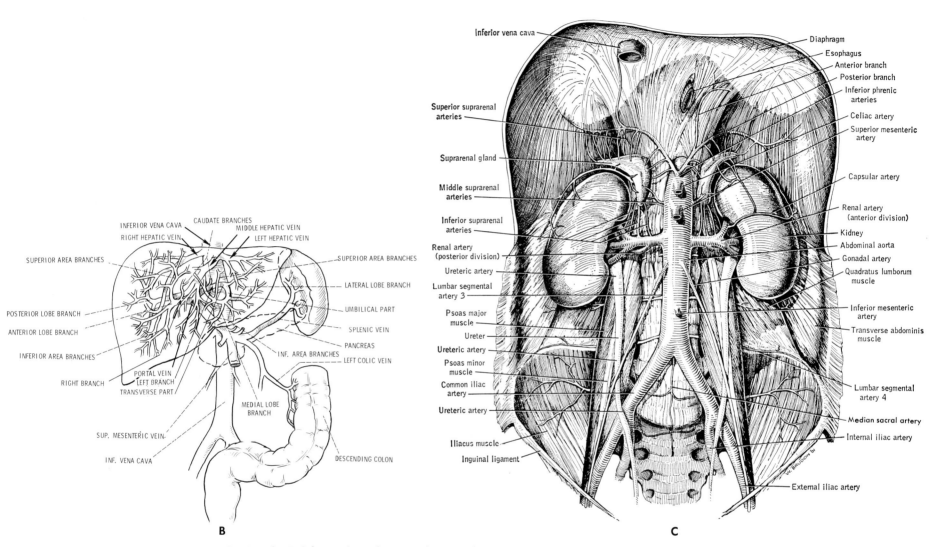

Figure 14–48 *Continued.* *B.* Schema of portal system of veins and its connections with systemic veins. It must be remembered that the systemic blood carried by the hepatic artery also enters the capillaries of the liver, and the hepatic veins contain therefore both portal and systemic blood. (Modified from Cunningham's Manual of Practical Anatomy, 11th ed. Vol. 2. London, Oxford University Press, 1949.) *C.* Abdominal aorta and its branches. (From Anson, B. J. (ed.): Morris' Human Anatomy, 12th ed. Copyright © 1966 by McGraw-Hill, Inc. Used by permission of McGraw-Hill Book Company.)

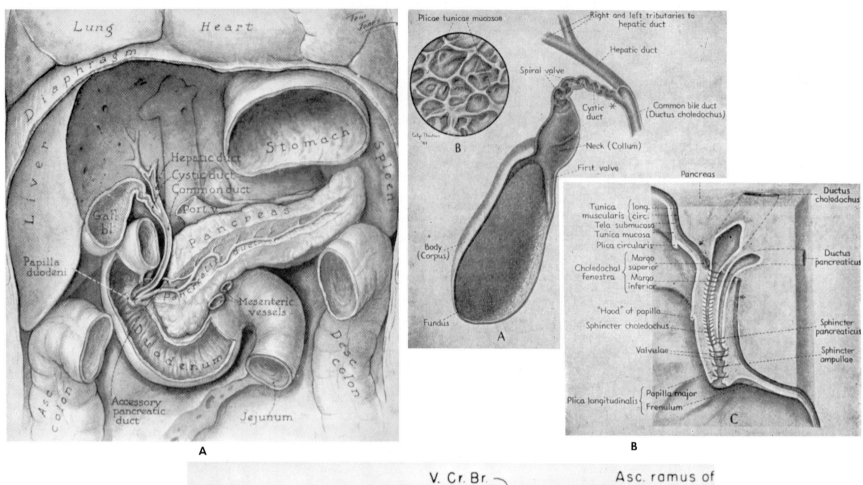

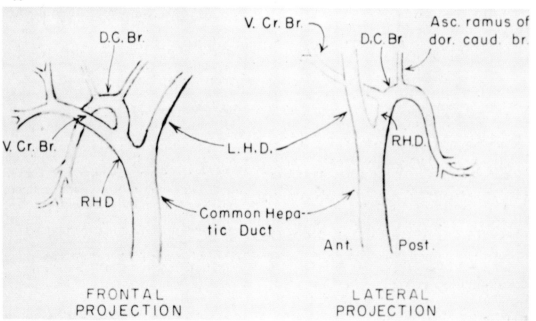

Figure 14–49. A. The gross anatomy of the biliary system. (From Jones, T.: Anatomical Studies. Jackson, Michigan, S. H. Camp and Co., 1943.) B. Gross anatomy of biliary tract. (A), Interior of the gallbladder and cystic duct; (B), surface of the mucosa of the gallbladder showing plicae; (C), diagram of frontal section through duodenum at the inferior duodenal flexure showing the structure and relations of the papilla major (duodenal papilla). (After Boyden in Surgery. From Jackson, C. M., and Blount, R. F., in Jackson (ed.): Morris' Human Anatomy. New York, The Blakiston Co.) C. Schematic composite of the roentgen anatomy of the hepatic ductal system in its most common configuration. (D.C.Br.) Dorsocaudal branch, (V. Cr. Br.) ventrocranial branch. (From Schein, C. J., Stern, W. Z., and Jacobson, H. G.: Surgery, 51:718–723, 1962.)

894

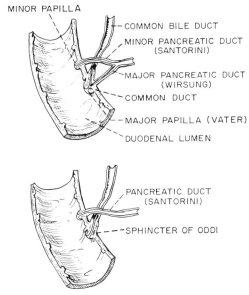

Figure 14–50. Anatomic sketch depicting the relationship of the major and minor papillae, the common bile duct, and the pancreatic duct. (After Daves.)

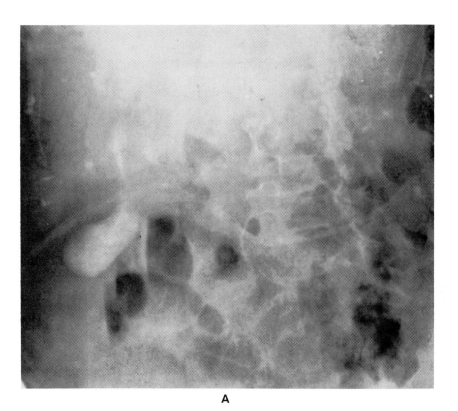

A

Variations of the Gallbladder (Fig. 14–51). The major variations of the gallbladder may be classified as follows:

1. *Variations in Shape.* The gallbladder may be ovoid, spherical or elongated.

2. *Variations in Position.* The gallbladder may be deeply embedded in the liver, or it may have a mesentery and lie in the iliac fossa. Its position also varies in relation to the spine. No definite pathologic function has been associated with these unusual locations.

3. *Construction by Mucosal or Serosal Folds.* These folds may produce a sacculation of the gallbladder and the so-called Phrygian cap. This does not have pathologic significance. Also, the gallbladder may be divided longitudinally into separate gallbladders and possess separate cystic ducts.

4. *Absence of the Gallbladder.* Rarely, the gallbladder is absent, and in such instances the hepatic ducts have usually been found to be dilated.

5. *Variations in Length of Ducts.* Variations in the length of the hepatic ducts, cystic duct and common bile duct may occur.

6. *Separate Openings.* The common bile duct and pancreatic duct may open separately into the duodenum.

Function of the Gallbladder. The functions of the gallbladder may be summarized as follows:

The Reservoir Function. A part of the bile secreted by the liver is stored in the gallbladder.

The Concentration Function. Water and salts are absorbed in the gallbladder, whereas the bile pigments are not, and as a result, bilirubin is concentrated about 20 times; cholesterol,

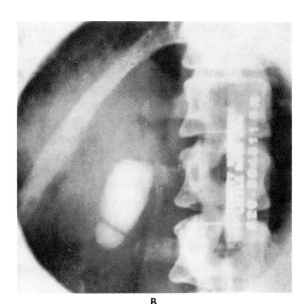

B

Figure 14–51. Variations in gallbladder of radiographic significance. A. Ptotic gallbladder lying in the iliac fossa. B. Mucosal or serosal fold of gallbladder, known as a Phrygian cap.

bile salts and calcium about 5 to 10 times (Rous and McMaster). In disease of the gallbladder, this concentration function is readily impaired. A contrast agent introduced in an inflamed gallbladder is reabsorbed in sufficient volume to prevent adequate concentration for visualization (Berk and Lasser). When a second dose of contrast agent is administered visualization may be possible. It has been postulated that many of the serum and tissue protein-binding sites are occupied in this second dose, thus leading to a more sustained elevation of the available opaque material in the blood and to an inhibition of reabsorption of the contrast material through the marginally inflamed gallbladder wall. As a result, more of the contrast agent is excreted in the bile and more remains in the gallbladder so that visualization may become possible (Rous and McMaster; Boyden).

The Emptying Mechanism. The exact mechanism involved is not completely understood. It is claimed by some that there is a reciprocal innervation of the gallbladder and sphincter of Oddi, so that vagal stimulation causes contraction of the gallbladder and relaxation of the sphincter. There is also a hormonal influence—when practically any acid or food substance, particularly fats and fatty acid, comes into contact with the duodenal mucosa, cholecystokinin is formed, which is absorbed into the blood stream and causes the gallbladder to contract (Boyden) (Fig. 14–52).

The Secretory Function. The gallbladder apparently secretes constituents of the bile, such as cholesterol and mucin.

Functions of Bile. The main functions of bile can be summarized as follows: (1) it is an important accessory agent in digestion because it accelerates the action of pancreatic enzymes; (2) it aids materially in the digestion of fats by decreasing surface tension, activating lipase, increasing the solubility of soaps and fatty acids, and materially aiding fatty absorption; (3) it forms a means of eliminating nitrogenous and toxic waste substances; (4) it helps to regulate acid-base and calcium balance in the blood stream.

(5) When fats are not absorbed adequately, the fat-soluble vitamins are not absorbed satisfactorily either. Therefore, in the absence of bile salts, vitamins A, E, D, and K are poorly absorbed. Vitamin K is usually not stored in the body and a deficiency of vitamin K results. This in turn leads to deficient formation by the liver of factor VII and prothrombin, which results in serious impairment of blood coagulation.

(6) Approximately 94 per cent of bile salts are reabsorbed from the intestine—on the average these salts make the circuit from intestine to liver and back to intestine some 18 times before being carried out in the feces (this is the enterohepatic circulation). The quantity of bile secreted by the liver is dependent on bile salts to a great extent, and hence, if there is a loss of bile salts

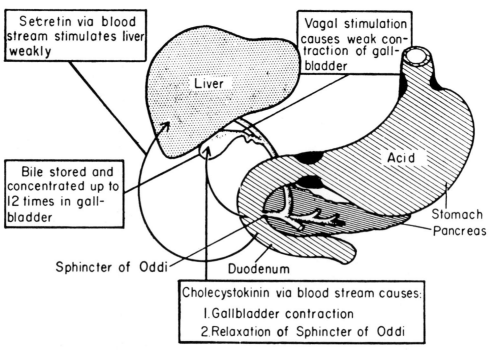

Figure 14–52. Mechanisms of liver secretion and gallbladder emptying. (From Guyton, A. C.: Textbook of Medical Physiology. 4th ed. Philadelphia, W. B. Saunders Co., 1971.)

TABLE 14-1 SELECTION OF PATIENTS FOR ORAL CHOLANGIOGRAPHY AND CHOLECYSTOGRAPHY

Test	Values	Probability of Success
Serum bilirubin		
(Mandel)	< 5 mg.%	{ Worth trying
	>10 mg.%	{ Failure
(Shehadi)	< 1 mg.%	Excellent
	< 2 mg.%	Satisfactory
	3 mg.% or	Poor or unlikely
	> 4 mg.%	Not possible
Bromsulphalein (BSP) retention		
(Etess and Strauss)	5–20%	Should not interfere
	>20–23%	Failure
(Blornstrom and Sandstrom)	>40%	Failure

through a fistula, for example, the volume of liver secretion is also depressed. (With a bile fistula, however, the liver increases its production of bile salts as much as ten-fold in an effort to increase bile secretion to normal.)

Jaundice. Jaundice causes a yellowish tint to the body tissues that results from large quantities of bilirubin in the extracellular fluids. The skin begins to appear jaundiced when the concentration rises to about three times normal, normal being 0.5 mg. per 100 ml. Borderline jaundice occurs at 1.5 mg. per 100 ml.

The common causes of jaundice are: (1) excessive destruction of red cells with release of bilirubin into the blood, or (2) obstruction of the bile ducts or damage to the liver cells so that bilirubin cannot be excreted by the liver.

Type 1 jaundice is *hemolytic* jaundice; Type 2 is *obstructive* jaundice. An understanding of these and other liver functions is inherent in the selection of patients for radiological gallbladder studies; Table 14–1 is presented as an aid in these judgments. Table 14–2 presents a battery of liver function studies helpful in the differential diagnosis of jaundice (Shehadi). It will be noted that generally gallbladder study by cholecystography is probably of no value when the serum bilirubin exceeds 10 mg. per cent; to insure reasonable success requires a serum bilirubin of less than 2 mg. per cent.

Gallstone Formation (Fig. 14–53). Bile salts are formed by

TABLE 14-2 LIVER FUNCTION STUDIES IN DIFFERENTIAL DIAGNOSIS OF JAUNDICE*

	Normal Values	Hemolytic Jaundice (Prehepatic)	Hepatocellular Jaundice (Hepatic) Medical	Obstructive Jaundice (Posthepatic) Surgical
Significant pathologic process	– –	Red blood cell destruction	Liver cell impairment	Bile flow interference
Cephalin cholesterol flocculation	0 to 1	Normal	Elevated	Normal or slightly elevated
Thymol turbidity	0 to 4	Normal	Elevated	Normal or slightly elevated
Zinc sulfate turbidity	0 to 4	Normal	Elevated	Normal or slightly elevated
Serum alkaline phosphatase	1 to 4 Bodansky units 5 to 13 King-Armstrong units	Normal	Normal or elevated	Markedly elevated
Brumsulfalein retention	5 per cent or less at 45 min.	Normal	Increased retention	Increased retention
Serum bilirubin	Up to 1.0 mg. per 100 ml.	Slight increase	Increase in proportion to degree of liver damage	Elevated
Icteric index	8 to 10	Elevated	Elevated	Elevated
Visualization of the gallbladder and bile ducts by means of cholecystography, oral and intravenous		Adequate Density may be slightly decreased	Possible but not satisfactory until B.S.P. retention is 5 per cent or below	None Sometimes possible in intermittent type, as jaundice is clearing, or between phases of obstruction

Icteric index 10 or below
Possible but faint up
   to 15
Bilirubin below 2 mg.,
preferably 1 mg.
Poor or unlikely above
   3 mg.
Not possible above 4 mg.

*From Shehadi, W. H.: Clinical Radiology of the Biliary Tract. New York, McGraw-Hill Book Company, 1963.

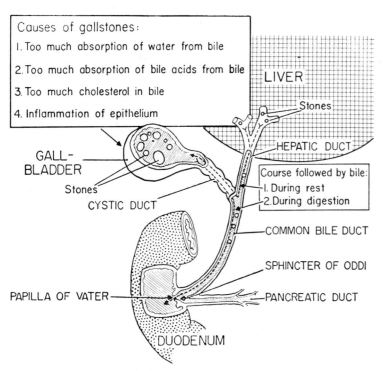

Causes of gallstones:

1. Too much absorption of water from bile

2. Too much absorption of bile acids from bile

3. Too much cholesterol in bile

4. Inflammation of epithelium

LIVER

Stones

HEPATIC DUCT

GALL-
BLADDER

Stones

CYSTIC DUCT

Course followed by bile:
1. During rest
2. During digestion

COMMON BILE DUCT

SPHINCTER OF ODDI

PAPILLA OF VATER

PANCREATIC DUCT

DUODENUM

Figure 14–53. Formation of gallstones. (From Guyton, A. C.: Textbook of Medical Physiology. 4th ed. Philadelphia, W. B. Saunders Co., 1971.)

ROENTGENOLOGIC EXAMINATION OF THE BILIARY TRACT

Introduction. Prior to the gallbladder examination, it is well to remove as much gas and fecal material from the gastrointestinal tract as possible. Cascara sagrada or enemas given at least 24 hours before the examination may be of considerable assistance. Pitressin may be employed intravenously (0.5 to 1 cc.) in those patients in whom it is not contraindicated on the basis of hypertension or arteriosclerosis.

It is also well to obtain a plain film of the entire right side of the abdomen in the posteroanterior projection prior to the administration of any dye. The gallbladder itself is not usually delineated with accuracy on such films, but if it should contain calcareous structure, this would immediately be evident from this preliminary study.

A visualization of the gallbladder requires that some form of contrast substance be introduced into it. Tetrachlorphenolphthalein had long been known as a bile secretion and had been used as a test for liver function. Graham and Cole (in 1924) introduced first the bromine radical and thereafter the heavier iodine radical

liver cells from cholesterol, and a small amount of cholesterol escapes with the bile salts in the bile. The bile salts, fatty acids, and lecithin in bile are responsible for the solubility of cholesterol in the bile. Abnormally, however, the cholesterol will precipitate and form gallstones (Fig. 14–53). As shown in this illustration, the causes of such precipitation are: (1) too much absorption of water from the bile, (2) too much absorption of bile acids from bile, (3) excessive cholesterol in bile, and (4) inflammation of the epithelium of the gallbladder. Inflammation permits excessive absorption of water, bile salts, and other substances through the epithelium of the gallbladder, and as a result cholesterol is no longer kept in solution.

Most cholesterol gallstones themselves are radiolucent (80 to 85 per cent) unless there are crevices in the gallstones, most likely containing excessive fat. These appear as "crow's feet" (Fig. 14–54). Calcium sometimes precipitates with some of the substances involved in the formation of cholesterol gallstones in the form of calcium carbonate—hence, these gallstones are radiopaque (Fig. 14–55). Since most stones in the gallbladder are radiolucent, however, special radiographic studies using iodinated contrast agents that may be concentrated in the gallbladder are necessary. These will be discussed shortly.

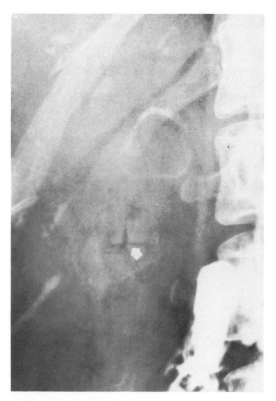

Figure 14–54. "Crowfoot" sign showing crevices which appear radiolucent in a gallstone, giving the appearance of a crow's foot.

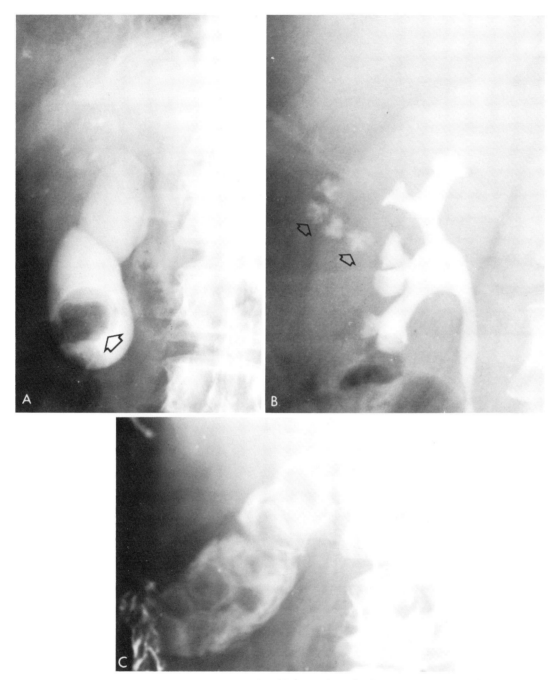

Figure 14–55.   *A.* Large cholesterol stone in the gallbladder. *B.* Calcified gallstones in the gallbladder, assuming a "mulberry" appearance. *C.* Partially calcified stones in a partially calcified gallbladder.

instead of the chlorine in this compound, and thus obtained a substance which was secreted by the liver in the bile, and concentrated with the bile in the gallbladder. This made it possible to render the bile radiopaque.

In recent years new compounds such as Priodax, Telepaque, Teridax, Monophen, and Cholografin (see Table 14–3) have been introduced which accomplish the same thing without many of the undesirable side effects attributed to the earlier contrast medium. Each of the newer compounds has certain contraindications and some adverse effects which are listed in Table 14–3.

TABLE 14–3 COMPARISON OF SOME OF THE MAJOR COMPOUNDS EMPLOYED FOR GALLBLADDER VISUALIZATION

Year of Introduction	Compound	Pharmacology	Contraindications	Accuracy and Adverse Effects
1940	Priodax	Phenylpropionic acid derivative Insoluble in water but soluble in alkali 51.38% iodine Excreted mostly by kidneys	Acute nephritis Uremia	35% less opacity than Telepaque 60% nausea, diarrhea, dysuria vs. 21.4% with Telepaque More patients require second dose (40%); fails to visualize 12% of gallbladders visualized with Telepaque
1949	Telepaque	Ethyl propanoic acid derivative Insoluble in water; soluble in alkali and 95% alcohol 66.68% iodine Excreted mostly via gastrointestinal tract	Acute nephritis Uremia Gastrointestinal diseases with disturbed absorption	Fails only in 3% of normal gallbladders or less with one dose Side reactions less than with Priodax Great opacity may obscure some gallstones
1953	Teridax	Triiodoethionic acid (ethyl propionic acid derivative) Insoluble in water; soluble in alkali 66.5% iodine Excreted mostly by kidneys	Acute nephritis Uremia	Failure after one examination not always indicative of disease; but after second dose approaches 100% accuracy Not as well worked out as to side reactions as Priodax or Telepaque Said to produce density intermediate between Priodax and Telepaque
	Monophen	Carboxylic acid derivative Insoluble in water 52.2% iodine Excreted mostly by kidneys	Acute nephritis Uremia	60% no adverse signs or symptoms 12% nausea 1% vomiting 9% diarrhea 9% cramps 3% dysuria Accuracy stated to be better (?) than Priodax
1953–1955	Cholografin	Iodipamide (triiodobenzoic acid derivative) For intravenous use (photosensitive) 64% iodine With normal liver 90% excreted in feces, 10% in urine With poor liver function: mostly excreted by kidneys (hence pyelograms)	Primary indication: Postcholecystectomy syndrome Contraindications: Iodine sensitivity Combined urinary and hepatic disease	Sensitivity high Side effects minimal with slow injection 77–85% successful biliary tree visualizations Visualization faint; usually gallbladder visualization too faint for significant accuracy Serious reactions: 2.5% Lesser reactions: 38.8%
	Orabilex (disapproved by Food and Drug Administration in U.S.A.)	Bunamiodyl (sodium acrylate derivative) 57% iodine Excreted in bile, but mainly by kidneys (70%): 30% by intestine	Renal disease Gastrointestinal diseases which would hamper absorption Double dose never to be used —may lead to acute renal failure	No advantage gained by second dose 12.5% nausea 8.9% vomiting 5.9% diarrhea 6.5% dysuria Approaches 100% accuracy
1959	Ipodate (Oragrafin) (Biloptin) (Solu-Biloptin)	Triiodohydrocinnamic acid derivatives (sodium or calcium salt) 61% iodine 42–48% excreted in bile in 24 hrs., equally in urine	Iodine sensitivity Combined renal-hepatic disease Severe kidney disorders Gastrointestinal disorders or liver disorders	Mild and transient nausea: vomiting; diarrhea

Methods of Study. There are several possible roentgenologic techniques that can be used to study the biliary system. These are:

1. Plain film of the abdomen.
2. Oral cholecystograms (including opacification of bile duct calculi).
   a. Rectal cholecystography.
3. Intravenous cholangiography.
4. Percutaneous transhepatic cholangiography.
5. Operative and postoperative cholangiography.
6. Biliary angiography.
   a. Liver.
   b. Gallbladder.

Plain Film of the Abdomen. The plain film of the abdomen should always precede contrast studies involving any organs contained in the abdomen.

In the case of the biliary tract, this should consist of: (1) KUB (kidney, ureter, bladder) film as described in Chapter 15, and (2) a 10×12 inch film of the right upper quadrant of the patient, with the patient in either the right posterior oblique or left anterior oblique projection (the same projection that is utilized subsequently in oral cholecystography). This film should extend from the iliac crest as close as possible to the right hemidiaphragm. The entire right lobe of the liver is usually included.

Oral Cholecystograms

Major Compounds Employed. Graham and Cole devised percutaneous, intravenous, and oral cholecystograms first, utilizing *tetrabromphenolphthalein* and later *sodium phenoltetraiodophthalein*. The compounds used later and some of the pharmacologic data are given in Table 14–3.

The pharmacodynamics of biliary contrast media have undergone considerable investigation (Shehadi, 1966a; Lasser et al.). By virtue of their chemical constitution, these agents are primarily "bile directed" rather than "urine directed."

The compound most frequently employed for oral study is *Telepaque,* a moderately lipid-soluble substance that is poorly soluble in an aqueous system. (*Cholografin,* the compound used in intravenous application, is freely soluble in an aqueous solution but is not appreciably absorbed from the gastrointestinal tract. This contrast agent will be discussed under intravenous cholangiography.)

After administration of Telepaque, there is a circulating level of 1 to 16 mg. per cent within 2 hours. Some patients, particularly those with less than 4 mg. per cent at 2 hours, show a rise at the 14 hour period. Shehadi has indicated that there are two distinct peaks in the absorption curve, one at 4 hours and a second, higher peak at 10 hours, and it is for this reason that the 10 hour interval is assumed to be the optimum time for film study for most patients.

Berk and Lasser have demonstrated the following cycle: the Telepaque is absorbed in the gastrointestinal tract, whereupon it is delivered to the liver. It is thereafter excreted in the bile, and if the extrahepatic biliary passages are open, it finds its way to the gallbladder. In the gallbladder the contrast agent and bile are concentrated above the level of the original bile. If, however, the gallbladder is inflamed or its mucosa is otherwise pathological, the contrast medium is absorbed from the gallbladder, and concentration of the agent does not occur sufficiently for roentgenologic visualization. When Cholografin is used, it accumulates in the gallbladder in the same form in which it is administered in sufficient concentration usually for visualization, although it is not as opaque as Telepaque. (For an understanding of the chemistry and conjugations involved, reference should be made to the original articles.)

Although many investigators may prefer one or another of these agents, preference in recent times has generally remained with Telepaque. There are some advantages and disadvantages of Telepaque versus *Oragrafin* (White and Fischer). The degree of opacification of the gallbladder and visualization of the biliary ducts is similar with both these oral cholecystographic agents. Calculi are more often demonstrated with Telepaque, but on the other hand, stones are not as often concealed by the lesser density of Oragrafin. The incidence of diarrhea is much higher and that of nausea and cramps slightly higher with Telepaque. There is also a lesser side effect with a double dose technique of Oragrafin as compared with Telepaque.

Technical Aspects of Oral Cholecystography

PREPARATION OF THE PATIENT. Prior to examination, it should be determined that: (1) the patient is not sensitive to iodine-containing contrast agents, and (2) the patient has been on a diet which might reasonably have produced previous evacuation of the gallbladder by fatty stimulation.

If possible, there should be at least one fat-containing meal the day prior to the cholecystographic examination in order to empty a distended gallbladder.

On the evening prior to the examination, the meal should be fat-free and may consist of fruit or fruit juice, fresh vegetables cooked without butter, a small portion of lean meat, toast or bread with jelly, coffee or tea but no milk, cream, butter, eggs, or any foods containing fat. Nothing should be eaten after the evening meal, although water may be taken in moderate amounts.

At about 10 P.M. six Telepaque tablets (3 grams) should be swallowed, each with one or two mouthfuls of water, a total of at least one full glass of water. To avoid nausea or vomiting, an interval of 5 minutes after each tablet may elapse. If roentgen examination is scheduled for 9 A.M., the best time for administration of Telepaque is between 9 and 11 P.M. on the night preceding the examination.

On the following morning, breakfast should be omitted.

The patient may be given an enema if it is discovered that

the contrast agent in the gastrointestinal tract interferes with adequate visualization of the gallbladder.

DOSE CONSIDERATIONS. It is probable that 3 grams of Telepaque are sufficient for all adults irrespective of weight (Whitehouse and Martin). With some patients we have used doses as high as 6 grams (12 tablets) within a period of 24 hours. Different studies on the renal toxicity of contrast medium in patients with hepatorenal damage have called attention to the danger of larger doses of oral cholecystographic media (Seaman, Cosgriff and Wells). It has therefore been recommended that a dose of 6 grams not be exceeded within a period of 24 hours, and if such a dose has been employed, that it not be repeated for a period of at least 1 week.

Pediatric patients may be given proportionately smaller doses (Harris and Caffey).

Salzman et al. have found that biliary stones can, at times, be visualized by administering 1 gram of Telepaque three times a day for 4 days, and this opacity may persist for as long as 2 to 14 days. It is thought that this gallstone opacification phenomenon is due to a reaction between biliverdin on the surface of the stones and the contrast medium in the bile.

Caution must be exercised not to use this technique in patients who have impaired hepatorenal function.

FILM AND FLUOROSCOPIC TECHNIQUES. On the morning after the patient has taken the contrast medium, films are repeated in the left anterior oblique projection (patient prone) with various degrees of obliquity. Each film should be studied until satisfactory visualization of the gallbladder is obtained. The gallbladder should be completely clear of interfering gas or other opaque shadows. Sufficient kilovoltage should be employed so that the contrast agent will not in itself obscure filling defects within the gallbladder (Fig. 14–56).

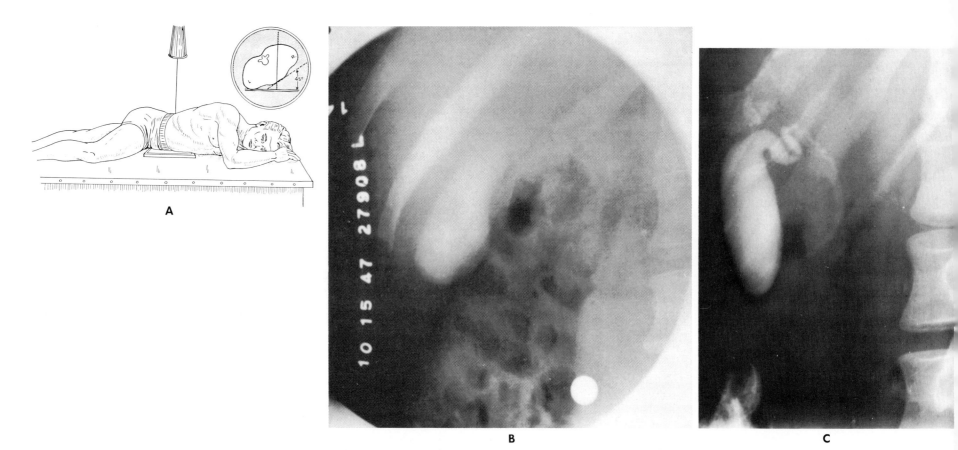

Figure 14–56. Radiograph of gallbladder before fatty stimulation. *A.* Position of patient. *B.* Radiograph. *C.* Representative scout film of the gallbladder region extending from the iliac fossa to the diaphragm and from the left portion of the spine to the outer flank region.

Upright or lateral decubitus films are also obtained routinely to determine possible stratification or mobility of filling defects within the gallbladder (Fig. 14–58). Fluoroscopy with compression spot-film studies may be employed for this purpose.

Following this first part of the examination, the patient is given a meal consisting of foods with a high fat content such as eggs, butter, toast or cream; or a synthetic cholagogue such as Bilevac may be employed.

After the fatty meal or fat stimulation is administered, the films of the right upper quadrant are repeated in identical positions (Fig. 14–57). Body section radiography may be employed at any time in the procedure to obtain better visualization of the gallbladder proper or of the ductal system.

When the customary dose of six tablets is used, visualization of the extrahepatic ducts can be obtained in most patients in 5 to 20 minutes after the fat meal. However, if visualization of the extrahepatic ducts is especially indicated a somewhat higher dose of Telepaque (6 grams) may be required.

Variations of this general procedure may be undertaken as follows: (1) The Telepaque may be taken earlier in the evening and castor oil may be administered five hours after the Telepaque tablets (Mauthe). However, if the gallbladder is not visualized the morning following administration of the Telepaque, the examination is repeated in a day or so without the castor oil. Repetition of the examination under these circumstances is important. (2) In order to overcome biliary stasis (one of the common causes of nonvisualization or delayed visualization of the gallbladder) the use of bile acid for 5 to 30 days before repeating the cholecystographic examination has been recommended (Berg and Hamilton).

SIDE EFFECTS. Whitehouse and Martin have reported the following side effects from 3 gram doses of Telepaque in 400 patients; diarrhea, 25.3 per cent (of which 2.5 per cent were severe); dysuria, 13.7 per cent; mild nausea, 5.8 per cent; and mild vomiting 1.5 per cent. There were other side effects in 2.8 per cent of the cases and no side effects were noted in 62.5 per cent of the cases.

Patients with hepatorenal dysfunction constitute a group subject to potential hazards from oral cholecystography. Doses of Telepaque larger than those recommended earlier should be employed with caution. There are advantages and disadvantages to each of the various compounds, and a careful choice must be

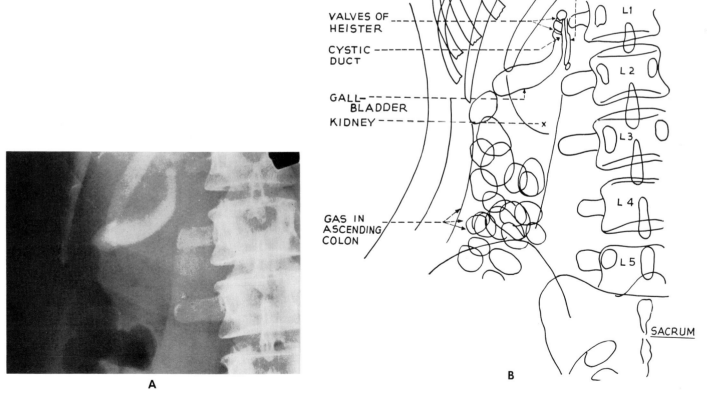

Figure 14–57. Gallbladder after fatty stimulation. *A.* Radiograph. *B.* Labeled tracing of *A.*

made with full knowledge of all aspects of the contrast agent employed as well as the importance of the clinical evaluation in the case at hand.

VISUALIZATION OR NONVISUALIZATION. It is well documented also that repeat examinations of the gallbladder following initial failures of visualization, or inadequate visualization, without evidence of gallstones will be interpreted as normal. In Rosenbaum's series of 450 consecutive patients examined by cholecystography, there were 66 visualizations in which evidence of gallstones was initially absent or inadequate. After the second dose of Telepaque and repeat roentgen study, findings were interpreted as normal in 10 per cent of those with initial nonvisualization and in 64 per cent of those with initially inadequate visualization.

A gallbladder that is consistently small or large but has good concentration and no other abnormalities is difficult to interpret. It is assumed, however, that a gallbladder that is visualized well and contains no stones is normal (Fig. 14–56). Distended gallbladders should be studied further.

VARIATION IN NUMBER. A double gallbladder and duplication of the cystic duct may occur (Fig. 14–59). Triplication of the gallbladder is a rare anomaly which has also been described (Ross and Sachs). The congenital folded fundus of the gallbladder or variation of a Phrygian cap gallbladder, which represents a mucosal or serosal fold of the gallbladder, must be carefully differentiated by a number of oblique views (Fig. 14–51 B).

THE SIGNIFICANCE OF NONVISUALIZATION OF THE GALLBLADDER IN PATIENTS WITH INTACT GALLBLADDER. ABNORMALITY OF FUNCTION. There are certain basic assumptions that must be verified as far as possible in order to interpret oral cholecystograms:

1. That the patient actually has taken the contrast agent.

2. That adequate absorption of the agent has occurred (no esophageal, gastric, or intestinal obstruction) (Fig. 14–60).

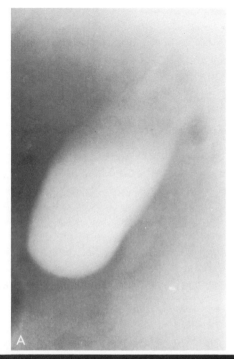

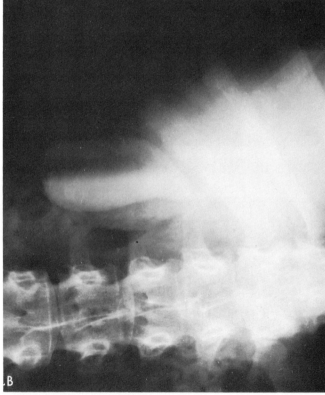

Figure 14–58. Layering of Telepaque that may occur normally in the gallbladder. A. Erect. B. Lateral decubitus with patient lying on left side.

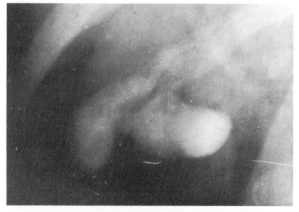

Figure 14–59. Cholecystogram demonstrating a double gallbladder. Note that even the cystic duct in this instance is duplicated.

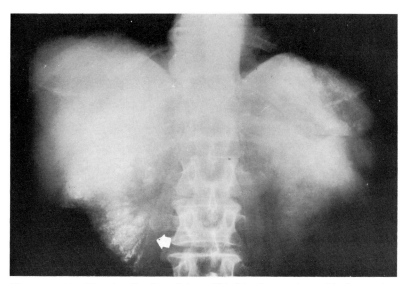

Figure 14–60. Nonvisualization of the gallbladder in a patient with obstruction of the duodenum. Note all of the contrast agent retained above the level of obstruction; this indicates inadequate absorption.

3. That the liver function is adequate for secretion of the test compound.

4. That the ductal system above the level of the gallbladder is not obstructed.

5. That the common bile duct is not obstructed (in which case there may be some associated gallbladder disease).

The oral cholecystogram is fundamentally a function test. It must not, however, be assumed that nonvisualization necessarily indicates abnormal function in certain rare instances. Complete absence of the gallbladder is a rare anomaly but can occur.

A surprisingly high proportion of men with cholelithiasis are asymptomatic (70 per cent of men with stones and 86 per cent of a control group have no symptoms) (Wilbur and Bolt). Of 30 per cent of patients with gallstones, two-thirds had only the unreliable signs and symptoms of dyspepsia and epigastric pain, symptoms which are found in 10 per cent of normal controls. Also, typical biliary colic can be a misleading description, since it is found in about 3.6 per cent of those with no stones and in 0.9 per cent of normal men.

Evaluation of Oral Cholecystography. Many investigators have compared the accuracy of the diagnosis following Telepaque cholecystography with the diagnosis established at surgery in patients undergoing surgery of the biliary tract.

In their series of 1207 cholecystographic examinations, in which all diagnoses were subjected to surgical and pathologic verification, Baker and Hodgson found only 1.9 per cent of all diagnoses to be in error. Of cases designated as normal preopera-

tively, 98.3 per cent were so found at surgery. Gallbladders designated as "poorly functioning" were found to be diseased. Of cases diagnosed as cholelithiasis, 98 per cent were confirmed. Gallbladders showing nonvisualization were found to be abnormal in 97.8 per cent of the cases. Alderson reported a 99 per cent accuracy in 315 patients.

Extrahepatic duct visualization was obtained in a high percentage of cases (85 per cent) when a synthetic cholagogue such as Bilevac was used (Norman and Saghapoleslami).

Dann et al. have reported that in 200 patients whose gallbladders were not visualized by oral cholecystography, the common bile duct was visualized in 30 per cent. Of this group, 28 patients were operated upon and all exhibited definite pathologic conditions in the gallbladder.

Rosenbaum, in a series of 400 consecutive patients examined by cholecystography, found that visualization was initially absent or inadequate without evidence of gallstones in 66. After a repeat dose and roentgen study, findings were normal in 10 per cent of those with initial nonvisualization and in 64 per cent of those with initially inadequate visualization.

Repeat dose, consecutive dose, or second dose cholecystography was also investigated by Berk. He studied 396 patients whose gallbladders were visualized poorly or not at all on initial cholecystograms employing Telepaque. Fifty per cent of these showed no improvement in concentration on the second study, 20 per cent showed moderate improvement, and 30 per cent showed marked improvement. Of these original 396 patients, 160 showed poor visualization on the initial study. Of these, a second or consecutive dose led to no improvement in 20 per cent, moderate improvement in 30 per cent, and marked improvement in 50 per cent. Of the 236 patients whose gallbladders were not visualized on the initial examination, 75 per cent showed no increase in opacification, 10 per cent showed moderate increase, and 15 per cent showed a marked increase. Hence, the "consecutive dose phenomenon" is more frequent in patients with initially faint visualization than in those with initial nonvisualization.

It is interesting to note that 38 of the 119 patients who demonstrated this phenomenon were restudied by follow-up cholecystograms 1 to 4 years later, and a majority of these failed to reproduce the same effect. Actually, in 33 of the 38 patients, the opacification of the gallbladder was normal with a single dose of Telepaque on the follow-up study.

It is thought by others, however, that if additional doses of Telepaque are justified, it may be best to follow the oral examination by an intravenous one to avoid some of the complications in relation to Telepaque (Whitehouse).

Morbidity Following Oral Cholecystography. Serious and even fatal reactions to gallbladder contrast media have been described by a number of authors. Increasing reports of renal complications have caused the withdrawal of Orabilex from active clinical use. Reports of renal insufficiency following the use of such a medium, especially in double dosage, have been made by a number of authors (Rene and Mellinkoff). The occurrence of thrombocytopenia following the administration of Telepaque was described by Bishopric in 1964. There would appear to be no way to predict the occurrence of thrombocytopenia despite the possibility of a previous similar reaction to another drug. Sensitivity to iodine may be a causative factor. Once again it should be emphasized that, as with all oral iodinated contrast media, these should not be administered in the presence of combined renal and hepatic disease or severe kidney impairment.

Modified Cholecystography. Various techniques have been devised for potentiating cholecystography.

1. The injection of cholecystokinin (75 Ivy dog units) intravenously has been advocated to enhance diagnostic accuracy in patients who apparently have gallbladder disease and yet are pronounced "normal" in routine cholecystography (Nathan et al.).

2. A rapid oral method for roentgenographic visualization has been investigated by Fischer et al., utilizing Oragrafin.

The student is referred to the original articles for further evaluation of these experimental techniques.

3. Certain pharmacologic agents are thought to enhance the diagnosis of biliary tract disease. For example, the combination of atropine and amyl nitrite may be utilized to differentiate a spasm of the sphincter of Oddi from an organic stenosis at this site. This is accomplished by the subcutaneous injection of 0.5 mg. of atropine sulfate about 1½ hours after the intravenous injection of contrast medium, with simultaneous inhalation of amyl nitrite. The two together may be used for relaxation of spasm of the sphincter of Oddi.

4. The intravenous or intramuscular injection of 0.01 gram of morphine may cause a contraction of the sphincter of Oddi and this, too, may prolong the persistence of the contrast agent in the bile duct. However, the routine use of morphine results in paralysis of the gallbladder and inhibits its contraction following administration of a cholagogue.

5. Prostigmine (0.5 mg. intravenously) has a less spastic effect on the sphincter of Oddi and does not affect the gallbladder.

6. Cholecystokinin may also be used. This agent causes contraction of the gallbladder and permits assessment of the dynamics of the biliary tract. Films are obtained approximately 5 to 35 minutes after the intravenous injection of this agent (75 Ivy units or 0.04 mg. of the dessicated material per kilogram of body weight). This time-span permits evaluation of gallbladder motility and sphincteric action.

7. Cholecystokinin may be combined with morphine also (Garbsch).

Rectal Cholecystography. This technique may be used when oral or intravenous methods are not practical or are contraindicated.

Orgrafin in a dose of 6 grams in a special rectal kit is utilized. The rectum must be thoroughly cleansed in advance. The contrast agent is dissolved in sterile distilled water immediately before use, and is slowly instilled in the rectum at bedtime over a period of 20 minutes. The examination of the gallbladder is carried forward as in the case of the oral cholecystogram 10 to 12 hours later. Calcium Oragrafin may be better for this purpose than the sodium preparation.

To be effective, the contrast agent must be retained by the patient. If expelled, the examination will be unsatisfactory.

The limiting factors for use of this technique are the relative unpredictability of rectal absorption and some rectal irritation.

Intravenous Cholangiography. *Contrast Medium.* The contrast agent, sodium iodipamide (Biligrafin in Germany), was replaced in 1955 by iodipamide methylglucamine and introduced in the United States under the trade name of Cholografin methylglucamine. The standard dose for the adult is 20 ml. of the latter compound. This dose contains approximately 5 grams of iodine. Approximately 90 per cent of the compound is excreted by the liver and 10 per cent by the kidneys. In patients with liver damage, a greater percentage will be excreted by the kidney. Wise has reported that in 12 years of experience with over 5000 injections, there have been no fatal reactions in the Lahey Clinic. Normal reactions such as nausea, vomiting, hypotension, or urticaria have, on occasion, occurred. (A dose greater than 20 ml. is contraindicated and may be toxic.)

Criteria and Indications for Intravenous Cholangiography. When serum bilirubin levels are 1 mg. per 100 ml. or less, opaci-

---

SITUATIONS JUSTIFYING USE OF INTRAVENOUS CHOLANGIOGRAPHY

1. Nonvisualization of gallbladder by oral route.
2. Need to distinguish gallbladder disease and obstructive disease of the distal common duct.
3. Evaluation of the postcholecystectomy syndrome.
4. Preoperative examination to demonstrate calculi in the common bile duct before cholecystectomy.
5. History of biliary abnormality in infants and children.
6. Emergencies in which speed is a factor.
7. Suspicion of a tumor near the porta hepatis.
8. Recent or subsiding jaundice in which bilirubin and BSP levels are appropriate to help differentiate infective hepatitis and common duct stones.
9. Functional biliary disorders in which a study of the duct system may help differentiate organic disease.

Figure 14–61.

fication of the ducts may be expected in 92.5 per cent of cases. If serum bilirubin values are above 4 mg. per 100 ml., opacification may be expected in only 9.3 per cent.

When BSP (bromsulphalein) retention level is below 10 per cent after 45 minutes, opacification may be expected in 96 per cent of injections, but if retention level is above 40 per cent, opacification may be expected in 26.2 per cent (Wise).

With these basic criteria in mind, *intravenous cholangiography is indicated in the following situations* (Fig. 14–61):

1. Nonvisualization by the oral route. According to Wise, 12 per cent of these patients were found to have gallbladders which appeared normal and in which no calculi were visualized. Of 201 patients with intact gallbladders not visualized by the oral route, visualization was accomplished in 70 by the intravenous method, and 24 of these were considered normal. All of those whose gallbladders were not visualized by the intravenous method were found later to be diseased.

2. Differentiation of gallbladder disease and obstructive disease of the distal common duct. (a) If the common duct is less than 7.0 mm. in diameter, nonvisualization of the gallbladder is due to cystic duct obstruction or primary gallbladder disease. (b) If the common duct is dilated, the cause of nonopacification may be common duct obstruction alone or a combination of cystic duct obstruction and common duct obstruction.

Further indications are listed in Figure 14–61.

Technique of Intravenous Examination. 1. Good catharsis on the night prior to the examination.

2. A plain film of the right upper quadrant in the right posterior oblique (and in some instances, left anterior oblique).

3. A preliminary subcutaneous injection of 5 mg. of parabromdylamine is given. The patient is examined in the hydrated and nonfasting state.

4. A test dose of 1 cc. of Cholografin is administered intravenously, and a 3 minute interval is allowed to elapse until the remaining 19 cc. are injected over a minimum period of 10 minutes ("minor" reactions occur in 4.3 per cent). Drip infusion may be employed.

5. The first film is obtained following the completion of the injection in the supine position with the left side elevated approximately 15 degrees. Low kilovoltage is used.

6. Repeat films are obtained at 10 to 20 minute intervals thereafter for 40 to 60 minutes.

7. If no visualization is obtained at 60 to 90 minutes in a patient in whom the gallbladder has not been removed, a film of the right upper quadrant is made at 4 hours and if possible at 24 hours for visualization of the gallbladder.

8. Once a film giving the best possible visualization is obtained, films are made at 20 minute intervals in order to evaluate radiodensity, particularly if it appears that the duct is dilated and partially obstructed. (If the density and retention of the contrast medium in the bile ducts is greater at 120 minutes than at 60 minutes, partial obstruction of the common bile duct or main biliary tract is present.) If the duct is normal in size without evidence of obstruction and good drainage is seen, the study may be terminated in 60 to 90 minutes.

9. *Body section radiography should be performed as an additional adjunct when ductal visualization is optimum* (Fig. 14–62 B).

10. In children with suspected anomalies of the extrahepatic biliary system, between 0.6 and 1.6 cc. of 20 per cent sodium iodipamide (Cholografin) per kilogram of body weight was injected slowly by Hays and Averbrook and exposures made at intervals over a 4 hour period. This intravenous injection was preceded by a test dose for sensitivity of 0.5 cc. (Methylglucamine iodipamide should require half this dosage.)

Some Radiographic Signs of Abnormality in Intravenous Cholangiography

ABNORMALITIES OF THE GALLBLADDER. When the gallbladder is visualized, the abnormalities previously described in respect to oral cholecystograms also apply here.

When, however, the biliary tree is not visualized, a specific interpretation is not possible. Wise has reported a visualization of bile ducts in approximately 90 per cent of cases after cholecystectomy in which patients' serum bilirubin levels have been below 1 mg. per 100 ml. and BSP retention has been 10 per cent or less after 35 minutes.

In patients with an intact gallbladder and nonvisualization by oral cholecystography, Wise visualized 35 per cent of 201 gallbladders. In 12 per cent the gallbladder was considered normal by this technique.

When the bile ducts were visualized but the gallbladder was not, approximately 70 per cent of the patients were shown to have primary gallbladder disease. Approximately 10 per cent were shown to have primary common duct or pancreatic disease, and 20 per cent had combined gallbladder and common duct or pancreatic disease.

ABNORMALITIES IN SIZE OF THE COMMON BILE DUCT. In a postmortem study of the common bile duct Nazareno et al. reported that, with the usual cholangiographic technique and with the inherent magnification in most radiographic procedures, the upper limit of the diameter of the magnified common bile duct was 10 mm. in 97.5 per cent of normal people. The actual anatomic measurement was approximately two-thirds of that obtained roentgenographically. Others have indicated slightly different measurements (Wise; Shehadi, 1963b; McClenahan et al.). In a postcholecystectomy state, a "normal" bile duct is less than 19 mm. in diameter (Wise). The size, therefore, is such a variable criterion that the physician, in caring for his patient, must first decide whether or not obstruction exists, and then make a judgment, on this basis, whether abnormality is indicated.

ABNORMALITY OF CONTOUR OF THE COMMON BILE DUCT. Or-

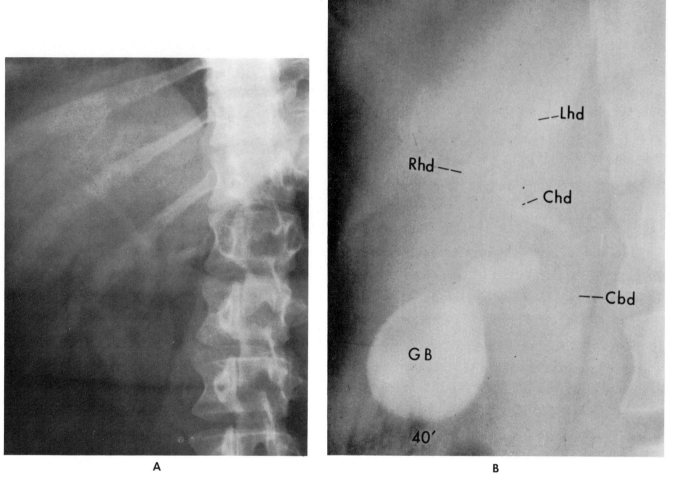

A   B

Figure 14–62. *A.* Faint visualization of the biliary tree by intravenous cholangiography with the aid of intravenous Cholografin. Ordinarily a visualization of this order of density is obtained. Enhancement of detail is obtained by tomography. *B.* Normal intravenous cholangiogram–tomogram.

Figure 14–62 continued on the opposite page.

dinarily the two hepatic ducts and common hepatic duct are approximately equal in size and do not taper significantly. However, the common bile duct begins to taper near its origin at the level of the cystic duct to the ampulla. Absence of tapering must be regarded with suspicion as indicative of possible abnormality.

Normally, the common bile duct is gently convex toward the left (Fig. 14–62). A reversal of this convexity suggests an abnormal contour and displacement.

In response to obstruction, the hepatic radicals may also change their normal contour and size and become progressively dilated and increasingly opacified (Fig. 14–63).

ABNORMALITIES OF FUNCTION.   Wise and O'Brien have proposed the time-density retention concept as applied to intravenous cholangiography and have shown a composite curve illustrating the relative density of contrast substance and drainage rates of unobstructed versus obstructed ducts (Fig. 14–64). In this curve maximum density in unobstructed cases is achieved at 45

minutes. Thereafter the density tends to diminish in unobstructed cases up to 2 hours after the beginning of the study. In obstructed cases, the density remains relatively constant at a maximum level during the 45 to 120 minute interval.

Evaluation of Intravenous Cholangiography in Patients with Intact Gallbladders.   Wise reports an overall accuracy of specific diagnoses based on intravenous cholangiography in 79.4 per cent of cases. False positive predictions were made in 8.6 per cent of cases.

Wise also analyzed 694 injections of patients with intact gallbladders and found that the duct was visualized in 621; the presence of common duct calculi was proved in 39 of these cases. In only one of these 39 cases was the common duct stone found to be associated with a normal gallbladder in an otherwise normal common duct.

The usefulness of the intravenous cholangiogram in patients with intact gallbladders was also investigated by Eckelberg et al.

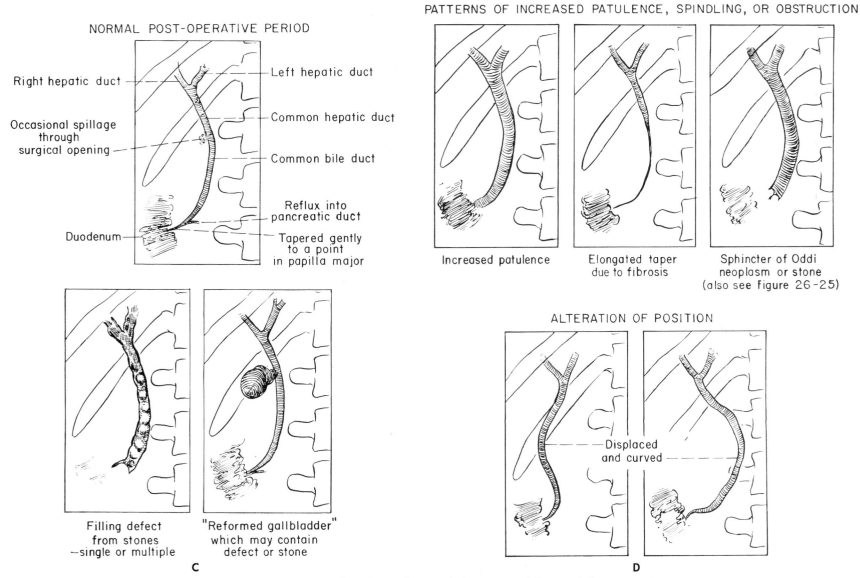

NORMAL POST-OPERATIVE PERIOD

Right hepatic duct

Left hepatic duct

Common hepatic duct

Occasional spillage through surgical opening

Common bile duct

Reflux into pancreatic duct

Duodenum

Tapered gently to a point in papilla major

PATTERNS OF INCREASED PATULENCE, SPINDLING, OR OBSTRUCTION

Increased patulence

Elongated taper due to fibrosis

Sphincter of Oddi neoplasm or stone (also see figure 26-25)

Filling defect from stones —single or multiple

"Reformed gallbladder" which may contain defect or stone

C

ALTERATION OF POSITION

Displaced and curved

D

Figure 14–62 *Continued.* *C* and *D.* Abnormalities in cholangiograms, following cholecystectomy.

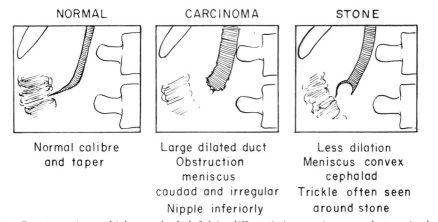

NORMAL

CARCINOMA

STONE

Normal calibre and taper

Large dilated duct Obstruction meniscus caudad and irregular Nipple inferiorly

Less dilation Meniscus convex cephalad Trickle often seen around stone

Figure 14–63. Roentgen signs which may be helpful in differentiating carcinoma and stone in the common duct in cholangiography.

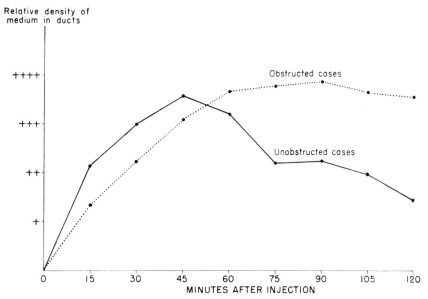

Figure 14–64. Composite curve illustrating the relative density of contrast substance, and drainage rates of an obstructed vs. a nonobstructed common bile duct. (From Wise, R. E., and O'Brien, R. G.: J.A.M.A., 160:822, 1956.)

They studied 133 patients and found that with intravenous cholangiography the gallbladder was visualized in 66 per cent. The longest interval before visualization was 135 minutes, and the average time for initial visualization was 33 minutes (but since 44 of the 133 examinations were terminated at 25 minutes, it is difficult to interpret this finding). The biliary ducts were visualized in 91 per cent, with the initial visualization occurring at 25 minutes in almost all patients. The longest interval for initial visualization of the ducts, however, was 50 minutes. The presence or absence of the contrast agent in the kidney-collecting system had no bearing upon the quality of visualization of the biliary tract.

Opacification of the bile duct accompanying nonvisualization of the gallbladder was found to be caused by complete mechanical obstruction of the cystic duct by stone or edema in about a third of the 57 patients for whom surgical exploration was done. Of the remaining patients most were found to have free gallstones at operation, but in about an eighth of the cases there was no discoverable anatomic reason to explain why the gallbladder had not filled with contrast media. Moreover, delay in opacification of the gallbladder beyond 25 minutes did not seem to be influenced by the presence or absence of stones in the gallbladder. In some cases, gallstones not demonstrated by oral cholecystography were disclosed by the intravenous examination.

Evaluation of Intravenous Cholangiograms in Postcholecystectomy Patients. Beargie et al. in 1962 presented their experience with intravenous cholangiography in the evaluation of 1956 patients with symptoms referable to the upper portion of the ab-

domen after cholecystectomy. They found, as did Wise, that a satisfactory visualization of the biliary tree correlated most closely with the results of serum bilirubin and bromsulphalein (BSP) retention studies. It was also reliably related to the values of alkaline phosphatase. They also concluded from a comparison of the radiologic cholangiographic findings with subsequent surgical findings that intravenous cholangiography provided an accuracy of diagnosis in 90 to 95 per cent of the patients. The diagnostic value of a delayed passage of contrast medium through the sphincter was a good sign of partial obstruction of the common bile duct.

Wise reported 1340 postcholecystectomy injections. Visualization of 1194 ducts was reported and common duct calculi were proved at surgery in 77 of these. In 51 of these there was no associated pathologic change. In 11 of those with calculi there were associated strictures; in 14, fibrosis of the sphincter of Oddi; and in 1, chronic pancreatitis. Of the 77 cases with proved common duct calculi 42 were visualized directly; in 29 the diagnosis was suspected by the indirect demonstration of abnormality in the common duct; and 6 were not diagnosed radiologically.

HAZARDS OF INTRAVENOUS CHOLANGIOGRAPHY. Accidents during gallbladder studies with Cholografin were studied by Frommhold and Braband. They collected data on 22 deaths attributed directly or indirectly to its administration. This death rate, even including doubtful and delayed deaths, represented a figure of 0.00035 per cent. This compares favorably with the death rate due to intravenous urography reported by Pendergrass—0.0009 per cent in a review of 12,200,000 excretory urograms performed over a 27 year period. The sensitivity tests were negative in 5 of the 22 recorded fatalities with intravenous cholangiography.

Percutaneous Cholangiography. Under normal circumstances, puncture of the liver with an exploratory needle will fail to produce bile. Bile is obtained if extrahepatic obstruction is present. Percutaneous cholangiography may be employed in the differential diagnosis of jaundice in certain selected cases, provided normal clotting factors are present and broad spectrum antibiotics are given for one day prior to the examination in case operation is necessary (Flemma et al; Mujahed and Evans). It is contraindicated in hemorrhagic diathesis and vitamin K-resistant hypoprothrombinemia or in patients with febrile cholangitis.

Information elicited by percutaneous cholangiography is of value mainly in the following situations (Mujahed and Evans):

1. Differentiation between obstructive and nonobstructive jaundice.

2. Demonstration of the presence and site of carcinoma of the biliary system.

3. Demonstration of the number of calculi in the biliary system and their location.

4. Study of the biliary tree in congenital biliary atresia.

5. Decompression of the biliary tree prior to surgery.

Procedure. The percutaneous puncture is performed under local anesthesia and proper asepsis, with a 7 inch, 20 or 21 gauge needle with a stylet. The patient lies supine on a fluoroscopy table.

Mujahed and Evans restrict the procedure to patients scheduled for surgery and it is performed an hour or two beforehand.

The stylet is removed when the liver has been entered and a 20 cc. syringe is applied to the needle. Gentle aspiration is applied as the needle is advanced until bile is withdrawn freely. As much bile is withdrawn as is necessary to decompress the liver and for bacterial culture. As much as 60 cc. of 50 per cent methylglucamine diatrizoate (Renografin) may be necessary to fill the obstructed biliary tree.

The aspiration syringe is then replaced by a syringe containing 20 cc. of Renografin-60 or 75 per cent Hypaque. A polyethylene catheter may be threaded over the needle in advance to minimize trauma to the liver. The injection is carried out under television monitor control and satisfactory spot filming is obtained.

Usually the needle reaches a bile duct about 4 to 5 inches below the skin. If bile appears in the syringe at a skin distance of 2 to 2.5 inches, the needle is probably in the gallbladder.

If no bile ducts are entered after four punctures over the liver, extrahepatic obstruction is probably excluded. Occasionally, emergency operative intervention is necessary in patients with extrahepatic jaundice when there is bile leakage or internal bleeding as a result of the procedure.

If the injection of test substance puddles, usually it is in the liver. Occasionally the test injection disappears very quickly, in which case the injection was made into a vein; when slow movement of the contrast agent is noted, the injection was probably made into nondilated, branching, and tubular ducts.

Roentgen Signs of Abnormality in Percutaneous Cholangiography. These can be divided into the following categories: (1) filling defects caused by calculi; (2) obstructed duct (convexity upward) is usually due to a calculus; (3) smooth narrowness of a short segment indicates stricture; (4) duct rigid and irregular indicates carcinoma; (5) dilatation of the duct with an uneven and ragged obstruction pattern indicates carcinoma of ampulla or pancreas (dilatation usually greater with pancreatic pathology; (6) smooth, flat, shallow obstruction with dilatation of the duct indicates ampullary carcinoma; (7) tortuous and marked dilatation of ducts indicates pancreatic carcinoma. Obstructed end may be rounded, bulbous, tapered, or notched.

Evaluation of Percutaneous Cholangiography (Mujahed and Evans). In this study of 140 patients, procedures were successful with 74 per cent. Carcinoma of the pancreas was detected correctly by cholangiography in 34 of 41 cases, or 87 per cent, whereas, in a gastrointestinal series, it was suspected in 15 of 41 cases, or 37 per cent. Carcinoma of the ampulla of Vater was diagnosed from cholangiograms in 7 of 7 cases (100 per cent), but in the gastrointestinal series the rate of success was 55 per cent (4 of 7 cases). Complications from the study can be summarized as follows: (1) one death occurred out of the 140 patients; the authors noted that, in 800 procedures performed by others, four deaths had occurred; (2) subphrenic abscess occurred in 2 patients; and (3) bile and blood (500 to 1000 cc.) in the peritoneum was noted in 7 patients.

Pain following transcutaneous cholangiography may persist in the right upper quadrant for 6 to 8 hours. Surgery is performed 1 to 5 days after the procedure when indicated.

In a report by Flemma et al. complications in a total group of 27 cases consisted of three cases of bile peritonitis and three of gram negative septicemia. The peritonitis patients underwent immediate surgery, and the infected ones responded well to antibiotic therapy.

Direct Cholangiography. There are two types of direct cholangiography: (1) operative cholangiography (at the time of operation); and (2) postoperative or T-tube cholangiography (during the postoperative period) (Fig. 14–65).

Cholangiography at the time of surgery, in the opinion of Edmunds et al., should be performed in all cholecystectomy patients without selection except in those with serious debility. Clinical indications for common duct exploration as presently accepted are not sufficiently accurate to reduce the number of negative explorations. There are, indeed, many reports of common duct stones revealed by operative cholangiograms when no clinical indications for exploration were present (Hight et al.). Fully 95 per cent of all secondary operations on the biliary tract are for intraductal stones that may have been overlooked.

Also, the performance of cholangiography at the time of operation gives the surgeon an opportunity to make certain that all calculi have been removed from, or are no longer present in, the biliary tree.

Cholangiography at the time of operation provides a means of recognizing noncalculus obstruction of the common duct also (Partington and Sachs).

The T-tube cholangiogram allows a study of the common bile duct in the postoperative period prior to removal of the T-tube. In this way, a determination of patency of the common bile duct is determined.

Technique. Twenty-five to 50 per cent methylglucamine diatrizoate or sodium diatrizoate (Renografin or Hypaque) is directly injected into the biliary tree (in approximately 5 ml. fractions) either at the time of operation by means of a polyethylene tube inserted into the common duct or through a T-tube that has been previously introduced into the common hepatic duct at surgery. The contrast agent is warmed to body temperature before use.

For the *operative cholangiogram*, the contrast agent may be injected in three or four fractions of approximately 5 cc. each, and films obtained in sequence during the injection of each fraction.

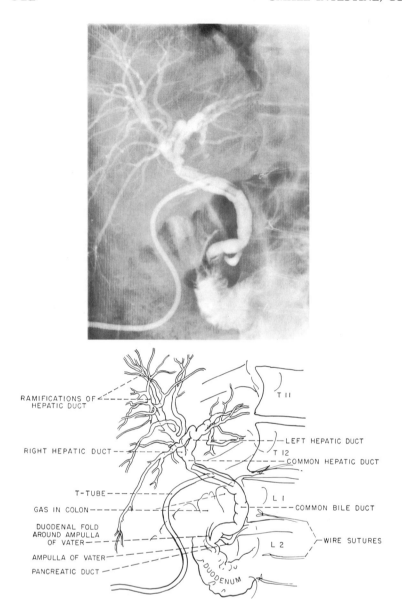

RAMIFICATIONS OF
HEPATIC DUCT

T II

LEFT HEPATIC DUCT

RIGHT HEPATIC DUCT

T 12

COMMON HEPATIC DUCT

T-TUBE

GAS IN COLON

L I

DUODENAL FOLD
AROUND AMPULLA
OF VATER

COMMON BILE DUCT

AMPULLA OF VATER

L 2

WIRE SUTURES

PANCREATIC DUCT

DUODENUM

Figure 14–65. Thirty-five per cent Renografin T-tube cholangiogram and its tracing. This contrast medium gives a more complete visualization of all hepatic radicles. This is extremely important since stones may be concealed in the hepatic radicles only to descend later and cause a recurrence of symptoms.

The films are numbered so that the sequence can be identified at the time of viewing. Care is exercised to remove all air bubbles from the syringe and connecting tube prior to injection. A cassette tunnel placed beneath the patient prior to surgery to allow proper positioning of the cassette under sterile conditions is important. A grid-cassette (or Bucky grid) beneath the table is also necessary to enhance detail. Diaphragmatic movement is suspended by the

anesthetist just prior to exposure and the exposures are made as rapidly as possible.

The films must be viewed immediately, so that additional studies may be taken as necessary.

The *postoperative cholangiogram* through the T-tube is performed as follows: a needle on the end of a long transparent catheter is carefully inserted into the end of the rubber T-tube and held vertically so that air that may not have been entirely expelled will rise to the surface. Every care must be exercised to avoid the injection of air into the biliary tree, since interpretation in respect to filling defects may thereby be complicated.

Approximately 5 cc. of the contrast agent is injected under fluroscopic control and a spot film is obtained in the anteroposterior projection. The patient is then rotated into the left posterior oblique position and the procedure repeated with an additional 5 cc. injection. A further injection is made when the patient is placed in the right posterior oblique, and finally, a fourth exposure is made with the patient supine once again in the straight anteroposterior. Ordinarily, a total of 20 to 25 cc. of the contrast agent is sufficient to obtain these several views. During this procedure the introduction of the fluid must be done gently and the rate slowed when necessary if resistance is met or if the patient complains of right upper quadrant discomfort. After the final injection, a right lateral film may be obtained if desired.

Also, if desired, another roentgenogram may be taken 15 minutes after the injection to visualize the emptying of the biliary tract. Depending upon the degree of delay, additional films may be taken at 15 minute or half-hour intervals until the patency of the biliary tract is determined (Hicken et al., 1959).

If an obstruction is encountered, it is recommended that withdrawal of as much of the contrast agent as possible be attempted prior to the removal of the injection apparatus.

An effort is made to visualize both the right and left hepatic ducts as well as the common bile duct in its entirety. At times, biliary calculi make their way into one or the other of the hepatic ducts after or during surgery and these would go unrecognized were it not for this procedure.

Complications. Edmunds et al. have reported that in 535 operative cholangiograms, there were four instances of complications which could possibly have been caused by these procedures. There were two cases of cholangitis, one case of acute hemorrhagic pancreatitis, and one case in which perforation of the common duct was thought to have occurred. All the patients survived their complications.

Value of Direct Cholangiography. Hampson and Petrie reported residual gallstones after cholecystectomy and common bile duct exploration in 7 per cent of primary operations and in 23 per cent of secondary operations for previously retained stones.

Hicken et al. (1950) reported the use of direct cholangiography with Hypaque in 350 patients. There were no local or constitutional reactions or complications which could be attributed to the contrast medium. Friesen has emphasized that the procedure is important in avoiding injury to the common duct at surgery. Operative cholangiography markedly decreases the risk of overlooking stones in seemingly normal common ducts at cholecystectomy. This possibility is estimated to occur in 10 to 18 per cent of cases (Vadheim and Rigos).

According to Chapman et al., normal operative cholangiographic findings are reliable evidence that the common bile duct does not contain stones or obstruction and therefore need not be explored.

Sachs has emphasized that unnecessary common duct exploration is reduced from 45 or 50 per cent to 4 or 5 per cent, and that overlooked stones are reduced from 16 or 25 per cent to 4 per cent.

Hess (1967) indicated an incidence of overlooked stones of 0.9 per cent in 650 cholangiograms.

Biliary Angiography (Deutsch; Farrell; Rösch et al.; Redman and Reuter). Selective celiac and mesenteric artery angiography for visualization of the gallbladder has been utilized for the diagnosis of gallbladder diseases which cannot be made by routine roentgenologic means.

Technique. The technique is similar to the Seldinger technique previously described for percutaneous transfemoral or brachial artery catheterization (see Chapter 10). Forty to 50 cc. of a contrast medium is injected directly into the celiac artery, or about half this quantity into the mesenteric artery. If selective catheterization of the cystic artery or hepatic artery can be accomplished, this route is desirable. Methylglucamine diatrizoate (Renografin) or sodium diatrizoate (Hypaque) is utilized. A pressure injector is employed so that the chosen volume is injected within 2 seconds, and exposures are made in rapid sequence—two per second for 4 seconds and one per second for 4 seconds thereafter. Thereafter ten exposures at 3 second intervals may be utilized. *Transjugular cholangiography* is a modification of the Seldinger technique, in which a catheter introduced via the jugular vein is directed into a hepatic vein (Weiner and Hanafee, for review). This technique avoids percutaneous liver entry and yet accomplishes a good visualization of an obstructed hepatic venous system (Fig. 14–66).

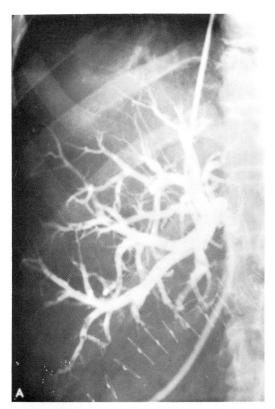
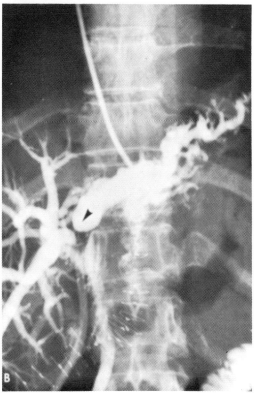

Figure 14–66. Operative exploration for obstructive jaundice in a 45 year old woman showed a mass obstructing the common hepatic duct near the bifurcation. A drainage catheter was placed from the common bile duct into the right ductile system, but the left system was completely obstructed and could not be entered. Biopsies were negative for neoplasm. Two weeks later she developed chills and fever.

One month postoperatively, transjugular cholangiogram was performed across a right hepatic vein, and showed visualization of the right ducts but no filling of the left system (A). The needle was then repositioned in a left hepatic vein; the left bile ducts were visualized and complete obstruction of the left system was demonstrated (B).

Subsequent biopsy at the time of surgery for reconstruction of the extrahepatic biliary tree revealed bile duct carcinoma. (From Weiner, M., and Hanafee, W. N.: Radiol. Clin. N. Amer., 8:61, 1970.)

Basic Anatomy. The basic anatomy of the cystic artery has already been described. It usually arises from the right hepatic artery near the origin from the common hepatic. Shortly after its origin it divides into an anterior branch, which is right-sided and peritoneal, and a posterior branch, which is left-sided and nonperitoneal. A rich capillary plexus communicates between these two main branches.

There are numerous variations of normal, well illustrated in the basic anatomy texts (Netter; Grant's *Atlas of Anatomy; Morris' Human Anatomy*). The most frequent of these are illustrated by Ruzicka and Rossi as shown in Figure 14–67. In about 25 per cent of the cases the two main branches of the cystic artery originate separately from the right hepatic artery. The cystic artery or one of its branches may also originate from the common

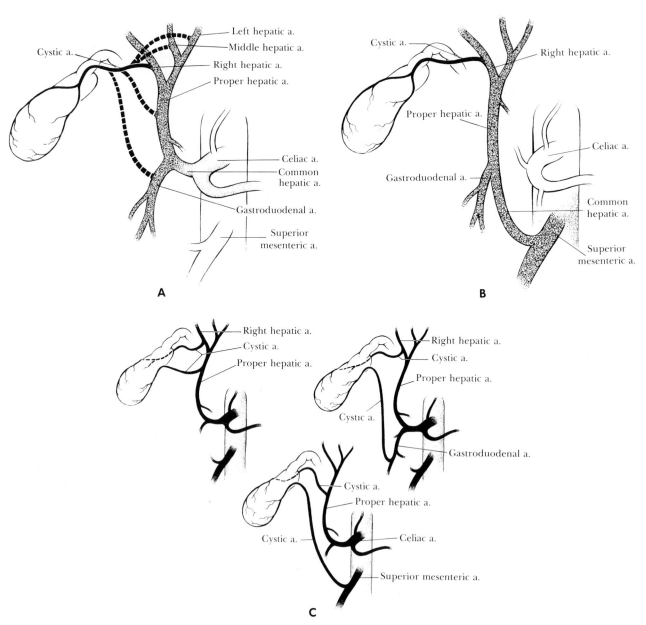

Figure 14–67. Cystic artery variations. In *A*, the solid vessel line indicates the most frequent site of origin of the cystic artery. The interrupted vessel lines show the more common variations. In *B*, the cystic artery arises from the right hepatic, which is a branch of the superior mesenteric artery. In *C*, three of the more common variations of double cystic arteries are shown. (From Ruzicka, F. F., Jr., and Rossi, P.: Radiol. Clin. N. Amer., 8:3–29, 1970.)

NORMAL GALLBLADDER MEASUREMENTS

The normal measurements of the gallbladder were derived angiographically by Redman and Reuter from 25 normal gallbladders as follows:

	Mean Measurement	Range	Standard Deviation
Area	21.1 sq. cm.	11.4 – 33 cm.	5 cm.
Width	3.6 cm.	1.9 – 5 cm.	0.77 cm.

Conclusions: Gallbladders measuring more than 35 sq. cm. or having a width of more than 5 cm. may be considered distended.

Figure 14–68.

hepatic artery, the left hepatic, the gastroduodenal, the celiac trunk itself, or the superior mesenteric.

Venous blood from the gallbladder is drained directly into the liver through a venous capillary plexus or into the portal venous system. Anastomoses with the choledochal and superior mesenteric veins occur.

Normal Gallbladder Measurements. The normal gallbladder has a wall thickness of 2 to 3 mm., 6 to 8 seconds after visualization of the cystic artery. Its measurements otherwise are shown in Figure 14–68. Generally, gallbladders measuring more than 35 sq. cm. or more than 5 cm. wide may be considered distended. An example of visualization of the gallbladder by cholecysto-angiography is shown in Figure 14–69.

Hepatic Angiogram. The basic anatomic variations of the hepatic artery have been previously described. These were shown to be closely related to variations of the celiac and superior mesenteric trunks (Fig. 14–67). The common hepatic artery is usually 3 to 6 cm. in length approximately, and is directed toward the right and superiorly toward the porta hepatis, where it divides into right and left hepatic arteries. These latter branches, in turn, divide into large interlobar arteries which follow along the connective tissue septa, subdividing repeatedly in the liver substance into smaller and smaller interlobular branches which run in the connective tissue between the lobules. Generally, the smaller vessels are straight and well defined, and approach the periphery of the liver in fairly predictable fashion. It will be recalled that the hepatic artery usually gives origin to the gastroduodenal, supraduodenal, and right gastric arteries. The hepatic artery then continues as the common hepatic artery before its division into right and left main branches. A middle hepatic artery sometimes arises from the left hepatic. The right hepatic passes behind the common hepatic duct to enter the "triangle of Calot" formed by the cystic duct, hepatic duct, and liver on its cephalad boundary.

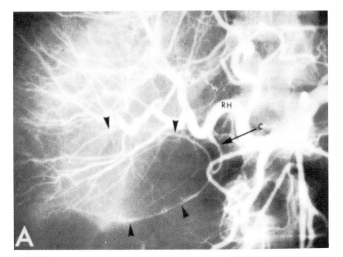

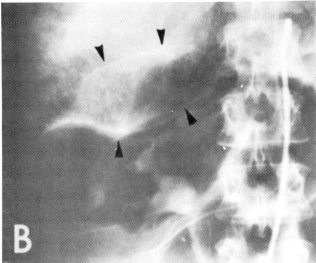

Figure 14–69. Celiac arteriogram. *A. (RH)* Right hepatic artery, *(C)* cystic artery. Arrowheads point out branches of cystic artery. *B.* Venous phase showing cystic veins. (From Ruzicka, F. F., Jr., and Rossi, P.: Radiol. Clin. N. Amer., 8:3–29, 1970.)

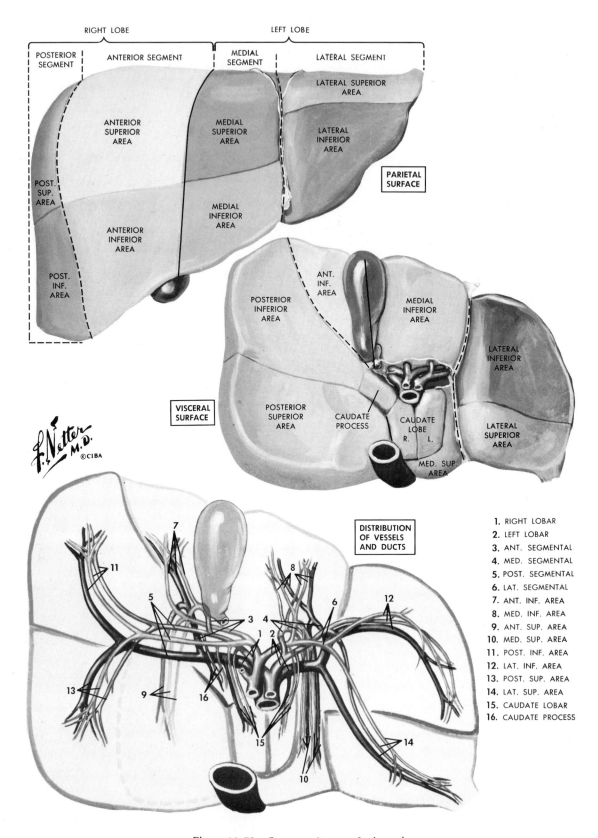

Figure 14–70.   *See opposite page for legend.*

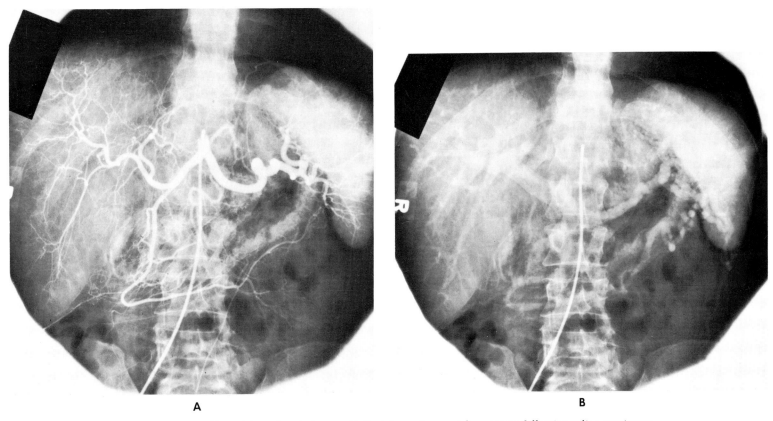

Figure 14-71. *A.* Normal hepatic arteriogram. *B.* Portal or splenoportal venogram following celiac arteriogram.

There is a distinct lobar and lobular composition of the liver, as illustrated in Figure 14-70, with the hepatic arteries, portal vein branches, and biliary ducts following parallel courses. The student is referred to Netter for a detailed description of the segmental division and lobar biliary ductal drainage of the liver.

An example of a normal hepatic arteriogram is shown in Figure 14-71. Hepatic arteriography is of significant value in the diagnosis and localization of a number of pathologic processes in the liver. These include malignancies, lymphomas, cirrhosis, cysts, hemangiomas, and vascular occlusions or aneurysm.

Visualization of the hepatic artery has also proven to be of considerable value in demonstrating the arterial blood supply as part of the management of continuous arterial infusion chemotherapy in the treatment of malignancies of the liver. The position of the infusion catheter is of great importance in that it must allow for selective chemotherapeutic treatment of the involved area. Also, hepatic arteriography provides a useful guide in determining the response of a lesion to this treatment.

Metastatic lesions or neoplasms may be better visualized by using epinephrine conjointly with the angiogram to obtain constriction of normal vessels, because abnormal vessels without vasomotor control do not respond to the adrenalin.

Portal Phlebography. The basic anatomy has been described previously (Fig. 14-48 *A*). The splenic and superior mesenteric veins comprise the main tributaries of the portal vein, with the inferior mesenteric usually draining into the splenic and the coronary vein terminating at the junction of the splenic and portal veins.

Techniques for Study. Percutaneous injection of the spleen results in opacification of the splenoportal trunk (Fig. 14-72).

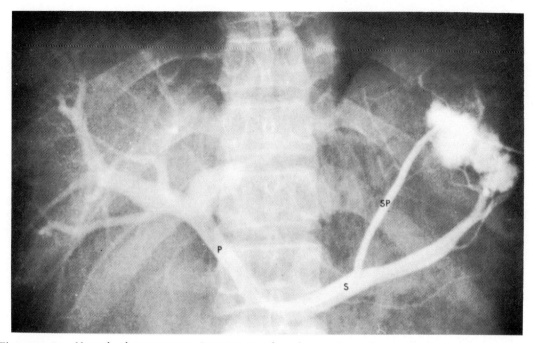

Figure 14–72. Normal splenoportogram. Injection into the splenic pulp results in visualization of splenoportal axis. Superior polar vein *(SP)* is part of splenoportal axis. Tributaries are not visualized normally by this technique. However, capsular veins of spleen and adjacent small vessels may fill during splenic injection in the normal patient. (S) Splenic vein, (P) portal vein. (From Ruzicka, F. F., Jr., and Rossi, P.: Radiol. Clin. N. Amer., 8:3–29, 1970.)

This procedure is performed by injection directly into the splenic pulp. Ordinarily 50 cc. of 70 per cent methylglucamine or sodium diatrizoate or its equivalent is employed. This volume is forcefully injected in 5 or 6 seconds, and exposures of one film per second for 12 to 15 seconds are usually adequate. The patient should be maintained in apnea during the injection and exposure. The following blood vessels are seen in rapid sequence: (1) the splenoportal trunk, (2) the intrahepatic portal branches, and (3) the sinusoidal system of the liver. The sinuosoidal phase reaches a maximum within 16 to 24 seconds and then fades, although it may persist for as long as 60 seconds.

The injection may be made directly into a cannulated branch of the portal system at surgery, and under these circumstances, the opacification is limited mostly to the vein injected along with the portal vein.

The splenic, superior mesenteric, and portal veins usually have approximately the same diameter and are confluent in the upper lumbar or lowermost thoracic region, which is usually projected over the spine. At the porta hepatis, the portal vein bifurcates into its two main branches. The coronary vein and the inferior mesenteric vein are also visualized, especially in the presence of increased resistance to flow within the liver (Fig. 14–73). Other tributaries of the portal system may also be shown, such as the gastroepiploic veins, the pancreatic veins, or even the

short gastric veins. The right main branch is usually readily detected along with its main ramifications, but there is a considerable superimposition of branches, making intimate detail difficult to obtain; the left main branch may be only partially visualized. It is thought that the better visualization of the right branch is due to its posterior position, and the effect of gravity of the contrast agent within the blood. The portal branches divide 5 to 7 times and almost any angle up to 90 degrees may be encountered, but branching occurs in a symmetrical manner and tapering of vessels is gradual. Although the more proximal vessels are straight, branches of the fourth to seventh order may be somewhat curved.

In the sinusoidal phase, the density of the contrast agent is fairly uniform. A spotted appearance is usually abnormal. There may, however, be some variation in density due to varying thicknesses of different parts of the liver. Since the left lobe is usually poorly opacified in this phase it cannot be evaluated accurately.

The other basic method of visualization of the extrahepatic portal venous system is by injection into the celiac artery and obtaining sequential studies during the venous phase. The splenoportal axis is usually fairly well defined (Fig. 14–74). Some of the veins that may be identified in this type of study are the gastric veins, coronary veins, gastroepiploic veins, and even the pancrea-

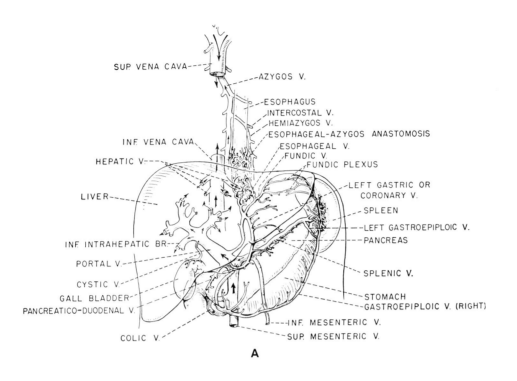

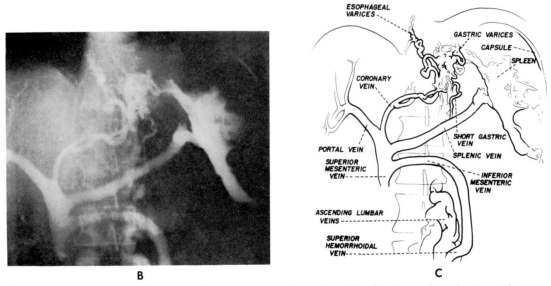

Figure 14–73. *A.* Anatomic diagram of the portal circulation and relationship to esophageal veins and azygos venous systems. *B.* Roentgenogram at 12 seconds demonstrates coronary vein, gastric and esophageal varices. The anastomosis between the inferior mesenteric vein and superior hemorrhoid plexus is demonstrated. The latter is also seen to drain into the vertebral venous plexus. *C.* Tracing of *B.* (From Evans, J. A., and O'Sullivan, W. D.: Amer. J. Roentgenol., *77*, 1957.)

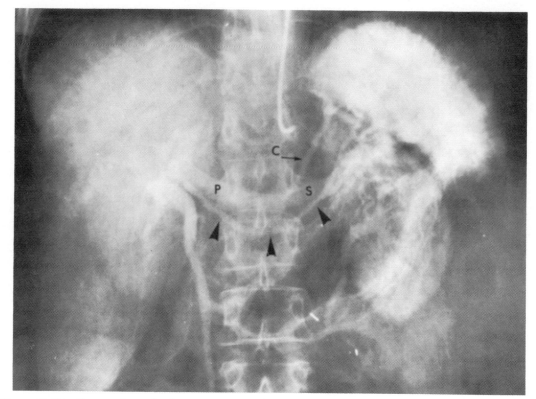

Figure 14–74. Venous phase of celiac artery injection. A double splenoportal axis is shown. The usual axis is made up of the splenic vein (S) and portal vein (P). Coronary vein (C) enters splenic vein. The anomalous axis (arrowheads) arises from a confluence of short gastric veins and splenic hilar radicles and passes parallel to the main S-P axis to enter the liver separately just below the portal vein. (From Ruzicka, F. F., Jr., and Rossi, P.: Radiol. Clin. N. Amer., 8:3–29, 1970.)

ticoduodenal veins. The rapidity of celiac injection and the volume of contrast agent employed will frequently determine the intensity of visualization. Usually the inferior mesenteric vein will not be seen unless the inferior mesenteric artery is selectively injected (Ruzicka and Rossi).

Diagrams illustrating the main routes of blood flow through regularly appearing tributaries of the portal system are shown in Figure 14–75. Thus, short gastric, pancreatic, inferior mesenteric, superior mesenteric, coronary, gastric, and esophageal dilated vessels become visible. This technique is particularly useful for demonstration of esophageal varices.

Summary of Circulation Through the Portal Venous System. Venous blood, carrying materials absorbed from the alimentary tract, passes into the liver through the portal vein and branches out progressively to reach the sinusoid in the individual liver lobules. The blood then reaches the central vein of the lobule. Arterial blood enters through the hepatic artery with oxygenated blood and it too enters the sinusoids to reach the central vein. The central veins are the actual beginnings of the hepatic venous system. The central veins from several lobules unite to enter sublobular veins, and these in turn merge to form increasingly larger trunks, finally converging to form three hepatic veins, which then enter the vena cava.

In the event of obstruction of the portal vein (Fig. 14–75 C) the most important collateral portal circulation is found in: (1) gastric veins of the portal and esophageal veins of the azygos system, (2) the inferior mesenteric of the portal and rectal veins of the internal iliac system, (3) branches along the falciform ligament which are tributaries of the portal vein and the superior and inferior epigastric veins, (4) intestinal veins of the portal system with retroperitoneal tributaries of the inferior vena cava. In the course of this collateral circulation, the region of anastomoses may become engorged and create esophageal varicosities, hemorrhoids, and a "caput medusae" owing to varicosities on the abdominal wall around the umbilicus.

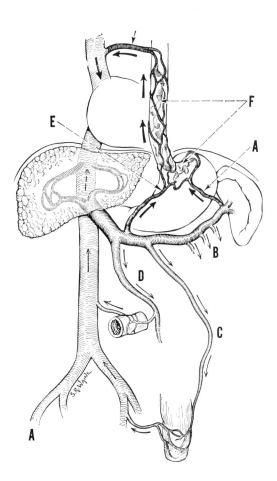

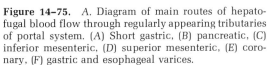

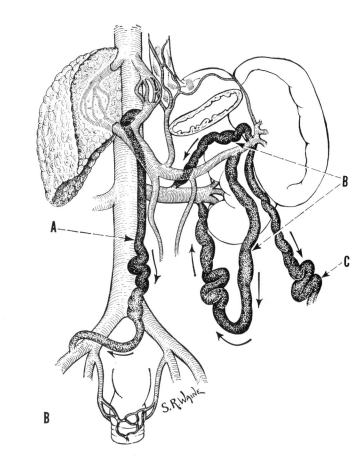

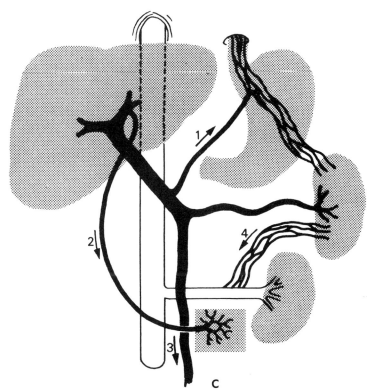

Figure 14–75. A. Diagram of main routes of hepatofugal blood flow through regularly appearing tributaries of portal system. (A) Short gastric, (B) pancreatic, (C) inferior mesenteric, (D) superior mesenteric, (E) coronary, (F) gastric and esophageal varices.

B. Diagram showing hepatofugal flow through newly utilized, persisting embryonic channels between portal and systemic systems. (A) Transhepatic (parumbilical) collateral, (B) splenorenal collaterals, (C) collateral arising from spleen and communicating with systemic veins of the abdominal wall and/or retroperitoneum. Only one of several possible sites of termination of parumbilical collateral shown. (Modified from Rousselot, L. M., et al.: Studies on portal hypertension. IV. The clinical and physiopathologic significance of self-established (non-surgical) portal systemic venous shunts. Ann. Surg., *150:3*, 1959.) (From Schobinger, R. A., and Ruzicka, F. F., Jr.: Vascular Roentgenology. New York, The Macmillan Company, 1964.)

C. The most important venous collaterals in portal vein occlusion: (1) the coronary vein, (2) the umbilical vein, (3) links between mesenteric and systemic systems, and (4) splenorenal and splenogastric anastomoses. (From Wenz, W.: Abdominal Angiography. New York, Springer-Verlag, 1974.)

REFERENCES

Alderson, D. A.: The reliability of Telepaque cholecystography. Brit. J. Surg., *47*:655–658, 1960.

Anson, B. J. (ed.): Morris' Human Anatomy. 12th edition. New York, McGraw Hill, 1966.

Ardran, C. M., French, J. M., and Mucklow, E. H. B.: Relationship of the nature of the opaque medium to the small intestine radiographic pattern. Brit. J. Radiol., *23*:697–702, 1950.

Baker, H. L., and Hodgson, J. R.: Further studies on the accuracy of cholecystography. Radiology, *74*:239–245, 1960.

Beargie, R. J., Hodgson, J. R., Huizenga, K. A., and Priestley, J. T.: Relation of cholangiographic findings after cholecystectomy to clinical and surgical findings. Surg. Gynec. Obst., *115*:143–152, 1962.

Berg, A. M., and Hamilton, J. E.: A method to improve roentgen diagnosis of biliary disease with bile acids. Surgery, *32*:948–952, 1952.

Berk, J. E.: Persistence of symptoms following gallbladder surgery. Amer. J. Digest. Dis., *9*:295–305, 1964.

Berk, R. N.: The consecutive dose phenomenon in oral cholecystography. Amer. J. Roentgenol., *110*:230–234, 1970.

Berk, R. N., and Lasser, E. C.: Altered concepts of the mechanism of nonvisualization of the gallbladder. Radiology, *82*:296–302, 1964.

Bierman, H. C.: Selective Arterial Catheterization. Springfield, Illinois, Charles C Thomas, 1969.

Bishopric, G. A.: Athrombocytosis following oral cholecystography. J.A.M.A., *189*:771–772, 1964.

Boyden, E. A.: Effects of natural foods on the distention of the gallbladder. Anat. Rec., *30*:333, 1925.

Caldwell, W. L., and Flock, M. H.: Evaluation of small bowel barium motor meal with emphasis on effect of volume of barium suspension ingested. Radiology, *80*:383–391, 1963.

Chapman, M., Curry, R. C., and LeQuesne, L. P.: Operative cholangiography. Brit. J. Surg., *51*:600–601, 1964.

Chrispin, A. R., and Fry, I. K.: The presacral space shown by barium enema. Brit. J. Radiol., *36*:319–322, 1966.

Clark, R. H., Schmidt, F. E., and Hendren, T.: Retroperitoneal extravasation of barium enema. J. Louisiana Med. Soc., *113*:90–92, 1961.

Cohen, W. N.: Roentgenographic evaluation of the rectal valves of Houston in the normal and in ulcerative colitis. Amer. J. Roentgenol., *104*:580–583, 1968.

Cook, G. B., and Margulis, A. R.: The use of silicone foam for examining the human sigmoid colon. Amer. J. Roentgenol., *87*:633–643, 1962.

Cunningham, D. J.: Textbook of Anatomy. Tenth edition. London, Oxford University Press, 1964.

Dann, D. S., Rubins, S., and Bauernfeind, A.: Significance of visualization of the common duct in the non-visualized gallbladder. Amer. J. Roentgenol., *82*:1016–1019, 1959.

Dassel, P. M.: Innocuous filling of the intestinal glands in the colon during barium enema (spiculation) simulating organic disease. Radiology, *78*:799–801, 1962.

Deutsch, V.: Cholecysto-angiography. Visualization of the gallbladder by selective celiac and mesenteric angiography. Amer. J. Roentgenol., *101*:608–616, 1967.

Eckelberg, M. E., Carlson, H. C., and McIlrath, D. C.: Intravenous cholangiography with intact gallbladder. Amer. J. Roentgenol., *110*:235–239, 1970.

Edling, N. P. G., and Eklöf, O.: A roentgenologic study of the course of ulcerative colitis. Acta Radiol., *54*:397–409, 1960.

Edmunds, M. C., Emmett, J. M., and Clark, W. D.: Ten year experience with operative cholangiography. Amer. Surg., *26*:613–621, 1960.

Eklöf, O., and Gierup, J.: The retrorectal soft tissue space in children: normal variations and appearances in granulomatous colitis. Amer. J. Roentgenol., *108*:624–627, 1970.

Emmanoulides, G. C., and Hoy, R. C.: Transumbilical aortography and selective arteriography in newborn infants. Pediatrics, *39*:337, 1967.

Farrell, W. J.: Angiography of the liver: practical applications and demonstration of color subtraction technique. Radiol. Clin. of N. Amer., *4*:571–582, 1966.

Fischer, H. W., Galbraith, W. B., and Schroeder, A. F.: Rapid cholecystography with pharmacological assistance. Amer. J. Roentgenol., *84*:484–490, 1965.

Flemma, R. J., Capp, P., and Shagleton, W. W.: Percutaneous transhepatic colangiography. Arch. Surg., *90*:5, 1965.

Frimann-Dahl, J.: The administration of barium orally in acute obstruction: advantages and risks. Acta Radiol., *42*:285–295, 1954.

Frommhold, W.: A new contrast agent for intravenous cholecystography. (German text). Fortschr. Geb. Röntgenstrahlen, *70*:283–291, 1963.

Frommhold, W., and Braband, H.: Accidents during gallbladder studies with Biligrafin and their treatment. Fortschr. Geb. Röntgenstrahlen, *92*:47–59, 1960.

Garbsch, H.: The intravenous roentgenologic function study of the extrahepatic biliary tree. Radiologia Austriaca, *14*:131–158, 1963.

Goldstein, H. M., Poole, G. J., Rosenquist, C. J., Friedland, G. W., and Zboralske, F. F.: Comparison of methods for acceleration of small intestinal radiographic examination. Radiology, 98:519–523, 1971.

Graham, E. A., and Cole, W. H.: Roentgenologic examination of the gallbladder: Preliminary report of a new method utilizing intravenous injection of tetrabromphthalein. J.A.M.A., 82:613–614, 1924.

Guyton, A. C.: Textbook of Medical Physiology. Fourth edition. Philadelphia, W. B. Saunders Co., 1971.

Hampson, L. G., and Petrie, E. A.: The problem of stones in the common bile duct with particular reference to retained stones. Canad. J. Surg., 7:361–367, 1964.

Harris, R. C., and Caffey, J.: Cholecystography in infants. J.A.M.A., 153:1333, 1953.

Haynes, W. F., Jr., and Pittman, F. E.: Application of fluorescein string test in 32 cases of upper gastrointestinal hemorrhage. Gastroenterology, 38:690–697, 1960.

Hays, D. M., and Averbook, B. B.: Experience with intravenous cholecystography in infants and children. Surgery, 42:638–641, 1957.

Henderson, S. G.: The gastrointestinal tract in the healthy newborn infant. Amer. J. Roentgenol., 48:302–335, 1942.

Henderson, S. G., and Briant, W. W., Jr.: The colon in the healthy newborn infant. Amer. J. Roentgenol., 39:261–272, 1942.

Hess, W.: Operative cholangiography. In Schinz, H. R., et al. (eds.): Roentgen Diagnosis. Vol. 1. New York, Grune and Stratton, 1967.

Hess, W.: Surgery of the Biliary Passages and Pancreas. Princeton, Van Nostrand, 1965.

Hicken, N. F., McAllister, A. J., Franz, B., and Crowder, E.: Technic, indications and value of postoperative cholangiography. Arch. Surg., 60:1102–1113, 1950.

Hicken, N. F., McAllister, A. J., and Walker, G.: The problem of retained common duct stones. Amer. J. Surg., 97:173–181, 1959.

Hicken, N. F., Stevenson, V. L., Franz, B. J., and Crowder, E.: The technic of operative cholangiography. Amer. J. Surg., 78:347–355, 1949.

Hight, D., Lingley, J. R., and Hurtubise, F.: An evaluation of operative cholangiograms as a guide to common duct exploration. Ann. Surg., 150:1086–1091, 1959.

Holt, J. F., Lyons, R. H., Neligh, R. B., Moe, G. K., and Hodges, R. J.: X-ray signs of altered alimentary function following autonomic blockade with tetraethylammonium. Radiology, 49:603–610, 1947.

Jacobson, G., Berne, C. J., Meyers, H. I., and Rosoff, L.: The examination of patients with suspected perforated ulcer using a water soluble contrast medium. Amer. J. Roentgenol., 86:37–49, 1961.

Kessler, R. E., and Zimmon, D. S.: Umbilical vein angiography. Radiology, 87:841–844, 1966.

Kleinsasser, L. J., and Warshaw, H.: Perforation of the sigmoid colon during barium enema. Ann. Surg., 135:560–565, 1952.

Krezanoski, J. Z.: Tannic acid: chemistry, analysis, and toxicology: an episode in the pharmaceutics of radiology. Radiology, 87:655–657, 1966.

Lasser, E. C., and Gerende, L. J. (and others in cooperative study): An efficacy study of Clysodrast. Radiology, 87:649–654, 1966.

Lonnerblad, L.: Transit time through the small intestine: Roentgenologic study of normal variability. Acta Radiol. (Suppl.), 88:1–85, 1951.

Lumsden, K., and Truelove, S. C.: Intravenous Pro-banthine in diagnostic radiology of the gastrointestinal tract with special reference to colonic disease. Brit. J. Radiol., 32:517–526, 1959.

Mandl, F.: Transcutaneous cholangiography in ichteric patients. Chirurg., 27:341–343, 1956.

Margulis, A. R.: Examination of the colon. In Margulis, A. R., and Burhenne, H. J. (eds.): Alimentary Tract Roentgenology. St. Louis, C. V. Mosby Co., 1967.

Margulis, A. R., and Jovanovich, A.: Roentgen diagnosis of submucous lipomas of the colon. Amer. J. Roentgenol., 84:1114–1120, 1960.

Marshak, R. H.: Regional enteritis: roentgenologic findings. In Bockus, H. L.: Gastroenterology. Vol. 2. Second edition. Philadelphia, W. B. Saunders Co., 1964.

Marshak, R. H., and Lindner, A. E.: Radiology of the Small Intestine. Philadelphia, W. B. Saunders Co., 1970.

Mauthe, H.: The accuracy of x-ray examination of the gallbladder. Wisconsin Med. J., 53:473–476, 1962.

McAlister, W. H., Anderson, M. S., Bloomberg, F. R., and Margulis, A. R.: Lethal effects of tannic acid in the barium enema. Radiology, 80:765–773, 1963.

McClenahan, J. L., Evans, J. A., and Braunstein, P. W.: Intravenous cholangiography in the postcholecystectomy syndrome. J.A.M.A., 159:1353–1357, 1955.

Meyers, M. A.: Roentgen significance of the phrenicocolic ligament. Radiology, 95:539–545, 1970.

Michels, A.: Blood Supply and Anatomy of the Upper Abdominal Organs. Philadelphia, J. B. Lippincott Co., 1955.

Miller, R. E.: Barium sulfate suspensions. Radiology, 84:241–251, 1965.

Moreton, R. D., Stevenson, C. R., and Yates, C. W.: Fictitious polyps as seen in double contrast studies of the colon. Radiology, 53:386–393, 1949.

Mujahed, Z., and Evans, J. A.: Percutaneous transhepatic cholangiography. Radiol. Clin. N. Amer., 4:535–545, 1966.

Nathan, M. H., Newman, A., Murray, D. J., and Camponovo, R.: Cholecystokinin cholecystography. Amer. J. Roentgenol., 110:240–251, 1970.

Nazareno, J. P., Studenski, E. V., and Pickren, J. W.: The cholangiogram: postmortem study. Radiology, 76:54–59, 1961 (14 ref).

Nelson, S. W., Christoforidis, A. J., and Roenigk, W. J.: Dangers and fallibilities of iodinated radiopaque media in obstruction of the small bowel. Amer. J. Surg., 109:546–559, 1965a.

Nelson, S. W., Christoforidis, A. J., and Roenigk, W. J.: A diagnostic physiologic sign of mechanical obstruction of the small intestine. Radiology, 84:881–885, 1965b.

Netter, F.: CIBA Collection of Medical Illustration. Vol. 3, Part 2. 1962.

Neuhauser, E. D. B., quoted in Sidaway, M. E.: The use of water soluble contrast medium in pediatric radiology. Clin. Radiol., 15:132–138, 1964.

Norman, A., and Saghapoleslami, M.: Oral extrahepatic cholangiography: a simple reliable technique. Radiology, 76:801–804, 1962.

Odnoralov, N. I.: Hepatic arteriography. In Schobinger, R. A., and Ruzicka, F. F., Jr. (eds.): Vascular Roentgenology. New York, The MacMillan Co., 1964. pp. 368–372.

Ostrum, B. J., and Heinz, E. R.: Small bowel obstruction versus adynamic ileus: A study using a water soluble oral contrast material (Hypaque sodium powder). Amer. J. Roentgenol., 89:734–739, 1963 (12 ref.).

Pansky, B., and House, E. L.: Review of Gross Anatomy. New York, The MacMillan Co., 1964.

Partington, P. F., and Sachs, M. D.: Routine use of operative cholangiography. Surg. Gynec. Obst., 87:299–307, 1948.

Pendergrass, E. P.: Symposium on contrast media reactions: introduction. Radiology, 91:61–62, 1968.

Reboul, J., Delorme, G., Marque, J., and Tavernin, J.: Results of the exploration of the colon by the double contrast method with Contalax lactose powder. Ann. Radiol., 6:283–296, 1963.

Redman,H. C., and Reuter, S. F.: The angiographic evaluation of gallbladder dilatation. Radiology, 97:367–370, 1970.

Rene, R. M., and Mellinkoff, S. M.: Renal insufficiency after oral administration of double dose of cholecystographic medium. New Eng. J. Med., 261:589–591, 1959.

Rösch, J., Grollman, J. H., Jr., and Steckel, R. J.: Arteriography in the diagnosis of gallbladder disease. Radiology, 92:1485–1491, 1969.

Rosenbaum, H. D.: The value of re-examination in patients with inadequate visualization of the gallbladder following a single dose of Telepaque. Amer. J. Roentgenol., 82:1111–1115, 1959.

Rosenbaum, H. D., Lieber, A., Hanson, D. J., and Pelligrino, E. D.: Routine survey roentgenogram of the abdomen on 500 consecutive patients over 40 years of age. Amer. J. Roentgenol., 91:903–909, 1964.

Rosenherg, L. S., and Fine, A. V.: Fatal venous intravasation of barium during a barium enema. Radiology, 73:771–773, 1959.

Ross, R. J., and Sachs, M. D.: Triplication of the gallbladder. Amer. J. Roentgenol., 104:656–661, 1968.

Rous, P., and McMaster, P. D.: The concentrating activity of the gallbladder. J. Exper. Med., 34:47, 1921.

Rubin, S., Dann, D. S., Ezekial, C., and Vincent, J.: Retrograde prolapse of the ileocecal valve. Amer. J. Roentgenol., 87:706–708, 1962.

Rudhe, U.: Roentgenologic examination of rectum in ulcerative colitis. Acta Paediat., 49:859–867, 1960.

Ruzicka, F. F., and Rossi, P.: Normal vascular anatomy of the abdominal viscera. Radiol. Clin. N. Amer., 8:3–29, 1970.

Sachs, M. D.: Routine cholangiography, operative and postoperative. Radiol. Clin. N. Amer., 4:547–569, 1966.

Salerno, F. G., Collins, O. D., Redmond, D., et al.: Transumbilical abdominal aortography in the newborn. J. Pediat. Surg., 5:40, 1970.

Salzman, E.: Opacification of bile duct calculi. Radiol. Clin. N. Amer., 4:525–533, 1966.

Salzman, G. F.: Solu-Biloptin (SH550) as a contrast medium for peroral cholegraphy. Acta Radiol., 52:417–425, 1960.

Sasson, L.: Entrance of barium into intestinal glands during barium enema. J.A.M.A., 173:343–345, 1960.

Schatzki, R.: Small intestinal enema. Amer. J. Roentgenol., 50:743–751, 1943.

Schlaeger, R.: Examination of the small intestine. In Margulis, A. R., and Burhenne, H. J. (eds.): Alimentary Tract Roentgenology. St. Louis, C. V. Mosby Co., 1967.

Schobinger, R. A., and Ruzicka, F. F., Jr.: Vascular Roentgenology. New York, The MacMillan Co., 1964.

Seaman, W. B., and Bragg, D. G.: Colonic intramural barium: complication of barium enema examination. Radiology, 89:250–255, 1967.

Seaman, W. B., Cosgriff, S., and Wells, J.: Renal insufficiency following cholecystography. Amer. J. Roentgenol., 90:859, 1963.

Seaman, W. B., and Wells, J.: Complications of the barium enema. Gastroenterology, *48*:728–737, 1965.

Shehadi, W. H.: Clinical problems and toxicity of contrast agents. Amer. J. Roentgenol., *97*:762–771, 1966a.

Shehadi, W. H.: Clinical Radiology of the Biliary Tract. New York, McGraw-Hill, 1963b.

Shehadi, W. H.: Oral cholangiography with Telepaque. Amer. J. Roentgenol., *92*:436–451, 1954.

Shehadi, W. H.: Intravenous cholecystocholangiography. J.A.M.A., *159*:1350–1353, 1955.

Shehadi, W. H.: Radiologic examination of the biliary tract: plain films of the abdomen; oral cholecystography. Radiol. Clin. N. Amer., *4*:463–482, 1966b.

Shehadi, W. H.: Simultaneous intravenous cholangiography and urography. Surg. Gynec. Obst., *105*:401–406, 1957.

Shehadi, W. H.: Studies of the colon and small intestines with water soluble iodinated contrast media. Amer. J. Roentgenol., *89*:740–751, 1963a.

Smith, C. A.: The Physiology of the Newborn Infant. Third edition. Springfield, Illinois, Charles C Thomas, 1959.

Smith, V. M.: String impregnation test for lesions of the upper digestive tract. Ann. Intern. Med., *54*:16–29, 1961.

Sovenyi, E., and Varro, V.: New method for x-ray studies of small bowel. Fortschr. Geb. Röntgenstrahlen, *91*:269–270, 1959.

Stacy, G. S., and Loop, J. W.: Unusual small bowel diseases: methods and observation. Amer. J. Roentgenol., *92*:1072–1079, 1964.

Steinbach, H. L., and Burhenne, H. J.: Performing the barium enema: equipment, preparation and contrast medium. Amer. J. Roentgenol., *87*:644–654, 1962.

Stern, W. Z., Schein, C. J., and Jacobson, H. G.: The significance of the lateral view in T-tube cholangiography. Amer. J. Roentgenol., *87*:764–771, 1962.

Templeton, A. W.: Colon sphincters simulating organic disease. Radiology, 75:237–241, 1960.

Tomenius, J.: A new instrument for gastric biopsies under visual control. Gastroenterology, *21*:544–546, 1952.

Traphagen, D. W., and Karlan, M.: Fluorescein string test for localization of upper gastrointestinal hemorrhage. Surgery, *44*:644–645, 1958.

Treves, V. F.: Anatomy of intestinal canal and peritoneum in man. Brit. Med. J., *1*:580–583, 1965.

Vadheim, J. L., and Rigos, F. J.: Cholangiography as an aid to biliary surgery. Northwest Med., *51*:400–402, 1952.

Weiner, M., and Hanafee, W. N.: Review of transjugular cholangiography. Radiol. Clin. of N. Amer., *8*:53–68, 1970.

Weintraub, S., and Williams, R. G.: A rapid method of roentgenologic examination of the small intestine. Amer. J. Roentgenol., *61*:45–55, 1949.

Weng, W.: Abdominal Angiography. Springer-Verlag, New York, 1974.

Whalen, J. P., and Riemenschneider, P. A.: An analysis of the normal anatomic relationships of the colon as applied to roentgenographic observations. Amer. J. Roentgenol., *99*:55–61, 1967.

White, W. W., and Fischer, H. S.: Double blind study of Oragrafin and Telepaque. Amer. J. Roentgenol., *87*:745–748, 1962.

Whitehouse, W. M., and Hodges, F. J.: Recent additions to radiographic techniques in biliary tract disease. Gastroenterology, *38*:701–705, 1956.

Whitehouse, W. M., and Martin, O.: Clinical and roentgenologic evaluation of routine 2-gram Telepaque dosage in cholecystography. Radiology, 65:422–424, 1955.

Wilbur, R. S., and Bolt, R. J.: Incidence of gallbladder disease in "normal" men. Gastroenterology, *36*:251–255, 1959.

Williams, I.: Diverticular disease of the colon without diverticula. Radiology, 89:401–412, 1967.

Wise, R. E.: Intravenous Cholangiography. Springfield, Illinois, Charles C Thomas, 1962.

Wise, R. E., and O'Brien, R. G.: Interpretation of the intravenous cholangiogram. J.A.M.A., *160*:819–827, 1956.

Wood, I. J., Doig, R. K., Motteram, R., and Hughes, A.: Gastric biopsy: report on 55 biopsies using the new flexible gastric biopsy tube. Lancet, *1*:18–21, 1949.

Zatzkin, H. R., and Irwin, G. H. L.: Nonfatal intravasation of barium. Amer. J. Roentgenol., *92*:1169–1172, 1964.

Zimmer, E. A.: Radiology of the small intestine. I. Studies on contrast media for the x-ray examination of the gastrointestinal tract. Brit. J. Radiol., *24*:245–251, 1951.

15

The Abdomen and Peritoneal Space

GROSS ANATOMY OF THE ABDOMINAL CAVITY

Boundaries and Subdivisions of the Peritoneal Cavity. The abdominopelvic cavity is that segment of the serous cavity of the trunk that lies below the diaphragm. The anterior wall is composed of the transversalis, internal oblique, and external oblique muscles, together with the rectus and pyramidal muscles, the skin and superficial fascia overlying these structures. The posterior wall is composed of the vertebral column, the posterior segment of the pelvis, the inferior portions of the diaphragm, and the quadratus lumborum and psoas muscles. The side walls of the abdomen are formed by the oblique and transverse muscles, and below by the iliacus muscles and the iliac bones.

The abdominal cavity is divisible into the abdominal cavity proper and the true pelvis or pelvis minor. The ribs cover approximately the same area of the abdomen as they do the thorax.

The true pelvis is bounded in front and at the sides by as much of the hip bones as lie below the level of the linea terminalis. These are partly clothed by the internal obturator muscle and pelvic fascia. The posterior wall is formed by the anterior aspect of the sacrum and coccyx, covered on each side by the pyriform muscle. The pyriform muscles pass out of the pelvis through the greater sciatic notch, thus closing these potential holes in the cavity. The floor of the pelvis is composed of the levator ani muscles, coccygeal muscles, and the endopelvic fascia.

There are certain openings in the abdominal walls that form potentially weak areas through which protrusions (herniations) may occur. These openings occur in the diaphragm to allow passage for the aorta, esophagus, and inferior vena cava; in the pelvic floor to allow passage for the urethra, rectum, and vagina; in the lower portion of the abdominal wall at the site of the inguinal canals through which the round ligaments and spermatic cords pass, and in the area of weakness formed by the femoral sheath, which contains the femoral arteries, veins, lymphatics, and femoral canal.

Ligaments and Mesenteric Folds of Peritoneum. The peritoneal cavity is, therefore, a potential space between the layers of the peritoneum. When all the viscera are cut away, there are

certain lines of reflection of the peritoneum that demonstrate that the peritoneum is a continuous covering on the dorsal and ventral walls of the abdomen as well as on the diaphragm.

On the dorsal abdominal wall, proceeding caudad, the following ligamentous structures are encountered. The *falciform ligament* is continuous with the ventral layer of the *coronary* and *triangular ligaments* of the liver (Fig. 15–1). The anterior layer of the coronary ligament of the liver is continuous with the right side of the falciform ligament, at the place where the peritoneum is reflected from the diaphragm to the right lobe of the liver. The posterior layer of the coronary ligament of the liver extends from the back of the right lobe to the right suprarenal gland and kidney. The left and right triangular ligaments of the liver are situated where the anterior and posterior coronary ligaments meet (Fig. 15–2). The *anterior layer* of the triangular ligament is continuous with the left side of the falciform ligament anteriorly; also, the peritoneum is here reflected from the diaphragm to the left lobe of the liver. The *posterior layer* of the triangular ligament is dorsal to the anterior layer and is situated where the peritoneum is reflected from the left lobe of the liver to the diaphragm. The two layers of the triangular ligament join in a sharp fold at the left (Fig. 15–2).

The *dorsal layer* of the coronary and triangular ligaments is continuous with the lesser omentum at the abdominal end of the esophagus. The *lesser omentum* splits around the esophagus and stomach and then reunites and becomes continuous with the dorsal mesentery as the *lienorenal (splenorenal) ligament.* The *dorsal mesentery* is actually the *greater omentum* and it is fused to the transverse mesocolon. The *hepatogastric* and *hepatoduodenal ligaments* are mesenteric folds of peritoneum that form the lesser omentum and extend from the porta hepatis to the stomach and duodenum respectively.

The greater omentum passes around the pylorus and unites with the free edge of the lesser omentum. The *transverse mesocolon* posteriorly is continuous with the peritoneum covering the ascending and descending colon. The peritoneum of the descending colon caudally merges with the *sigmoid mesocolon* (Fig. 15–2). There is a *bare area of liver* which is not covered by peritoneum lying between the layers of the coronary ligament (Fig. 15–2).

926

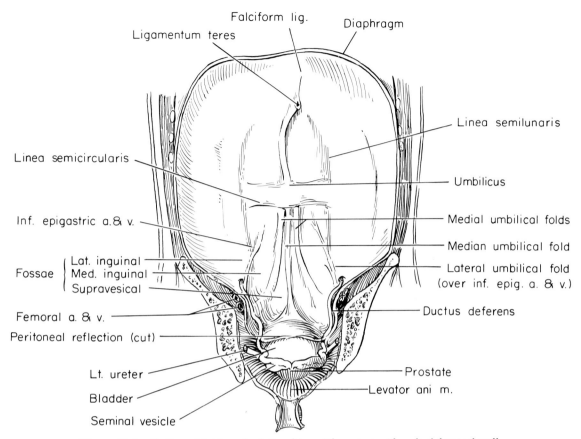

Figure 15–1.   Peritoneal folds and relationships of the anterior (dorsal) abdominal wall.

The *greater omentum* is a double layer of peritoneum hanging from the greater curvature of the stomach, crossing over the transverse colon and descending in front of the abdominal viscera. There are three extensions from the greater omentum: (1) the *gastrocolic ligament,* which is the omentum between the stomach and transverse colon; (2) the *lienorenal ligament,* which is the mesentery from the left kidney to the spleen; and (3) the *gastrolienal ligament,* which is the dorsal mesentery joining the spleen to the stomach.

The *transverse mesocolon* is the dorsal mesentery of the transverse colon (see sagittal section, Figure 15–5). The *phrenicocolic ligament* is that fold of peritoneum extending between the left colic flexure to the diaphragm and helping to support the spleen (*sustentaculum* of the spleen). The *mesentery proper* is a broad fanlike fold of peritoneum extending from the posterior wall of the abdomen and suspending the entire jejunum and ileum from the dorsal body wall (Fig. 15–3).

The *omental bursa* or *lesser sac* is situated behind the stomach and communicates with the main cavity of the peritoneal space through the *epiploic foramen* (Figs. 15–4 and 15–5). As shown in the diagrams, the lesser sac is bounded

ventrally by the caudal lobe of the liver, the stomach, the greater omentum, and the lesser omentum; dorsally it is bounded by the greater omentum, transverse colon, and mesocolon as well as the left suprarenal and left kidney. To the right it opens into the greater sac. To the left are the phrenicocolic ligament, the hilum of the spleen, and the gastrolienal ligament (Fig. 15–4).

On the anterior abdominal wall moving cephalad above the umbilicus there is the *falciform ligament* containing the *ligamentum teres* (Fig. 15–1). On the ventral abdominal wall moving caudad to the umbilicus there is a fold extending from the umbilicus to the apex of the urinary bladder called the *median umbilical fold* which contains the obliterated urachus (Fig. 15–6). On either side of this middle umbilical plica or fold are *lateral folds* or *plicae* which cover ligamentous structures beginning at the umbilicus and extending to join the superior vesical branch of the internal iliac artery. These folds are remnants of the fetal umbilical arteries. More laterally and convexly toward the lateral abdominal margin are the *epigastric folds* or *plicae,* which are folds of peritoneum covering the inferior epigastric vessels (Fig. 15–1).

The *pelvic peritoneum* extends downward from the abdominal

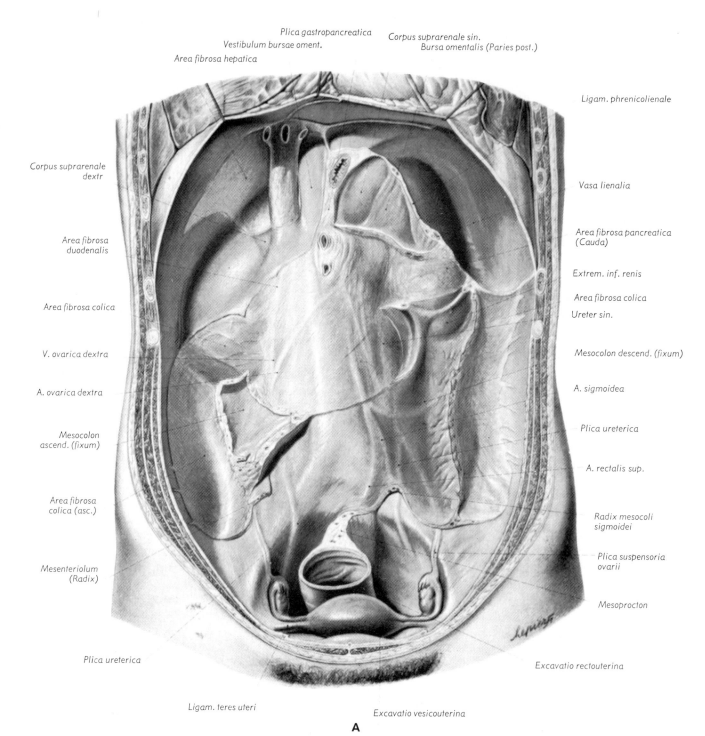

Plica gastropancreatica
Vestibulum bursae oment.
Corpus suprarenale sin.
Bursa omentalis (Paries post.)
Area fibrosa hepatica

Ligam. phrenicolienale

Corpus suprarenale dextr

Vasa lienalia

Area fibrosa duodenalis

Area fibrosa pancreatica (Cauda)

Extrem. inf. renis

Area fibrosa colica

Area fibrosa colica
Ureter sin.

V. ovarica dextra

Mesocolon descend. (fixum)

A. ovarica dextra

A. sigmoidea

Plica ureterica

Mesocolon ascend. (fixum)

A. rectalis sup.

Area fibrosa colica (asc.)

Radix mesocoli sigmoidei

Plica suspensoria ovarii

Mesenteriolum (Radix)

Mesoprocton

Plica ureterica

Excavatio rectouterina

Ligam. teres uteri

Excavatio vesicouterina

A

Figure 15–2.   A. Peritoneal relationships on the posterior abdominal wall.

Figure 15–2 continued on the opposite page.

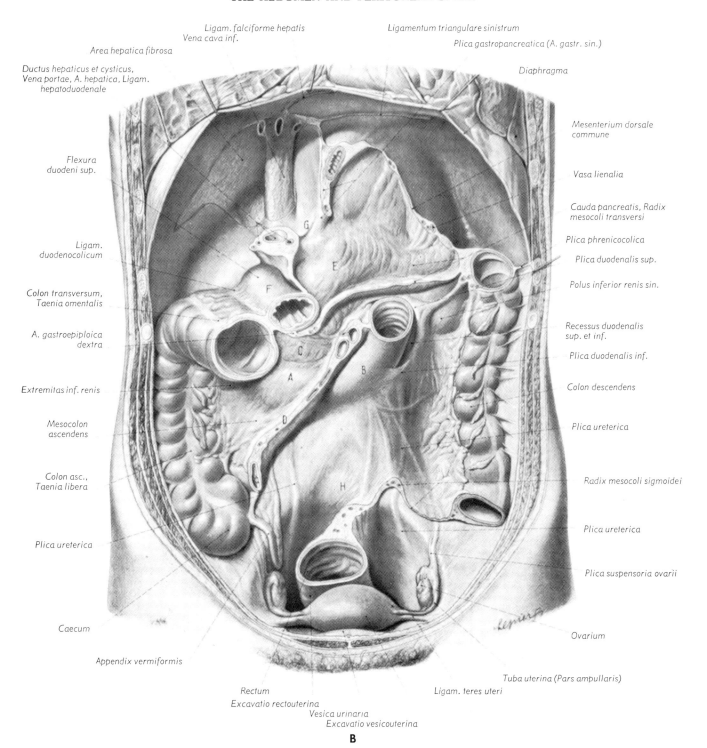

Ligam. falciforme hepatis
Vena cava inf.
Area hepatica fibrosa
Ductus hepaticus et cysticus,
Vena portae, A. hepatica, Ligam.
hepatoduodenale
Ligamentum triangulare sinistrum
Plica gastropancreatica (A. gastr. sin.)
Diaphragma
Flexura
duodeni sup.
Ligam.
duodenocolicum
Colon transversum,
Taenia omentalis
A. gastroepiploica
dextra
Extremitas inf. renis
Mesocolon
ascendens
Colon asc.,
Taenia libera
Plica ureterica
Caecum
Appendix vermiformis
Mesenterium dorsale
commune
Vasa lienalia
Cauda pancreatis, Radix
mesocoli transversi
Plica phrenicocolica
Plica duodenalis sup.
Polus inferior renis sin.
Recessus duodenalis
sup. et inf.
Plica duodenalis inf.
Colon descendens
Plica ureterica
Radix mesocoli sigmoidei
Plica ureterica
Plica suspensoria ovarii
Ovarium
Tuba uterina (Pars ampullaris)
Rectum
Excavatio rectouterina
Vesica urinaria
Excavatio vesicouterina
Ligam. teres uteri

B

Figure 15–2 *Continued.*　B. Peritoneum on the posterior abdominal wall with the roots of the mesenteries and the posterior wall of bursa omentalis. Peritoneum covering duodenum, pancreas, and colon ascendens and descendens with mesocolon asc. and desc.

　　A, Pars tecta duodeni　　　　　E, Corpus pancreatis
　　B, Pars ascendens duod.　　　　F, Pars horizontalis superior duod.
　　C, Caput pancreatis　　　　　　G, Vestibulum bursae omentalis
　　D, Radix mesenterii　　　　　　H, Promontorium

(From Pernkopf, E.: Atlas of Topographical and Applied Human Anatomy. Vol. 2. Philadelphia, W. B. Saunders Co., 1964.)

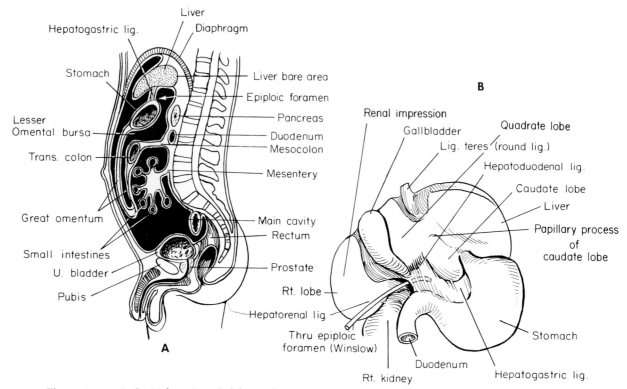

Figure 15–3. *A.* Sagittal section of abdominal cavity showing greater and lesser omental sacs with adjoining mesenteric attachments. *B.* View of hepatogastric ligament and epiploic foramen into lesser omental bursa, with adjoining structures.

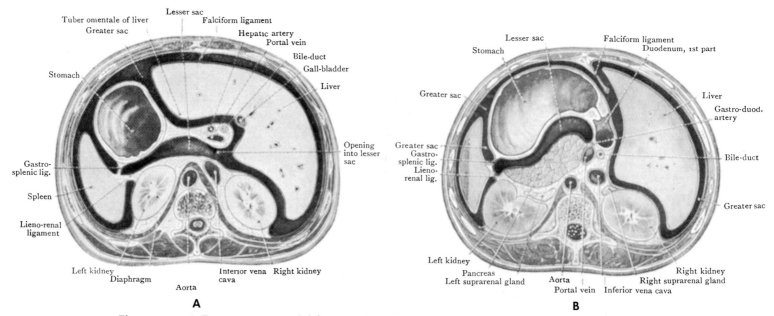

Figure 15–4. *A.* Transverse section of abdomen to show the arrangement of peritoneum at the level of the opening into lesser sac. *B.* Transverse section of abdomen to show the arrangement of the peritoneum immediately below the opening into the lesser sac.

Figure 15–4 continued on the opposite page.

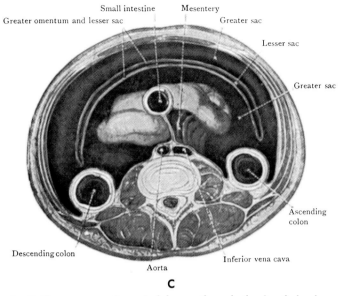

Figure 15-4 *Continued.* C. Transverse section of abdomen through the fourth lumbar vertebra, to show the arrangement of the peritoneum. (From Cunningham's Manual of Practical Anatomy, 12th ed. London, Oxford University Press, 1958.)

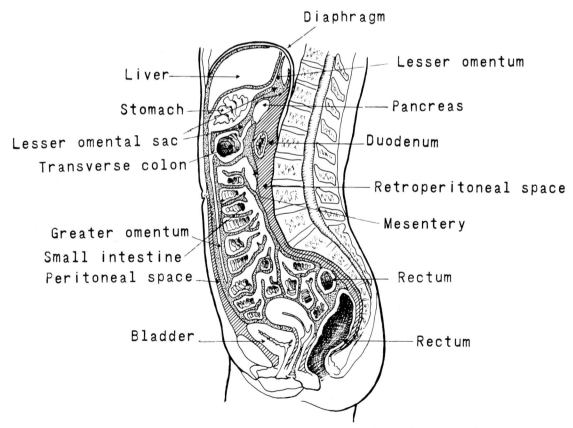

Figure 15-5.   Sagittal diagram of abdomen showing relationships of lesser omental sac.

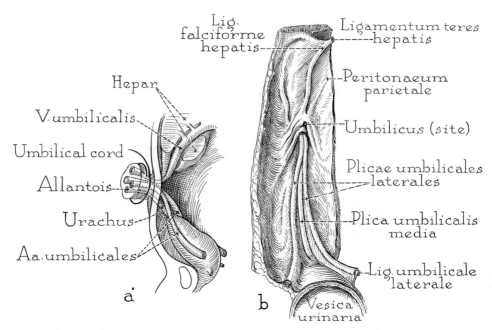

Figure 15–6. Plicae on the inner aspect of the anterior wall occasionally visualized in the posteroanterior view. Umbilical blood vessels and remnant of the urachus, and the serous folds caused by their presence on the internal aspect of the anterior abdominal wall. The obliterated umbilical vein occupies a fold of peritoneum, the falciform ligament of the liver, which, arising from the upper part of the anterior abdominal wall, runs to the umbilical incisura of the liver. Below the level of the umbilicus the urachus, persisting as a ligamentous strand, lifts the peritoneum in the median plane to produce a middle umbilical fold. Over the umbilical arteries the peritoneum projects, to each side of the midline, as a lateral umbilical fold. These *plicae*, together with lesser serous elevations over the functional inferior epigastric vessels, form boundaries of *foveae* on the internal aspect of the wall. (From Anson, B. J.: An Atlas of Human Anatomy. Philadelphia, W. B. Saunders Co., 1963.)

walls, covering the pelvic viscera and the anatomic structures contained therein. There is a vesicouterine pouch in the female between the urinary bladder and the uterus and a rectouterine pouch (pouch of Douglas) between the uterus and the rectum posteriorly. The relationship of these pouches to the vagina is evident in Figure 15–7. In the male the pelvic peritoneum extends on the posterior aspect of the urinary bladder into the rectum, creating a rectovesical pouch (Fig. 15–8).

Contents of the Abdomen. The following structures are found within the abdominopelvic cavity: (1) the peritoneum, mesenteries, omenta, and ligaments, (2) the liver, (3) the spleen, (4) the pancreas, (5) the adrenal glands, (6) the urinary tract, (7) the reproductive organs, (8) the gastrointestinal tract and (9) the blood vessels, lymphatics, and nerves.

The gastrointestinal tract, genitourinary tract, and cardiovascular system are considered separately.

RADIOLOGIC ANATOMY OF THE PERITONEAL SPACE

Lesser Peritoneal Sac. Anatomic drawings illustrating the anterior wall of the lesser sac and the posterior wall with the stomach partially removed are shown in Figures 15–9 and 15–10. The *anterior wall* is composed of the lesser omentum, the posterior surface of the stomach and duodenal bulb, and the gastrocolic ligament (Fig. 15–9). The *posterior wall* is bounded by peritoneum covering the pancreas, left adrenal gland, a part of the upper anterior surface of the left kidney, and portions of the posterior diaphragm (Fig. 15–10). Note the large fold of peritoneum raised from the posterior abdominal wall by the left gastric and left hepatic arteries. This fold divides the lesser sac into two compartments. The upper recess on the right is limited by the diaphragm and is caudad to the liver (also see Fig. 15–5). On the left aspect of

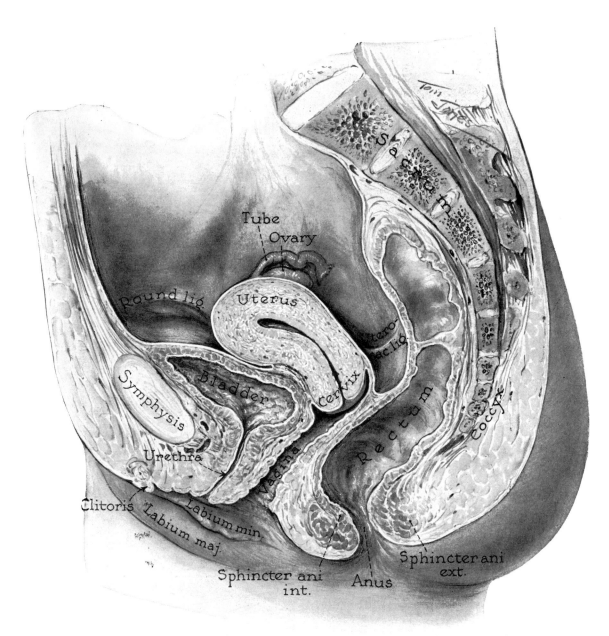

Figure 15–7. Female pelvis, sagittal section, showing the relations of the organs and the course of the peritoneum. The peritoneum ascends over the bladder to cover the vesical surface of the body of the uterus, from which it is continued lateralward as the anterior layer of the broad ligament; the shallow trough-like recess thus formed is the vesicouterine excavation (uterovesical pouch). The peritoneal layer next covers the fundus of the uterus, investing all of the posterior uterus and a small upper segment of the vaginal wall; from the uterus it is again draped lateralward to form the posterior layer of the broad ligament of the uterus. From the uterus and the ligament the peritoneum passes to the front of the rectum, forming a deeper sac, the rectouterine excavation. The peritoneum reaches the rectum approximately at the junction of its lower and middle thirds; in the middle third it covers only the front of the tube, while in the upper third it clothes the sides as well; the layers of the two sides then meet above to form a mesenteric support for the sigmoid colon. In partially investing the rectum the peritoneum forms paired pouches, the pararectal fossae, bounded on each side by a crescentic fold of peritoneum, the rectouterine fold (fold of Douglas). (From Anson, B. J.: An Atlas of Human Anatomy. Philadelphia, W. B. Saunders Co., 1963.)

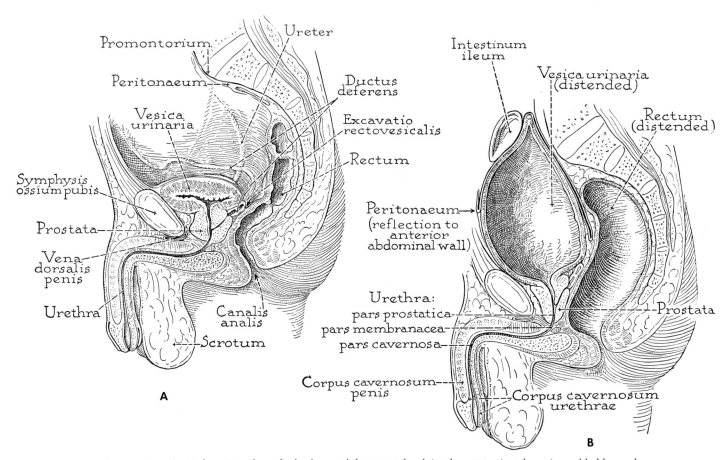

Figure 15–8. Sagittal section through the lower abdomen and pelvis, demonstrating the urinary bladder and rectum. *A.* Showing the organs in the empty condition. In sagittal section the bladder is three-sided. The superior surface faces upward; the posterior surface is directed both backward and downward; inferiorly, the bladder rests upon the pelvic floor, the levitor ani muscles, and the pubic symphysis. *B.* The bladder and rectum distended. The distended bladder rises above the space just described, projecting into the true abdominal cavity. It assumes a bulbous form and loses its triangular configuration. (From Anson, B. J.: An Atlas of Human Anatomy. Philadelphia, W. B. Saunders Co., 1963.)

this recess, the peritoneum of the posterior wall of the lesser sac is reflected from the diaphragm onto the posterior surface of the fundus of the stomach. This reflection is called the *gastrophrenic ligament* and is continuous laterally with the gastrosplenic and lienorenal ligaments. Inferiorly the lesser peritoneal space is limited by the transverse mesocolon, the root of which crosses the head of the pancreas and extends along its inferior margin (Fig. 15–10). The *right margin* of the lesser sac is formed by the peritoneal reflection over the inferior vena cava. The *foramen of Winslow* described previously in Chapter 13 is only large enough to admit one finger but this size may vary.

In the living, the lesser sac is very distensible but it can expand only to the left inferiorly and anteriorly, since the liver, diaphragm, and posterior abdominal wall prevent expansion in the other directions (Walker and Weens). Pneumoperitoneum of the lesser sac, herniations, and abscesses may be responsible for such distention and may be recognized by the anatomic boundaries given.

Differentiation of Peritoneal Organs from Retroperitoneal Organs. An organ only partly covered by peritoneum is referred to as a "retroperitoneal" organ. An organ that is completely covered by peritoneum except for entrance of vessels is called a "peritoneal" organ. The various ligaments or folds of mesentery previously described connect the completely peritonealized organs to the abdominal wall. The opening from the general peritoneal cavity into the lesser peritoneal cavity through the foramen of Winslow has been described earlier. In addition, in the female there are two minute apertures in the peritoneal cavity at the openings of the uterine tubes. As will be shown in Chapter 17, injections into the uterine cavity and uterine tubes communicate with the pelvic peritoneal space.

Some of these relationships of peritoneal and retroperitoneal organs are best seen in cross-sectional diagrams of the abdomen. For example, at about the *level of the fourth lumbar vertebra* or the umbilicus (Fig. 15–4 *C*): the descending and ascending colon are only partially peritonealized and therefore are partially retroperitoneal. There is a mesenteric band extending approximately from the midline to the small intestine which contains the major mesenteric vessels and nerves; hence the small intestine is completely peritonealized. The aorta and inferior vena cava are retroperitoneal and are posterior to the mesentery containing the major blood vessels to the small intestine.

At the level of the *first and second lumbar vertebrae* (Fig. 15–4 *B*), the reflections of the peritoneum are somewhat more complex. Here the epiploic foramen of Winslow connecting the general peritoneal cavity and omental bursa can be identified. The omental bursa is just dorsal to the stomach; its vestibule is that portion of this space that lies just dorsal to the hepatoduodenal ligament. The omental bursa is limited ventrally by the liver, the lesser omentum, the stomach, and the greater omentum; dorsally by the abdominal wall, the left suprarenal glands, the pancreas,

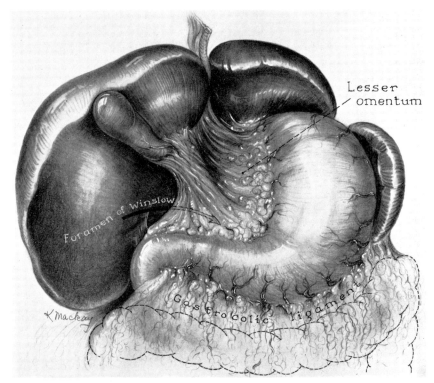

Figure 15–9. Anatomic drawing illustrating anterior wall of lesser sac; composed of lesser omentum, posterior surface of stomach and duodenal bulb, and gastrocolic ligament. (From Walker, L. A., and Weens, H. S.: Radiology, *80*:727, 1963.)

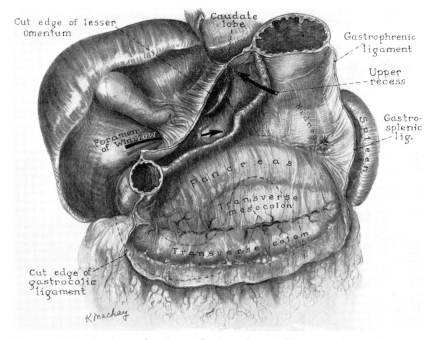

Figure 15–10. Anatomic drawing with stomach partially removed, exposing posterior wall of lesser sac. Note fold of peritoneum raised by left gastric and hepatic arteries. (From Walker, L. A., and Weens, H. S.: Radiology, *80*:727, 1963.)

the transverse mesocolon, and at times the dorsal portion of the greater omentum. At this level, the spleen is largely peritoneal, although there is a small segment dorsally adjoining the kidney which is not completely invested by peritoneum. The spleen is connected with the stomach by a ligamentous mesenteric structure called the gastrosplenic ligament (gastrolienal). The pancreas, both kidneys, the aorta, and superior vena cava are all retroperitoneal structures. On the ventral aspect of the pancreas at this level is the lesser omental bursa.

Along the *right aspect of the lesser omental bursa* are the root structures of the liver or portal triad which are invested partly by peritoneum from the greater peritoneal cavity and partly by the lesser omental bursa. These structures are mainly the *portal vein*, *hepatic artery*, and *common bile duct*—the structures of the portal triad. The foramen of Winslow in cross section is situated on the dorsal aspect of the kidney adjoining the liver, which at this level is completely invested by peritoneum and lies in the peritoneal space. The falciform ligament appears to suspend the liver from the anterior abdominal wall.

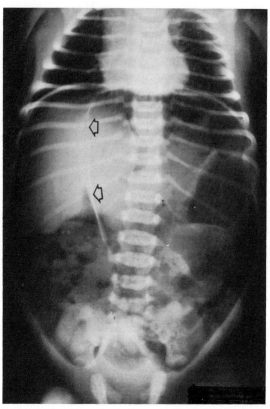

Figure 15–12. "Air dome" or "football sign" indicating a large amount of free air in the abdomen. Arrows point to falciform ligament—the "lacing" on the "football."

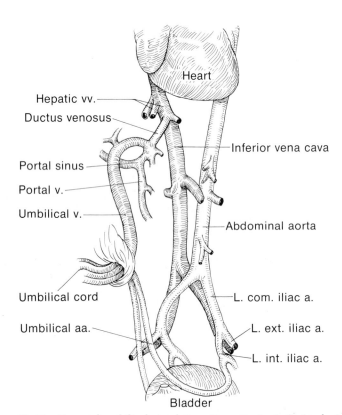

Figure 15–11. Neonatal umbilical circulation. (From Sapin, S. O., Linde, L. N., and Emmanouilides, G. C.: Pediatrics, *31*:946–951, 1963.)

In sagittal section, Figure 15–5, other special relationships can be noted. The liver is almost completely invested by peritoneum except for a small area on its superior and posterior aspects. The omental bursa in part lies posterior to the liver, whereas the general peritoneal cavity is otherwise anterior to the liver and the hepatogastric ligament. The stomach is partially invested by the peritoneum of the omental bursa dorsally, and by the peritoneum of the general peritoneal cavity ventrally. The bands of mesentery extending to the colon and small intestine from the posterior abdominal wall are also shown in diagram. The greater omentum is a sac-like structure which extends down from the greater curvature of the stomach and then folds back upon itself to continue with the posterior wall of the lesser omental bursa and the anterior aspect of the transverse colon.

The *general peritoneal cavity* continues downward to the upper aspect of the urinary bladder and the uterus in the female, and it dips down once again between the uterus and the rectum, investing the anterior aspect of the rectum. Since the sigmoid colon is completely surrounded by peritoneum it is connected by a mesentery with the posterior wall of the abdomen, and is called the "mesosigmoid" or "mesocolon." We have previously noted the vesicouterine pouch and the rectouterine pouch between the uterus and anterior abdominal wall, and the uterus and colon respectively (Figs. 15–7 and 15–8).

The falciform ligament previously described contains the remains of the left umbilical vein of the fetus, and, as pointed out in Chapter 14, it is an important route for venous catheterization in the newborn (Fig. 15–11). The falciform ligament is readily identified in pneumoperitoneum of the infant (Fig. 15–12).

When air is introduced into the peritoneal space the abdominal organs separate from the abdominal wall and the cavity becomes visible.

The Folds of Peritoneum and Fossae of the Pelvis in the Female. The folds and fossae of the pelvis, especially that of the female, are of considerable significance in radiologic anatomy. The *transverse vesicle fold* extends from the urinary bladder lat-

erally to the pelvic wall (Fig. 15–13; this is the same in the male and female). Likewise, there is a *ureteral fold* overlying the ureter in both sexes. In the female, however, there is a *broad ligament* which incompletely divides the pelvic cavity into anterior and posterior compartments by folds of peritoneum draped over the uterine tubes and ovaries (Fig. 15–13). This will be described further in Chapter 17. A third fold in the female is the *rectouterine fold,* which extends from the rectum to the uterus. There is also a strong ligamentous structure extending between the uterus and the sacrum called the *uterosacral ligament* (see Chapter 17).

Potential Peritoneal Spaces. The various reflections in the peritoneal cavity described above create certain potential spaces which can be considerably significant, particularly with inflammatory processes. Thus, the supraomental region contains four recesses: (1) a *right subphrenic recess,* which lies between the right lobe of the liver and the diaphragm and is bounded by the

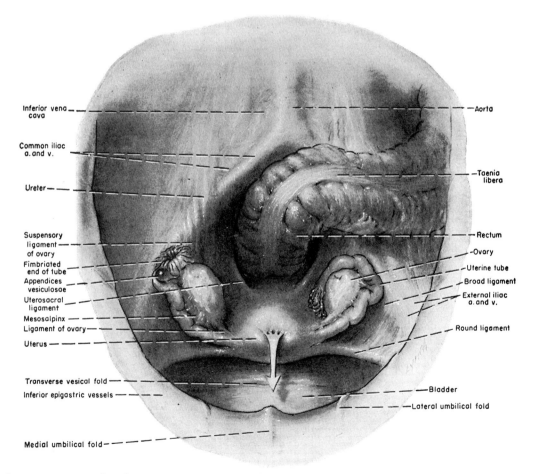

Figure 15–13. Female pelvic organs, anterior view. The uterus is retracted slightly ventrad in the direction of the arrow. (From Anson, B. J. (ed.): Morris' Human Anatomy, 12th ed. Copyright © 1966 by McGraw-Hill Inc. Used by permission of McGraw-Hill Book Company.)

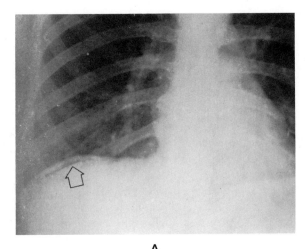

A

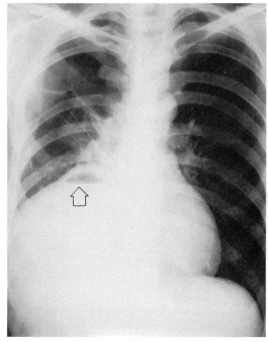

B

Figure 15–14. *A.* Free air beneath the right hemidiaphragm producing a crescentic shadow. *B.* Greater elevation beneath the right hemidiaphragm due to a subphrenic abscess, likewise with free air.

falciform ligament and the coronary ligament. A subphrenic abscess or free air from a ruptured hollow viscus may accumulate here (Fig. 15–14 *A* and *B*); (2) a *subhepatic recess,* which lies between the liver and the other abdominal viscera. Abscess accumulation is prone to occur here also (Fig. 15–15); (3) a *left subphrenic recess,* which is anterior and perigastric and lies between the dome of the diaphragm, the left lobe of the liver, the stomach, the spleen, and the greater omentum. It is also bounded

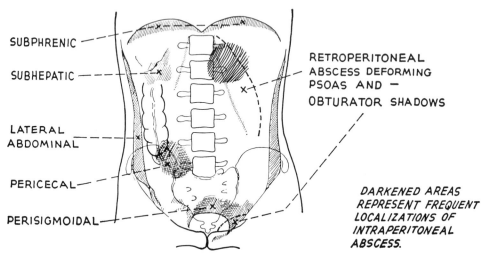

Figure 15–15. Diagram illustrating the various localizations of intraperitoneal and retroperitoneal abscesses.

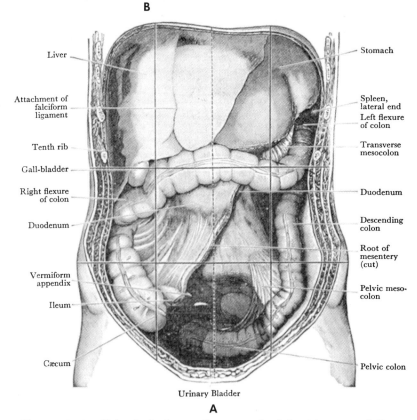

A

Figure 15–16. Abdominal viscera after removal of the jejunum and ileum, demonstrating the three infraomental potential spaces: two created by the root of the mesentery (cut), and the third being the pelvic cavity proper. (From Cunningham's Manual of Practical Anatomy, 12th ed. Vol. 2. London, Oxford University Press, 1958.)

Figure 15–16 continued on the opposite page.

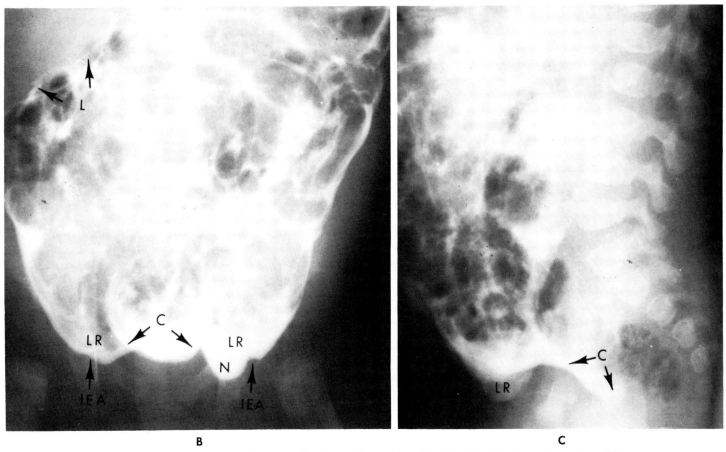

B

C

Figure 15–16 *Continued.* B and C. Normal study. *B.* Note good coating of the lateral peritoneal margins and liver edge (*L*). The contrast material has pooled in the normal lateral recesses (*LR*) and cul-de-sac (*C*). Note the notch due to the inferior epigastric artery (*IEA*) and the normal extension of the peritoneal sac medial to it (*N*).

C. Lateral view (not a necessary part of the examination) showing location of the lateral recesses (*LR*) and cul-de-sac (*C*). (From Swischuk, L. E., and Stacy, T. M.: Radiology, *101*:139–146, 1971.)

by the falciform ligament; (4) the *omental bursa,* which some anatomists regard as a diverticulum from the subhepatic fossae, communicating with the general peritoneal cavity through the epiploic foramen.

The infraomental region contains three potential spaces; two of these spaces are created by the division of the posterior abdominal cavity along the root of the mesentery extending from the duodenojejunal flexure to the right iliac fossa (Fig. 15–16). The infraomental compartment communicates with the supraomental compartments in the neighborhood of the hepatic or splenic flexures of the colon on the right and left sides respectively. The third infraomental potential space is the pelvic cavity proper.

Position of Abdominal Viscera. The usual position of the abdominal viscera as visualized roentgenographically is illustrated in Figures 15–16, 15–17 and 15–18. There is a wide normal range in both form and position of abdominal viscera in the liv

ing. These may be altered by gravity, physiologic changes, or constitutional variations. Even with retroperitoneal structures considerable variation may be noted during life. The urinary and genital tracts will be described in greater detail in Chapters 16 and 17, and the alimentary tract has already been described in Chapters 13 and 14. These organs may all be visualized in part in plain film surveys of the abdomen without additional contrast media by virtue of the fatty envelope or tela subserosa, which surrounds these various organs, or by gas which may be found normally or abnormally in the hollow viscera. Abnormally, calcification in some form may further intensify the image of one or another of these several organs.

The Properitoneal Fat Layer or Tela Subserosa. Between the transverse fascia, which covers the inner surfaces of the abdominal muscles, and the peritoneum lies a considerable quantity of extraperitoneal areolar tissue, which contains a variable amount of fat (Fig. 15–19). This is called the *tela subserosa* and

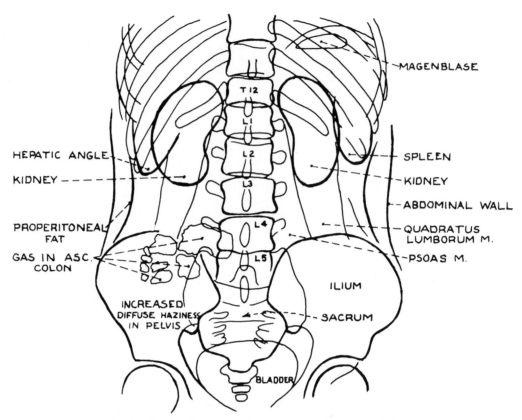

Figure 15–17. Routine for examination of the recumbent film of the abdomen.

its parietal component is called the *properitoneal fat layer*. At times an intraperitoneal fat component is visualized as well. These layers are of considerable importance radiologically, since their identification may reflect intra- or extrainflammatory or neoplastic processes of the abdomen. Moreover, the tela subserosa continues posteriorly, and is particularly abundant around the kidneys, giving rise to a considerable perirenal fat layer. It is this continuation of the tela subserosa around the kidneys ("Gerota's" capsule) that permits a fairly accurate visualization of these organs without the necessity for contrast media (Figs. 15–17, 15–19, and 15–20).

The introduction of a gas such as air in the tela subserosa often separates the fatty layer from the corresponding organ and allows a clear depiction of this organ (Fig. 15–21). Thus, the kidneys and the suprarenal glands can be accurately identified. Somewhat similar depiction, although not as clearly defined, may be obtained by retroperitoneal tomography (Fig. 15–22).

Further Correlative Studies of the Properitoneal Fat Layer (extraperitoneal perivisceral fat pad [EPFP]) (Whalen et al., 1969). Whalen et al. have demonstrated schematically, by comparative cross sections with cadavers, the relationships of the extraperitoneal perivisceral fat pad ("properitoneal fat layer" in other terminology). In Figure 15–23 the extraperitoneal perivis-

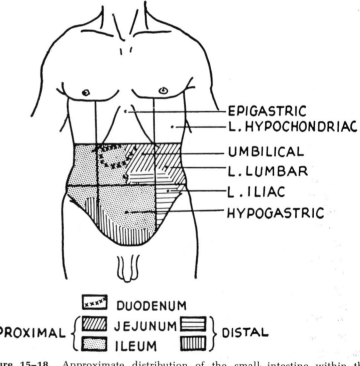

Figure 15–18. Approximate distribution of the small intestine within the abdomen.

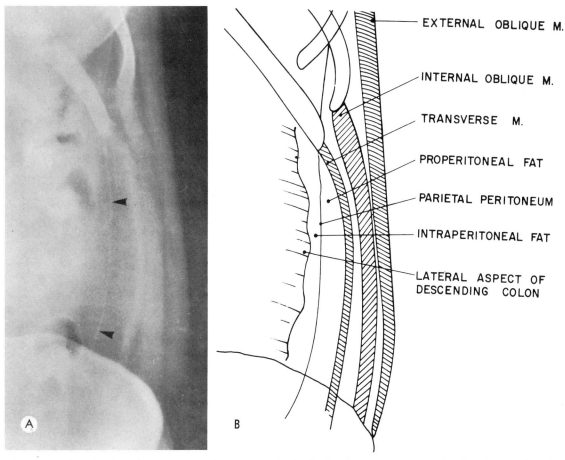

EXTERNAL OBLIQUE M.

INTERNAL OBLIQUE M.

TRANSVERSE M.

PROPERITONEAL FAT

PARIETAL PERITONEUM

INTRAPERITONEAL FAT

LATERAL ASPECT OF
DESCENDING COLON

Figure 15–19. *A.* Normal roentgenographic anatomy in the flank. There is unusually extensive visualization of parietal peritoneum (arrows). *B.* Diagram of roentgenogram. (From Budin, E., and Jacobson, G.: Amer. J. Roentgenol. 99:62, 1967.)

ceral fat pad is shaded, showing an intimate contact of the posterior portions of the liver and spleen with the perivisceral fat. The structures in Figure 15–23 *A* and *B* which are not in contact with this fatty layer are rarely visualized on plain films of the abdomen, whereas those below the indicated horizontal line are consistently identifiable on plain films in older children and adults. The associated schematic frontal view of the liver is also shown.

Schematic frontal and lateral views of the liver (Fig. 15–24) show the fatty layer behind the liver and between it and the right kidney. Whalen and his associates believe that the anterior portions of the right lobe and the entire left lobe are not related to the extraperitoneal perivisceral fat pad, but do relate closely to the colon and stomach respectively. Similarly, in Figure 15–25, a schematic frontal view of the spleen demonstrates the relationship of anterior and posterior margins of the spleen to the fatty layer as well as the splenic angle. The reason for poor correlation between radiological and clinical evaluation of liver and spleen size is explained by the fact that the fatty layer delineates the posterior margin but not the anterior margin of these organs.

The Hepatic Angle and Splenic Angle. The tela subserosa and properitoneal fat not only delineate the flank regions as shown in Figure 15–19 but normally surround the liver and spleen, creating the so-called hepatic angle and splenic angle as shown diagrammatically in Figure 15–23. As shown in diagrams in previous discussions of the anatomy of the liver and spleen, these organs are almost completely enclosed by peritoneum and may therefore be clearly identified by the properitoneal fatty envelope of tela subserosa.

The flank not only has a specific structural pattern but is generally concave between thorax and iliac crest; asymmetry in this shape is clinically significant, since mass or inflammatory lesions may cause a bulging of the flank on one side or the other. Indeed, accurate measurements of the spleen and liver may be made for demonstration of possible abnormalities contained in these organs (see later discussions of the spleen and liver).

A representative abnormality of the right flank and hepatic angle is illustrated in Figure 15–27. In this instance irregularity of the properitoneal fat line and fracture of the right lower ribs in-

(Text continued on page 945.)

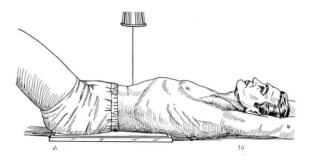

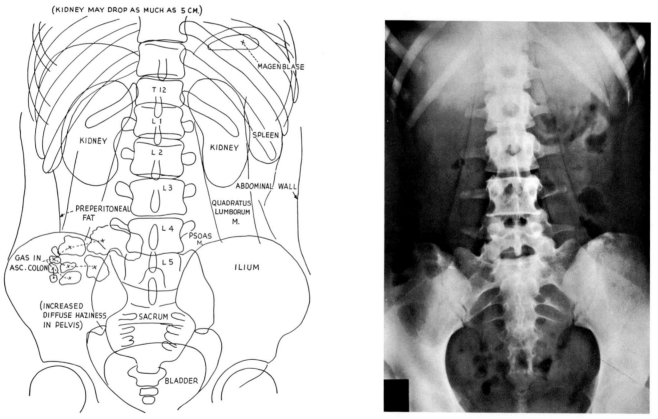

Figure 15–20.   Anteroposterior view of abdomen (KUB film).

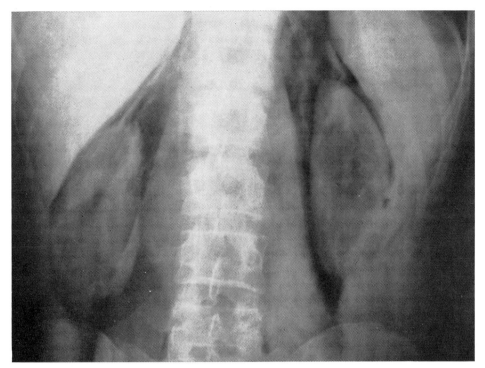

Figure 15–21. Normal retroperitoneal pneumogram. (From McLelland, R., Landes, R. R., and Ransom, C. L.: Radiol. Clin. N. Amer., 3:115, 1965.)

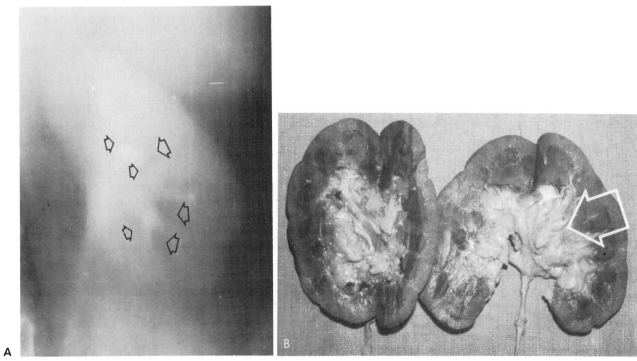

Figure 15–22. Renal fibrolipomatosis. *A.* Excretory urogram (tomogram) showing excessive fat around renal pelvis and calyces. *B.* Specimen.

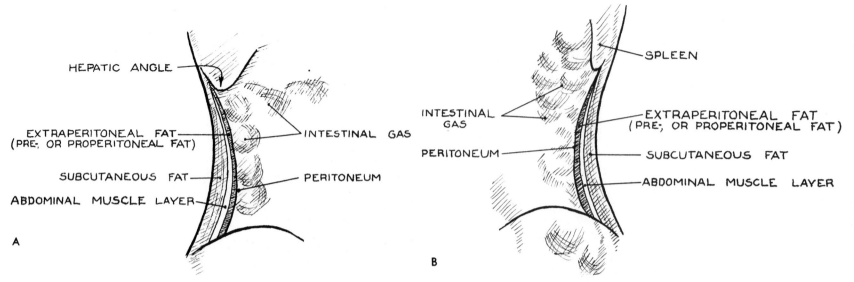

Figure 15–23. *A* and *B.* Diagrams demonstrating flank anatomy, showing the relationship of the properitoneal fat layer to the rest of the abdominal wall.

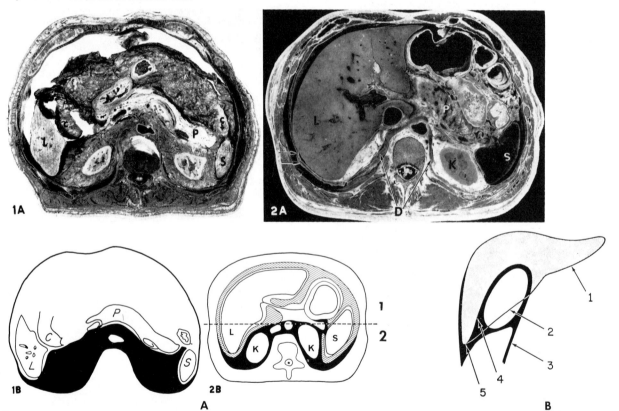

Figure 15–24. *A.* Horizontal cross section (1A) and tracing (1B) of cadaver at the level of the lower border of liver. The "extraperitoneal perivisceral fat pad" is shaded. Note the deep indentation and intimate contact of the posterior portions of liver and spleen with the perivisceral fat. Code: (L) Liver, (S) spleen, (P) pancreas, (C) colon, (D) diaphragmatic crura, (K) kidney.

Horizontal cross section (2A) and schematic drawing (2B) of another cadaver at the level of the upper portion of liver. The structures above the horizontal line (1) which are not in contact with e.p.f.p. are rarely visualized on plain films. The structures below this line (2) and intimate with e.p.f.p. are consistently identifiable on plain films.

Note the diaphragmatic crura buried in the e.p.f.p. (A) and the large fat pad adjacent to the posterior liver and spleen, which is well shown in this specimen.

Observe paucity of e.p.f.p. where diaphragm (↪) contacts the liver. The properitoneal fat lines terminate here.

B. Schematic frontal view of liver. E.p.f.p. shown in black. (1) Left lobe of liver, (2) anterior portion of right lobe of liver, (3) e.p.f.p. outlining psoas muscle, (4) posterior portion of liver, (5) hepatic angle.

Figure 15–24 continued on the opposite page.

year have at least some fat present (Fig. 15–28). Likewise, the splenic outline was not noted in neonates but it was seen in 50 per cent of children over 1 year of age. The psoas muscle margin (to be discussed below) was seen in only one of 23 neonates, but in 56 per cent of the 1 to 5 year age group and in 100 per cent of the 11 to 15 year age group.

The Roentgenology of the Paracolic Gutter. The ascending and descending colon are partially retroperitoneal as shown in Figure 15–4 *C*. When the patient is in the supine position a "paracolic gutter" is created. Normally, the peritoneal gutter either is empty or may contain intestine or omentum; the lines of contrast in the anteroposterior projection are shown in Figure 15–29 *A*. The opposing visceral and parietal peritoneal surfaces may be visualized radiographically as a hair line separating the serosal and retroperitoneal structures. Figure 15–29 *B* shows what happens in the anteroposterior projection when a small amount of fluid is free within the gutter. When increasing amounts of fluid in the gutter (c) spill over into the main peritoneal cavity these roentgen appearances are further modified. Figure 15–29 *C* and *D* illustrates the result of turning the patient first on one side and then on the other, allowing gravity to move the fluid that is free within the peritoneal space out of the gutter; the fluid that is fixed in the retroperitoneal tissues remains immobile (Fig. 15–30). Somewhat similar demonstrations are shown in Figure 15–30 *B* and *C*. "Dog ears" in the pelvis refers to mass densities superior and lateral to the urinary bladder that are sec-

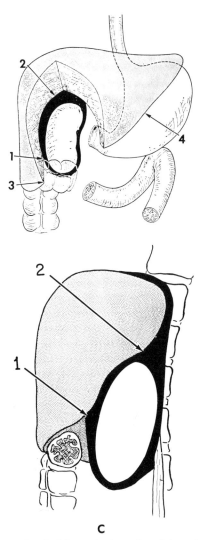

C

Figure 15–24 *Continued.* *C*. Schematic frontal and lateral views of the liver. *Upper*, a section of the liver is absent to show the e.p.f.p. behind the liver and between it and right kidney.

Any surface of the liver between points 1 and 2 may cast a recognizable shadow, depending upon the path of the central ray and the shape of the renal fossa of the liver.

The anterior portions of the right lobe (3) and the entire left lobe (4) are *not* related to the e.p.f.p. and do relate to colon and stomach respectively. (*A*, *B*, and *C* from Whalen, J. P., Berne, A. S., and Riemenschneider, P. A.: Radiology, 92:466–472, 1969.)

dicate an impact over the liver with blood presenting itself in the flank between the fat line and the ascending colon.

Hepatic Angle and Splenic Angle as a Function of Age. Franken has demonstrated that our ability to visualize these angles in children varies depending upon their age. The visualization is related directly to the extent of development of extraperitoneal fat. Only 47 per cent of neonates have a demonstrable properitoneal flank stripe, whereas all children above the age of 1

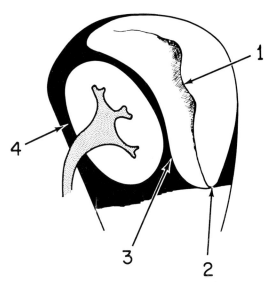

Figure 15–25. Schematic frontal view of spleen. E.p.f.p. shown in black. (1) Anterior portion of spleen, (2) splenic angle, (3) posterior portion of spleen, (4) e.p.f.p. outlining psoas muscle. (From Whalen. J. P., Berne, A. S., and Riemenschneider, P. A.: Radiology, 92:466–472, 1969.)

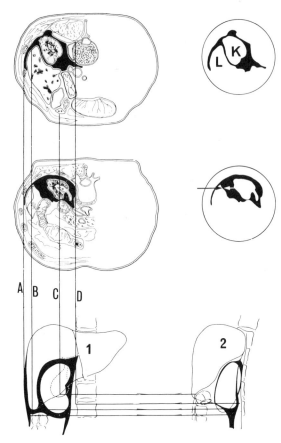

Figure 15–26. Cross-section drawings of normal right upper quadrant, showing that the contour of the pliable e.p.f.p. (black) conforms to the shape and size of the organs indenting it. The roentgen shadows which represent the e.p.f.p. in conventional anteroposterior and lateral views are diagrammed below (1 and 2).

(→ ←) demonstrates the significant anterior-posterior fat-soft-tissue interface which occurs normally. (K) Kidney, (L) liver, (A) properitoneal fat line, (B) posterior portion of liver, (C) anterior portion of liver, (D) spine. (From Whalen, J. P., and Berne, A. S.: Radiology, 92:473–480, 1969.)

ondary to intra-abdominal fluid in the peritoneal recesses lateral to the rectum (Fig. 15–30 D).

Importance of Peritoneal Reflections and Mesenteric Attachments. As discussed earlier, the transverse mesocolon is a major barrier dividing the abdominal cavity into supra- and inframesocolic compartments. The root of the small bowel mesentery further divides the lower compartment into two unequal infracolic spaces.

The external paracolic gutters represent potential channels of spread between the upper and lower abdominal compartments. The left infracolic space is more anatomically continuous with the pelvic cavity. The right paracolic gutter is continuous with the right subhepatic space. This is called "Morrison's pouch," in its posterosuperior extension. The right paracolic gutter may also be continuous with the right subphrenic space, in which case Mor-

rison's pouch is more dependent when the body is in a supine position. The most dependent recess in Morrison's pouch is formed by a peritoneal groove between the lateral aspect of the descending duodenum and the underlying right kidney just above the transverse mesocolon.

The falciform ligament separates the right and left subphrenic spaces. The left subphrenic and subhepatic spaces communicate with one another freely around the smaller left lobe of the liver (Meyers, 1970). This space is also continuous with the perisplenic space.

Variations in the position of the appendix, as pointed out in

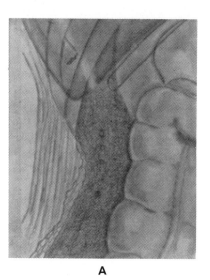

A

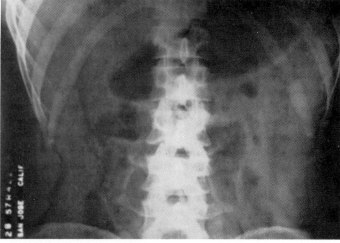

B

Figure 15–27. A and B. Irregularity of the properitoneal fat line and fracture of the right lower ribs indicating impact over the liver. Blood is present in the flank between the fat line and the ascending colon. A mild adynamic ileus is present. At operation there were three lacerations of the liver and a large amount of free blood in the peritoneal cavity. (From McCort, J. J.: Radiology, 78:49, 1962.)

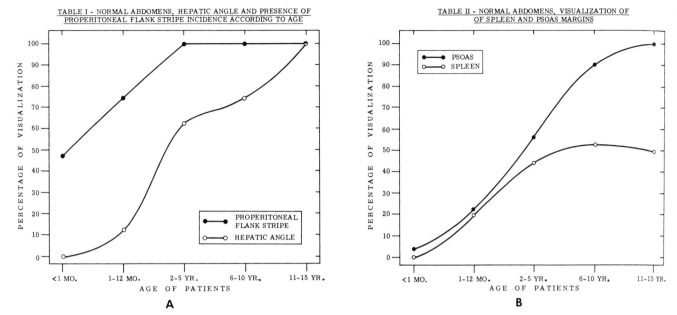

Figure 15–28. *A.* Table showing normal abdomens, hepatic angle and presence of properitoneal flank stripe incidence according to age. *B.* Normal abdomens, visualization of spleen and psoas margins. (From Franken, E. A.: Radiology, *102*:393–398, 1972.)

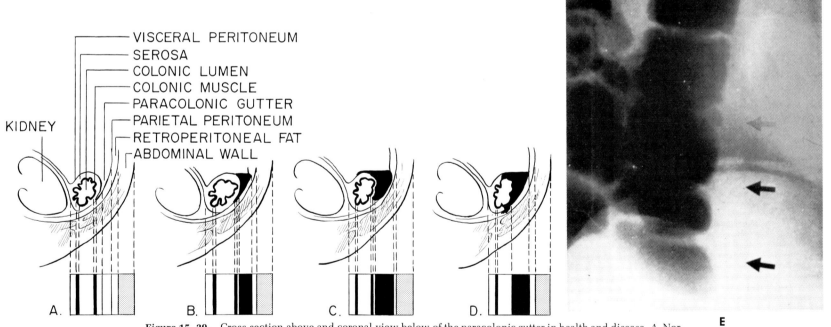

Figure 15–29. Cross section above and coronal view below of the paracolonic gutter in health and disease. *A.* Normal. The peritoneal gutter either is empty or may contain intestine or omentum. The opposing visceral and parietal peritoneal surfaces may be visualized radiographically as a hair line separating the serosal and retroperitoneal masses, both of which may vary greatly in thickness. *B.* Small amount of fluid free within the gutter. *C.* More fluid within the gutter spilling over into the main peritoneal cavity (as with rupture of the spleen or liver). *D.* The fluid (or blood) arising from the retroperitoneal tissues infiltrating the serosa gives a radiographic picture similar to *C*, but should be differentiated from free fluid by various gravity techniques. *E.* Thickened "wall" of colon between gas medially suggested free peritoneal fluid from injured spleen. Surgery demonstrated that the thickened "wall" originated in serosal infiltration from a massive retroperitoneal hematoma. Scoliosis of spine, present in this patient, is not characteristic of ruptured spleen and points more to a retroperitoneal irritation. (*A–E* from Cimmino, C. V.: Radiology, *90*:761, 1968.)

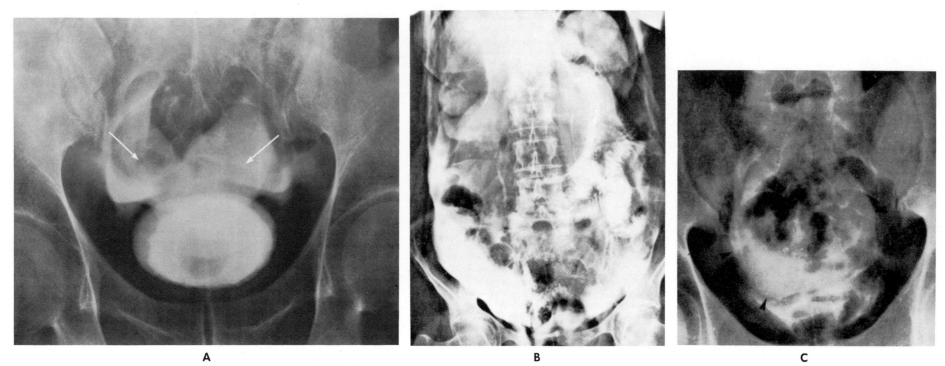

Figure 15–30. *A.* Roentgenogram of the pelvis in a patient with ascites demonstrates the "dog ears" sign. Fluid in peritoneal recesses on either side of the rectum produces "ears" superior and lateral to the bladder shadow. *B.* Extensive leakage of Hypaque during examination of perforated duodenal ulcer demonstrates extent of peritoneal cavity in abdomen; lateral borders represent margins of paracolonic fossae. *C.* Spill of Hypaque during study of ruptured bladder demonstrating pelvic fossa (arrows) just above bladder. (From Budin, E., and Jacobson, G.: Amer. J. Roentgenol., 99:62, 1967.)

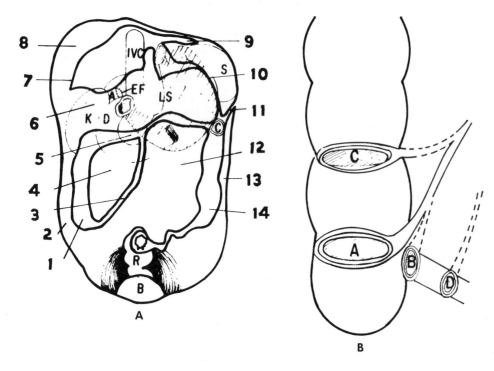

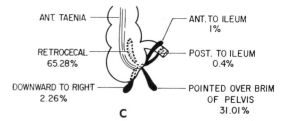

Figure 15–31. *A.* Diagram of posterior peritoneal reflections and recesses. (S) Spleen, (LS) lesser sac, (IVC) inferior vena cava, (EF) epiploic foramen, (K) right kidney, (D) duodenum, (A) adrenal gland, (C) splenic flexure of colon, (R) rectum, (B) urinary bladder, (1) attachment of peritoneal reflections of ascending colon, (2) right paracolic gutter, (3) root of mesentery, (4) right infracolic space, (5) root of transverse mesocolon, (6) area of Morrison's pouch, (7) right triangular ligament, (8) right subphrenic space, (9) left triangular ligament, (10) gastrolienal ligament, (11) phrenicocolic ligament, (12) left infracolic space, (13) left paracolic gutter, (14) attachment of peritoneal reflections of descending colon.

B. Diagram showing variations in the insertion of the lower end of the small-bowel mesentery. The commonest insertion is at the cecocolic junction (A), but possible variations include the ileocecal valve (B), the ascending colon (C) or the terminal ileum (D). (After Testut and Latarjet).

C. Diagram showing the incidence of variations in position of the appendix, as determined by Wakeley. The majority of the retrocecal appendices are also intraperitoneal. (*A, B,* and *C* from Meyers, M. A.: Radiology, 95:547–554, 1970.)

Chapter 14, are also important from the standpoint of determining potential inflammatory foci in the peritoneal space. These relationships are documented by Meyers in Figure 15–31 *A* and *B*. Thus, a knowledge of these basic anatomic attachments becomes of considerable significance in plotting the diagram of pathways of flow of intraperitoneal fluid or exudates.

Displacement of Abdominal Organs by Mass Lesions. A knowledge of the cross-sectional anatomy of the abdomen is particularly important in evaluation of displacement phenomena (Whalen et al., 1971, 1972). Displacement of abdominal organs by

mass lesions is an important indicator in differential diagnosis. Analysis of mass displacements that can occur in the left upper quadrant reveals the following distinguishing characteristics (Fig. 15–32):

1. *Enlargements of the spleen* displace the stomach medially when the enlargement involves the anterior aspect of the spleen, but when the posterior aspect is enlarged, the kidney is depressed.

2. *Suprarenal enlargements* ordinarily increase the size of the triangular space above the kidney, depress the kidney, and

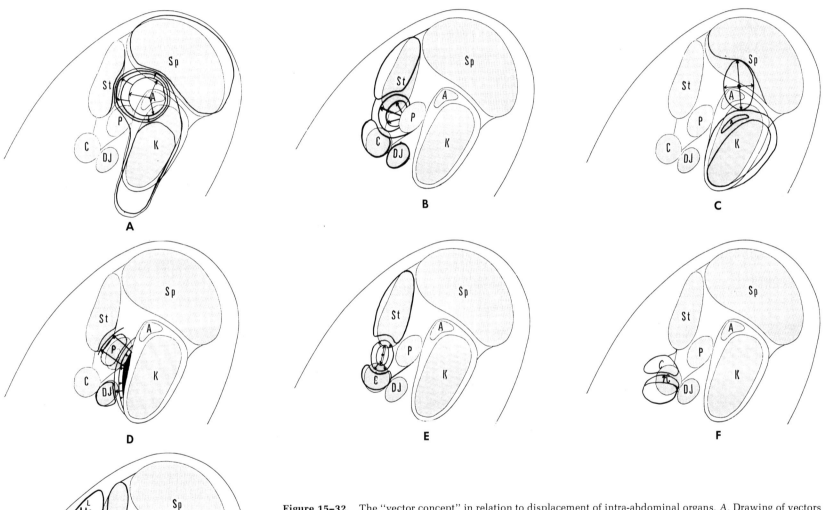

Figure 15–32. The "vector concept" in relation to displacement of intra-abdominal organs. *A.* Drawing of vectors involved with an adrenal mass. *B.* Drawing of vectors involved with a mass lesion of the pancreas. *C.* Drawing of vectors involved with a high extraperitoneal lesion. *D.* Drawing of vectors of a low extraperitoneal mass lesion. *E.* Drawing of vector showing the displacement of an anterior mass lesion, such as a hemorrhagic cyst of the gastrocolic ligament. *F.* Drawing of the vector force of an inframesocolic anterior mass. *G.* Drawing of vectors involved showing the anterior mass effect of an enlargement of the left lobe of the liver. (Sp) spleen, (St) stomach, (A) suprarenal gland, (P) pancreas, (C) colon, (DJ) duodenal-jejunal juncture, (K) kidney. (From Whalen, J. P., Evans, J. A., and Shanser, J.: Amer. J. Roentgenol., 113:104, 1971.)

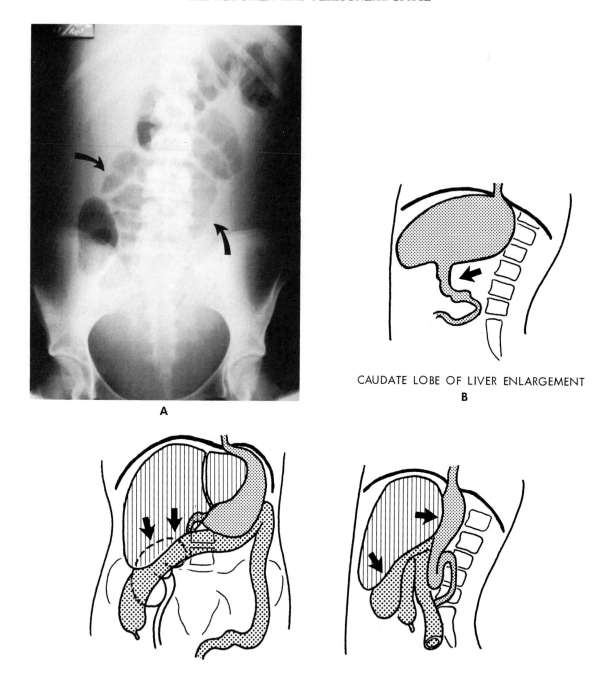

CAUDATE LOBE OF LIVER ENLARGEMENT

B

RIGHT LOBE OF LIVER ENLARGEMENT

DISPLACEMENT OF STOMACH TO LEFT AND POSTERIORLY
DOWNWARD DISPLACEMENT OF RIGHT KIDNEY
NO DISPLACEMENT OF SECOND PART OF DUODENUM
DOWNWARD DISPLACEMENT OF TRANSVERSE COLON
DOWNWARD AND POSTERIOR DISPLACEMENT OF HEPATIC FLEXURE
NO DISPLACEMENT OF DUODENOJEJUNAL FLEXURE

B

Figure 15–33.   *A.* Anteroposterior view of the abdomen: hepatoma with ascites and floating loops of bowel. *B.* Diagrams showing changes with enlargement of the right lobe and caudate lobe of the liver.

possibly impress or elevate the spleen. The splenic artery may be elevated on arteriography but the renal artery may or may not be depressed.

3. *Pancreatic masses* are more anterior than renal or adrenal masses, and they do not usually separate the kidney and spleen unless there is an unusually large pseudocyst or cyst of the pancreas. The duodenojejunal junction is depressed and the stomach is elevated. The splenic artery is not elevated but flattened.

4. *Renal enlargements* produce a variable appearance depending upon the portion of the kidney from which enlargement arises.

5. *Extraperitoneal mass lesions* that are high in the left abdomen simulate adrenal tumors but not as predictably. The kidney is often displaced laterally or downward, and the spleen and kidney may be separated by an inordinate distance.

6. *Low extraperitoneal masses* may simulate superficially pancreatic masses. The stomach is pushed forward and the duodenum is displaced forward, but the duodenojejunal junction may not be depressed.

7. *Mass lesions arising in the gastrocolic ligament* displace the stomach upward and the colon downward without displacement of any posterior structures such as the kidney.

8. *Masses arising in the intraperitoneal cavity* that are *inframesocolic* and tend to elevate the colon, are often near the midline and displace only anterior structures.

9. The *left lobe of the liver* is the most anterior structure in the abdomen. It displaces the stomach posteriorly or downward when enlarged; occasionally the colon will also be displaced downward and posteriorly as well.

10. *Generally, the properitoneal fat or extraperitoneal fat layer defines posterior structures better than the anterior structures;* thus, the suprarenal portion of the spleen, the adrenal, renal, and some extraperitoneal mass lesions are better defined than those that are anteriorly situated.

11. Similarly, Figure 15–33 demonstrates what might occur *when the right lobe of the liver enlarges.* Usually the stomach is displaced to the left and posteriorly, and the hepatic flexure is displaced downward. With caudate lobe of liver enlargement, the pyloric antrum and adjoining duodenal bulb are displaced anteriorly.

There are many other indicators that are outside the scope of this text. These few, however, emphasize the importance of a careful knowledge of the anatomy of the abdomen for radiologic interpretation.

Gas Patterns of the Abdomen. Normally, except in the very young and the very old, gas is not contained in the small intestines. However, it can readily be visualized in the region of the stomach and colon. Often intermixed with the gas shadows in the colon are shadows representing fecal material. In the newborn, gas is ordinarily visualized throughout the gastrointestinal tract by at least 24 hours after birth, but early in the newborn period

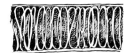 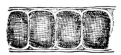 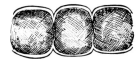

JEJUNUM (NO INDENTED SEROSA; COILED SPRING APPEARRANCE)   ILEUM (NO INDENTED SEROSA)   COLON (NOTE INDENTED SEROSA BY HAUSTRA)

Figure 15–34. Schematic illustration of distended bowel, showing differences between jejunum, ileum, and colon.

such is not the case. The schematic illustrations applying to barium-containing loops of bowel (Chapters 13 and 14) also apply to loops containing only gas. Thus, the valvulae conniventes impart a spiral appearance to the gas shadows of the jejunum, and the spiral loops tend to be close to one another high in the small intestine. In the ileum, however, the valvulae are more widely separated, but can be differentiated from the haustrations of the colon because of the lack of indented serosa at these sites (Fig. 15–34). The gas pattern of the stomach follows closely that pattern that might be expected from our previous descriptions of the barium-filled stomach (Fig. 15–35). Mass lesions impressing themselves on the gas-filled stomach may produce outright roentgen evidence of abnormality resembling the barium-filled stomach (Fig. 15–36).

Abnormal gas patterns in the abdomen are an important indicator of disease, either when they are found outside the usual distribution in the gastrointestinal tract (Fig. 15–37, for example), or when they are so bizarre that they suggest some other pathologic process (Fig. 15–38).

CHANGES IN APPEARANCE OF
GAS-CONTAINING STOMACH

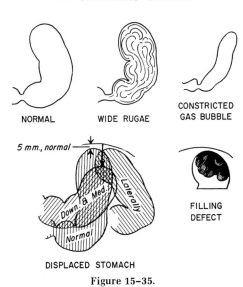

Figure 15–35.

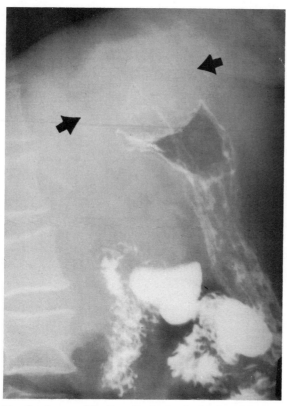

Figure 15–36. Carcinoma of the liver displacing the fundus of the stomach downward from the left hemidiaphragm. This carcinomatous involvement of the liver was thought to be secondary to a carcinoma of the pancreas.

Abnormal gas patterns in the abdomen are of course outside the scope of the present text but are shown here as examples of this important appearance.

Erect or Lateral Decubitus Films for Study of Gas Patterns (horizontal x-ray beam study). As will be shown in our description of films obtained in study of the abdomen, a horizontal x-ray beam is employed with the patient either erect or lying on one side or the other (lateral decubitus) to allow gas to rise to the uppermost level and fluid to gravitate to a lower level, thus frequently giving better definition of (1) free air in the abdominal cavity, or (2) gas-to-fluid interfaces. Moreover, unusual mobility is an indication at times of abnormality, and fixation may likewise indicate the presence of an inflammatory or neoplastic process.

For example, gas bubbles contained in an abscess will move very little when the patient moves, and thus can be differentiated from gas intermixed with feces which will tend to gravitate dependently. When air has escaped into the peritoneal space, it will rise to the highest possible level, and unless there are adhesions preventing such a rise, this gas will accumulate under the diaphragm in relation to its point of origin as described in previous sections (Fig. 15–39). In the upright film, the soft tissue structures of the pelvis minor are less clearly defined, and, in general, structural detail is less distinct than in the recumbent film.

However, in the recumbent film, a large fluid-containing mass with only a very small amount of gas may not be indicated at all because its water density blends with adjoining structures. In the erect position, the fluid level is an important indicator of this mass lesion. A comparison of these appearances is shown in Figure 15–40.

At times gas can be demonstrated in the cecum and ascending colon in an abnormal position in the abdominal cavity, providing an important clue to an abnormality in rotation of the gastrointestinal tract. When the midgut is first withdrawn into the abdominal cavity from the umbilical cord, it occupies a position in the left half of the abdomen with the cecum and ascending colon in the left lower quadrant. Normally, the cecum and ascending colon gradually ascend toward the right to their final position (Fig. 15–41). In a child abnormality of gastrointestinal rotation is a particularly important finding since it may be associated with intermittent or markedly debilitating episodes of intestinal obstruction. Even in the adult it may be an important indicator of such pathology. (The barium-filled gastrointestinal tract is shown in Figure 15–41.)

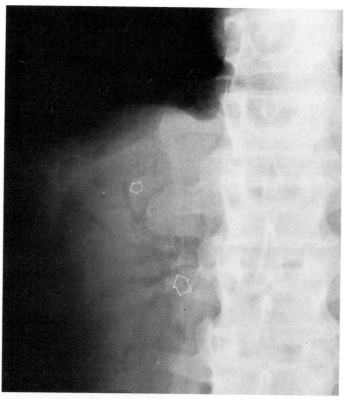

Figure 15–37. Free air in the biliary tract resulting from a surgical communication produced between the gallbladder and the duodenum.

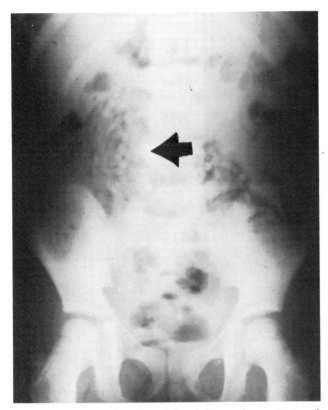

Figure 15-38. Anteroposterior view of the abdomen demonstrating the coiled gas appearance of worm infestation in the gastrointestinal tract.

Prone Position in Study of Gas Patterns. The prone position, particularly in a child, may at times be more advantageous for diagnostic purposes than the supine (Berdon et al.). Marked gaseous distention of the small intestine is frequent in infants due to air swallowing. The prone position may result in markedly improved visualization of the small intestine and the retroperitoneal structures such as the kidneys. In the supine position, sometimes a fluid-filled fundus of the stomach has the appearance of a left suprarenal mass. Likewise, in an infant, the duodenal bulb, when full of fluid, may simulate a mass. When the infant is prone, on the other hand, gastric air fills the fundus (Fig. 15-42) and other posterior loops of alimentary tract, and the central abdomen appears relatively free of gas. The kidneys and adrenal areas may be better seen.

The Psoas Shadows. The fatty tissue contained in the capsule of the iliac and psoas muscles as well as in the region of the obturator fascia permits an accurate delineation of these retroperitoneal structures in most instances (Fig. 15-43). The quadratus lumborum muscle is usually also visible. The aortic shadow, in an adjoining retroperitoneal location, is ordinarily not seen unless it is aneurysmal or contains abnormal calcium deposits from atherosclerosis. Identification of these fascial planes is particularly significant in determination of certain types of retroperitoneal mass lesions such as hemorrhage, inflammation, neoplasm, and aneurysm.

Obliteration of the psoas shadow is likewise important. When the fascial envelope of the psoas muscle is infiltrated by an

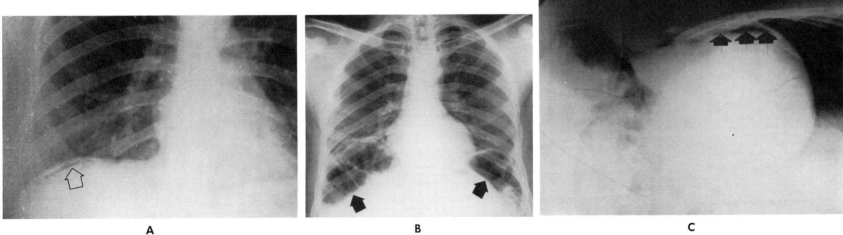

A   B   C

Figure 15-39. *A.* PA film of the chest indicating the rather typical semilunate type of shadow which is produced under the right hemidiaphragm by free air under the diaphragm. *B.* PA film of the chest demonstrating the appearance of interposition of colon under the right hemidiaphragm. This appearance must not be confused with free air under the diaphragm and can usually be distinguished by the appearance of haustrations within the gas pattern. *C.* Free air on the lateral decubitus film study. The free air is above the liver and beneath the right hemidiaphragm.

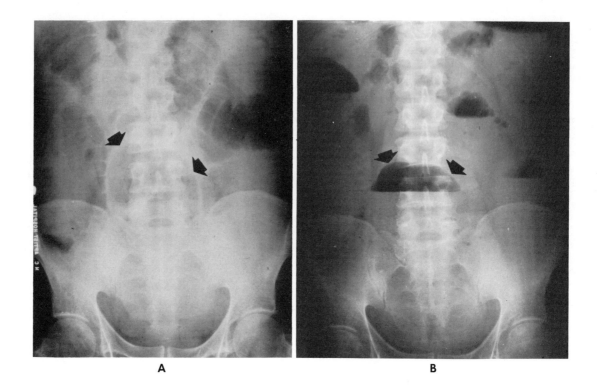

A   B

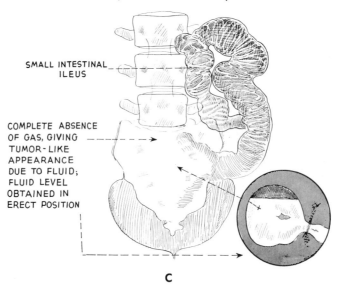

STRANGULATION
(SUPINE APPEARANCE)

SMALL INTESTINAL
ILEUS

COMPLETE ABSENCE
OF GAS, GIVING
TUMOR-LIKE
APPEARANCE
DUE TO FLUID;
FLUID LEVEL
OBTAINED IN
ERECT POSITION

C

Figure 15–40.   Strangulation of a loop of small intestine producing mechanical obstruction. The strangulation was due to internal herniation. *A.* Supine study. *B.* Erect study. *C.* Line tracing. Note the complete absence of gas in the pelvis minor (pseudotumor appearance). The gas in the strangulated bowel is best seen in the erect position.

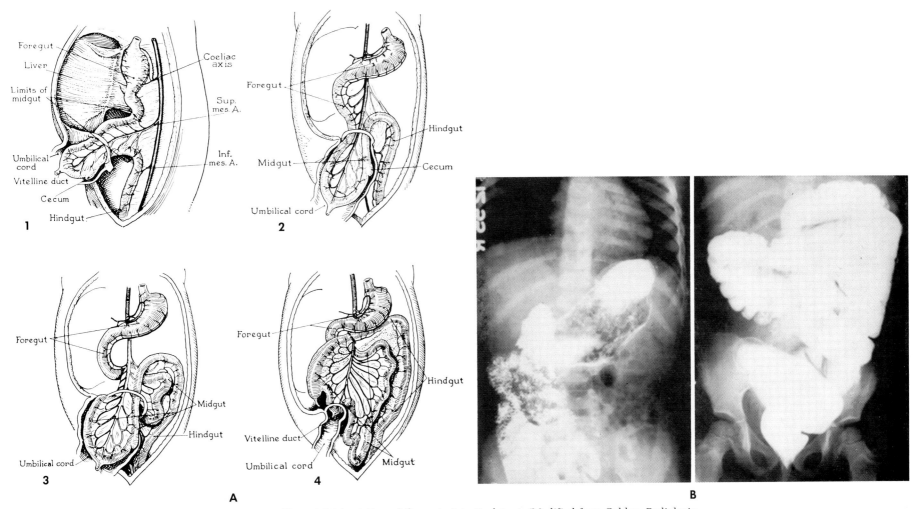

Figure 15–41 *A. 1* to *4.* Normal fetal rotation of the gastrointestinal tract. (Modified from Golden: Radiologic Examination of the Small Intestine; *in* Caffey, J.: Pediatric X-ray Diagnosis, 4th ed. Chicago, Year Book Medical Publishers, 1961.) *B.* Barium-filled gastrointestinal tract demonstrating nonrotation of the small intestine and colon.

inflammatory or neoplastic process, the normal psoas stripe may be obscured. This sign, of course, must be interpreted with caution since overlying gas or intestinal content may give the false impression of such obliteration. A diagram and radiograph illustrating the normal and abnormal obturator fascial planes are shown in Figure 15–43.

Hernia. Hernia may be defined as "the protrusion of any organ or part of an organ from its normal enclosure." Abdominal hernias are quite frequent, and although they are in the realm of the pathological, a brief word about their roentgen anatomy is in order here.

Abdominal hernias may involve any of the abdominal viscera and any of the actual or potential foramina surrounding the general peritoneal cavity. Internal hernias are formed by protrusion

of the gut, usually into certain peritoneal fossae within the abdominal cavities. Usually this is related to a faulty fixation of the mesentery. Thus, there may be a hernia of intestine through the epiploic foramen into the omental bursa. Retroperitoneal hernia may occur at the site of the inferior duodenal recess, and intersigmoid hernia may protrude through the sigmoid mesocolon. Likewise, hernia may occur between unfused components of the transverse mesocolon as well as in the retrocecal or retrocolic region. The incidence of internal herniation as given by Hansmann and Morton is: paraduodenal fossae, 53 per cent; pericecal, 13 per cent; transverse mesocolon, 8 per cent; epiploic foramen into omental bursa, 8 per cent.

The most usual presentation of internal hernias is that of partial or complete obstruction of the small intestine, although

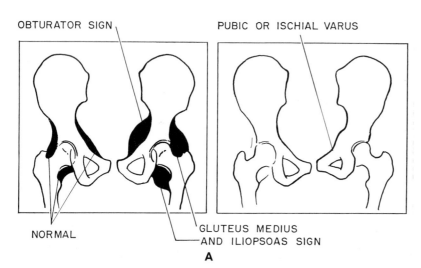

Figure 15–42.   *A.* Diagram of supine abdomen showing localization of air. Note obscuration of renal areas leading to confusion of the transverse and sigmoid colon with the small bowel. *B.* Diagram of prone abdomen showing shift of air with resultant clearing of the renal areas, and improved separation of the colon gas from the small bowel gas. (From Bendon, W. B., Baker, D. H., and Leonidas, J.: Amer. J. Roentgenol., *103*:444, 1968.)

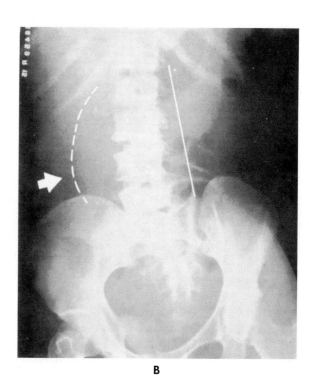

Figure 15–43.   *A.* Diagram illustrating the normal and abnormal obturator and iliopsoas fascial planes of the pelvis and hips. *B.* Radiograph demonstrating the appearance of the widened psoas shadow resulting from a large retroperitoneal abscess. Note the loss of detail in the flank shadow region. (Lines added to show psoas margins.)

the patient may be asymptomatic and diagnosed incidentally during the evaluation of other abdominal symptoms. With a right paraduodenal hernia, almost all of the small intestine is imprisoned in a peritoneal sac behind the ascending and transverse colon, occupying the right half of the abdomen and opening just to the left and near the duodenojejunal junction at the ligament of Treitz. A left paraduodenal hernia occurs on the left side of the abdomen in the mesentery of the transverse descending and sigmoid colon, with the mouth of the sac opening to the right. The left paraduodenal hernia occurs much more frequently than the right in the ratio of approximately 3 to 1. Paraduodenal hernias, in most series, account for more than half of internal hernias.

External hernias are protrusions through gaps or weaknesses in the muscular wall, usually covered by parietal peritoneum. Thus, hernia may occur externally through the diaphragm into the chest, through the lumbar triangle, the greater sciatic foramen, the perineum in the pelvic diaphragm, the obturator foramen, the umbilicus, the inguinal canal, the femoral canal, and ventrally, through surgical defects or through the linea alba above the umbilicus. Of these, the inguinal, femoral, diaphragmatic, and umbilical hernias are the most frequent types.

The Kidneys, Ureters, or Urinary Bladder Without Adequate Contrast. On the plain film, the kidneys are studied from the standpoint of size, position, radiodensity, contour, architecture of the renal fascia, and the presence or absence of calcific shadows. The normal features of these aspects of the kidney as well as the special identification of collecting structures following the introduction of contrast media are postponed for a full description to Chapter 16 (Fig. 15–44).

BLOOD SUPPLY OF THE ABDOMEN

The Abdominal Aorta. The abdominal aorta has been shown in cross section at various levels in Figure 15–4. Its main branches have been described in Chapters 13 and 14. The longi-

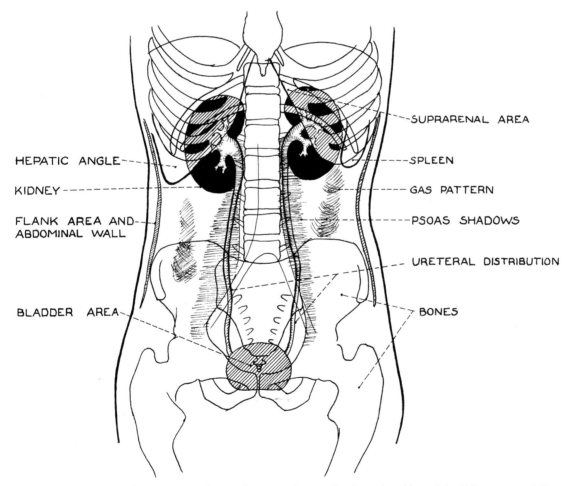

HEPATIC ANGLE

KIDNEY

FLANK AREA AND ABDOMINAL WALL

BLADDER AREA

SUPRARENAL AREA

SPLEEN

GAS PATTERN

PSOAS SHADOWS

URETERAL DISTRIBUTION

BONES

Figure 15–44. Areas where roentgen abnormalities may be visualized on plain films of the kidney, ureteral distribution, and bladder region, apart from calcification (shown later).

tudinal appearance of the abdominal aorta and its primary proximal branches are shown in Figure 15–45. Since the branches have already been described in considerable detail, Table 15–1 is included here as a summary of the arterial supply of the abdomen. The abdominal aorta begins at the aortic hiatus of the diaphragm, usually at the lower level of the twelfth thoracic vertebra, and extends caudad just to the left of the midline. It ends opposite the L4 vertebra by dividing into right and left common iliac arteries. At its origin the aorta is approximately 20 mm. in diameter; just below the renal arteries it is 16.5 mm. in diameter; and at its termination opposite the L4 vertebral body it reduces slightly to 15.9 mm. On its right aspect lies the inferior vena cava, which is ventral to it at the level of L1 and dorsal to it at L4. The aorta is retroperitoneal throughout.

Throughout its length it lies on the anterior longitudinal liga-

ment of the lumbar spine, L1 to L4. The lumbar segmental arteries and the middle sacral artery are all dorsal to the aorta. There are numerous para-aortic lymph nodes along its entire length (the lymphatics will be described more fully later).

The branches of the aorta are shown in Table 15–1 and usually occur in the following descending order: right and left inferior phrenic, celiac, right and left middle suprarenal, right and left first lumbar, superior mesenteric, right and left renal, right and left testicular or ovarian, right and left second lumbar, inferior mesenteric, right and left third lumbar, right and left fourth lumbar, median sacral, and right and left common iliac.

Measurements of the abdominal aorta in the living obtained during the course of intravenous aortography in adults are shown in Table 15–2. In this table, the degree of magnification is not clearly described, and it is suggested that body surface area deter-

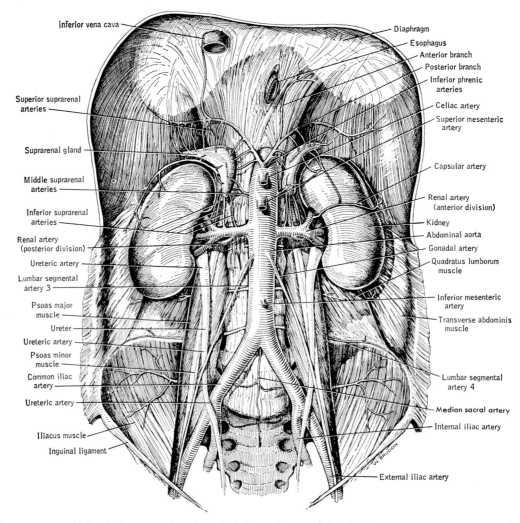

Figure 15–45. Abdominal aorta and its branches. (From Anson, B. J. (ed.): Morris' Human Anatomy, 12th ed. Copyright © 1966 by McGraw-Hill, Inc. Used by permission of McGraw-Hill Book Company.)

TABLE 15-1 ARTERIAL SUPPLY OF THE ABDOMEN*

Distribution	Artery	Origin	Distribution	Artery	Origin
Phrenic Artery, Right and Left			Spleen, pancreas, stomach, greater omentum	Splenic	Celiac
Right crus of diaphragm, central tendon of diaphragm	Inferior phrenic (right and left)	Abdominal	Left portion, greater curvature of stomach	Short gastric	Splenic
Anastomoses with left phrenic, internal mammary and pericardiophrenic arteries	Anterior branch (right and left)	Phrenic	*Superior Mesenteric Artery*		
Anastomoses with intercostals	Posterior branch (right and left)	Phrenic	Pancreas, duodenum	Inferior pancreaticoduodenal	Superior mesenteric
Suprarenal gland, branches to vena cava, liver and pericardium	Superior suprarenal (right and left)	Phrenic	Ileum, jejunum	Intestinal	Superior mesenteric
			Transverse colon	Middle colic	Superior mesenteric
			Ascending colon	Right colic	Superior mesenteric
Suprarenal Arteries, Right and Left			Cecum, appendix, ascending colon	Ileocolic	Superior mesenteric
Suprarenal gland (right and left)	Middle suprarenal (right and left)	Aorta	Mesentery of vermiform appendix	Appendicular	Ileocolic
Lumbar Arteries, I, II, III, IV			*Renal Arteries, Right and Left*		
Bodies of vertebrae and ligaments	Vertebral	Lumbar	Kidney	Renal	Abdominal aorta
Psoas, quadratus lumborum, oblique muscles of abdomen	Muscular	Lumbar	Suprarenal gland	Inferior suprarenal	Renal
			Kidney capsule and perirenal fat	Capsular	Renal
			Upper end of ureter	Ureteral	Renal
Longissimus dorsi and multifidus spinae	Dorsal	Lumbar	Kidney	Terminal branches	Renal
Multifidus	Lateral branch	Dorsal	*Internal Spermatic and Ovarian Arteries*		
Sacrospinalis	Medial branch	Dorsal	Testis	Internal spermatic	Abdominal aorta
Vertebral canal	Spinal	Dorsal	Ureter, adjacent retroperitoneal tissue	Ureteral	Internal spermatic
Celiac Axis			Cremaster muscle	Cremasteric	Internal spermatic
Esophagus, lesser curvature of stomach	Left gastric	Celiac	Epididymis	Epididymal	Internal spermatic
			Terminal branches to testis	Testicular	Internal spermatic
Anastomoses with branches from thoracic aorta	Esophageal branches	Left gastric	Ovary, ureter, uterus, tubes	Ovarian	Abdominal aorta
Stomach, greater omentum	Left gastroepiploic	Splenic	*Inferior Mesenteric Artery*		
Pancreas	Pancreatic	Splenic	Lower half of descending colon, sigmoid, rectum	Inferior mesenteric	Abdominal aorta
Stomach, pancreas, liver, duodenum	Common hepatic	Celiac	Descending colon	Left colic	Inferior mesenteric
Lesser curvature of stomach	Right gastric	Hepatic	Sigmoid flexure of colon	Sigmoid	Inferior mesenteric
Right lobe of liver	Right hepatic	Hepatic proper	Upper part of rectum	Superior hemorrhoidal	Inferior mesenteric
Left lobe of liver	Left hepatic	Hepatic proper			
Gallbladder, undersurface of liver	Cystic	Hepatic proper			
Stomach, duodenum, pancreas	Right gastroepiploic	Gastroduodenal			

*From Bierman, H. C.: Selective Arterial Catheterization. Springfield, Ill., Charles C Thomas, 1969. Table 11.1.

TABLE 15-2 AVERAGE AGE AND DIAMETER IN MM. OF ABDOMINAL AORTA AT SITES MEASURED*

Sex	No. of Cases	Age	At 11th Rib	Above Renal Arteries	Below Renal Arteries	At Bifurcation of Aorta	Difference between 11th Rib and Bifurcation of Aorta
Male	29	53.9 ± 13.7	26.9 ± 3.96	23.9 ± 3.92	21.4 ± 3.65	18.7 ± 3.34	8.14 ± 2.14
Female	44	56.9 ± 14.3	24.4 ± 3.45	21.6 ± 3.16	18.7 ± 3.96	17.5 ± 2.52	6.80 ± 4.54

*From Steinberg, C. R., Archer, M., and Steinberg, I.: Measurement of the abdominal aorta after intravenous aortography in health and arteriosclerotic peripheral vascular disease. Amer. J. Roentgenol., *95*:703, 1965.

Element of magnification not indicated. Target-film distance is 48 inches.

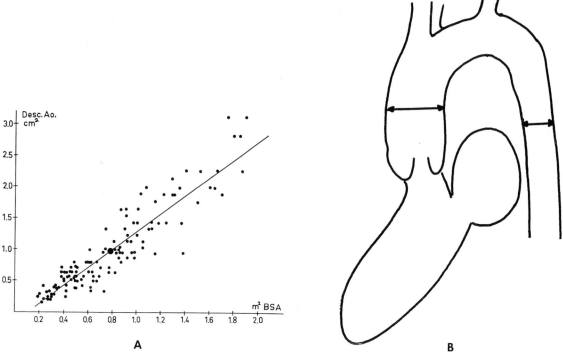

Figure 15–46.   *A.* Descending aorta in cm² plotted against body surface area in m². All diagnostic groups are plotted together since no statistical difference between the groups was found in the co-variance analysis. *B.* Schematic drawing of lateral angiocardiogram. The points of measurements for the ascending and descending aorta are marked by horizontal lines. All measurements were performed on films exposed in systole. (From Arvidsson, H.: Acta Radiol. (Diag.), 1:981–994, 1963.)

minations are not significant. The average of the abdominal aorta was larger for men than for women in this study (Steinberg et al.). For comparison, the measurements of the descending thoracic aorta recorded by Arvidsson are shown in Figure 15–46. Here, the measurements in square centimeters are plotted against body surface area in square meters, resulting in virtually a straight line regression. Thus, a measurement of the descending thoracic aorta of approximately 2.25 sq. cm. is indicated for an average body surface area of 1.7 sq. meters. (It should be noted that this measurement is in square centimeters, in contrast to the measurements by Steinberg et al. which are in linear millimeters.)

Collateral Circulation of the Abdominal Aorta.   There are two general anatomic systems of collateral circulation which develop in response to the gradual occlusion of the abdominal aorta (Bron). These have been designated as collaterals extending between the viscera and systemic circulation as well as from one systemic vessel to another. Schematic illustrations of the more common anastomotic channels are presented in Figure 15–47. The main anastomotic pathway from the viscera to the systemic circulation is a single vessel continuing from the superior mesenteric artery to the internal iliac arteries, via the middle colic artery through the left colic branch of the inferior mesenteric arte-

ry. This vessel passes into the pelvis as the superior hemorrhoidal artery and communicates ultimately with the internal iliac artery.

The anastomotic channels allowing for communication from one systemic branch to another around the aorta are also shown in this figure. This is a rich plexus of vessels involving the flanks, back, and abdominal wall, and consisting of intercostal, lumbar, internal mammary, deep circumflex iliac, and inferior epigastric arteries—all providing blood to the internal and external iliac arteries. In contrast with these vessels are the arterial collaterals (Fig. 15–48 *A, B*) which develop during high and low obstruction of the thoracic aorta (Grupp et al.).

The Inferior Vena Cava.   The inferior vena cava has been shown in cross section in Figure 15–4 *A, B,* and *C.* It is formed by the union of the right and left common iliac veins opposite the L5 vertebral body, passing cranially ventral to the lumbar vertebrae to the right of the abdominal aorta through the caval opening in the diaphragm, and ending in the inferior part of the right atrium of the heart usually opposite the T8 vertebra. In the lower abdomen it is slightly dorsal to the aorta but in the upper abdomen it is on a plane ventral to the aorta, separated from it by the right crus of the diaphragm and the caudate lobe of the liver.

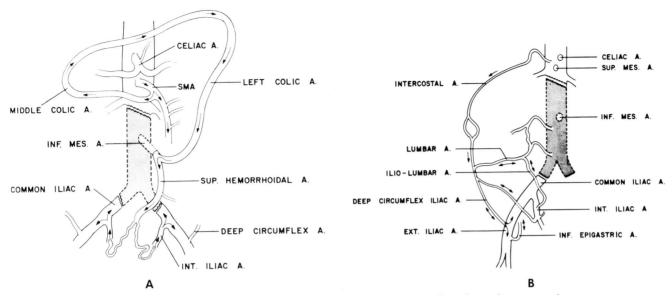

Figure 15–47. *A.* Composite schematic drawing of the viscerosystemic collateral circulation in eight patients with aortic occlusion at the renal level. The shaded area represents the occluded portion of the aorta. *B.* Composite schematic drawing of the systemic–systemic collateral pathways in abdominal aortic occlusion. The shaded area represents the occluded portion of the aorta. (From Bron, K. M.: Amer. J. Roentgenol., 96:887–895, 1966.)

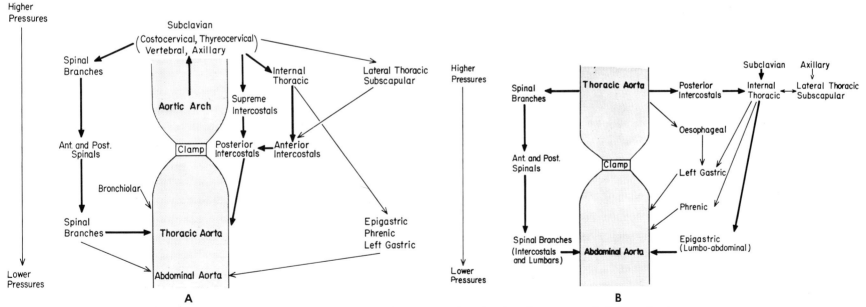

Figure 15–48. *A.* Diagrammatic representation of the arterial collaterals when the aorta is occluded just distal to the left subclavian artery (high occlusion). Heavy lines indicate the direction of preferred flow. *B.* Diagrammatic representation of the arterial collaterals when the aorta is occluded between the origin of the 8th and 9th posterior intercostal arteries (low occlusion). Heavy lines indicate the direction of preferred flow. (From Grupp, G., Grupp, I. L., and Spitz, H. B.: Amer. J. Roentgenol., 94:159–171, 1965.)

Lymphatic channels draining the pelvis and abdomen are in close apposition to the inferior vena cava throughout its course in the retroperitoneal space.

Tributaries to the inferior vena cava generally correspond with branches of the abdominal aorta except for those contributing to the portal vein. The following are the main tributaries:

right testicular or ovarian, renal, right suprarenal, inferior phrenic, and hepatic (which indirectly receives blood from the portal vein). It also receives other smaller tributaries.

A schematic representation of the relationships of the inferior vena cava with surrounding anatomic structures in frontal and lateral views is shown in Figure 15–49 *A* and *B*.

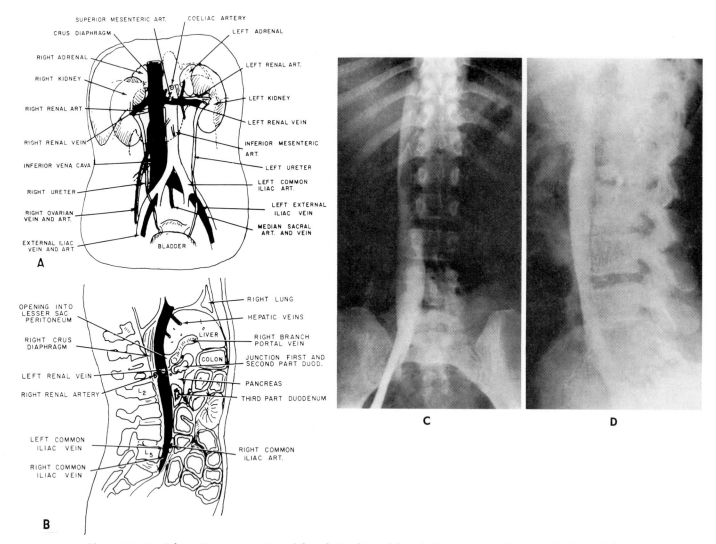

Figure 15–49. Schematic representation of the relationships of the inferior vena cava (shown in black) with the surrounding anatomic structures. *A.* In the anteroposterior view notice the relationships of the vena cava to the course of the external iliac vein and artery, the right ureter, and the relation of the right renal artery, as it crosses from the aorta behind the vena cava, to the right kidney. *B.* In the lateral view the compression of the vena cava by the right renal artery is demonstrated at the level of the interspace between L-1 and L-2. A slight anterior indentation at the lower end of the vena cava caused by anterior compression from the right common iliac artery is also shown. The pancreas and third portion of the duodenum lie just anterior to the vena cava. *C* and *D.* Anteroposterior and lateral inferior vena cavograms in a normal subject. *C.* Note that the course of the right external iliac vessel is smooth and straight and the lateral border of the inferior vena cava in the anteroposterior projection is smoothly outlined. The column of Hypaque shows some dilution from the renal vessels on the left. *D.* In the lateral projection there is a small indentation at the level of the L/1–2 interspace, where the right renal artery indents the vena cava as it crosses from the aorta to enter the right kidney. A slight anterior compression of the upper end of the vena cava is caused by the liver mass. (From Hillman, D. C., Tristan, T. A., and Bronk, A. M.: Radiology, *81:*416, 1963.)

In view of the low pressure and thin wall of the inferior vena cava it is rather readily displaced, distorted, or obstructed by external pressure from adjoining masses. Hence, investigation of the inferior vena cava has a significant place in the diagnostic armamentarium.

The inferior vena cava can be readily examined by means of an injection of approximately 30 cc. of 50 per cent methylglucamine diatrizoate or sodium diatrizoate (Hypaque), manually injected during a 3 second period into a femoral vein, a blood pressure cuff having occluded the opposite femoral vein. The femoral vein may be catheterized, if desired, percutaneously. Alternatively, both femoral veins may be catheterized percutaneously by the Seldinger method and 30 cc. of the contrast agent injected simultaneously through each catheter. The bilateral injection probably gives better results than unilateral injection.

Anteroposterior and lateral views may be obtained simultaneously or in sequence. Six exposures are made, one every three-fourths of a second with a film changer, during which time the patient is directed to suspend breathing and expiration and not to perform a Valsalva maneuver.

The column of contrast medium may appear slightly diluted, particularly opposite the renal region, because blood containing no contrast enters the inferior vena cava at these levels.

These studies are particularly helpful in detecting abnormal mass lesions involving lymph nodes or contiguous organs.

The Inferior Vena Cava After Ligation (Ferris et al.; Grupp et al.).   Surgical procedures to obstruct or filter the blood returning to the heart via the inferior vena cava have been utilized to prevent thrombi from moving through the inferior vena cava into the heart in the course of recurrent embolization. The anatomic routes of venous return after occlusion of the inferior vena cava are numerous, and Ferris et al. have divided these into the following groups:

1. CENTRAL CHANNELS (Fig. 15–50 *A*).   The central channels consist of the ascending lumbar, internal and external vertebral venous plexuses, hemiazygos-azygos system, and the inferior vena cava above the level of occlusion.

2. INTERMEDIATE CHANNELS.   These consist of the ovarian-testicular veins, the ureteric veins, and the left renal–azygos system (Fig. 15–50 *B*). The ureteric veins under these circumstances may attain such a large size that they produce a notching of the ureters radiographically.

3. THE PORTAL SYSTEM (Fig. 15–50 *C*).   The portal system fills via the superior hemorrhoidal anastomoses with the middle and inferior hemorrhoidal plexus. Also, abdominal wall veins may communicate with a patent umbilical vein, thus forming another means of filling the portal veins.

4. SUPERFICIAL ROUTES.   These are very extensive (Fig. 15–50 *C*) and involve many veins, such as the inferior epigastric draining into the internal mammary; the superficial epigastric and circumflex iliac veins draining into the thoraco-abdominal veins; and the lateral thoracic draining into the axillary veins.

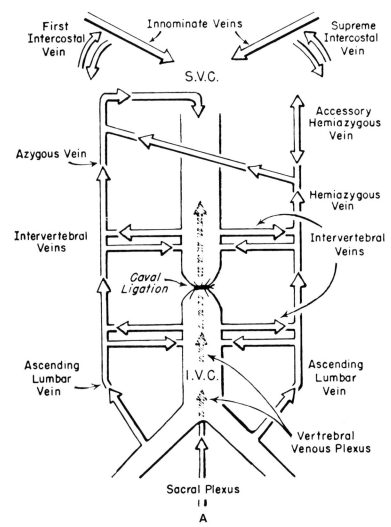

Figure 15–50. *A.* Central channels. The semidiagrammatic sketch shows the central routes of venous return after caval occlusion. The ascending lumbar veins and the vertebral venous plexus are connected at multiple levels by intervertebral veins. These latter permit flow in either direction. (From Ferris, E. J. et al.: Radiology, 89:1–10, 1967.)

Figure 15–50 continued on the following page.

Another diagrammatic representation of the collaterals between the inferior and superior vena cava is shown in Figure 15–50 *E*.

ABDOMINAL LYMPHATICS

The abdominal lymphatics may be discussed under two main categories: (1) the parietal lymph nodes, and (2) the lymphatic drainage of viscera.

Parietal Lymph Nodes. The parietal lymph nodes are largely divided into two main groups: (1) the *epigastric parietal* lymph nodes, which are situated along the inferior epigastric vessels, and (2) the *lumbar parietal* lymph nodes, which are situated

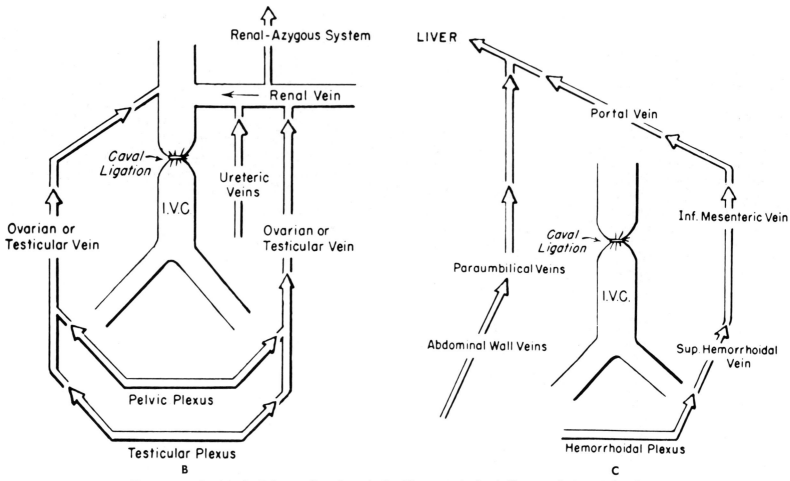

Figure 15–50 *Continued.* B. Intermediate channels. Semidiagrammatic sketch illustrates the intermediate bypass routes of the occluded inferior vena cava. The ovarian or testicular veins usually drain into the renal vein on the left and into the cava on the right. Ureteric veins are included in the intermediate group.
C. Portal route. Semidiagrammatic sketch of the routes of the portal vein filling in obstruction of the inferior vena cava. (From Ferris, E. J. et al.: Radiology, 89:1–10, 1967.)

Figure 15–50 continued on the opposite page.

to the right or left of the aorta, in front of it (preaortic), or behind it (retroaortic). Those to the right of the aorta are generally ventral to the inferior vena cava or dorsal to it, with afferent channels coming from common iliac nodes, gonads, kidneys, and suprarenal and abdominal muscles. Those situated to the left of the aorta are similar to these except that their origins are in the region of the left psoas muscle and left crus of the diaphragm. Those lymph nodes in front of the aorta are mainly clustered around the three major arterial branches: celiac, superior mesenteric, and inferior mesenteric. Those behind the aorta are found largely on the bodies of the third and fourth lumbar vertebrae.

Other groups of lymph nodes of the ilio-pelvic-aortic region are divided as follows: (1) an *external iliac group* situated around the external iliac vessels, (2) a *hypogastric group* near the origin of the different branches of the hypogastric artery in the angles formed by their separation, (3) a *common iliac group* around the common iliac artery, and (4) the *abdominoaortic group* located around the abdominal aorta as described earlier. All of these form the four chains to the right and left, in front of, and behind the aorta (Fig. 15–51).

Lymphatic Drainage of the Pelvic Organs. Figure 15–51 illustrates not only the usual basic anatomy of lymphatics and lymph nodes but also the primary lymphatic drainage of the urinary bladder and testicle. In most instances, the drainage will find its way to the juxta-aortic group. A somewhat similar general pattern of lymphatic drainage exists for the ovary and body of the uterus. The important primary echelon for the pelvic organ is the external iliac, common iliac, and juxta-aortic lymph nodes.

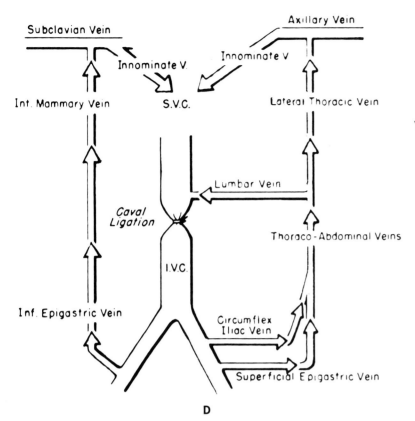

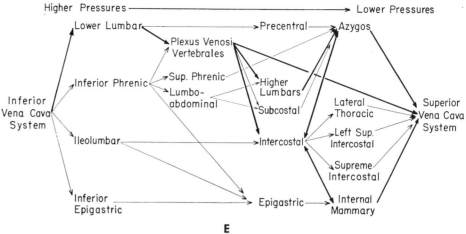

D

E

Figure 15-50 *Continued. D.* Superficial routes. Semidiagrammatic sketch depicts some of the superficial routes of venous return of the occluded inferior vena cava. (From Ferris, E. J. et al.: Radiology, *89:*1–10, 1967.) *E.* Diagrammatic representation of the venous collaterals when the inferior vena cava is occluded just above the diaphragm. Heavy lines indicate the direction of preferred flow. (From Grupp, G., Grupp, I. L., and Spitz, H. B.: Amer. J. Roentgenol., 94:159–171, 1965.)

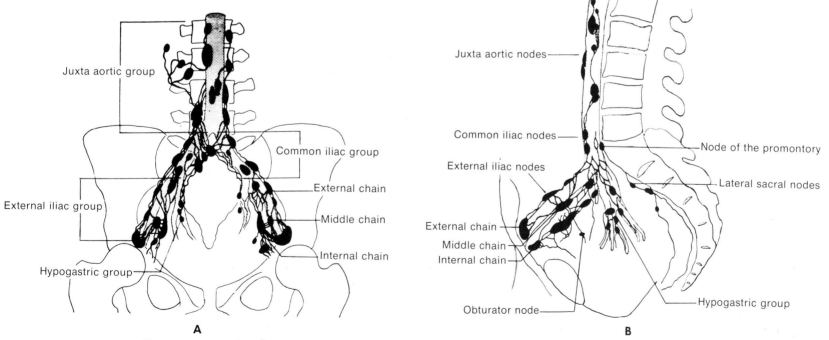

A

B

Figure 15-51. *A.* Semidiagrammatic anterior view based on the anatomical studies of Cunéo and Marcille. The three-chain arrangement of the iliac groups is well shown, and the major node groupings are outlined. *B.* Semidiagrammatic lateral view of the right iliopelvic lymphatic system, again showing the three-chain arrangement of the external and common iliac groups. A small satellite node, which is the true anatomical "obturator" node, is designated. (From Herman, P. G., Benninghoff, D. L., Nelson J. H., Jr., and Mellins, H. Z.: Radiology, 80:82–193, 1963.)

Figure 15–51 continued on the following page.

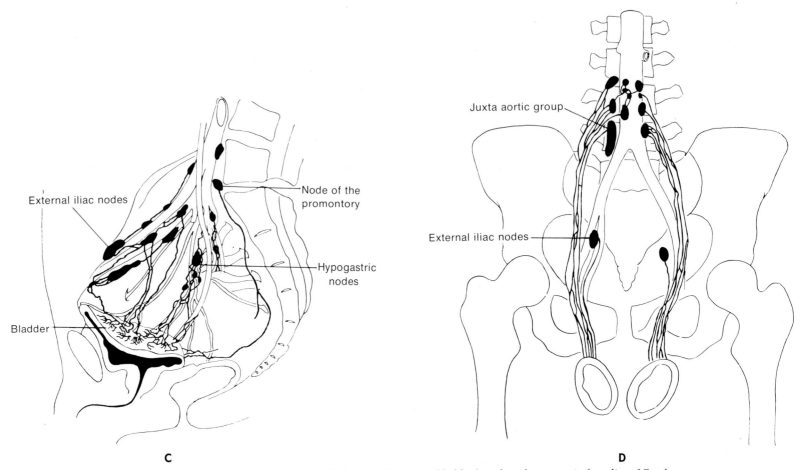

Figure 15–51 *Continued.*   C. Lymphatic drainage of the urinary bladder based on the anatomical studies of Cunéo and Marcille. Note the three lymphatic pedicles leading to the primary echelon of lymphatic drainage of the bladder. The major pedicle leads to the external iliac, while accessory pedicles lead to the common iliac and the hypogastric groups. The same pattern of lymphatic drainage applies to the prostate, rectum, cervix, and the vagina above the hymen. *D.* Lymphatic drainage of the testicle based on the anatomical studies of Rouvière. Note two lymphatic pedicles: a major pedicle leading to the juxta-aortic group and a minor pedicle leading to an external iliac node. (From Herman, P. G., Benninghoff, D. L., Nelson, J. H., Jr., and Mellins, H. Z.: Radiology, *80:*82–193, 1963.)

Figure 15–51 continued on the opposite page.

Generally, the hypogastric nodes are less important in this respect.

The *uterine cervix* has additional clinical significance because the lymphatic drainage is achieved by three main pathways leading to: (1) the *external iliac lymph nodes,* (2) the *hypogastric lymph nodes,* and (3) the *common iliac lymph nodes.* A middle node of the internal chain of the external iliac group has been named by some the *principal node,* and by others the *obturator node* because of its location between the iliac vein and the obturator nerve in the "obturator fossa." This usually adjoins the acetabulum on its inner aspect, or is close to it (Herman et al.).

It is interesting to note that the radiologic demonstration of

lymph nodes corresponds very closely to the classical anatomic descriptions.

Lymphatic Drainage of Viscera (Fig. 15–52). As previously pointed out in the description of the *stomach* (Chapter 14), there are three major zones and flow of the lymphatics in this region: (1) to the superficial gastric lymph nodes, (2) along the inferior gastric, and (3) to the splenic nodes. These in turn drain to the preaortic celiac nodes.

The main drainage of the *liver* is to retrosternal and anterior thoracic nodes, to hepatic nodes, and to preaortic nodes as well as to nodes along the inferior vena cava.

The *pancreas* drains to pancreaticosplenic nodes and from

(Text continued on page 973)

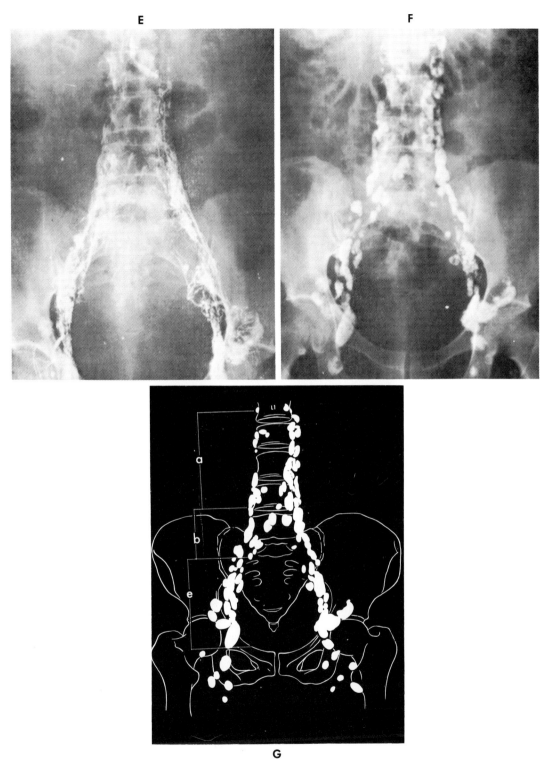

Figure 15–51 *Continued.* *E.* Anteroposterior roentgenogram made immediately after completion of injection of contrast medium. Lymphatic channels are primarily filled, while the lymph nodes are incompletely opacified.

F. Anteroposterior roentgenogram showing the lymph nodes, taken 24 hours after *E.* The striking similarity to Fig. 15–51 *A* is apparent.

G. Tracing of *E,* illustrating the major node groups. (a) Juxta-aortic, (b) common iliac, (e) external iliac. (From Herman, P. G., Benninghoff, D. L., Nelson, J. H., Jr., and Mellins, H. Z.: Radiology, *80:*82–193, 1963.)

Figure 15–51 continued on the following page.

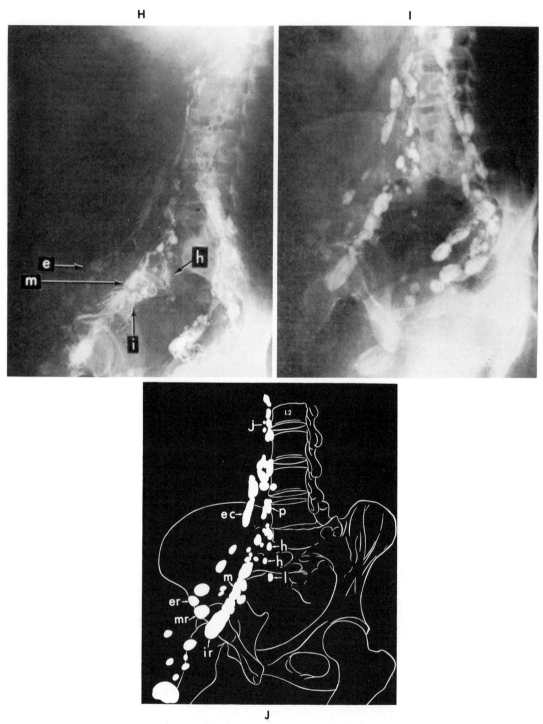

Figure 15–51 *Continued.* *H.* Right posterior oblique roentgenogram made immediately after completion of injection. Lymphatic channels are filled, while the lymph nodes are incompletely opacified. (e) External chain of the external and common iliac groups, (m) middle chain of the external and common iliac groups, (i) internal chain of the external and common iliac groups, (h) channels connecting hypogastric with external and common iliac groups.

I. Right posterior oblique roentgenogram showing lymph nodes as they appeared 24 hours after *H.*

J. Tracing of *I.* (er) External retrocrural node, (mr) middle retrocrural node, (ir) internal retrocrural node, (m) middle node of the internal chain, (l) lateral sacral node of the hypogastric group, (h) hypogastric nodes, (j) juxta-aortic nodes, (p) node of the promontory, (ec) common iliac node. (From Herman, P. G., Benninghoff, D. L., Nelson, J. H., Jr., and Mellins, H. Z.: Radiology, 80:82–193, 1963.)

Figure 15–51 continued on the opposite page.

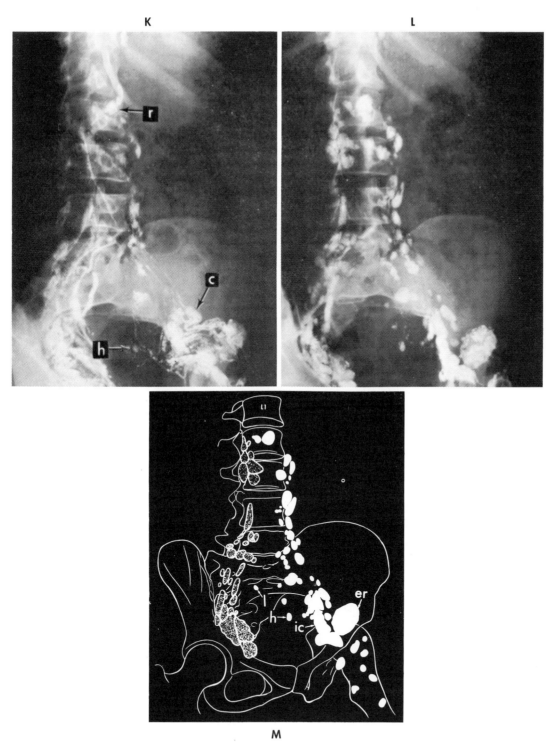

Figure 15–51 *Continued.* K. Left posterior oblique roentgenogram made immediately after completion of injection. Lymphatic channels again dominate the picture, while the nodes are incompletely filled. (h) Hypogastric tributaries connecting with the external and common iliac chains, (c) communications between external and middle chains of the external iliac group, (r) receptaculum chyli.

L. Left posterior oblique roentgenogram showing lymph nodes as they appear 24 hours after K.

M. Tracing of L. (er) External retrocrural node, markedly enlarged. (ic) internal chain, represented by a closely packed group of nodes, (h) hypogastric nodes, (l) lateral sacral nodes of hypogastric group. (From Herman, P. G., Benninghoff, D. L., Nelson, J. H., Jr., and Mellins, H. Z.: Radiology, *80*:182–193, 1963.)

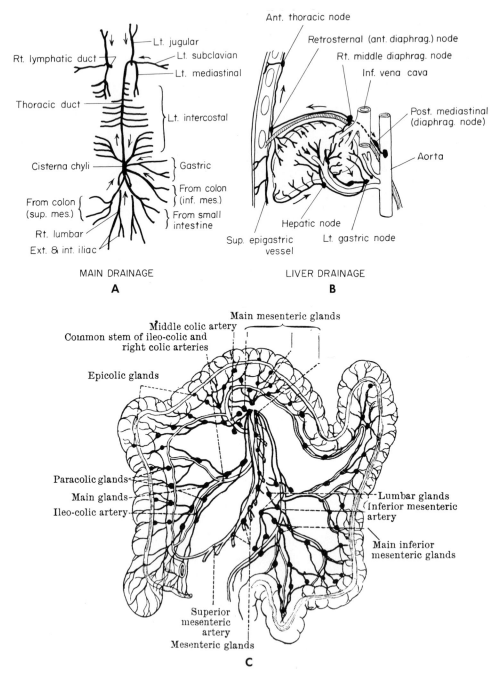

Figure 15–52. *A.* Diagram illustrating the main lymphatic drainage from the lumbar region to the jugular. *B.* Lymphatic drainage of the liver. *C.* Diagram of the lymph glands and lymph vessels of the large intestine. (After Jamieson and Dobson.) (From Cunningham's Textbook of Anatomy, 6th ed. London, Oxford University Press, 1931.)

Figure 15–52 continued on the opposite page.

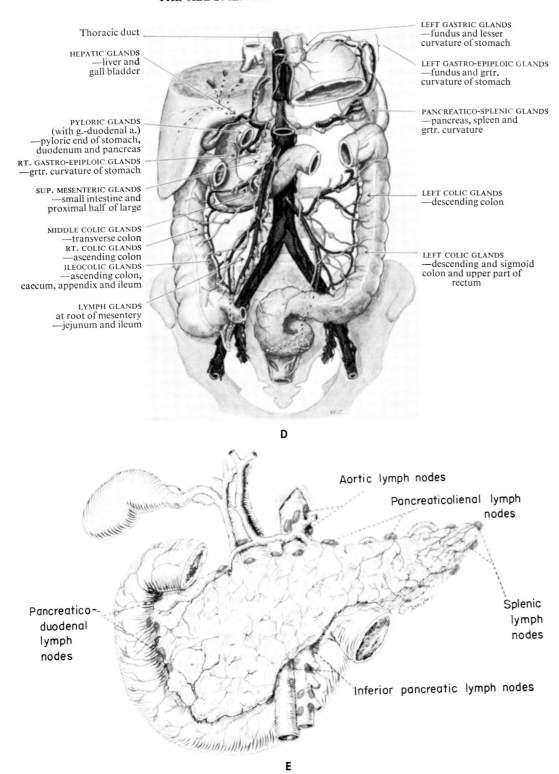

Thoracic duct

HEPATIC GLANDS
—liver and
gall bladder

PYLORIC GLANDS
(with g.-duodenal a.)
—pyloric end of stomach,
duodenum and pancreas

RT. GASTRO-EPIPLOIC GLANDS
—grtr. curvature of stomach

SUP. MESENTERIC GLANDS
—small intestine and
proximal half of large

MIDDLE COLIC GLANDS
—transverse colon
RT. COLIC GLANDS
—ascending colon
ILEOCOLIC GLANDS
—ascending colon,
caecum, appendix and ileum

LYMPH GLANDS
at root of mesentery
—jejunum and ileum

LEFT GASTRIC GLANDS
—fundus and lesser
curvature of stomach

LEFT GASTRO-EPIPLOIC GLANDS
—fundus and grtr.
curvature of stomach

PANCREATICO-SPLENIC GLANDS
—pancreas, spleen and
grtr. curvature

LEFT COLIC GLANDS
—descending colon

LEFT COLIC GLANDS
—descending and sigmoid
colon and upper part of
rectum

D

Aortic lymph nodes

Pancreaticolienal lymph
nodes

Pancreatico-
duodenal
lymph
nodes

Splenic
lymph
nodes

Inferior pancreatic lymph nodes

E

Figure 15–52 *Continued.* D. Abdominal lymph nodes with their main drainage areas. Lumbar and iliac lymph vessels, and nodes, black; portion of aorta removed to show cisterna chyli. (Reprinted by permission of Faber and Faber Ltd. from Anatomy of the Human Body, by Lockhart, Hamilton, and Fyfe: Faber & Faber, London, J. B. Lippincott Company, Philadelphia.) E. Lymphatics of pancreas and duodenum. (From Anson, B. J. (ed.): Morris' Human Anatomy, 12th ed. Copyright © 1966 by McGraw-Hill, Inc. Used by permission of McGraw-Hill Book Company.)

Figure 15–52 continued on the following page.

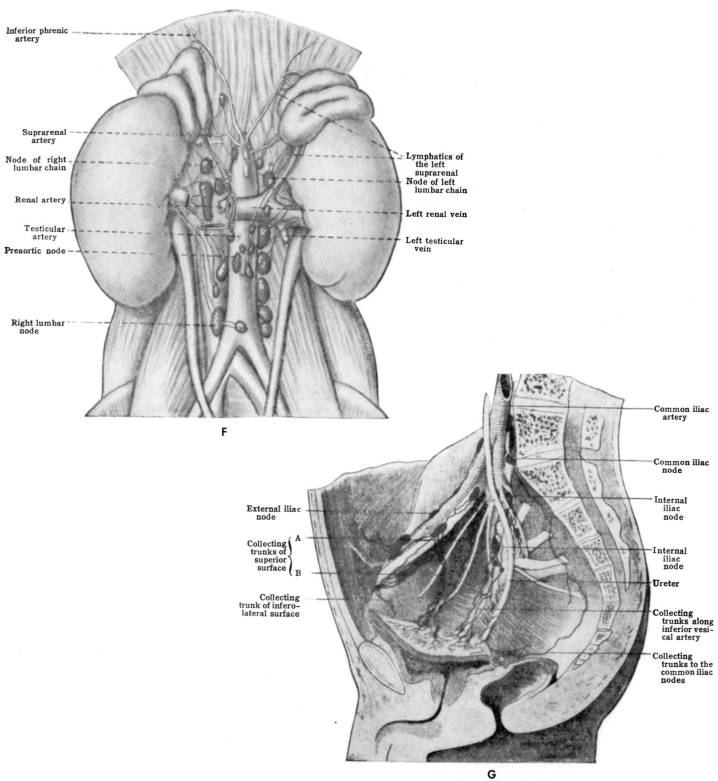

Figure 15–52 *Continued.* *F.* Lymphatics of kidneys and suprarenal glands. (After Poirier and Cunéo.) *G.* Lymphatics of bladder. (After Cunéo and Marcille.) (From Anson, B. J. (ed.): Morris' Human Anatomy, 12th ed. Copyright © 1966 by McGraw-Hill, Inc. Used by permission of McGraw-Hill Book Company.)

Figure 15–52 continued on the opposite page.

there to celiac nodes of the preaortic group, to pancreaticoduodenal nodes, and to superior mesenteric nodes in the preaortic group.

The lymphatics of the *small intestine* are the lacteal to mesenteric nodes in the mesentery; from these lymph flows on to the superior mesenteric group of preaortic nodes.

The *colon* has a lymphatic drainage corresponding closely to its blood supply, with the ascending and transverse colon draining to the superior mesenteric group of preaortic lymph nodes, and the descending and sigmoid colon draining ultimately to the inferior mesenteric group of preaortic lymph nodes.

The *cisterna chyli* is located in front of the second lumbar vertebra behind and to the right of the aorta, just beside the right crus of the diaphragm. It is formed by the right and left lumbar trunks and intestinal trunk. At its termination it narrows down and passes through the aortic hiatus of the diaphragm to become the *thoracic duct* (see Chapter 12).

Diagnostic Criteria for Normal Lymph Nodes

Architecture of Nodes. Lymph nodes generally have a very fine reticular internal architecture. They should normally have no significant filling defects. In the presence of some of the lymphomas (malignant lymphosarcomas), a lymph node often will take on a marked foaminess in its architecture—this must be regarded as abnormal. Moreover, the replacement of more than one-third of a lymph node by a filling defect is an indicator of abnormality.

Lymphatic Channels. The persistence of multiple channels on the 24 hour film is an indicator of lymphatic obstruction. Moreover, excessive filling of channels is sometimes an indicator of partial obstruction.

Measurements. Abrams has advocated three measurements to aid diagnosis of normal lymph nodes (Fig. 15–53). The right lateral spine-to-node distance (measurement B) is the measurement from the right lateral border of a lumbar vertebral body at its midpoint to the most lateral border of the right juxtacaval node group. Measurement C is the left lateral spine-to-node distance similarly obtained. Measurement A is obtained from the lateral view and represents the distance to the most anterior margin of the lymph node chain from the twelfth to the second lumbar vertebrae.

Single lymph nodes were also measured for size, care being taken not to measure clusters but rather isolated nodes. These measurements, as recommended by Abrams, are shown in Table 15–3. The 95 per cent confidence limit for the maximum size of a lymph node is shown to be 2.7 cm.; for measurement A it is 3.2 cm.; for measurement B it is 1.8 cm.; and for measurement C it is 2 cm. Abrams has proposed a maximum normal measurement for lymph node size of 2.6 cm.; a maximum for A of 3 cm.; for B of 2 cm.; and for C of 2 cm. These measurements are based upon 60 normal and 60 abnormal cases.

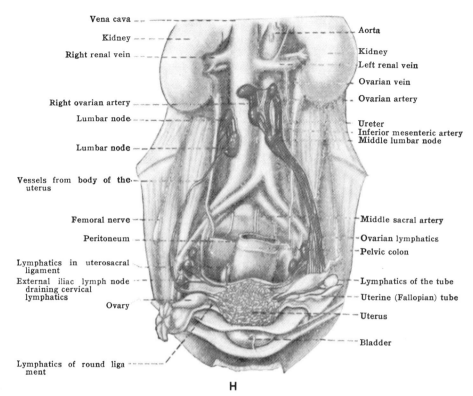

Figure 15–52 *Continued.* *H.* Lymphatics of internal genital organs in the female. (After Poirier.) (From Anson, B. J. (ed.): Morris' Human Anatomy, 12th ed. Copyright © 1966 by McGraw-Hill, Inc. Used by permission of McGraw-Hill Book Company.)

Lymphographic Technique. This technique has been previously described in Chapter 5. A superficial lymphatic vessel on the medial aspect of the dorsum of the foot is cannulated and the contrast material, usually Ethiodol, is slowly injected over a period of approximately 2 hours. (Ethiodol is the ethyl ester of poppyseed oil and contains approximately 37 per cent iodine.) Usually 5 cc. (but as much as 10 cc. can be used on occasion) is injected on each side by a special pumping device.

Generally, 6 to 24 hours after the injection, the Ethiodol concentrates in the lymph nodes, and disappears from the lymphatic channels proper. The lymph nodes retain the contrast material for several months.

Roentgenograms are taken immediately after the injection and then 24 and 48 hours later. The roentgenograms obtained are the anteroposterior, oblique, and lateral projections as well as a posteroanterior view of the chest. At times, at the 24 or 48 hour period it may be desirable to combine this study with intravenous pyelograms. Pelvic arteriograms or venograms may be obtained following the lymphograms for better topographic evaluation.

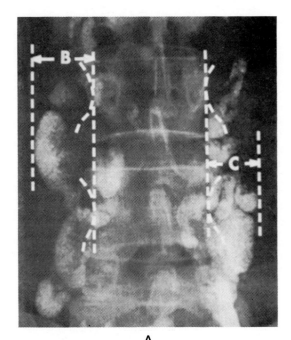

A

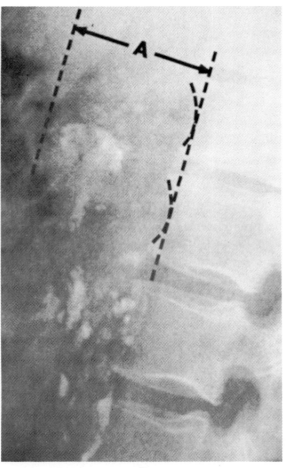

B

TABLE 15–3   SIZE AND POSITION OF LYMPH NODES IN LYMPHOMA*

(a comparison of 60 normal and 60 abnormal cases)

	Mean	± 1 S. D.	± 2 S. D.	Proposed Maximum Normal
Size of Node				
Normal	1.9	0.42	2.7	2.6
Abnormal	3.1	0.96		
Measurement A				
Normal	2.0	0.61	3.2	3.2
Abnormal	3.3	1.32		
Measurement B				
Normal	0.9	0.47	1.8	2.0
Abnormal	1.8	1.24		
Measurement C				
Normal	1.0	0.52	2.0	2.0
Abnormal	2.2	1.17		

*From Abrams, H. L.: Angiography, Vol. 2. 2d ed. Boston, Little, Brown & Co., 1971. Table 80–4.

Radiographic Study of the Peritoneal Space and Abdominal Wall

1. **Anteroposterior Film of the Abdomen, Recumbent.** This is also commonly referred to as a "KUB" film, since it is usually employed in examinations of the urinary tract, and the letters symbolize "kidney, ureter, and bladder." The structures delineated in this examination are shown in Figures 15–54 and 15–56. It will be seen that several layers can be identified in the lateral abdominal wall above the iliac crests: the skin and subcutaneous tissues, the muscular layer, the properitoneal fat layer, and finally the abdominal viscera. The tela subserosa is continued around the kidney, permitting the outline of that organ to be seen; the psoas muscle shadow and quadratus lumborum muscle shadows are likewise differentiated on both sides. The posterior inferior margin of the liver casts a rather well-defined shadow beneath both lower poles of the kidneys and under the peritoneum above the iliac crests. The obturator fascial planes can be clearly delineated on the inner aspect of the pelvic inlet, and often the dome of the urinary bladder, when distended with urine, can be clearly demonstrated by its tela subserosa.

Figure 15–53. *A* and *B.* Three of the four basic measurements that are obtained to show lymphatic size. The fourth measurement is the maximum size of individual lymph nodes. (From Abrams, H.: Angiography, Vol. 2. 2d ed. Boston, Little, Brown & Co., 1971.)

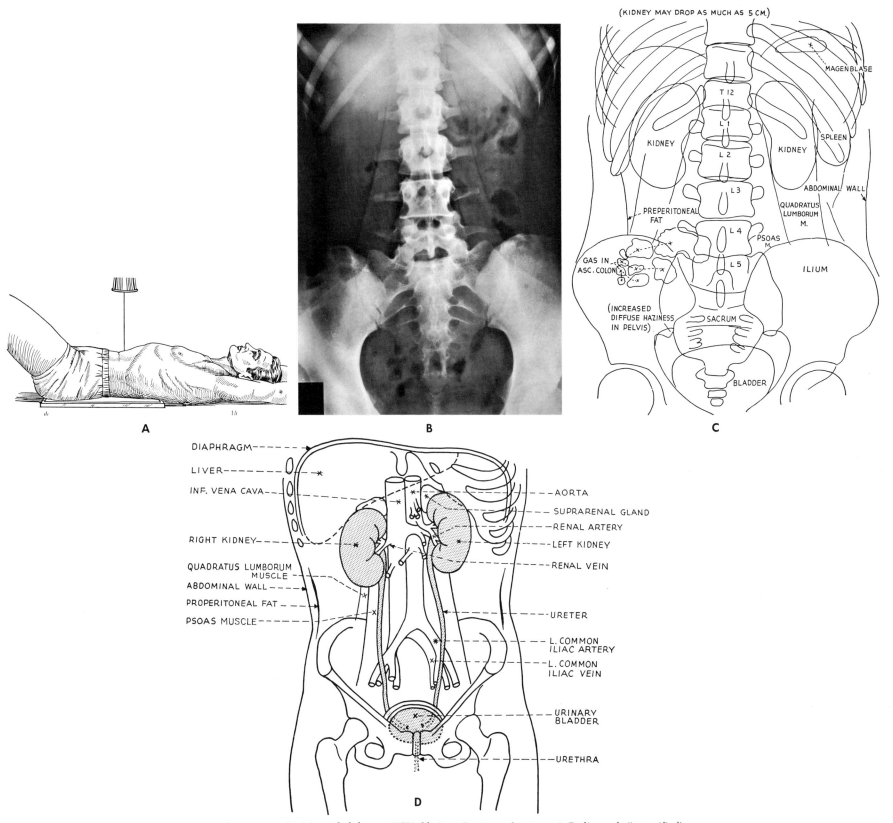

Figure 15–54. Anteroposterior view of abdomen (KUB film). *A.* Position of patient. *B.* Radiograph (intensified). *C.* Labeled tracing of *B.* *D.* Diagram intensifying the urinary tract and indicating other anatomic relationships.

There are variable gas shadows and fecal shadows in the colon and stomach in the adult, and in the small intestine as well in the infant. These tend to obscure soft tissue detail considerably, as well as the detail of the bony structure of the lumbar spine and pelvis. For that reason, if it is desired that such interference be eliminated, and if the patient can be prepared for this examination, it is well to give the patient a good cathartic such as 2 tablespoonfuls of castor oil the night before the examination. If the examination is an emergency, such preparation is of course impossible.

2. **Anteroposterior Film of the Abdomen, Erect.** In this study, most of the abdominal viscera tend to descend owing to the action of gravity. Unusual mobility is an indication of abnormality, but the limits of normal in this respect are fairly great. If there is fluid in the gastrointestinal tract as well as gas, fluid levels are obtained. In the small intestine, such fluid levels are frequently an indication of mechanical obstruction. Abnormally, also, air which has escaped into the peritoneal space may be present, in which case it will rise to the highest possible level. Unless there are adhesions which prevent such rise, this gas will usually accumulate under the diaphragm. In obtaining this film, it is important that the diaphragm be absolutely motionless—otherwise a thin stripe of free air will be obscured and may escape detection. *A rapid exposure technique should always be employed if free air under the diaphragm is suspected, and in our laboratory we employ a separate chest exposure, or lateral decubitus film of the abdomen* (patient lies on his side and a horizontal x-ray beam is employed to obtain a frontal view of the abdomen), as well as the upright film of the abdomen. The chest film allows for simultaneous examination of that portion of the trunk and helps to exclude referred disease—a very important consideration whenever one is confronted with abdominal complaints.

In the upright film, the soft tissue structures in the anatomic pelvis are less clearly defined, and in general, structural detail is less distinct than in the recumbent film.

3. **Patient Supine; Horizontal X-ray Beam.** In this film study, the patient lies supine, and a horizontal x-ray beam is directed at the abdomen from the patient's side. The main purpose of this examination is to demonstrate free air under the xiphisternum, and also to see any fluid levels which may be present in the small or large intestine. All other detail is generally obscured.

4. **Patient on Side; Horizontal X-ray Beam.** In this examination, the patient lies on one side, and a horizontal x-ray beam is directed at the abdomen from the anterior aspect. Ordinarily, a Potter-Bucky diaphragm is employed, if possible, to obtain better detail. The viscera tend to drop by gravity, but if there are fluid levels present, once again they can be readily demonstrated, and any free air in the peritoneal space rises to the uppermost part of the abdomen where it can be seen. This examination is also helpful when it is desired to eliminate gaseous shadows from one side of the abdomen, since the gas-containing loops of bowel will tend to drop away from the side which is uppermost. Kirklin has shown that this can be used efficaciously in gallbladder studies.

Recommended Routine for Study of the Acute Abdomen (Fig. 15–55). The pathologic abdomen is out of the realm of this text, but in this connection it may be pointed out that in the study of a patient for acute abdominal disease, it is well to obtain both a recumbent and an erect film of the abdomen, a chest film, and frequently an additional study with the patient on his side, employing a horizontal x-ray beam.

It is also important to note the degree of separation of the gas-containing loops of bowel, since peritoneal disease will often widen the space between adjoining loops of bowel, which is normally about 2 mm. Indeed, this phase of the study is just as important, if not more so, as the examination for the relative clarity of the properitoneal fat line.

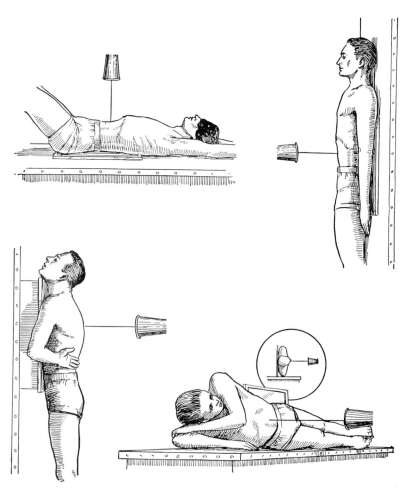

Figure 15–55. Routine film studies obtained for plain film survey of abdominal disease. Note that a PA chest film is part of this routine. (Decubitus left lateral may be preferable.)

A useful routine to follow in examining a KUB film is summarized in Figure 15–56. The following sequence may be used: (1) the kidneys are studied for size, position, contour, density and architecture; (2) the ureteral distribution is postulated and outlined, and any opacities are particularly noted; (3) the urinary bladder area is identified and also the adjoining obturator fascia; (4) the psoas shadows and shadows of the quadratus lumborum muscles are clearly identified; (5) the flank area and abdominal

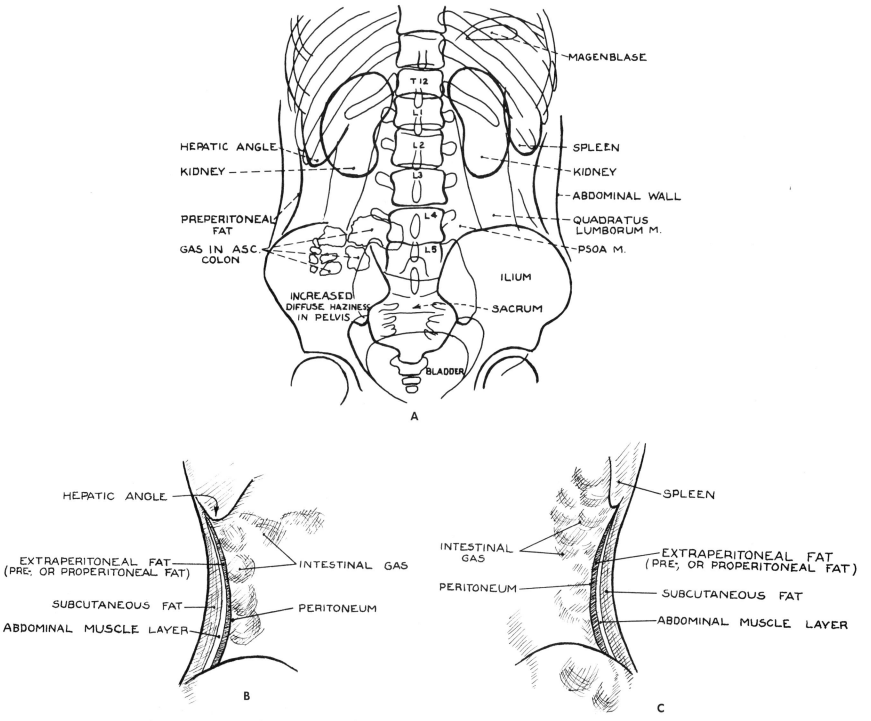

Figure 15–56. Routine for examination of the recumbent film of the abdomen. *B* and *C*. Diagrams demonstrating flank anatomy, showing the relationship of the properitoneal fat layer to the rest of the abdominal wall.

wall are carefully studied (see Fig. 15–56 *B* and *C*); (6) the bony structures are carefully examined for intricate detail and configuration as well as density; (7) the gas pattern is carefully defined; (8) the hepatic and splenic angles are clearly defined if possible; (9) any abnormal masses are described, with particular attention to their size, position, contour, density, and architecture; (10) any opaque shadows in the abdomen are noted and identified etiologically, if possible.

THE LIVER

The basic and radiologic anatomy of the liver and pancreas have been described in Chapter 14 because of the close relationship of these structures to the alimentary tract. Only those aspects pertinent to this section on the abdomen without added contrast will be included here.

Surface Topography; Gross Anatomy. A line connecting the lower border of the fifth rib on the left with the upper border of this rib on the right usually forms the upper border of the superior surface of the liver. This border is ordinarily slightly concave under the xiphisternum. As seen from the front, the lower margin of the liver is found under the costal margin on the right and passes obliquely upward to the eighth or ninth costal cartilage on the left (Fig. 15–54 *D*).

The liver maintains this relationship in the recumbent position, but when erect it drops a variable distance of several centimeters. The position of the liver also varies with the body habitus and the position of the patient.

The falciform ligament on the anterior and superior surface of the liver divides the liver into a large right lobe and a small left lobe. The quadrate and caudate lobes on the inferior surface of the liver are subdivisions of the right lobe, and are important in that they impart an irregularity to the inferior margin of the liver as it is seen on the plain radiograph of the abdomen.

The left lobe of the liver is contained under the cupola of the left diaphragm and overlies the stomach and the spleen.

Although the liver can be moderately well outlined on the plain radiograph, nevertheless it is rather difficult to detect with certainty even with moderate degrees of enlargement.

Areas of calcification as well as bronchovascular markings from the lung may be projected into the liver area from the posterior costophrenic angle of the chest. These must not be misinterpreted as liver abnormalities.

Pneumoperitoneum (Fig. 15–57). The introduction of air into the peritoneal space provides a means of delineating the viscera separately from the abdominal wall. The location, size, mobility, outline, and attachments of the various abdominal organs can be detected in this manner.

Normally, there is a fairly wide range of mobility of the liver,

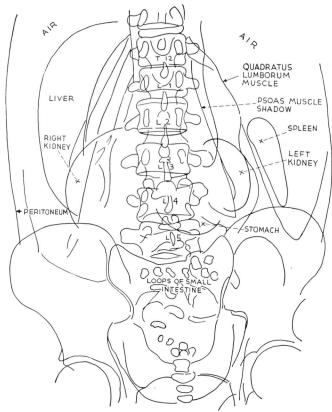

Figure 15–57. Tracing of a radiograph demonstrating pneumoperitoneum in the erect anteroposterior view of the abdomen.

spleen, and other intra-abdominal organs, and any restriction in motion can be readily detected. Examination of the patient while on his left side allows the air to rise over the right lobe of the liver, and the liver drops into the left abdomen, allowing a clear visualization of the right kidney. When the patient lies on his right side, the left kidney, spleen, splenic flexure, and descending colon are visible. When the patient lies prone, with the abdomen suspended between two supports under the thigh and chest, the air rises to the prevertebral space, outlining the structures here.

In the erect position, the liver drops away from the diaphragm and any subphrenic space-occupying lesion becomes readily demonstrable.

Pelvic pneumoperitoneum will be described separately (Chapter 17).

Pneumoperitoneum is somewhat painful and even somewhat dangerous if there is a communication through the diaphragm into the chest. A pneumothorax may result when a marked shift of the mediastinum produces considerable respiratory and cardiovascular embarrassment. Immediate relief of such a pressure pneumothorax is a necessity. There is some question as to whether the information gained is worth the inconvenience of the examination.

Peritoneography. Peritoneography is the double contrast examination of the peritoneal cavity and its contents using a water-soluble positive contrast medium and gas. The technique proceeds as follows (Meyers, 1973a): The patient is given a laxative on the night prior to the examination to cleanse the gastrointestinal tract; cleansing enemas and emptying of the bladder are performed just prior to positioning the patient for examination. The patient should be supine at the time the local anesthetic is administered and during the transabdominal puncture, which is performed in the left supraumbilical area, lateral to the border of the left rectus abdominis muscle. A Rochester needle with a stylet is employed. After the needle has been appropriately inserted and it is certain that a blood vessel or bowel has not been punctured, the inner metallic needle is withdrawn and the flexible plastic outer cannula is allowed to remain in place. Under fluoroscopic control, a small amount of air or meglumine diatrizoate is injected to document the position of the needle in the peritoneal cavity. Approximately 1200 to 1500 ml. of nitrous oxide, recommended as the gas of choice, is introduced during a period of several minutes into the peritoneal cavity. Thereafter, 150 to 200 ml. of 60 per cent meglumine diatrizoate diluted with 50 to 75 ml. of normal saline is instilled into the abdominal cavity. A test dose is first introduced and the patient is observed for any adverse reactions. An open intravenous drip is maintained throughout the procedure and vital signs are monitored. An obturator is then inserted into the cannula, which is taped to the skin to prevent dislodgement.

Roentgenograms of the abdomen are obtained in various positions, supplemented by image amplifier fluoroscopic observation. Increments of 50 to 75 ml. of meglumine diatrizoate can be utilized thereafter to enhance visualization.

Following radiography, as much gas as possible is withdrawn from the abdomen; thereafter the patient remains recumbent for about 30 minutes to 1 hour to allow further absorption of the gas and to minimize abdominal distress.

This examination may be combined with simultaneous upper gastrointestinal study with barium sulfate or intravenous cholangiography. It may also be combined with tomography for more accurate visualization of a given anatomic area.

The structures routinely visualized include the peritoneal reflections and ligaments, such as the parietal peritoneum, greater omentum, lesser omentum, and transverse mesocolon, and the ligaments of the upper abdomen and those surrounding the liver, such as the coronary, falciform, splenorenal, gastrosplenic, phrenicocolic, and umbilical ligaments. No contrast medium apparently gains entrance to the lesser peritoneal sac. The thickness of the wall of portions of the alimentary tract can be described in detail.

Some illustrative radiographs are shown here: (1) In the prone position, peritoneography shows the right lobe of the liver, the gallbladder, greater omentum, the walls of bowel loops, falciform ligament, and spleen (Fig. 15–58 A).

The double contrast examination provides clear visualization of the perisplenic compartment and structures since the spleen is suspended in the left upper quadrant posteriorly by its ligamentous reflections (see Chapter 14 and Figure 15–58 B, C, D). The anterior notched border of the spleen is well outlined (Fig. 15–58 E). The tail of the pancreas may also thereby be seen.

The contrast medium may also gravitate to the pelvic cavity where visualization of the urinary bladder and female reproductive organs may be obtained.

The films recommended by Meyers are: frontal and both oblique projections in the prone Trendelenburg position (20 to 30 degrees), posteroanterior, anteroposterior, right and left lateral with the table horizontal, and frontal and both oblique views in the supine Trendelenburg position. Since the contrast medium gravitates to the pelvic recesses, the earlier phases of the examination are carried out in the prone Trendelenburg position.

About 80 per cent of the nitrous oxide is absorbed within 2 hours. Experimentally, the ascites induced by this intraperitoneal injection of the hypertonic water-soluble contrast agent is completely resorbed in 2 to 24 hours.

Related study of the pelvic structures will be described in Chapter 17.

Herniagram in an Infant (White et al.; Swischuk and Stacy, 1971). Hernias have already been described; they are of primary interest in this text from the standpoint of their anatomic and roentgen presentations. Demonstration of an inguinal hernia in an infant is often difficult. The technique of the herniagram is carried out as follows: With the patient in the supine position, 10 to 15 ml. of 60 per cent meglumine diatrizoate is injected transperitoneally. The injection is usually made in the midline about 1 to 2 cm. below the umbilicus, after a trial aspiration for possible penetration of the bowel or urinary bladder is made. The contrast medium is thereafter instilled and the child is held erect until a single upright anteroposterior roentgenogram of the lower abdomen, penis, and upper thighs is obtained about 5 to 10 minutes later (Fig. 15–59).

There are several advantages to this procedure: (1) It accomplishes the demonstration of occult bilateral hernias. (2) It provides a full delineation of the anatomy of the peritoneal sac before it is distorted by operative manipulation. (3) In addition to the inguinal herniagram, an excretory urogram can be obtained because the contrast agent is so readily absorbed from the peritoneal space. The excretory urogram can be obtained approximately 45 minutes following the instillation of the contrast material into the peritoneal cavity. (4) It requires only a single pelvic roentgenogram with its consequent radiation. (5) It demonstrates at an early age a cryptorchid testis (abdominal testis) associated with the hernia.

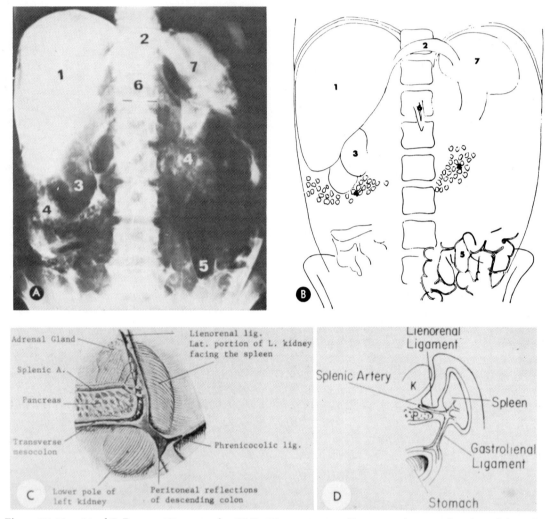

Figure 15–58. *A* and *B*. Prone peritoneography. (1) Positive contrast medium coats the ventral surface of the right lobe of the liver. (2) The arcuate collection resides within the median subphrenic space, anterior to the stomach beneath the central tendinous portion of the diaphragm. (3) The gallbladder displaces the positive contrast medium and is outlined as a "filling defect." (4) The greater omentum presents a characteristic honey-combed appearance. (5) The walls of bowel loops are outlined by contrast medium in the peritoneal cavity and intraluminal gas. (6) The falciform ligament. (7) The spleen. *C.* Posterior peritoneal attachments of the left upper quadrant (after Corning). The spleen has been removed. *D.* Diagrammatic transverse section with emphasis on the peritoneal attachments. The tail of the pancreas (P), anterior to the left kidney (K), resides within the lienorenal ligament. The perisplenic space is bounded by this and the gastrolienal ligament. (From Meyers, M. A.: Amer. J. Roentgenol., *117*:353–363, 1973.)

Figure 15–58 continued on the opposite page.

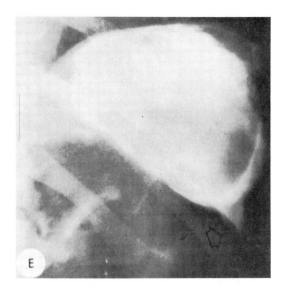

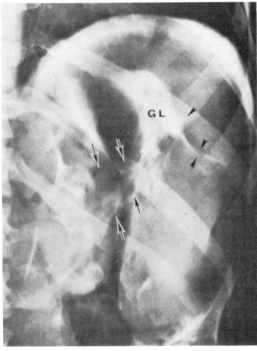

F

Figure 15-58 *Continued.* E. Supine peritoneography. Selective opacification outlines the margins of the spleen to the level inferiorly of the phrenicocolic ligament (arrow). (From Meyers, M. A.: Radiology, *95*:539–545, 1970.) *F.* Prone peritoneography. The tail of the pancreas, ensheathed within the leaves of the lienorenal ligament, is outlined (arrows). It is directed toward the splenic hilus, between the anterior notched border of the spleen (arrowheads) indicated by contrast medium apposing the gastrolienal ligament (GL) and the more medial posterior margin in relationship to the left kidney. Compare to diagram in C. (From Meyers, M. A.: Amer. J. Roentgenol., *117*:353–363, 1973.)

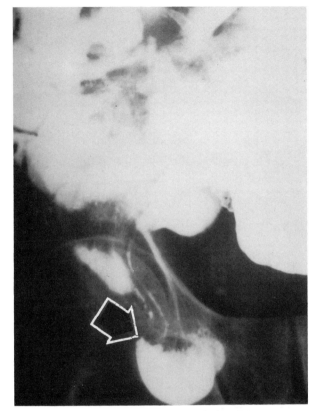

Figure 15-59. Inguinal hernia filled with barium.

In most cases, absorption of the meglumine diatrizoate from the peritoneal cavity occurs within 4 to 8 hours.

It is probably prudent to test for sensitivity to the contrast agent as if it were being injected intravenously.

A normal study is shown for comparison (Fig. 15–60). There is usually a good coating of the lateral peritoneal margin and even the liver edge. The contrast material collects in a pool in normal lateral recesses and cul-de-sacs. A notch caused by the inferior epigastric artery and the normal extension of the peritoneal sac medial to it may be noted.

SPECIAL RADIOGRAPHIC STUDY OF THE LIVER

Hepatolienography with Thorotrast. This is now a historic method since the Food and Drug Administration no longer permits the use of Thorotrast, owing to its inherent alpha radiation and toxicity (Rösch). However, because some patients may have Thorotrast in the liver and spleen even at the present time, it is of clinical interest and utility to recognize its appearance in the abdomen.

Thorotrast is a stable suspension of 25 per cent thorium dioxide which, when introduced intravenously, is stored in the re-

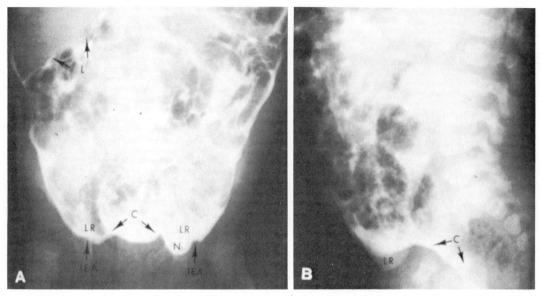

Figure 15–60. *A* and *B*. Normal study. *A*. Note good coating of the lateral peritoneal margins and liver edge (*L*). The contrast material has pooled in the normal lateral recesses (*LR*) and cul-de-sac (*C*). Note the notch due to the inferior epigastric artery (*IEA*) and the normal extension of the peritoneal sac medial to it (*N*).

B. Lateral view (not a necessary part of the examination) showing location of the lateral recesses (*LR*) and cul-de-sac (*C*). (From Swischuk, L. E., and Stacy, T. M.: Radiology, *101*:139–146, 1971.)

ticuloendothelial system. *Because of its long-lived radioactivity, it had the potential to induce late degenerative, fibrotic, and even malignant changes in the liver and spleen.* It was supplied in 25 cc. ampules, and was freely miscible with water or saline. A total dose of 50 to 75 cc. was necessary over a period of several days, given intravenously. The initial dose did not exceed 10 or 15 cc., but in the absence of symptoms, this was increased to 25 cc. intravenously in 1 day. The radiographic examination was made 1 or 2 days after the last dose.

Because the thorium salts were fixed by the reticuloendothelial cells of the liver and spleen, these organs were clearly outlined on the radiograph (Fig. 15–61). Lymph nodes near the porta hepatis may also be seen. Any space-occupying lesions within the liver or spleen were clearly demarcated since they did not become impregnated.

The injection of short-lived radioactive material such as technetium-99m-labeled sulfur colloids has replaced long-acting radioactive material for visualization of the spleen and liver following the advent of various imaging devices in nuclear medicine. The student is referred to textbooks in Nuclear Medicine for further detail.

Hepatic Angiogram. See Chapter 14.

THE SPLEEN

The spleen lies in the left upper quadrant posterior to the stomach and immediately under the diaphragm. It varies in size considerably, but ordinarily does not project significantly below the horizontal plane at the level of the left costal margin. The diaphragm separates it from the ninth, tenth, and eleventh ribs on the left. The medial surface of the spleen is in contact with the tail of the pancreas (Fig. 15–4), and the lower pole of the spleen is in contact with the splenic flexure of the colon. The anteromedial portion of the spleen is in contact with the greater curvature of the stomach (Fig. 15–4 *A* and *B*).

The spleen is supported by *three main ligamentous attachments:* (1) the *phrenicosplenic* ligament, which is a reflection of the peritoneum running from the diaphragm and ventral aspect of the left kidney to the hilum of the spleen, and which contains splenic vessels; (2) the *gastrosplenic* (or gastrolienal), which is actually a dorsal mesentery between the spleen and the stomach, and contains the short gastric and left gastroepiploic artery; and (3) the *phrenicocolic* ligament, which lies beneath the caudal end of the spleen.

The *primary functions* of the spleen are: (1) the *storage of red*

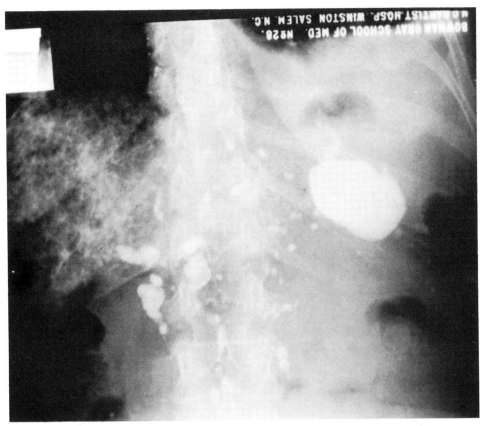

Figure 15–61. Thorotrast hepatolienography following intravenous injection of 60 cc. of Thorotrast in 3 days. This film was obtained 1 week following the last injection. Note deposition in upper abdominal lymph node caudad to the liver. (The use of Thorotrast is no longer permitted for these purposes by the FDA.)

blood cells that may be forced back into the circulation in a respiratory crisis by contraction of the smooth muscle in the capsule and trabeculae; (2) *destruction of worn-out red blood cells;* (3) *removal of foreign material* from the blood stream; (4) *production of mononuclear leukocytes;* and (5) it is an important part of the reticuloendothelial defense mechanism and system.

Normal Blood Supply (Fig. 15–62). The normal vascular supply of the spleen is extremely varied, to the extent that, in one study of 100 dissections, no two vascularization patterns were exactly alike (Michels, 1942). Measurements of the splenic artery have revealed an average length of 13 cm., with a range of 8 to 32 cm., and an average width of 7.5 mm., with a range of 5 to 12 mm. Tortuosity is frequent. There are four main segments of the *splenic artery:* (1) the *suprapancreatic*—the first 1 to 3 cm.; (2) the *pancreatic,* which is usually found in the dorsal surface of the pancreas and supplies small pancreatic branches; (3) *prepancreatic,* which runs obliquely along the anterior surface of the tail of the pancreas and usually branches into a superior and an inferior ter-

minal artery, but occasionally into a medial terminal artery as well; (4) *prehilar,* which is found between the tail of the pancreas and the spleen.

The *dorsal pancreatic artery* originates from the splenic artery in about 40 per cent of dissections. It may arise from the celiac, hepatic, or superior mesenteric artery, and it supplies the dorsal and ventral surfaces of the pancreas in the region of the neck. It has two branches, one which anastomoses with the superior pancreaticoduodenal artery and one which supplies the uncinate process.

A left branch of the splenic artery, the *transverse pancreatic,* runs along the inferior surface of the pancreas until it anastomoses with the arteria pancreatic magna and the caudal pancreatic vessels.

An additional branch may arise from the dorsal pancreatic which communicates with the superior mesenteric artery and provides a collateral pathway between celiac and superior mesenteric channels.

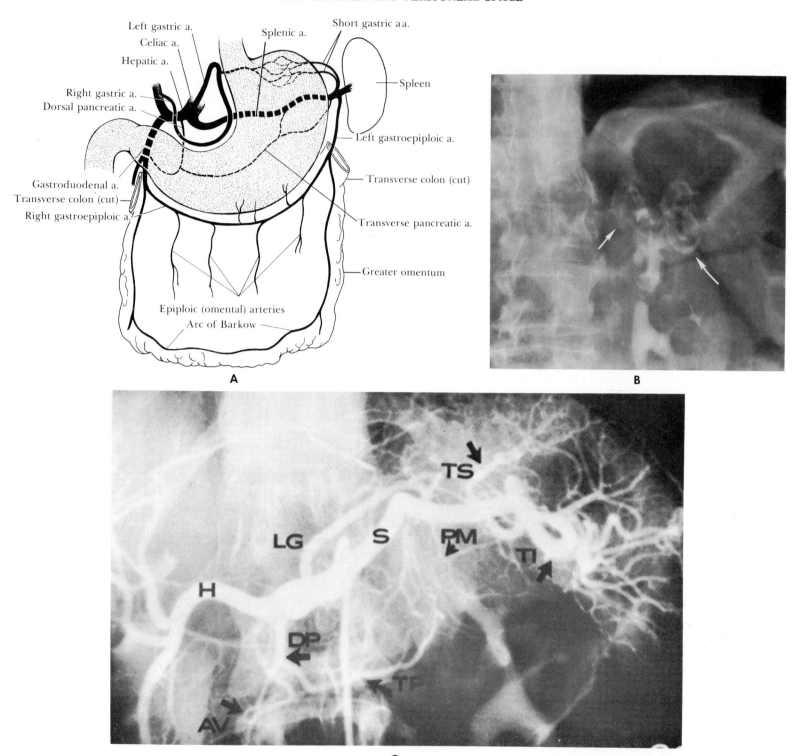

Figure 15–62. *A.* Line drawing representing celiac arterial axis as related to stomach and greater omentum. (Modified from Ruzicka, F. F., Jr., and Rossi, P.: Radiol. Clin. N. Amer., 8:3–29, 1970.) *B.* Dilated and tortuous calcified splenic artery. *C.* Normal splenic arterial anatomy. This 40-year-old female patient was investigated for abdominal pain. Hepatic artery (*H*); left gastric artery (*LG*); splenic trunk (*S*). Superior terminal (*TS*) and inferior terminal (*TI*) vessels supply numerous branches to the splenic parenchyma. The dorsal pancreatic branch (*DP*) is well visualized originating from the proximal splenic and divides into the transverse pancreatic (*TP*) and anastomotic vessels (*AV*) which supply the head of the pancreas and anastomose with the pancreaticoduodenals. The pancreatica magna (*PM*) originates from the second segment of the splenic trunk. (*C* from Abrams, H. L.: Angiography, 2d ed. Vol. 2. Boston, Little, Brown & Co., 1971.)

The *arteria pancreatic magna* is the largest arterial branch of the pancreas, measuring about 2 to 4 mm. in width and arising from the distal third of the splenic artery. It supplies the tail of the pancreas and anastomoses with the transverse pancreatic and with the caudal pancreatic vessels.

The *caudal pancreatic artery* originates from the distal splenic trunk or from the left gastroepiploic artery. It supplies the tail of the pancreas or a small accessory spleen when present. It anastomoses with the transverse pancreatic and arteria pancreatic magna.

There is considerable variation in the terminal splenic branches. They average about 4 cm. in length but may vary from 1 to 12 cm.

The *left gastroepiploic* arises from the splenic artery in about 72 per cent of dissections, 1 to 4 cm. proximal to the primary terminal division. It descends along the right aspect of the greater curvature of the stomach, anastomosing with the right gastroepiploic. There are various branches to the spleen from this vessel. An important branch is the *left epiploic* which originates from the left gastroepiploic near the spleen and descends in a posterior layer of the greater omentum below the transverse colon.

A *superior polar artery* is found in about 65 per cent of dissections, most commonly arising from the splenic trunk proximal to its primary division. It may vary in length from 2 to 12 cm. and in width from 1 to 5 mm. Occasionally, it arises directly from the celiac artery, forming a double splenic artery.

An *inferior polar branch* is found in 82 per cent of dissections, most frequently originating from the left gastroepiploic artery. It varies in length from 3 to 8 cm.

For a detailed discussion of angiographic analysis of normal vessels, their origin and incidence of visualized branches, the student is referred to Abrams' comprehensive review of this subject. The vessel diameters recorded by Abrams were as follows:

Tortuosity and increased length of the pancreatic artery increases somewhat with age but is not necessarily associated with atherosclerosis (Michels, 1955).

TABLE 15-4 DIAMETER OF THE SPLENIC ARTERY
IN ITS VARIOUS PORTIONS

Vessel	Average Diameter in mm.	Maximum Diameter in mm.	Minimum Diameter in mm.
Celiac origin	10.9	21	8
Splenic origin	8.2	14	6
Splenic midportion	7.3	11	5
Splenic hilum	6.5	10	3

TABLE 15-5 THE LENGTH OF THE SPLENIC ARTERY
AND ITS SEGMENTS

Splenic Artery	Average Length in cm.	Maximum Length in cm.	Minimum Length in cm.
Total	17.3	33	8.5
Suprapancreatic segment	2.5	7	1
Pancreatic segment	10.4	22.5	5
Prepancreatic segment	2.5	6	0.4
Prehilar segment	1.5	4.5	0.3

The *splenic vein* emerges from the hilum of the spleen, runs in a groove on the dorsum of the pancreas below the splenic artery, and usually joins the superior mesenteric vein behind the neck of the pancreas to form the portal vein (see Chapter 14).

The *lymphatics of the spleen* drain into the pancreaticosplenic lymph nodes.

The splenic artery and vein run in the phrenicolienal ligament to the hilus and, as noted previously, the artery's course is often tortuous.

To summarize, the significant branches from the splenic artery and vein are: (1) a *left gastroepiploic,* which may or may not anastomose with the right gastroepiploic; (2) *pancreatic branches;* and (3) *short branches to the stomach;* and all of these may provide collateral circulation for the spleen. Because of the end-organ relationship of the arteries, the spleen is subject to infarction.

Ordinarily, the spleen creates a slight impression upon the splenic flexure of the colon and the greater curvature of the stomach.

Calcification (Fig. 15–63) is frequent in the region of the spleen, and this may be due to phleboliths, tubercles, calcified infarcts, splenic artery aneurysms, and certain cysts (hydatid), but this subject is outside the scope of this text. Subcapsular calcification may also occur, but this is also most likely a pathologic degenerative change.

Apart from lobulation, accessory spleens are not infrequently found. These are usually in the neighborhood of the main organ but sometimes they may be distributed elsewhere in the abdominal cavity.

A congenital absence of the spleen may also occur, particularly in relation to some types of congenital heart disease.

Techniques of Examination. The usual techniques of visualization of the spleen are: (1) *plain film studies,* especially anteroposterior or posteroanterior views of the left upper quadrant; (2) *contrast visualization* of the *stomach, kidneys,* or *splenic flex-*

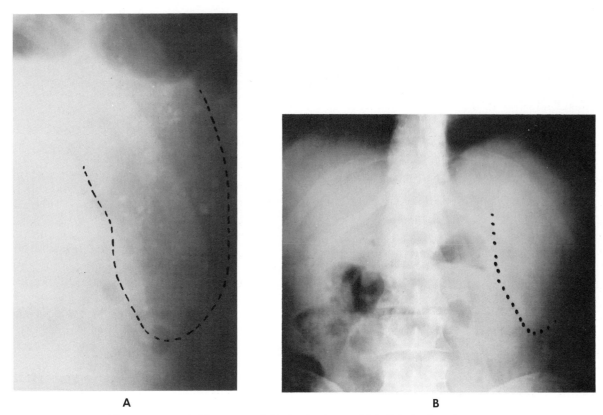

A   B

Figure 15–63. *A.* Numerous calcified tubercles or phleboliths in the spleen.

ure of the colon, together with a visualization of the *diaphragm;* (3) *pneumoperitoneum;* (4) *angiography* (arteriography and venography) through an aortic route; (5) *splenoportography;* (6) *radioisotopic scanning techniques,* using labeled compounds that are taken up selectively by the reticuloendothelial system, such as technetium-99m sulphur colloid (which is also taken up by the liver), crenated red cells labeled with chromium-51, or colloidal gold.

Retroperitoneal air studies with laminagraphy in the anteroposterior projection may be helpful. The spleen is seen best at a distance of 4 to 11 cm. from the back.

The Spleen in the Anteroposterior Film of the Abdomen. The splenic shadow can usually be identified along the left upper lateral aspect of the stomach as a tonguelike structure, the tip of the tongue normally extending to the left costal margin (Fig. 15–17). Only the inferior one-half or one-third of the spleen is visible radiographically on a plain film of the abdomen. Small 3 to 5 mm. calcific tubercles or phleboliths may frequently be recognized within the spleen. Rarely, the splenic capsule itself is calcified (Fig. 15–63). In older age groups, the splenic artery is often seen

as a tortuous calcific aneurysmal structure arising from the celiac trunk medial to the spleen and projected over the stomach.

Measurement of Splenic Size. The caudal tip of the splenic shadow forms a good basis for measurement, as shown in Figure 15–63 *B.* Measurement of the spleen 2 cm. above its tip should not exceed 3.5 cm. (Wyman).

Whitley et al. have demonstrated by means of a computer approach to the prediction of splenic weight from routine films, that the parameters L and W, as indicated on a routine film, provide the most accurate basis for predicting the weight of the spleen (Fig. 15–64 *B*). L is estimated by a vertical line from the tip of the spleen to the intercept with the diaphragm, and W is the width of the spleen at the midpoint of L or as close to this point as this measurement can be made. In their study, the measurement of the spleen 2.5 cm. above the tip was the least accurate and has the lowest correlation coefficient. The product of L and W alone offered a fairly accurate first approximation of splenic weight. Actually, the measurement of L alone is in itself quite accurate and was the single best indicator found by these investigators: "On a routine abdominal film in an average sized adult, an L of more than 11.3 cm. can give a 70 per cent probability, and an L above 15 cm., a 98 per cent probability of the spleen being enlarged. . . .

"If the product of L and W is obtained, correcting for magnification: if this product is 50 or more, the probability is 75 per cent that the spleen's weight is more than 200 grams; and if this product is 75 or more, the probability is 98 per cent that the spleen's weight is more than 200 grams."

THE PANCREAS

Gross Anatomy (Figs. 15–65, 15–66). The pancreas has already been described in relation to the stomach and duodenum (see Chapter 13). It lies transversely and obliquely on the posterior abdominal wall, its right end in the concavity of the duodenum and its left end touching the spleen. The greater part of the pancreas lies behind the stomach.

Anatomically, it is subdivided into a head, body, and tail having the following relationships. The head, which is largely retroperitoneal, is in contact superiorly with the pylorus and proximal portion of the duodenum; on the right with the descending duodenum and terminal portion of the common bile duct; caudally with the horizontal portion of the duodenum; and on the left with the terminal ascending portion of the duodenum. The inferior vena cava and abdominal aorta lie behind it. The body crosses to the left where it tends to pass upward slightly and posteriorly as it traverses the spine, left kidney, and adrenal gland.

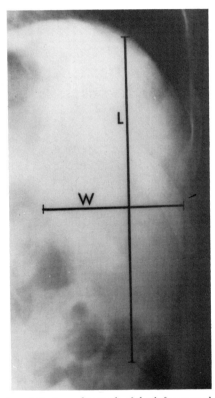

Figure 15–64. Anteroposterior radiograph of the left upper abdomen illustrating the parameters L and W superimposed on the image of the spleen. (From Whitley, J. E., Maynard, C. D., and Rhyne, A. L.: Radiology, *86*:73–76, 1966.)

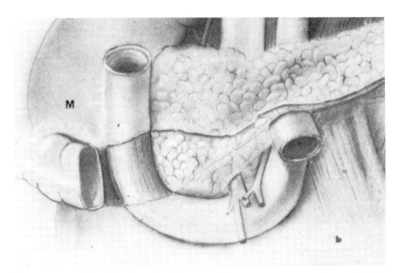

Figure 15–65. Drawing showing the root of the transverse mesocolon, extending across the infra-ampullary portion of the duodenum and the lower border of the pancreas. Note the relationships of the anterior hepatic flexure of the colon and of the duodenojejunal junction. M marks the location of Morison's pouch, the intraperitoneal posterior extension of the right subhepatic space. (From Meyers, M. A., and Whalen, J. P.: Amer. J. Roentgenol., *117*:263–274, 1973.)

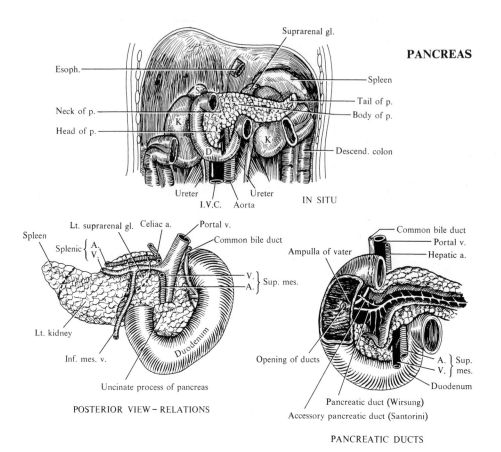

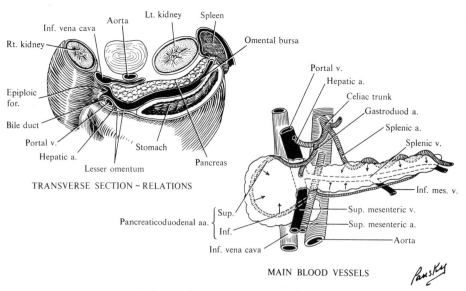

Figure 15–66.   Summary of anatomic details of the pancreas: *in situ*, from posterior view, pancreatic ducts, transversely, and main arterial supply and venous drainage. (K) kidney, (D) duodenum, (I.V.C.) inferior vena cava, (a.) artery, (v.) vein, (aa) arcades. (From Pansky, B., and House, E. L.: Review of Gross Anatomy. New York, Macmillan Company, 1964.)

It forms the posterior wall of the lesser omental bursa. The tail of the pancreas projects into the splenorenal ligament and is in contact laterally with the medial aspect of the spleen, and caudally with the splenic flexure of the colon.

As noted previously, the pancreaticoduodenal arteries are situated on the ventral aspect of the head of the pancreas along with pancreaticoduodenal veins and superior mesenteric vessels. The splenic artery runs along the superior margin or border of the body of the pancreas. The root of the transverse mesocolon extends across the middle of the head of the pancreas and lower border of the body. The splenic vessels cross ventral or dorsal to the tail of the pancreas on their way to join the spleen (Fig. 15–66).

These relationships of the pancreas are important radiographically since it is only by displacement of contiguous structures that abnormalities of this organ can be recognized.

The relationships of the pancreatic duct and accessory pancreatic duct have been previously described in conjunction with the biliary system (Chapter 13).

Accessory or supernumerary nodules of pancreatic tissue are not rare, and they may occur anywhere in the foregut. They are most common in the duodenum and are usually situated in the postbulbar region on the right aspect of the second part of the duodenum.

At times a ring of glandular tissue from the head of the pancreas surrounds the descending duodenum, forming an annular pancreas. The aberrant pancreas can usually be recognized by the smoothness of the filling defect produced and by the dimple centrally related to a supernumerary pancreatic duct draining into the adjoining gastrointestinal tract.

METHODS OF EXAMINATION OF PANCREAS

Plain Posteroanterior Film of the Abdomen. This is useful only if the pancreas contains abnormal calcific deposits, or if there is obvious displacement of the stomach as seen by the gas contained within it.

Barium Meal. The stomach and duodenum are outlined with barium, and displacement of these organs as seen in the posteroanterior and lateral projections is of significance in detecting abnormality in the pancreas.

Passage of Radiopaque Tube into the Stomach and Duodenum. This method basically involves the same principle as the barium meal in that displacements of the tube are interpreted in the light of enlargement of the pancreas or lesser omental bursa. This method has the advantage of not requiring the introduction of an opaque medium; thus, interference with the presence of calcium in the pancreas is avoided. The stomach and duodenum are not outlined as accurately as they are with barium, however.

Introduction of Air into the Stomach. Air may also be used to outline the stomach, but it does not provide as clear visualization as does barium. Posteroanterior and lateral views of the abdomen are taken as before, and displacements of the stomach detected by this means.

Other Methods

Laminagraphy with retroperitoneal air, combined with gaseous distention of the stomach and duodenum. This technique has not received wide acceptance.

Hypotonic duodenography (see Chapter 13).

Angiography (see Chapter 13).

Radioisotopic techniques are generally considered of only moderate usefulness and are outside the scope of this text.

Peroral pancreaticobiliary ductography (see Chapter 13).

Transduodenal pancreatic ductography (see Chapter 13).

THE ADRENAL GLANDS (SUPRARENALS)

Gross Anatomy. The adrenal glands are two small glands that lie upon the superior poles of each kidney, and are 3 to 5 cm. in height, 3 cm. in width, and 1 to 2 cm. in anteroposterior thickness. Each is composed of a thick cortex, a medulla of chromaffin tissue, and each lies within Gerota's capsule, which also surrounds the kidney.

The right adrenal is rather pyramidal in shape, having its anterior surface laterally in contact with the liver and with the inferior vena cava, its posterior surface with the diaphragm, and its base with the kidney below. Both of its sides are concave and its general appearance is that of a "cocked hat."

The left gland is more semilunar in shape. Anteriorly it is in contact with the stomach above, the pancreas below, and the diaphragm posteriorly; its base touches the left kidney below it. The left adrenal lies as much medial to the left kidney as above it, in contrast to the right adrenal, which caps the kidney. The amount of peritoneum covering the gland is variable. The right gland is more medial and lower in relation to the spine than the left.

The dimensions, weight, and area of the suprarenal gland as gathered from the literature are summarized in Table 15–6. It is

TABLE 15–6 DIMENSIONS, WEIGHT, AND AREA OF THE SUPRARENAL GLAND

Reference	Length	Width	Thickness	Weight	Area Right	Left
Herbut	3–5 cm.	2–4 cm.	0.4–0.6 cm.	3.5–5 Gm.		
Soffer	4–6 cm.	2–3 cm.	0.2–0.8 cm.	3–5 Gm.		
Steinbach and Smith					2.0–7.8 (aver. 4.2) sq. cm.	2.0–8.7 (aver. 4.3) sq. cm.

apparent from these tabular notations that although the normal suprarenal gland may vary considerably in size, its shape is fairly well preserved and its margins are practically always concave (Meyers, 1963). Occasionally, the normal medial border of the left suprarenal gland may be minimally convex.

The adrenals, unlike the kidneys, are firmly fixed at their apices and hence, in the erect position there is a tendency for the renal structures to separate from the suprarenal.

In the infant, the adrenal gland is relatively large—the fetal cortex in particular is larger in proportion to the rest of the gland during the prenatal months, beginning with approximately the seventh month. The cortex gradually diminishes proportionately to age 2, when its relationship to the medulla is stabilized and remains relatively constant thereafter. The decrease in weight of the gland is rapid during the first months of extrauterine life but it slows down after this period. After the first postnatal year the glands enlarge slowly and continue to grow progressively until puberty, with final weights of approximately 5 gm. (Warwick

and Williams). The female suprarenal gland usually is slightly larger than that of the male. The left gland is usually slightly larger than the right (Anson).

Blood Supply (Fig. 15–67). The suprarenal glands receive an abundant blood supply, and this has become increasingly important clinically. There are three arteries or groups of arteries supplying the glands: (1) single or multiple branches *from the phrenic artery,* (2) single or multiple branches directly *from the aorta* (the middle suprarenal), and (3) single or multiple renal branches directly *from the renal arteries* on each side.

Most of the branches are short. The middle suprarenal arising from the aorta may be absent and there may be variable branches from the gonadal arteries or arteries from the renal pelves or cortex as well.

One large vein arises from a central part of the medulla of each gland and drains most of the blood from each suprarenal gland. Blood from the left gland empties into the left renal vein, whereas blood from the right gland empties directly into the infe-

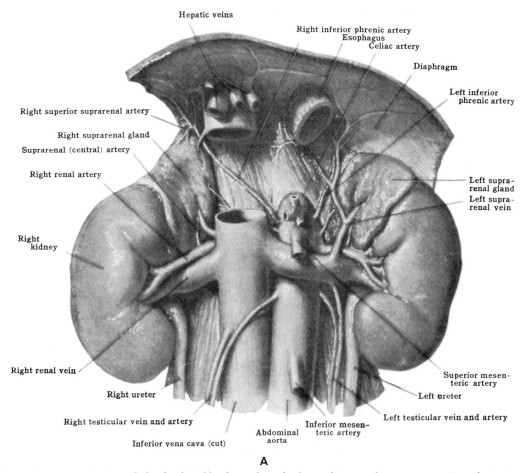

A

Figure 15–67. *A.* Suprarenal glands, their blood supply and relationships to adjacent retroperitoneal structures. (From Anson, B. J. (ed.): Morris' Human Anatomy, 12th ed. Copyright © 1966 by McGraw-Hill, Inc. Used by permission of McGraw-Hill Book Company.)

Figure 15–67 continued on the opposite page.

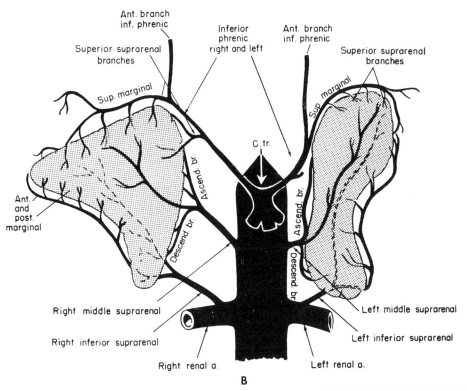

B

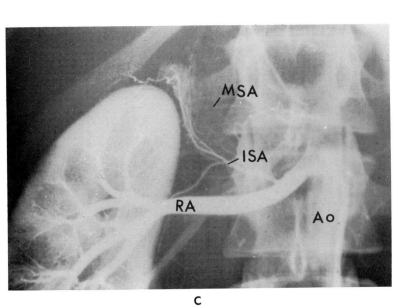

C

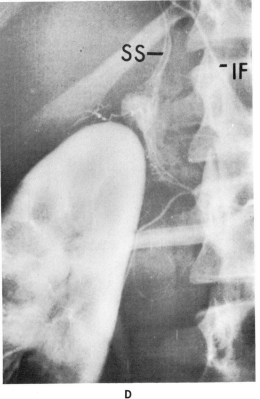

D

Figure 15–67 Continued. B. Schematic diagram of adrenal circulation. After Gérard. Some of the variations are discussed in the text. (From Kahn, P. C., and Nickrosz, L. V.: Amer. J. Roentgenol., 101:739–749, 1967.) C to E. Close-up views of adrenal arterial supply and capillary phase.

Figure 15–67 continued on the following page.

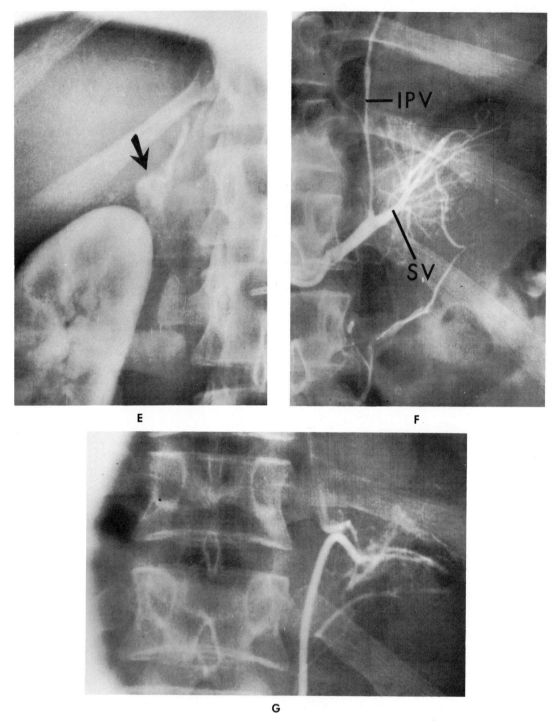

Figure 15–67 *Continued.*   *F* and *G*. Close-up views of adrenal vein.

rior vena cava. Because of the greater constancy and relative simplicity of the topography of the suprarenal veins, they are considered by some investigators to be more significant for investigation than the arteries. Displacement of these vessels or alterations in the branching pattern or types of vessels provide clues to the abnormal morphology of the suprarenal gland.

Method of Study by Perirenal Air Insufflation (Fig. 15–68). This method involves the introduction of air, oxygen, or carbon dioxide directly into the perirenal areolar tissue by needle puncture through the lumbar triangle. Several hundred cubic centimeters are usually necessary, and 12 to 24 hours must elapse to allow for proper distribution of air around the kidney and adrenal gland. Stereoscopic anteroposterior and lateral films are obtained at 24 hour intervals for approximately 3 days. Occasionally, the gas diffuses over to the opposite side, and a bilateral visualization is obtained.

When oxygen is used, the examination must be carried out more quickly, since most of this gaseous medium will be absorbed in about 6 hours. Carbon dioxide has been proposed as the safest gaseous medium to employ, since large volumes of this gas can be introduced directly into the blood stream without untoward results. However, the absorption of carbon dioxide is so rapid that diagnostic radiographic detail is impaired. With proper technique, carbon dioxide may well be the best medium to employ for this purpose.

The presacral route has achieved greater popularity for insufflation of gases around the renal and suprarenal areas (Fig. 15–68). In this technique, the needle is inserted through the skin outside the anus into the tela subserosa between the rectum and the sacrum. A finger is placed in the rectum during the needle insertion to help guide its positioning. Approximately 1000 cc. of gas are introduced. During the next 2 hours, the patient is rotated frequently.

When air is used, an initial film of the suprarenal area is obtained at the 2 hour interval and hourly thereafter until maximal visualization is obtained. At this time, it is well to perform intravenous pyelograms, and once again appropriate films of the suprarenal area are obtained. Oblique and stereoscopic films as well as body section radiographs (5 to 10 cm. from posterior) are now used to aid in the diagnosis.

The adrenal gland on the right is thereafter seen as a pyramidal structure capping the right kidney, and the left adrenal as a semilunar-shaped structure partially capping and medial to the left kidney.

Gas embolism has been described as one of the unfortunate complications of this procedure and, for that reason, it cannot be used indiscriminately as it is never completely without hazard.

In the survey reported by McLelland et al., in a total of 11,422 procedures there were 122 cases of severe gas embolism, of which 58 ended fatally (Ransom et al.).

With *retroperitoneal pneumography* the films recommended by Meyers are: (1) both supine posterior obliques, (2) anteroposterior erect, (3) body section radiographic cuts at 1 cm. intervals between 6 and 12 cm. from the posterior, and (4) a 24 hour film if oxygen is used. If air or oxygen is used, a scout film centered over the suprarenals is obtained 2 hours after the injection and hourly thereafter until maximum visualization is obtained. Excretory urograms and nephrotomograms may be combined with this procedure at this time.

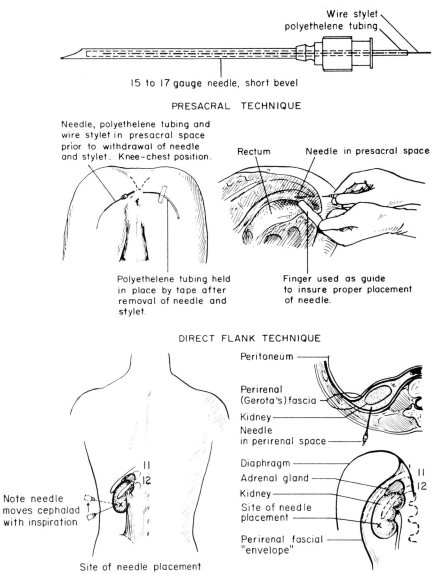

Figure 15–68. Diagrams illustrating the direct flank and presacral techniques for retroperitoneal pneumography. (From McLelland, R., Landes, R. R., and Ransom, C. L.: Radiol. Clin. N. Amer., 3:116, 1965.)

Normal retroperitoneal pneumograms are illustrated in Figure 15–69.

Adrenal Arteriography. Although generally the three adrenal arteries already described represent the main blood supply of the adrenal gland, more than one adrenal branch arises directly from the aorta in approximately 30 per cent of cases. There are a number of other variations (Gagnon). The *middle* adrenal artery traverses laterally to the posterior surface of the adrenal gland where it breaks up into a number of twigs (4 or 5) just barely visible on the radiograph. The *superior* adrenal arteries supply the

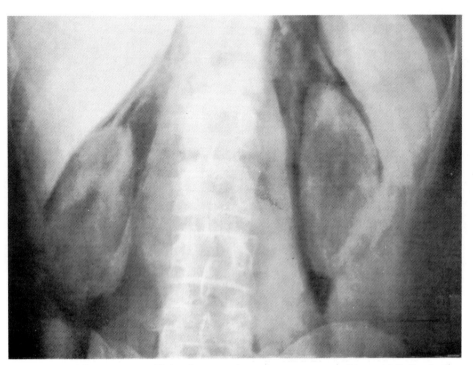

Figure 15–69. Normal retroperitoneal pneumogram. (From McLelland, R., Landes, R. R., and Ransom, C. L.: Radiol. Clin. N. Amer., 3:115, 1965.)

upper pole of the adrenal gland and arise principally from the inferior phrenic arteries. These branch off the aorta just above the celiac axis usually. At times, however, the inferior phrenic arises below the celiac or even from the renal artery itself. The adrenal arteries are actually a number of twigs arising from the inferior phrenic and its posterior division. The inferior adrenal arteries arise from the renal arteries either directly or with the superior renal capsular branch. Other adrenal branches may arise from the gonadal arteries.

Technique. Midline abdominal aortograms may be sufficient for opacification of the adrenal arteries and glands. The Valsalva maneuver improves this visualization by slowing down the aortic blood flow, and by separating to some extent the kidneys and adrenals. Intra-arterial epinephrine or norepinephrine may also improve visualization. This is particularly helpful because it reduces the vascularization of surrounding organs that might interfere. Unfortunately, epinephrine may produce undesirable effects by constriction of the spinal arteries.

Selective catheterization of the three main blood vessels of supply is feasible.

A series of 6 to 8 films spaced over 8 to 12 seconds is usually sufficient for the purpose and the frontal projection may be supplemented by a right posterior oblique for the right adrenal gland, and left posterior oblique for the left.

The Normal Adrenal Arteriogram. The cortex of the adrenal gland can usually be identified as a dense blush about 2 mm. wide. The medulla is relatively less opaque, and the adrenal vein appears later in the film sequence. Examples are shown in Figure 15–67. Multiple injections are usually required to opacify the entire adrenal gland. Unfortunately, confusing shadows caused by opacification of surrounding organs may occur.

Adrenal Venography. Since each adrenal gland drains by only one vein (Figs. 15–67 and 16–70) injection of the adrenal veins is a valuable study, particularly for demonstration of filling defects within these glands.

There are no valves in adrenal veins. On the right side there are three main tributaries to the renal vein—inferolateral, ventromedial, and posterior. The junction of these three veins occurs near the top or the middle of the gland, thus forming the adrenal vein, usually about 3 mm. in diameter and rarely exceeding 10 mm. in length. The right adrenal vein usually drains into the inferior vena cava about 3 to 4 cm. above the right renal vein and near the T12 vertebra. This occurs in very close proximity to or in conjunction with the hepatic vein. On the left side there are four main venous trunks: inferolateral, ventral, medial, and posterior. The left adrenal vein is usually 20 to 40 mm. long, and it is joined by the left inferior phrenic vein about 15 to 20 mm. below the left adrenal gland. A renal capsular vein often joins the adrenal, and communications occur to other veins such as the gonadal, lumbar, and hemiazygos. The left adrenal vein therefore empties into the left renal vein on its upper surface to the left of the aorta near the point at which the renal vein crosses the lateral border of the vertebral body.

Technique. Superselective adrenal vein catheterization is different on each side and special configuration of the catheter has to be devised. For percutaneous femoral catheterization, two catheters each different in design must usually be employed (Kahn). For specifics of technique the student is referred to Kahn.

The contrast agent should be injected gently to avoid rupture of the gland, even though this causes some inevitable discomfort to the patient. The volume varies from 0.5 to 5 ml., depending on the location of the catheter tip. Single films or short serial sequential films are utilized. Frontal and oblique projections are recommended. On the right side in the right oblique view, the inferior vena cava is superimposed over the gland and in the left oblique, the spine is superimposed, unfortunately. Adrenal vein ruptures may occur in 5 to 10 per cent of cases, even in experienced hands.

Normal Adrenal Venograms. The adrenal veins are very thin and sinuous. The adrenal glands can be measured by means of venography—normally the area should be less than 17 sq. cm. (Reuter et al.). Usually some veins outside the adrenal are also seen. Unfortunately, also, a hepatic vein may be injected by mistake and great care must be exercised so that a false interpretation does not result.

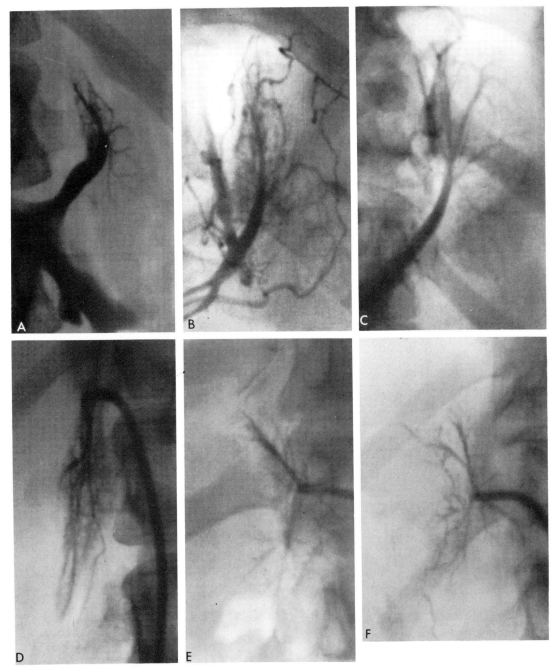

Figure 15–70. Adrenal venography in the anteroposterior projection. Appearance of normal left adrenal glands. *A.* Small normal gland (4 cm.²) in a 90 lb. woman without biochemical evidence of adrenal abnormality. *B.* Larger normal gland with single central vein (9.4 cm.²) in a 165 lb. man. The gland was removed because of primary aldosteronism. A nodule 2 mm. in diameter was found. The gland weighed 9.3 g. The large vein medial to the adrenal gland is the inferior phrenic vein. *C.* Large normal gland with two central veins (16.7 cm.²) in a 209 lb. woman without biochemical evidence of adrenal abnormality.

Adrenal venography in the anteroposterior projection. Appearance of normal right adrenal glands. *D.* The main adrenal vein drains the length of the gland and exits at the top. *E.* A main adrenal vein exiting at the mid-portion of the gland receives two primary branches. *F.* A main adrenal vein exiting at the mid-portion of the gland receives three primary branches. (From Reuter, S. R., Blair, A. J., Schteingart, D. E., and Bookstein, J. J.: Radiology, *89*:805–814, 1967.)

REFERENCES

Abrams, H. L. (ed.): Angiography, Vol. 2. Second edition. Boston, Little, Brown & Co., 1971.

Anson, B. (ed.): Morris' Human Anatomy, 12th edition. New York, McGraw-Hill, 1966.

Arvidsson, H.: Angiocardiographic measurements in congenital heart disease. Acta Radiol. (Diag.), *1*:981–994, 1963.

Berdon, W. E., Baker, D. H., and Leonidas, J.: Advantages of prone positioning in gastrointestinal and genitourinary roentgenologic studies in infants and children. Amer. J. Roentgenol., *103*:444–455, 1968.

Bierman, H. C.: Selective Arterial Catheterization. Springfield, Ill., Charles C Thomas, 1969.

Bron, K. M.: Thrombotic occlusion of the abdominal aorta. Amer. J. Roentgenol., *96*:887–895, 1966.

Budin, E., and Jacobson, G.: Roentgenographic diagnosis of small amounts of intraperitoneal fluid. Amer. J. Roentgenol., *99*:62–70, 1967.

Campbell, R. E.: Roentgenologic features of umbilical vascular catheterization in the newborn. Amer. J. Roentgenol., *112*:68–76, 1971.

Cimmino, C. V.: Further experiences with the roentgenology of the paracolonic gutter. Radiology, *90*:761–764, 1968.

Coopwood, T. B., and Bricker, D. L.: Paraduodenal hernias. South. Med. J., *65*:1138–1141, 1972.

Cunningham, D. J.: Manual of Practical Anatomy, Vol. 2. 12th edition. London, Oxford University Press, 1959.

Ferris, E. J., Vittimberga, F. J., Byrne, J. J., Nabseth, D. C., and Shapiro, J. H.: The inferior vena cava after ligation and plication. Radiology, *89*:1–10, 1967.

Franken, E. A.: Ascites in infants and children. Radiology, *102*:393–398, 1972.

Gagnon, R.: The arterial supply of the human adrenal gland. Rev. Canad. Biol., *16*:421, 1957.

Gagnon, R.: Middle suprarenal arteries in man: a statistical study of 200 human adrenal glands. Rev. Canad. Biol., *23*:461, 1964.

Grupp, G., Grupp, I. L., and Spitz, H. B.: Collateral vascular pathways during experimental obstruction of aorta and inferior vena cava. Amer. J. Roentgenol., *94*:159–171, 1965.

Hansmann, G. H., and Morton, S. A.: Intra-abdominal hernia, report of a case and review of the literature. Arch. Surg., *39*:973–986, 1939.

Herbut, P. A.: Urologic Pathology, Vol. 2. Philadelphia, Lea and Febiger, 1952.

Herman, P. G., Benninghoff, D. L., Nelson, J. H., Jr., and Mellins, H. Z.: Roentgen anatomy of the ilio-pelvic-aortic lymphatic system. Radiology, *80*:182–193, 1963.

Hillman, D. C., and Tristan, T. A.: Inferior cavography in the detection of abdominal extension of pelvic cancer. Radiology, *81*:416–427, 1963.

Kahn, P. C.: Adrenal venography. *In* Abrams, H. L. (ed.): Angiography, Vol. 2. Second edition. Boston, Little, Brown & Co., 1971. Pp. 941–950.

Kahn, P. C., and Nickrosz, L. V.: Angiography of the adrenal glands. Amer. J. Roentgenol., *101*:739–749, 1967.

McLelland, R., Landes, R. R., and Ransom, C. I.: Retroperitoneal pneumography: A safe method using carbon dioxide. Radiol. Clin. N. Amer., *3*:113–128, 1965.

Meyers, M. A.: Diseases of the Adrenal Gland: Radiological Diagnosis. Springfield, Ill., Charles C Thomas, 1963.

Meyers, M. A.: Peritoneography. Amer. J. Roentgenol., *117*:353–363, 1973.

Meyers, M. A.: The spread and localization of acute intraperitoneal effusions. Radiology, *95*:547–554, 1970.

Meyers, M. A., and Whalen, J. P.: Roentgen significance of the duodenal colic relationships: an anatomic approach. Amer. J. Roentgenol., *117*:263–274, 1973.

Michels, N. A.: The variational anatomy of the spleen and splenic arteries. Amer. J. Anat., *70*:21, 1942.

Michels, N. A.: Blood Supply and Anatomy of the Upper Abdominal Organs. Philadelphia, J. B. Lippincott Co., 1955.

Pansky, B., and House, E. L.: Review of Gross Anatomy. New York, Macmillan, 1964.

Ransom, C. L., Landes, R. R., and McLelland, R.: Air embolism following retroperitoneal pneumography: a nationwide survey. J. Urol., *76*:664, 1956.

Reuter, S. R., Blair, A. J., Schteingart, D. E., and Bookstein, J. J.: Adrenal venography. Radiology, *89*:805–814, 1967.

Rösch, J.: Roentgenologic possibilities in spleen diagnosis. Amer. J. Roentgenol., *94*:453–461, 1965 (27 references).

Soffer, L. S.: Diseases of the Endocrine Glands. Philadelphia, Lea and Febiger, 1951.

Steinbach, H. L., and Smith, K. L.: Extraperitoneal pneumography in diagnosis of retroperitoneal tumors. Arch. Surg., *70*:161–172, 1955.

Steinberg, C. R., Archer, M., and Steinberg, I.: Measurement of the abdominal aorta after intravenous aortography in health and arteriosclerotic peripheral vascular disease. Amer. J. Roentgenol., *95*:703–708, 1965.

Swischuk, L. E., and Stacy, T. M.: Herniography: radiologic investigation of inguinal hernia. Radiology, *101*:139–146, 1971.

Walker, L. A., and Weens, H. S.: Radiological observations on the lesser peritoneal sac. Radiology, *90*:727–737, 1963.

Warwick, R., and Williams, P. L.: Gray's Anatomy. 35th British edition. London, Faber and Faber, 1973.

Whalen, J. P., Berne, A. S., and Riemenschneider, P. A.: The extraperitoneal perivisceral fat pad. 1. Its role in the roentgenologic evaluation of abdominal organs. Radiology, *92*:466–472, 1969.

Whalen, J. P., Berne, A. S., and Riemenschneider, P. A.: The extraperitoneal perivisceral fat pad. 2. Roentgen interpretations of pathologic alterations. Radiology, *92*:473–480, 1969.

Whalen, J. P., Evans, J. A., and Shanser, J.: Vector principle in the differential diagnosis of abdominal masses. 1. The left upper quadrant. Amer. J. Roentgenol., *113*:104–124, 1971.

Whalen, J. P., Evans, J. A., and Meyers, M. A.: Vector principle in the differential diagnosis of abdominal masses. 2. Right upper quadrant. Amer. J. Roentgenol., *115*:318–333, 1972.

White, J. J., Parks, L. C., and Haller, J. A.: The inguinal herniagram: a radiologic aid for accurate diagnosis of inguinal hernia in infants. Surgery, *63*:991–997, 1968.

Wyman, A. C.: Traumatic rupture of the spleen. Amer. J. Roentgenol., *72*:51–63, 1954.

16

The Urinary Tract

The urinary tract consists of the following major structures: (1) the kidneys—one on each side, (2) the ureters, (3) the urinary bladder, and (4) the urethra.

CORRELATED GROSS AND MICROSCOPIC ANATOMY OF THE URINARY TRACT

The Kidneys

The kidneys are paired, retroperitoneal, bean-shaped organs lying on each side of the vertebral column. The exact relationships of the kidney to the vertebral column are indicated in Figure 16–1. Thus, the distance in centimeters cranially and caudally of the poles of normal adult kidneys from the middle of L2 vertebra in plain roentgenograms is shown for both male and female (plus or minus two standard deviations). Usually the left kidney is slightly higher than the right and the upper pole is approximately 4 cm. closer to the midline than the lower pole. The angle between the longitudinal axis of the kidneys and the midline within two standard deviations is shown in Figure 16–1 C for both male and female. On the right side in the male this approximates 19.4 degrees; on the left side, 18.9 degrees. For the female, on the right side, the angle of the longitudinal axis of the kidneys to the midline approximates 17.1 degrees, and on the left side, 15.8 degrees.

Normal Kidney Size. The right kidney is usually slightly smaller than the left. A number of different methods of measurement of the kidneys are available.

Table 16–1 shows the normal adult renal size in absolute measurements, plus or minus two standard deviations.

Simon has reported the ratio of renal adult cephalocaudad lengths to height of the second lumbar vertebral body (plus disk) to be 3.7 ± 0.37, with a statistical range of normal values between 3.0 and 4.4 cm. (Meschan, Martin).

Normal measurements in adults and children in relation to body height and age are indicated in Table 16–2. Kidney length increases with age until approximately age 20 in both men and women, and begins to diminish somewhat in the cephalocaudad

dimension from about age 50. In children, kidney length increases progressively with body height; and in adults, similarly, kidney length is related to body height but with a lesser angle of inclination.

These data summarize renal size as studied by Hodson in normal children. The mean kidney length in children varies from 6 cm. with a body height of 24 inches to 12 cm. with a body height of 72 inches. The size of the kidney depends largely on the size of the child. Body height is probably the most reliable guide, since it is less liable to rapid fluctuation than is body weight. Between 4 and 15 years, there is a steady mean increase per year of 0.35 cm. and 5 cm. in kidney length and body height, respectively.

Friedenberg et al. utilized a *renal index* for measurement of kidney size, as shown in Figure 16–2. The renal index in this instance is defined as the product of the length and width of the kidney divided by the body surface area of the patient in square meters.

The left and right renal indices for children are shown in Figure 16–3 A and B. The left-minus-right renal index for children is shown in Figure 16–3 C. Similarly, the left and right renal indices and the left-minus-right index for adult males are shown in Figure 16–4. Figure 16–5 contains similar information for adult females.

Currarino related the length in centimeters of four lumbar vertebral bodies to kidney length for various age groups in children and found (Fig. 16–6) that the length of each kidney corresponded closely to the length of this segment of the lumbar spine plus or minus 1 cm. throughout childhood, with the exception of the first 1 to 1½ years of life in which the length of a normal kidney was greater.

It is important to compare the kidney size on each side of the patient. Discrepancies between the two kidneys of greater than 1 cm. are of considerable significance. Generally, a difference in length of the two kidneys up to 1 cm. may occur normally, especially in children (Currarino). Elkin, in comparing the kidneys of the two sides, found that the average left kidney measurement is greater than the right—the difference between the two sides varying from 1 to 9 per cent. This calculation is based upon the product of the horizontal and vertical measurements of the

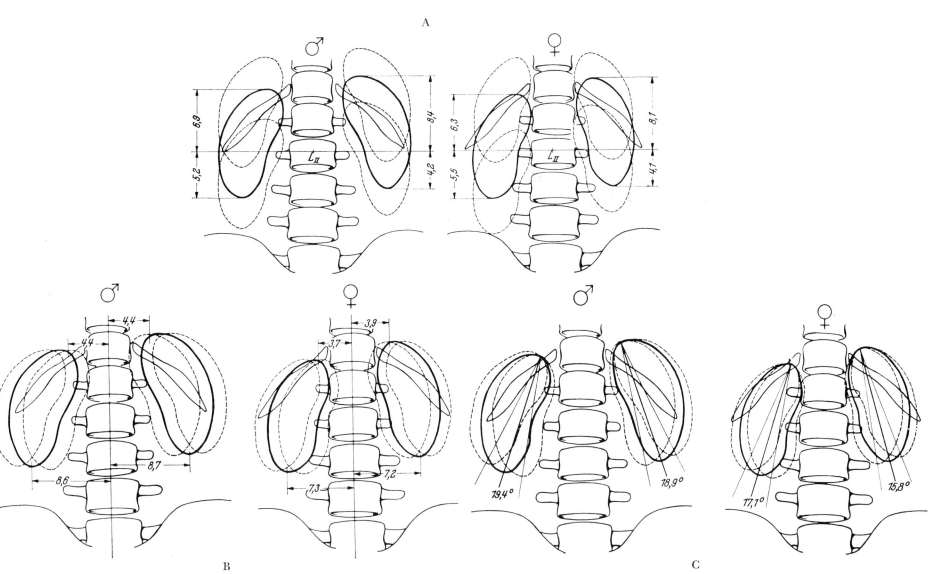

Figure 16–1. *A.* Distances in centimeters cranially and caudally from the middle of vertebra L-II, of the poles of normal adult kidneys in plain roentgenograms. Dotted lines indicate ± 2s. *B.* Distances in centimeters of the cranial and caudal poles of normal adult kidneys from the midline in plain roentgenograms. Dotted lines indicate ± 2s. *C.* The angle between the longitudinal axis of the kidneys and the midline. Dotted lines indicate ± 2s. (After Moell, H.: Acta Radiologica, 46:640–645, 1956.)

TABLE 16–1 NORMAL ADULT RENAL SIZE
(THE MEAN PLUS OR MINUS TWO STANDARD DEVIATIONS)[a]
(Modified after Moell)

Male:	Right kidney	Vertical: 11.3–14.5 cm.
		Width: 5.4– 7.2 cm.
	Left	Vertical: 11.6–14.8 cm.
		Width: 5.3– 7.1 cm.
Female:	Right kidney	Vertical: 10.7–13.9 cm.
		Width: 4.8– 6.6 cm.
	Left	Vertical: 11.1–14.3 cm.
		Width: 5.1– 6.9 cm.

[a]Standard deviation = 0.8 cm. for vertical dimension.

two kidneys in centimeters. Because this measurement was developed particularly to note kidney size in acute ureteral obstruction, it was arbitrarily determined that differences of greater than 11 per cent were significant. However, if the right kidney were larger than the left by a smaller percentage, this could also present a criterion for enlargement.

Kidney Mobility. There is considerable mobility of the kidneys during respiration. Normally, the range of movement is about 3 cm. less on the right side than on the left and is somewhat larger for women than for men. However, on deeper inspiration excursion up to 10 cm. may be recorded.

TABLE 16–2*

RADIOGRAPHIC SIZE OF THE KIDNEY

Department of X-ray Diagnosis
University College Hospital
London, England

NORMAL MEASUREMENTS IN ADULTS AND CHILDREN

This chart is published in response to considerable demand by radiologists and clinicians for graphic data on the size of normal kidneys as determined from radiographs. The size of a normal kidney varies widely from person to person, depending on the number and distribution of calyces and the actual shape of the organ, making accurate estimation of the size of an individual kidney difficult. However, knowledge that a kidney is larger or smaller than average has considerable significance.

Good radiographic definition of the renal outline of a majority of patients is a simple matter, provided the patient is prepared properly.
Good definition of the renal outline of infants and bedridden patients is more difficult to obtain, however, and usually tomography or localized abdominal compression must be used.

The graphs have been found useful in the interpretation of radiographs, especially those of children. Statistically, the graphs are valid.
In particular, the one relating to children shows an unusually close relation between the length of the kidney and the height of the body throughout the period of growth. The simple relation of length of kidney to height of body or to age and sex was chosen because statistically this measurement is as satisfactory as others more complicated.[1,2]

TECHNICAL POINTS

A. The data were derived using a target-film distance of 36 inches (91.5 cm). Radiographs made at a target-film distance of 40 inches (101.8 cm) would show a 2 percent reduction in the size of the kidney.

B. For the normal kidney, 68 percent of the readings lie within the range of mean plus or minus 1 standard deviation; 99.5 percent lie within the range of mean plus or minus 2½ times the standard deviation.

REFERENCES

1. Karn, M. N.: Radiographic Measurements of Kidney Section Area. **Ann. Hum. Genet.**, 25:379-385, May, 1962.

2. Hodson, C. J.; Drewe, J. A.; Karn, M. N.; and King, A.: Renal Size in Normal Children. A Radiographic Study During Life. **Arch. Dis. Child.**, 37:616-622, December, 1962.

BIBLIOGRAPHY

Hodson, C. J.: Radiology of the Kidney. In Black, D. A. K. (editor): **Renal Disease.** Published by F. A. Davis Company, Philadelphia, Pennsylvania, and Blackwell Scientific Publications, Oxford, England, 1962, pp. 388-417.

Möell, H.: Kidney Size and Its Deviation from Normal in Acute Renal Failure. A Roentgenographic Study. **Acta Radiol.**, Supp. 206, 1961, pp. 5-74.

Panichi, S., and Bonechi, I.: Il volume del rene in condizioni normali. **Boll. Soc. Medicochir. Pisa,** 26:611-614, November-December, 1958.

Vuorinen, P.; Anttila, P.; Wegelius, U.; Kauppila, A.; and Koivisto, E.: Renal Cortical Index and Other Roentgenographic Renal Measurements. **Acta Radiol.**, Supp. 211, 1962, pp. 5-54.

EASTMAN KODAK COMPANY
Radiography Markets Division
Rochester, N.Y. 14650

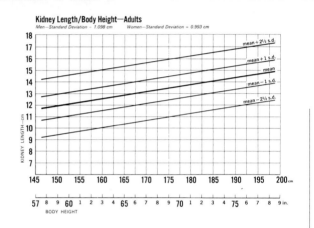

Kidney Length/Body Height—Adults
Men—Standard Deviation ~ 1.098 cm   Women—Standard Deviation ~ 0.993 cm

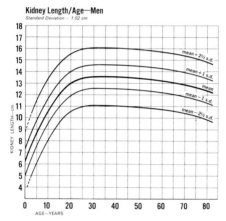

Kidney Length/Age—Men
Standard Deviation ~ 1.02 cm

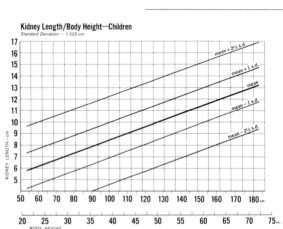

Kidney Length/Body Height—Children
Standard Deviation ~ 1.529 cm

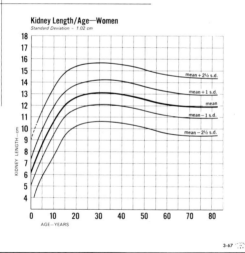

Kidney Length/Age—Women
Standard Deviation ~ 1.02 cm

M4-8A   3-67

*Courtesy Radiography Markets Division, Eastman Kodak Company.

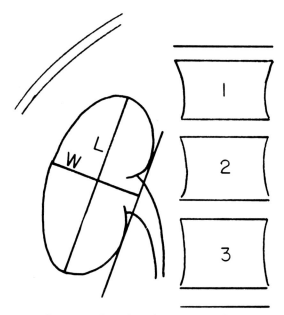

Figure 16–2. Line drawing of the right kidney region to demonstrate the method of measuring renal size (see text). Length of kidney in centimeters is indicated by *L* and width in centimeters by *W*. Renal index is calculated as follows: $RI = L \times W/BSA$, where *BSA* is the body surface area of the patient in square meters. (From F.iedenberg, M. J. et al.: Radiology, 84:1022–1029, 1965.)

A maximum excursion of 5 cm. (or 1½ vertebral bodies) occurs in the change from the recumbent to the erect position.

Gondos has recommended that measurements of the kidneys be made from a film taken with the patient prone, suggesting that in this position renal rotation is reduced or eliminated.

Renal Shape. Normally, the kidney is bean-shaped. Fetal lobulation (Fig. 16–7), however, is frequently encountered in children and tends to occur in three basic patterns, as illustrated in Figure 16–12 *A* (Cooperman and Lowman): (1) there may be a local bulge of the lateral border of the left kidney; (2) the left kidney may be triangular, and somewhat enlarged; (3) there may be a diffuse multilobulated form that is either unilateral or bilateral.

Additionally, lobulation may indicate partial or complete duplication of one kidney that may be without special pathologic significance. To make absolutely certain of this, usually complete study, sometimes including nephrotomography and arteriography, is necessary.

The medial border of the kidney is concave and contains a slitlike aperture, the hilus. This is the orifice of a cavity called the *renal sinus*, which is about 2.5 cm. in depth and contains the following structures: (1) the renal *pelvis* and *calyces;* (2) the branches of the *renal artery* before their entrance into the actual substance of the kidney, and the tributaries of the *renal vein* after their exit; (3) the *lymph vessels* and *nerves* of the kidney; and (4) small amounts of *fat* around and among the other structures (Fig. 16–8).

There are usually 8 to 10 *renal papillae* which protrude into the renal sinus, but there may be as few as 4 or as many as 18 (Anson).

The "Edge Pattern" of the Kidney. The surface of the kidney is invested by a thin but strong fibrous capsule. External to it is a considerable quantity of fat tissue known as the *adipose capsule* (Gerota's capsule). It is this fatty tissue envelope that permits identification of the kidney on plain radiographs, since it is considerably more radiolucent than the surrounding muscular structures. On the other hand, perirenal inflammations or neo-

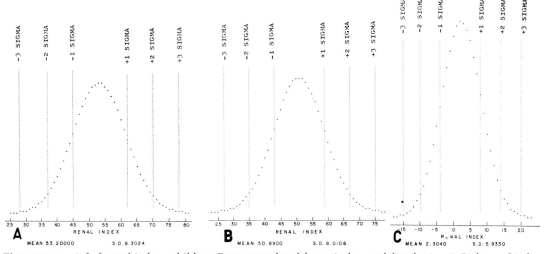

Figure 16–3. *A.* Left renal index—children. Frequency plot of theoretical normal distribution. *B.* Right renal index—children. Frequency plot of theoretical normal distribution. *C.* Left minus right renal index—children. Frequency plot of theoretical normal distribution. (From Friedenberg, M. J. et al.: Radiology, 84:1022–1029, 1965.)

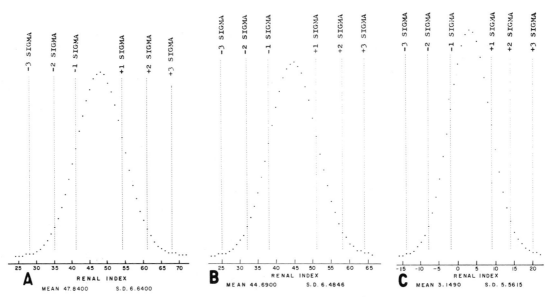

Figure 16–4. *A.* Left renal index—adult males. Frequency plot of theoretical normal distribution. *B.* Right renal index—adult males. Frequency plot of theoretical normal distribution. *C.* Left minus right renal index—adult males. Frequency plot of theoretical normal distribution. (From Friedenberg, M. J. et al.: Radiology, *84*:1022–1029, 1965.)

plasms may invade this fatty envelope and impair good detail, and this is a roentgen sign of abnormality. It is this adipose capsule which is continuous with the tela subserosa and which is insufflated with air or oxygen in the performance of perirenal air insufflation studies.

Relationship of the Kidney to Other Retroperitoneal Structures. Each kidney is retroperitoneal alongside the last thoracic and upper three lumbar vertebrae, the left usually being higher than the right.

Posteriorly, the kidneys lie on a muscle bed composed of the

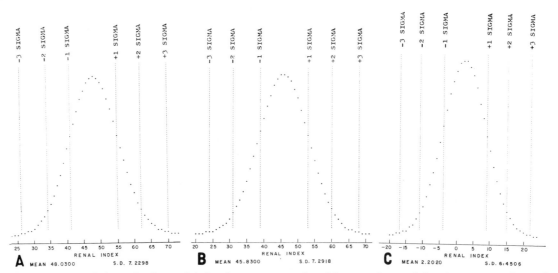

Figure 16–5. *A.* Left renal index—adult females. Frequency plot of theoretical normal distribution. *B.* Right renal index—adult females. Frequency plot of theoretical normal distribution. *C.* Left minus right renal index—adult females. Frequency plot of theoretical normal distribution. (From Friedenberg, M. J. et al.: Radiology, *84*:1022–1029, 1965.)

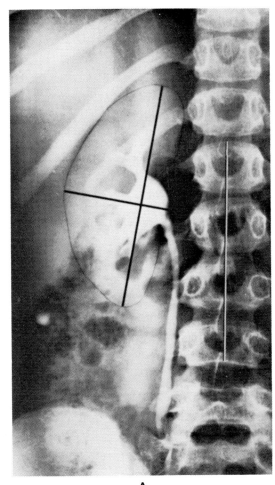

A

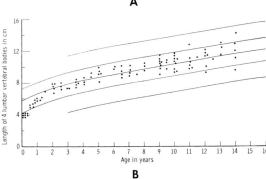

B

Figure 16–6. *A.* Comparative measurement of the length of the kidney and the length of a segment of the lumbar spine, comprising the four upper lumbar vertebral bodies and the three intervertebral spaces between them. *B.* Graph of the length of the comparative lumbar spine segment, as measured by the method shown in *A*, superimposed on the graph for kidney length of Hodson et al. (*A* and *B* from Currarino, G.: Amer. J. Roentgenol., *93*:464, 1965.)

diaphragm, the psoas major, quadratus lumborum, and transversus abdominis muscles. The structures intervening between the quadratus lumborum and the kidney are the subcostal vessels and nerves such as the ilio-hypogastric and ilio-inguinal. The dia-

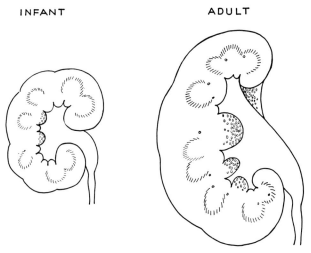

Figure 16–7. Infantile renal lobulation and its comparison with the adult renal contour. (After Caffey.)

phragm separates the upper part of the kidney from the pleura and the twelfth rib.

Anteriorly, the right kidney has the following relationships: the suprarenal gland overlaps its upper end, especially medially, and the duodenum overlaps it along its hilus. The hepatic flexure

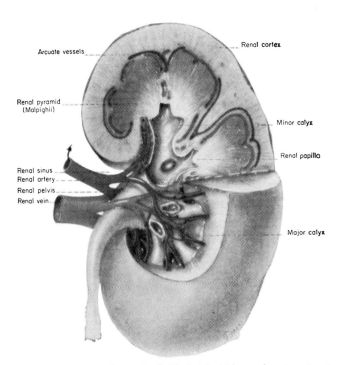

Figure 16–8. Dissection of anterior half of right kidney, showing structures in the renal sinus. (From Anson, B. J. (ed.): Morris' Human Anatomy, 12th ed. Copyright © 1966 by McGraw-Hill, Inc. Used by permission of McGraw-Hill Book Company.)

of the colon covers a considerable part of the lower end of the kidney. Between the colon and the lower part of the duodenum, a small part of the lower end of the kidney is contiguous to the jejunum (Fig. 16–9). The right lobe of the liver tends to overlie the right kidney as well as the other structures named.

The *left kidney anteriorly* has the following relationships (Fig. 16–9 C): the suprarenal gland caps its upper and medial portion, and the spleen borders upon its upper lateral aspects. The body of the pancreas with the splenic vessels lies across the kidney at or near its midsection. The left half of the transverse colon crosses the kidney below the pancreas, and the descending colon overlaps its lower part laterally. A small portion of the lower pole of the left kidney is in contact with the colon but the rest of its anterior surface is covered by the peritoneum. The stomach, the transverse colon, and the jejunum are all separated from the kidney by the peritoneum, and although the spleen is also separated by peritoneum it is attached at one point by the lienorenal ligament.

Longitudinal Section Through the Kidney (Coronal Section) (Fig. 16–10).   The substance of the kidney as revealed by

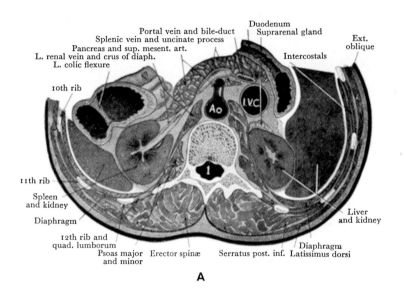

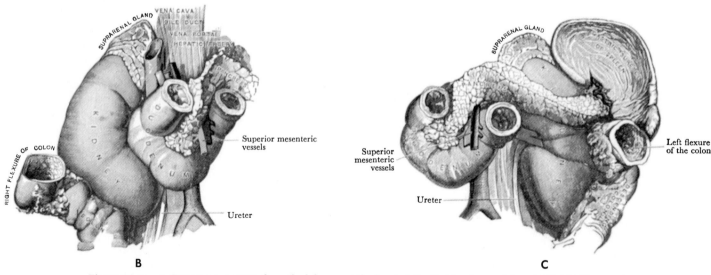

Figure 16–9.   *A.* Transverse section through abdomen at the level of the first lumbar vertebra. *B.* Right kidney and duodenum. The relation of the duodenum and the right flexure to the kidney is not so extensive as usual. *C.* Relations of left kidney and pancreas. (From Cunningham's Manual of Practical Anatomy, 12th ed., Vol. 2. London, Oxford University Press, 1958.)

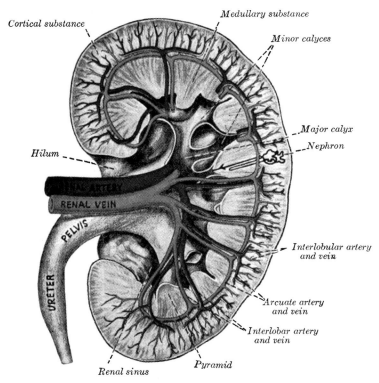

Figure 16–10. Longitudinal section through a normal kidney. (From Gray's Anatomy of the Human Body, 29th ed. Goss, C. M. (ed.) Philadelphia, Lea & Febiger, 1973.)

this section has three main parts—an external cortex, an internal medulla, and the renal tubules. The *external cortex* is approximately 12 mm. thick and contains numerous renal corpuscles, convoluted tubules, and minute vessels. The cortex is actually composed of two portions: (1) a *peripheral layer*, the cortex proper; and (2) processes called *"renal columns"* which dip inward between renal pyramids to reach the bottom of the sinus of the kidney (Fig. 16–8).

The *internal medulla* contains approximately eight structures called *renal pyramids*. The apices of these pyramids project into the bottom or side of the renal sinus, and into minor calyces of the renal pelvis (Fig. 16–8). The bases of the pyramids form a margin with the cortical substance. Each pyramid contains strandlike structures which converge upon the apex, called the *papilla*, which in turn protrudes into a calyx. The papilla contains a variable number of minute apertures which represent the terminations of *papillary ducts*. The urine passes from these ducts into the renal calyces and thereafter, into the renal pelvis.

The *renal tubules* with their associated glomeruli of blood vessels constitute the essential units of the kidney (Fig. 16–11). Each tubule is composed of a *glomerular capsule* invaginated by a *glomerulus* of blood vessels; the glomerulus and its capsule

together are spoken of as a *renal (malpighian) corpuscle*. The renal corpuscles are found only in the cortex and renal columns of the kidney. Extending inward from the glomerular capsule is a *proximal convoluted tubule* which twists considerably before it passes into the *descending limb of Henle's loop* (Fig. 16–11 *B*). Henle's loop extends into the medullary pyramid, but thereafter it reverses its direction, increases in size, and becomes the *ascending limb of Henle's loop*. It then leaves the pyramid to re-enter the cortex and once again twists about as the *distal convoluted tubule*. The tubule becomes narrower and opens with other similar tubules into a *straight* or *collecting tubule*, which descends into the medullary pyramid and unites with other collecting tubules, and then finally it opens as a *papillary duct* into a *renal calyx* at the summit of a papilla.

The *renal pelvis* is a reservoir contained within the renal sinus. Usually it contains two main subdivisions or *major calyces*. The major calyces divide into *minor calyces*, each of which terminates in relation to one, two, or sometimes three renal papillae. The protrusion of papillae into the calyces impart a characteristic cup-shaped appearance to the calyces. Considerable variation occurs in the number of major and minor calyces and shape of the renal pelvis (Fig. 16–12); the pelvis may be *intrarenal* where it lies entirely within the renal sinus, or *extrarenal* where it lies like a dilated sac largely outside the kidney proper (Fig. 16–12 *B*).

Blood Vessels of the Kidney

Arteries. The renal arteries arising from the aorta usually divide into *two main branches* directed anteriorly and posteriorly to the kidney (Fig. 16–13). The *posterior* or *dorsal* branch usually arises first and is somewhat smaller in caliber than the *anterior* or *ventral* branch. Secondary branches from the dorsal and ventral branches supply the *five main renal arterial segments* of the kidney as shown in Figure 16–14. The *apical segment* is usually supplied largely by the posterior or dorsal branch of the renal artery, whereas the *lower segment* is supplied mostly by the anterior or ventral branch. Furthermore, *upper and middle branches* of the anterior segment can usually be identified. This segmental distribution within the kidney takes on practical significance if a surgeon contemplates removal of a small part of the kidney. The renal arteries thereafter branch into *interlobar arteries* between the pyramids (Fig. 16–10). At the bases of the pyramids, the interlobar arteries unite to form the *arcuate* arteries. The arcuate arteries, in turn, send branches into the cortex as the *interlobular arteries*, and these give rise to *afferent glomerular arteries* and some *nutrient* and *perforating capsular arteries*. Arising out of the glomerulus are the *efferent glomerular arteries* which form a capillary network around the nephrons but also give rise to a few *arteriolae rectae*, which enter the medulla and run directly toward the pelvis.

Measurements of the Renal and Splenic Arteries. The renal and splenic arteries may be measured at the place where they in-

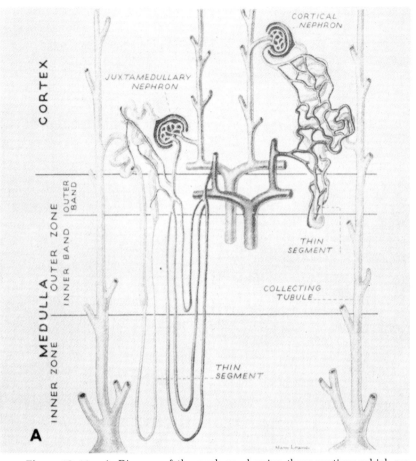

CORTEX

JUXTAMEDULLARY
NEPHRON

CORTICAL
NEPHRON

OUTER ZONE
OUTER BAND
INNER BAND

THIN
SEGMENT

COLLECTING
TUBULE

INNER ZONE

MEDULLA

THIN
SEGMENT

A

Figure 16–11. *A.* Diagram of the nephron showing those portions which are situated in the cortex as against those situated in the medulla. The cortical nephron and juxtamedullary nephron are separately shown. (From Smith, H. W.: Principles of Renal Physiology. New York, Oxford University Press, 1956.)

Figure 16–11 continued on the opposite page.

tersect a line 2 cm. from, and parallel to, the lateral border of the aorta, as shown in Figure 16–13 *B.* When the renal artery bifurcates at a point closer than 2 cm. from the aorta it is measured just proximal to this bifurcation. When a kidney receives more than one artery from the aorta, the equivalent diameter (D) is obtained from the equation:

$$D = 4 \times \sqrt{D1^4 + D2^4 + \ldots Dn^4}$$

in which D1 and D2 are the diameters of two such arteries, and Dn the diameter of the nth such artery.

The *ratio of the internal diameter of the renal artery* to the splenic artery is indicated in the accompanying table. The normal ratio of the renal artery to the splenic artery should be greater than 1. The tabular values are shown within one standard deviation (Maluf).

A narrow renal artery is always indicative of reduced renal function but not renal ischemia; an artery of normal caliber does not necessarily imply normal renal function.

Veins. The renal veins (Fig. 16–13 *C*) begin in the plexuses around the tubules and correspond closely to the arteriolae rectae and the interlobular, arcuate, and interlobar arteries. There are, however, some veins contained in the fibrous capsule of the kidney known as the *stellate venules* that open into the interlobular veins, and communicate with the veins of the fatty capsule around the kidney.

Anastomoses between the renal and systemic vessels occur in the fat around the kidney where the perforating capsular arteries join branches from suprarenal, gonadal, superior, and inferior mesenteric arteries. The renal veins terminate in the inferior vena cava. The *left* renal is longer than the right, crossing the ventral side of the aorta just below the superior mesenteric artery and opening into the inferior vena cava above the right renal vein. It receives as tributaries the *left inferior phrenic,* the *left internal spermatic,* and the *left suprarenal.* It usually lies above the level of the right renal vein, and dorsal to the renal vein, the body of the pancreas, and splenic vein; the inferior mesenteric vein crosses it ventrally.

The *right* renal vein is short and lies in front of the renal artery with no extrarenal tributaries ordinarily.

Blood Vessels of the Adrenal Glands

As indicated previously, the *arteries of the adrenal glands* are derived from three sources: a *superior* artery *from the phrenic;* a *middle* artery *from the aorta;* and an *inferior* artery *from the renal* itself on each side (see Chapter 15).

The veins generally follow the arteries with *one main vein* from each suprarenal gland derived from its medullary portion.

Lymphatic Channels of the Kidney (Rawson; Lilienfeld et al.). The distribution of the lymphatic channels of the human kidney is shown diagrammatically in Figure 16–13 *C.* The lymphatic vessels generally follow closely the arterial and venous channels, with the exception of the afferent and efferent arterioles

Figure 16–11 *Continued.* *B.* Scheme of tubules and vessels of the kidney. (From Anson, B. J. (ed.): Morris' Human Anatomy, 12th ed. Copyright © 1966 by McGraw-Hill, Inc. Used by permission of McGraw-Hill Book Company.)

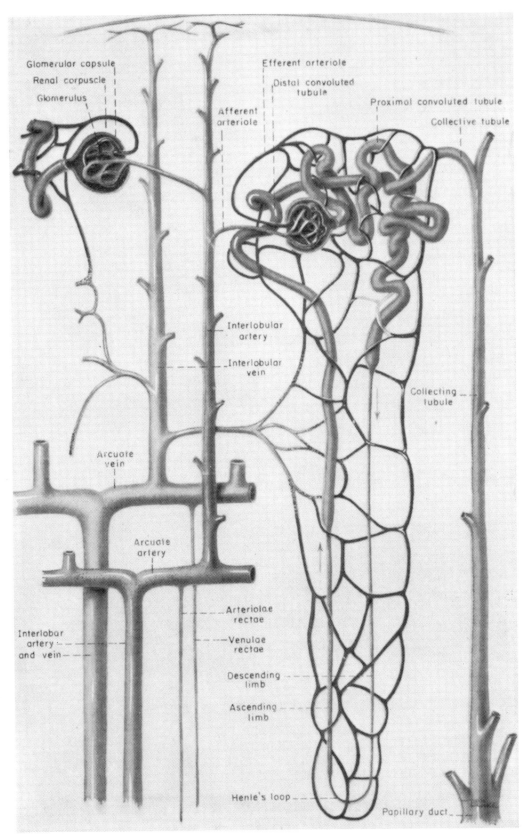

Figure 16–11. *See opposite page for legend.*

B

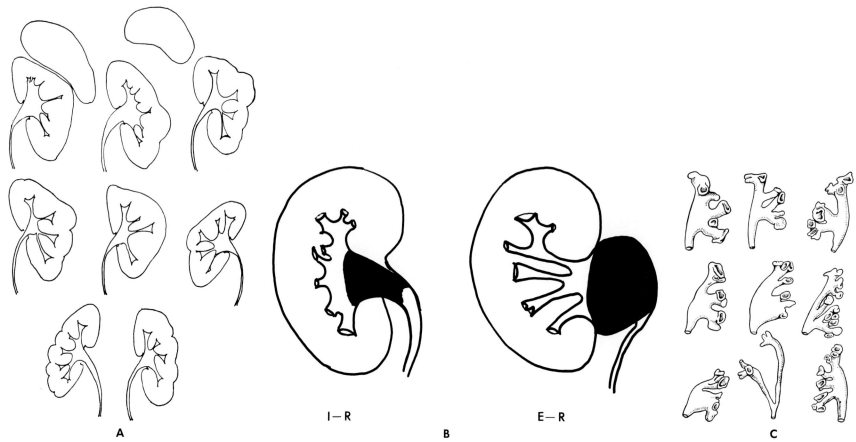

A   I–R   E–R   C
                                                              B

Figure 16–12. *A.* Various types of lobulated renal contours. (From Cooperman, L. R., and Lowman, R. M.: Amer. J. Roentgenol., *92*:273, 1964.) *B.* Intrarenal (I-R) and extrarenal (E-R) pelvis of kidney (pelvis in solid black). The demarcation of the junction of the intrarenal pelvis and the ureter is not distinct. *C.* Variations in configuration of normal renal pelves and calyces.

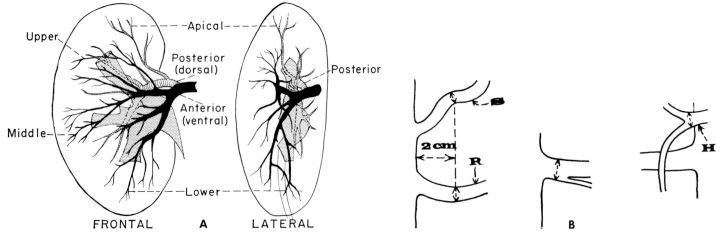

Figure 16–13. *A.* Diagram illustrating the renal artery and its segmental branches in frontal and lateral perspectives, showing the relationship to the pelvocalyceal system. (After Boijsen, E.: Acta Radiol. (Suppl.), *183*:51, 1959.) *B.* Drawings illustrating method of measuring internal diameter of renal, splenic, and hepatic arteries. *Left,* The renal (R) and splenic (S) arteries are measured where they intersect a line 2 centimeters from and parallel to the lateral border of the aorta. The measurements are made at right angles to the longitudinal axis of the vessel at the 2 centimeter intersection. *Center,* When the renal artery bifurcates at a point closer than 2 centimeters from the aorta it is measured proximal to this bifurcation. *Right,* The hepatic artery (H) is measured proximal to its bifurcation into the hepatic artery, proper, and into the pancreaticoduodenal artery. Target-to-film distance 32 inches. Measurements are reduced by 10% for distortion. (From Atlas of Roentgenographic Measurement, 3rd ed., by Lusted, L. B., and Keats, T. E. Copyright © 1972 by Year Book Medical Publishers, Inc., Chicago. Used by permission. [Redrawn from Maluf, N. S. R.: Surg., Gynec., & Obstet. *107*:415, 1958.])

Figure 16–13 continued on the opposite page.

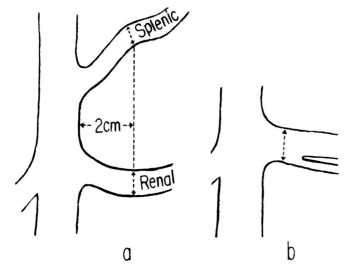

INTERNAL DIAMETER OF RENAL ARTERY

		S.D.
Two normal kidneys	6.5 − 6.7 mm.	0.75 − 0.88
One healthy hyper-trophied kidney	8.4 − 8.6 mm.	0.71 − 0.83

Normal ratio: $\dfrac{\text{Diameter of renal artery}}{\text{Splenic artery}} = >1$

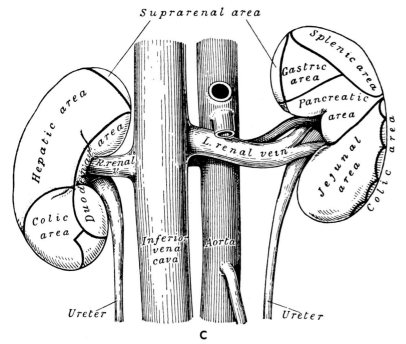

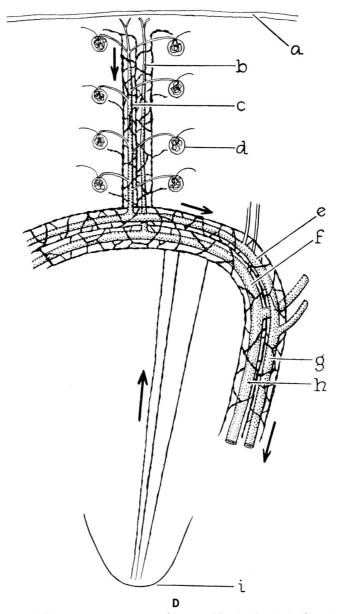

grammatic). Two separate systems are demonstrable. One begins in the cortex and accompanies the interlobular vessels toward the corticomedullary junction; the other starts at the papilla and ascends to join the cortical system at the cortico-medullary junction. From there large trunks follow the arcuate and interlobar vessels to leave the kidney at the hilus. Arrows show the probable direction of the lymph flow. The structures shown are: (a) tunica fibrosa, (b) interlobular vein, (c) interlobular artery, (d) glomerulus, (e) arcuate artery, (f) arcuate vein, (g) inter-lobar artery, (h) interlobar vein, and (i) papilla. (From Rawson, A. J.: Arch. Path., 47:283–292, 1949. Copyright 1949, American Medical Association.)

Figure 16–13 *Continued.*   C. Gross relationships of renal veins to inferior vena cava and anterior surface relationships of the kidneys. (From Warwick, R., and Williams, P. L.: Gray's Anatomy. 35th British edition. London, Longman [for Churchill-Livingstone], 1973.) D. Lymphatic channels of the human kidney (dia-

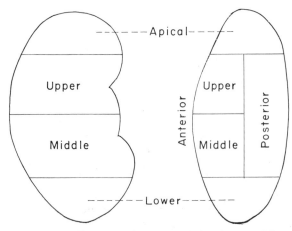

Figure 16–14. Diagram illustrating the segmental distribution of the renal artery. The apical segment is usually supplied largely by the posterior or dorsal branch of the renal artery, whereas the lower segment of the kidney is supplied by the anterior or ventral branch of the renal artery for the most part. (After Boijsen, E.: Acta Radiol. (Suppl.), *183*:10, 1959.)

of the glomeruli, which apparently are not accompanied by lymphatic vessels. The lymphatic channels are more plentiful in the cortex than in the medulla. *Two separate systems* of channels are present: one system begins as tiny blind-ending vessels lying in close contact with Bowman's capsule. These channels gradually enlarge, forming a network around the arterial and venous vessels of the cortex beginning near the terminal branching of both arteries and veins. Lymphatic channels wind loosely around the arteries and veins, frequently coming in chance contact with a convoluted tubule. Those channels that lie in close proximity to large thin-walled venous vessels are prominent, particularly in the outer half of the cortex. The lymphatic channels accompany the interlobular vessels and progress toward the hilus, winding around the arcuate vessels and interlobar arteries and veins. They finally leave the kidney at the hilus, terminating in lymph nodes on either side of the aorta.

Another system of lymphatic channels begins blindly as a network beneath the mucosa of the papilla. These channels ascend in a rather straight line, gradually increasing in size and running parallel to the small blood vessels of the medulla. They empty into the larger lymphatic channels that surround the arcuate arteries and veins.

Generally, increased renal blood flow augments urinary output and increases lymph flowing from the kidneys.

In some respects this double renal lymphatic system corresponds closely to the two hemic circulations demonstrated in the kidney by Trueta et al. These two hemic systems, a greater and a lesser, originate close to the arcuate arteries. The *greater circulation for blood* consists of: interlobular arteries, afferent arterioles, glomerular capillaries, efferent arterioles, capillaries of the medullary rays, capillaries around the convoluted tubules, collecting veins, and interlobular veins.

The *lesser circulation for blood* consists of afferent arterioles of the juxtamedullary glomeruli, these glomeruli themselves, their efferent arterioles, and the vasa recta, arterial and venous, of the medulla.

Variations of the Normal Kidney. The kidneys of different individuals vary considerably as to *size* as noted previously, but generally they are proportional to the size of the body (with numerous exceptions, however).

Variations in *shape* of the kidney are numerous also: they may be elongated or lobulated; they may appear double or may actually be completely duplicated on one side, each with a separate renal pelvis and ureter. In the infant or fetus lobulations are frequent—being found much less frequently in the adult.

Variations in *position* of the kidney have already been described (see Figure 16–1).

There may be *multiple renal arteries* in approximately 25 per cent of normal individuals.

Absence of one kidney is quite rare, occurring on an average of only once in 2400 persons (Anson). Likewise, an extra kidney may sometime be found caudal to the normal one and either attached to it or completely separate (Fig. 16–15). When there are two ureters arising from such a duplex kidney, they usually cross so that the ureter draining the upper renal portion implants itself in the urinary bladder at a lower level than the other.

VARIATIONS IN RENAL SIZE OR NUMBER

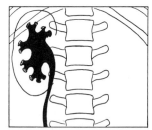
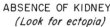
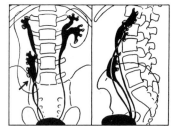

ABSENCE OF KIDNEY
(Look for ectopia) SUPERNUMERARY KIDNEY

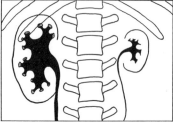
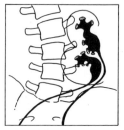

COMPENSATORY HYPERPLASIA
OF ONE KIDNEY WITH APLASIA
OF THE OTHER UNILATERAL FUSED
KIDNEY

Figure 16–15.

Ureters

Introduction. The ureter is a tubular connection between the kidney and the urinary bladder, extending downward from the renal pelvis in extraperitoneal tissue. It is approximately 5 mm. in diameter and 25 cm. in length. It is fairly uniform in size except for three slight constrictions: (a) at the *ureteropelvic junction* (superior isthmus); (b) at the place where the *ureter crosses the pelvic brim* (inferior isthmus); and (c) at the extreme lower end of the ureter as it passes through the urinary bladder wall (called an *intramural constriction*) (Fig. 16–16). The ureter is slightly longer on the left side than on the right, and longer in the male than in the female. It has two portions—the *superior abdominal portion* and the *inferior pelvic portion.*

The *abdominal portions* of the ureters on both sides are embedded on the medial aspect of the psoas major muscles and pass ventral to the common or external iliac artery to enter the true pelvis. They lie ventral to the transverse processes of the third, fourth, and fifth lumbar vertebrae, and both are crossed by the spermatic or ovarian vessels. The right abdominal portion of ureter is covered by descending duodenum and is situated to the right of the inferior vena cava. It is crossed by right colic and ileocolic vessels, the mesentery, and terminal ileum. The left abdominal ureter is crossed by left colic vessels and sigmoid mesocolon. The left ureter is ordinarily separated from the aorta by a space which ranges from 2.5 cm. cranially to 1.5 cm. opposite the bifurcation of the aorta.

The *pelvic portion* of the ureters must be described separately for males and females. In the *male,* this portion of the ureter begins at the pelvic brim, courses caudad close to the internal iliac artery along the ventral border of the greater sciatic notch. It lies medial to the obturator, inferior vesicle, and middle rectal arteries. It turns medially to reach the lateral angle of the urinary bladder at the level of the lower part of the greater sciatic notch. Here, it lies ventral to the seminal vesicles. The vas deferens crosses over it as it approaches the urinary bladder.

In the *female,* the pelvic ureter forms the dorsal boundary of the ovarian fossa. It runs medially and ventrally on the lateral aspect of the cervix and upper part of the vagina to the fundus of the urinary bladder. As it runs ventrally it passes inferior to the uterine artery.

At the level of the urinary bladder the two ureters on each side are about 5 cm. apart in both male and female.

The *intramural* portion of the ureters runs obliquely through the urinary bladder for a distance of approximately 2 cm. and opens into the urinary bladder through two slitlike apertures, the *ureteral ostia,* which are about 2.5 cm. apart in the empty bladder but may be as much as 5 cm. distant from each other when the bladder fills. The ureteral ostia together with the urethral opening of the urinary bladder consitute the *bladder trigone.*

The ureters are not provided with a definite valve at their junction with the urinary bladder, but these slitlike openings ap-

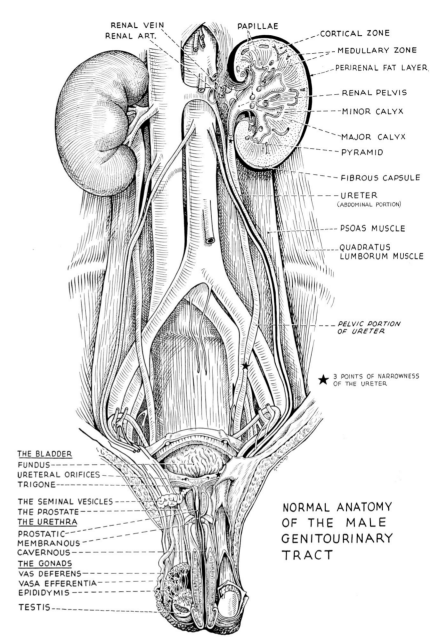

Figure 16–16. Gross anatomy of the urinary tract.

pear to have a valvelike action, so that ureteral reflux from the urinary bladder is considered abnormal. However, on occasion, reflux of urine from bladder to ureter probably takes place normally. Reflux is particularly important in the presence of recurrent infection, in which case pyelonephritis may ensue. The ureter is constantly undergoing peristalsis and hence its lumen is variable in size.

The course of the ureter varies somewhat and tends to be redundant in some individuals, particularly following pregnancy.

Vessels of the Ureter

Arteries. The arteries of the ureter are branches of the renal, internal spermatic, superior, and inferior vesicle arteries.

The *veins* follow correspondingly named arteries and terminate in correspondingly named veins.

The *lymphatics* pass to the lumbar and internal iliac nodes (Fig. 16–17).

Variations of Normal. Apart from variations in length and diameter, the ureter varies with body height, sex, and variations in the positions of the kidneys and urinary bladder. Unilateral absence is usually accompanied by absence of the kidney on the same side. At times there are supernumerary or double ureters that may be complete or incomplete, unilateral or bilateral.

As noted previously, if a ureter is duplicated on one side, the ureter from the superior pelvis terminates inferior to that from the inferior pelvis. Duplication of the ureter occurs in approximately 3 per cent of all individuals (Anson). It occurs slightly more often in females than in males and is more frequently unilateral than bilateral. It is more often complete than incomplete.

Congenital kinking of the ureter is infrequent but may occur, particularly as an accompaniment to ectopia of a kidney. However, kinking of the ureter may also occur over an anomalous vessel.

Anomalies of implantation of the ureteral ostium also occur, most frequently in the female urethra. In the male this formation may occur in the ejaculatory ducts, seminal vesicles, ductus deferens, prostatic utricle, or vestibule. In the female, abnormalities of implantation may also occur in the vagina, uterus, or uterine tubes.

The Urinary Bladder

Introduction. The urinary bladder is a strong, muscular hollow viscus which receives the urine from the kidneys through the ureters, retains it for a period of time, and ultimately expels it through the urethra by micturition. It lies anteriorly, posterior and superior to the pubic symphysis, below the peritoneum and surrounded by extraperitoneal fatty tissue. In the adult, when empty, it lies in the pelvis, but when distended, it balloons upward.

In a *child,* even when empty, it is in contact with the abdominal wall, and is located almost entirely in the abdomen proper. By 6 years of age the greater part of the urinary bladder is ordinarily accommodated by the pelvis, but it is not wholly a pelvic organ until shortly after puberty.

In the male, the seminal vesicles and deferent ducts lie on the lower part of the *posterior surface* of the urinary bladder (Fig. 16–18 *A, B*). The bladder is separated from the rectum by the rectovesical septum, seminal vesicles, and vas deferens (bilaterally).

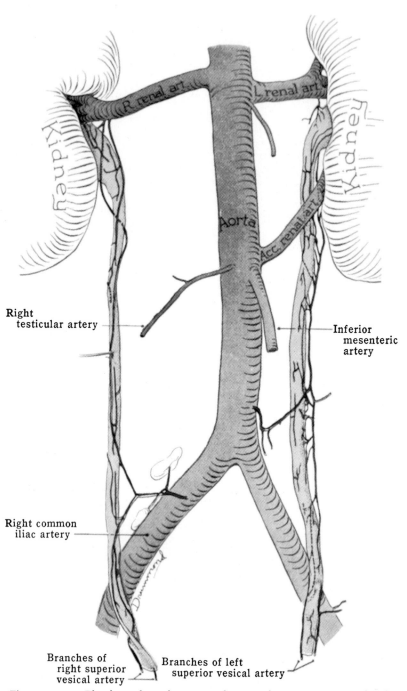

Figure 16–17. Blood supply to the ureter. The arterial system was injected with latex by way of the femoral artery. (Dissection by W. R. Mitchell.) (Reproduced by permission from J. C. B. Grant: An Atlas of Anatomy, 5th ed. Copyright © 1962, The Williams and Wilkins Company.)

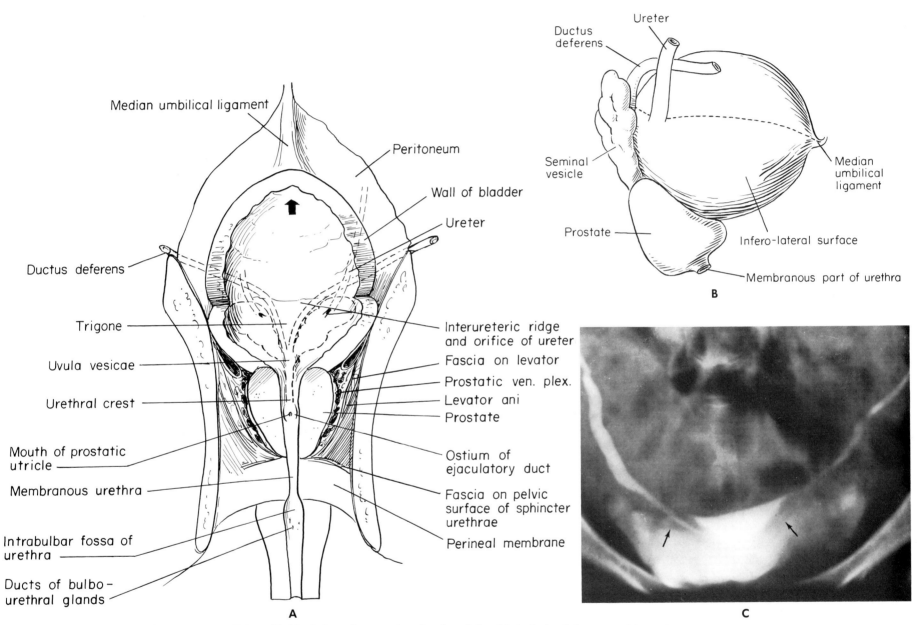

Figure 16–18. *A*. Urinary bladder in frontal perspective, showing relationship to ductus deferens, prostate, ureters, and male urethra. *B*. Urinary bladder hardened in situ showing relationship to ureters, ductus deferens, seminal vesicles, and prostate in lateral view. (From Cunningham's Manual of Practical Anatomy, 12th ed., Vol. 2. London, Oxford University Press, 1958.) *C*. Radiograph of urinary bladder cystogram showing interureteric ridge.

In the *female,* the posterior surface is separated from the uterus by the peritoneum.

In the male, the pelvic colon and coils of the distal ileum rest on the *upper surface* of the urinary bladder, whereas in the female, the upper surface is related closely to the overhanging uterus and a loop of ileum.

In the *infant,* a median umbilical ligament extends up the abdominal wall from the apex of the urinary bladder to the umbilicus. This represents the urachus.

The *neck* of the urinary bladder is about 2 to 3 cm. behind the pubic symphysis, a little above its lower border. Pubovesical ligaments are attached in front and at the sides. In the female it narrows abruptly to become continuous with the urethra. In the male it is continuous with the prostate which surrounds the first part of the urethra, and posteriorly it is in contact with the commencement of the ejaculatory ducts (Fig. 16–18 *A*).

The *inferolateral surface* of the bladder is separated from the pubis by a prevesical cleft and is spoken of as the *retropubic space of Retzius.*

In the female, the *fundus* of the urinary bladder is separated from the ventral surface of the uterus by a vesicouterine pouch below; behind, it is proximal to the cervix and the upper vaginal wall. The inferior surface of the bladder rests on pelvic and urogenital diaphragms.

Interior of Urinary Bladder. When the bladder is full its mucous coat is smooth. When empty, it is wrinkled except over the *trigone,* which is a smooth triangular area above the urethral orifice. The three points of reference for the trigone are the two *ureteric orifices* dorsolaterally and the *internal urethral orifice* ventrally. The base of the triangle is formed by the *interureteric ridge* between the orifices (Figs. 16–18 *A* and 16–19). The internal urethral orifice, placed at the apex of the trigone, presents a very slight elevation, the *uvula vesicae,* caused by the middle lobe of the prostate (Fig. 16–18 *A*).

Vessels and Nerves. The arteries supplying the bladder are the superior, middle, and inferior vesical, which are derived from the anterior trunk of the hypogastric artery (Fig. 16–19). The obturator and inferior gluteal arteries also supply small visceral branches to the bladder. In the female additional branches are derived from the uterine and vaginal arteries.

The *veins* consist largely of a plexus on the inferolateral surface, the plexus communicating with the prostatic plexus. Several veins drain this plexus and pass into the internal iliac vein.

The *lymphatics* drain toward the external, internal, sacral, and median common iliac lymph nodes.

The nerves on the bladder are supplied *via* the inferior hypogastric and vesical plexuses.

Variations of Normal. The urinary bladder varies in shape considerably in different individuals—it may be ellipsoid, triangular, conical, or spherical. At times, the urinary bladder is deformed by adjoining tissues or masses.

The Male Urethra

The male urethra extends from the internal urethral orifice of the urinary bladder to the external urethral orifice at the end of the penis. It is divided into three portions: *prostatic, membranous,* and *cavernous* (Fig. 16–20 *B*).

The *prostatic portion* is somewhat dilated, measuring about 3 cm. in length. In transverse section it is horseshoe shaped with a convexity directed forward. The *urethral crest* (verumontanum) is a longitudinal ridge on its posterior wall. It is about 3 mm. in height and 15 to 17 mm. long. A depressed fossa, the *prostatic sinus,* lies on either side of the crest. These fossae are perforated by numerous apertures which are the orifices of the prostatic ducts from the lateral lobes of the prostate. The ducts of the middle lobe open behind the crest.

At the distal end of the urethral crest is another elevation, the *colliculus seminalis,* which contains the orifices of the prostatic utricle and the slitlike openings of the ejaculatory ducts.

The *membranous portion* of the urethra is short and narrow with a very slight anterior concavity between the apex of the prostate and the bulb of the urethra. It represents that portion of the urethra which perforates the urogenital diaphragm about 2.5 cm. below and behind the pubic symphysis. The membranous portion of the urethra is surrounded by a sphincter.

The *cavernous portion* is approximately 15 cm. long and extends from the membranous portion to the external urethral orifice. It begins just below the urogenital diaphragm and bends downward and forward, measuring about 6 mm. in diameter. It is slightly dilated proximally within the bulb and again distally within the glans penis, where it forms the *fossa navicularis* of the urethra.

The *external urethral orifice* is a vertical slit about 6 mm. long bounded on either side by two small labia.

There are numerous mucous glands which open on the floor of the cavernous portion of the urethra called the *urethral glands of Littré.* There are small pitlike recesses or lacunae of different sizes between these glands. One of the lacunae is larger than the rest and situated in the fossa navicularis (Fig. 16–20).

The Female Urethra

The *female urethra* is about 4 cm. long and extends from the internal to the external urethral orifice. Located behind the pubic symphysis and embedded in the wall of the vagina, it is approximately 6 mm. in diameter and perforates the urogenital diaphragm. Its external orifice is situated in front of the vaginal opening about 2.5 cm. from the glans of the clitoris. A prominent feature is a slight elevation or fold which is called the *urethral crest.* Many small urethral glands open into the urethra, the largest of which are the *paraurethral glands of Skene* (Fig. 16–21).

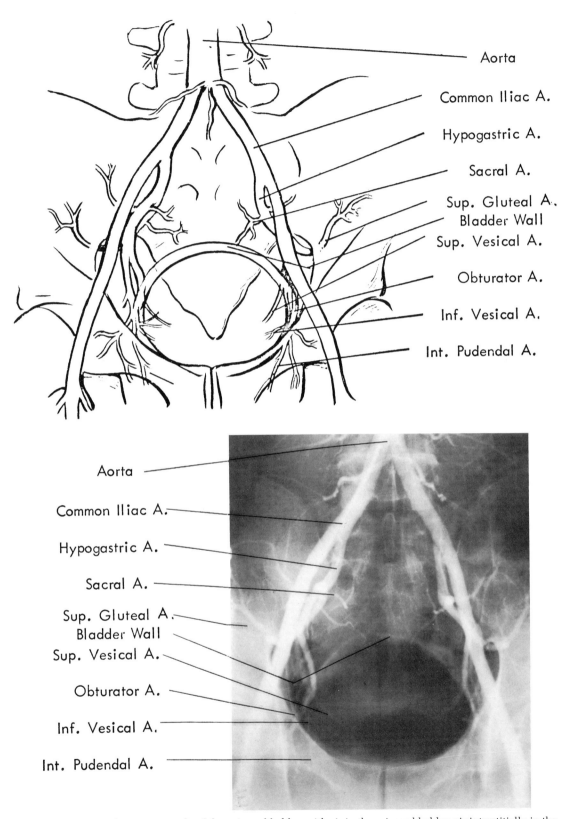

Aorta

Common Iliac A.

Hypogastric A.

Sacral A.

Sup. Gluteal A.
Bladder Wall
Sup. Vesical A.

Obturator A.

Inf. Vesical A.

Int. Pudendal A.

Aorta

Common Iliac A.

Hypogastric A.

Sacral A.

Sup. Gluteal A.
Bladder Wall
Sup. Vesical A.

Obturator A.

Inf. Vesical A.

Int. Pudendal A.

Figure 16–19. Triple contrast study of the urinary bladder, with air in the urinary bladder, air interstitially in the urinary bladder wall, and arterial angiograms for demonstration of the urinary bladder arterial blood supply.

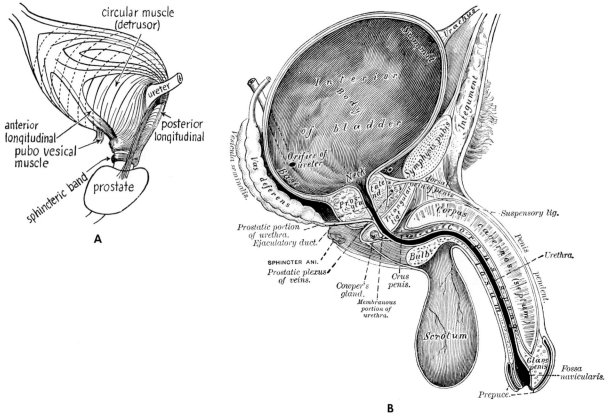

Figure 16–20. *A.* Diagram of the muscles of the bladder (after McCrea). *B.* Vertical section of bladder, penis, and urethra. (*A* from Gray's Anatomy of the Human Body, 29th ed. Goss, C. M. (ed.) Philadelphia, Lea & Febiger, 1973. *B* from 24th ed., 1942, edited by W. H. Lewis.)

GENERAL COMMENTS REGARDING URINARY BLADDER FUNCTION

The Trigonal Canal (Shopfner and Hutch). Radiologic study during the late stages of voiding of the bladder base and urethra in an oblique or lateral position has revealed two primary anatomical units of the bladder: the *vault* and the *base plate*. The *base plate* extends from a point 2 cm. anterior to the internal urethral orifice to another point about 2 cm. posterior to the interureteric ridge (Fig. 16–22 *A*). As indicated by Shopfner and Hutch, a slight constriction or contraction ring is present at the superior margin of the base plate in some patients (Fig. 16–22 *F*). This represents the division between the base plate below and the vault above. There is considerable variation in the contour of the base plate. The internal urethral orifice is slightly anterior to its center, and its anterior edge is the most dependent part of the urinary bladder. That portion of the base plate extending from its anterior edge to the urethrovesical junction is designated the *an-terior trigonal plate*, whereas the part between the urethrovesical junction and the interureteric notch is the *posterior trigonal plate*. The base plate is flat regardless of the degree of bladder distention but increases slightly in length as bladder filling increases. The segment above the interureteric notch is the *nontrigonal portion* of the base plate and this corresponds to the fundus ring (Fig. 16–22). The nontrigonal portion may droop over the flat posterior trigonal plate if the bladder is not maximally filled or is not contracting vigorously (Figs. 16–23, 16–24).

Physiologically it would appear that the base plate functions independently of the vault of the urinary bladder. The base plate appears to dilate slightly in the early stages of voiding, apparently to receive the contents of the vault. It appears first to be shaped like a funnel, and then finally, a tube. After voiding, the trigonal canal gradually returns to its normal flat position to await refilling of the urinary bladder.

In *children under two years of age*, the base plate is convex inferiorly and funnel-shaped rather than flat as in the older child.

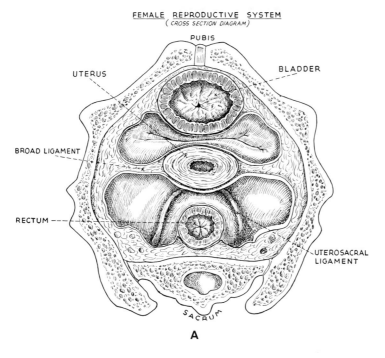

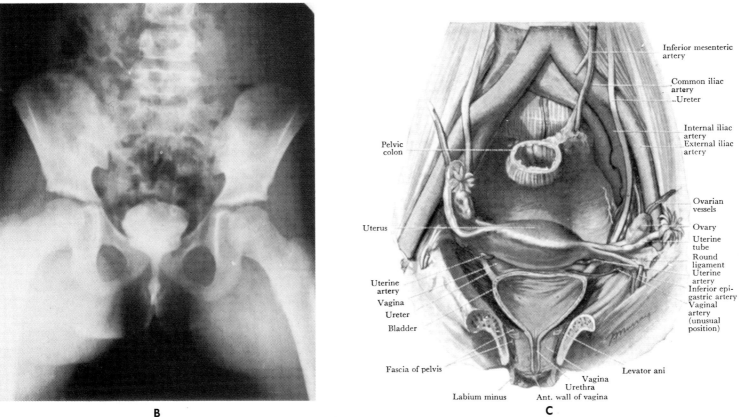

Figure 16–21. *A.* Gross anatomy of the female reproductive system. Superior cross-sectional diagram. *B.* Normal female urethrogram. *C.* Dissection of pelvis of a multiparous female, showing the relations of bladder to uterus and vagina, of vagina to urethra and broad ligaments, and of ureters to broad ligaments and vagina. (From Cunningham's Manual of Practical Anatomy, 12th ed., Vol. 2. London, Oxford University Press, 1958.)

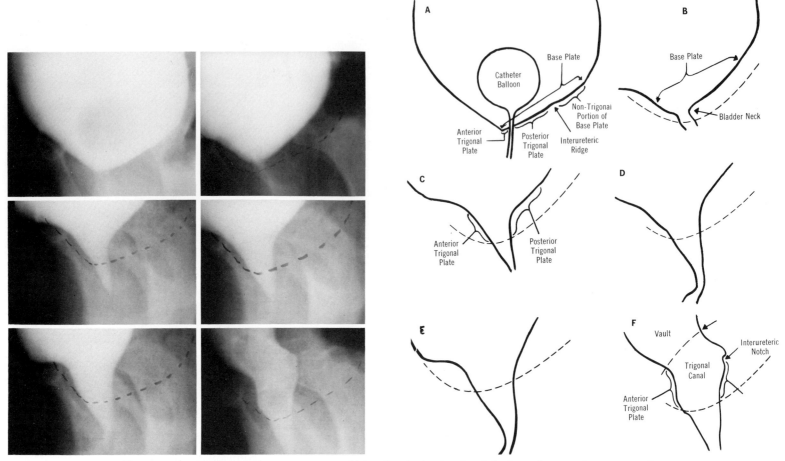

Figure 16–22. Voiding sequence in a 4 year old female. The landmarks of the base plate are shown in *A*. The contraction ring in *F* indicates the division between the base plate below and the vault above. Progressive cephalic movement of the anterior and posterior trigonal plates creates the trigonal canal which is continuous with the posterior urethra. The contraction ring is above the interureteric ridge, indicating that the trigonal canal is formed by the entire base plate and not by the trigonal plates alone. (From Shopfner, C. E., and Hutch, J. A.: Radiology, *88*:209–221, 1967.)

The specific demonstration of the trigonal canal is feasible in perhaps only 55 per cent of patients (Shopfner and Hutch). However, it may be demonstrated in higher percentages in those with mature bladder bases.

Anatomic Changes in the Normal Urinary Tract in the Change from the Supine to the Prone Position (Riggs et al.). Although individual variations occur, the majority of patients show the following changes in the prone position as compared with the supine (Fig. 16–25). (1) There is a bilateral increase in renal length due to magnification and transverse axial rotation. (2) The right kidney tends to move cephalad and medially while the left kidney tends to move caudad. (3) Both kidneys tend to become more parallel to the spine in both frontal and lateral perspectives. (4) Both kidneys tend to rotate about their long axes with the renal pelves moving posteriorly. (5) Both kidneys tend to move anteriorly except in infants. (6) The contrast medium in the urinary bladder gravitates cephalad and anteriorly, creating a more convex, denser, and higher dome. (7) Although many adults

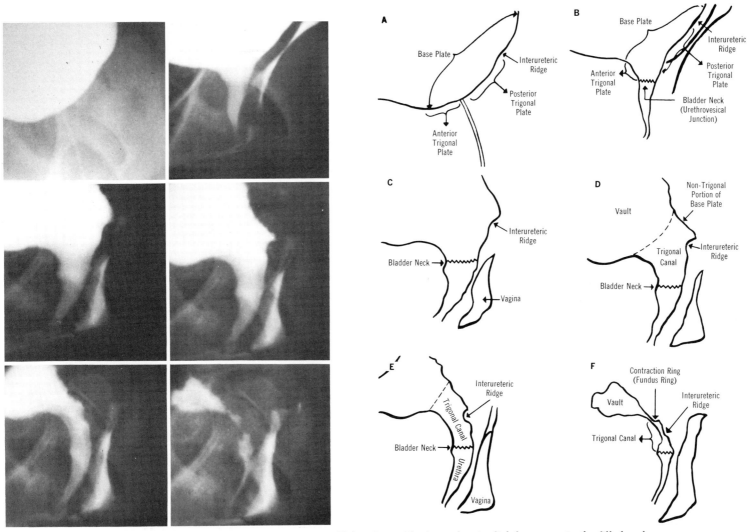

Figure 16–23.   Voiding sequence in a 5 year old female. *A.* The base plate is slightly convex in the filled and resting bladder. *B.* During early voiding, the trigonal plates have moved to an oblique position but the base plate has changed little in size. *C* and *D.* Progressive decrease in the size of the vault and base plate is occurring. In *D*, the trigonal canal is beginning to develop and extends well above the interureteric notch. A distinct difference in caliber exists between the base and the vault. *E.* The trigonal plates are vertical and the trigonal canal is well-developed and continuous with the posterior urethra. *F.* Voiding has almost ceased and the canal has reduced in width during the urethral stripping process. A distinct constriction exists between the base plate and the vault, above the interureteric ridge. (From Shopfner, C. E., and Hutch, J. A.: Radiology, *88:*209–221, 1967.)

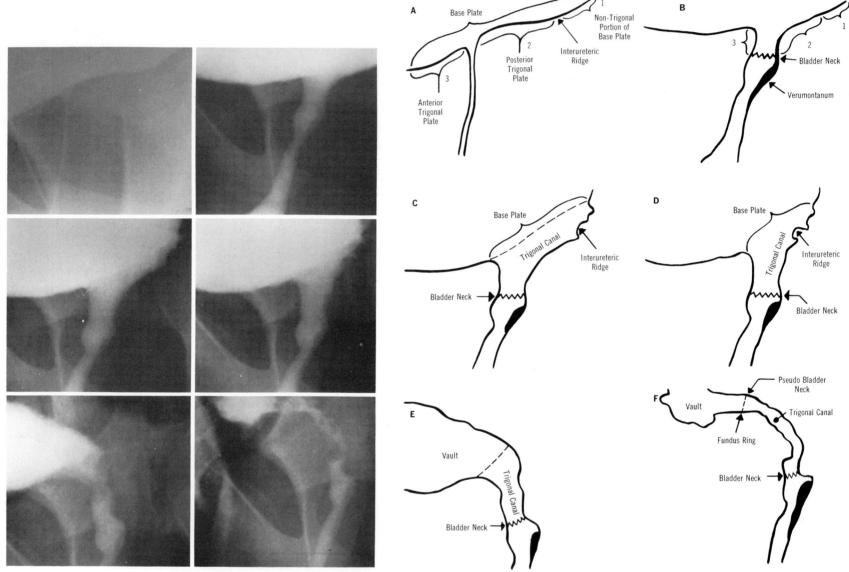

Figure 16–24.   Voiding sequence in a 13 year old male. *A.* The trigonal plates are flat in the filled and resting bladder. The nontrigonal portion of the base plate droops over the posterior trigonal plate (bracket #1). *B.* Voiding has started and the trigonal plates have moved to an oblique position. *C* and *D.* The vault and base plate are becoming smaller as voiding progresses and the trigonal canal is already well-developed. *E.* During the late stages of voiding, the trigonal canal has become narrower and longer as the plates have moved to a vertical position. *F.* A contraction ring marks the division between the trigonal canal and the vault and acts as a pseudo-bladder neck. The canal has decreased in width but increased in length during urethral stripping. (From Shopfner, C. E., and Hutch, J. A.. *Radiology, 88:*209–221, 1967.)

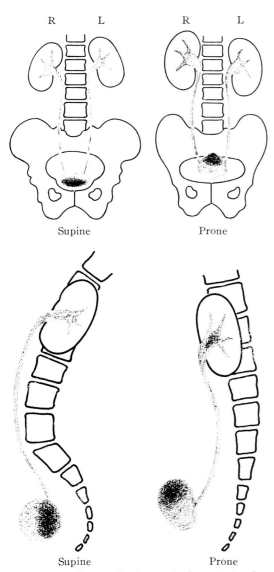

Figure 16–25. Summary of anatomic changes in the majority of cases. *Upper,* In the prone view both kidneys appear larger and are more parallel to the spine. The profile of the renal pelves is better, i.e., wider. Right kidney is higher and more medial, but the left kidney is slightly lower. Dome of the bladder is higher and more convex.

Lower, In the prone view the spine shows straightening of lumbar lordosis. Both kidneys are more parallel to the spine. There is a slight tendency to anterior movement. Pelves appear more true lateral. Bladder appears higher and more anterior. (From Riggs, W., Jr., Hagood, J. H., and Andrews, A. E.: Radiology, 94:107–113, 1970.)

show only minimal change, the findings are most pronounced and consistent in infants. (8) The upper portion of the left kidney in adults is often better seen on the prone film.

GENERAL URINARY TRACT VARIANTS

1. *Suprahilar bulge.* There may be a localized bulge of renal parenchyma just above the hilus continuous with the medial sur-

face of the upper pole. This is more common on the left side. It is thought to be caused by a knuckle of renal cortex of indefinite size which bulges down into the upper pole of the renal sinus (Fig. 16–26).

2. There may be a *"normal" large kidney* with unilateral localized renal enlargement and without contralateral diminution of renal size.

3. The liver and spleen may alter the "normal" renal shape by *pressure.* A renal bump in the midsegment has been described in approximately 10 per cent of patients that is caused by pressure from the spleen (Frimann-Dahl). This has been called the "dromedary kidney" by Harrow and Sloane and has also been described by Doppman and Shapiro.

4. *Double renal hilus.* The renal hilus is usually central but may on occasion be eccentric, lying closer to either the upper or lower pole. When there is a duplication of the collecting system, two hili can be visualized, especially by nephrotomography. There is apparently no relationship between the double hilus and multiple renal arteries.

5. There may be *venous impressions* on the calyceal system as shown in Figure 16–27. Generally, these are wide, smooth filling defects involving the proximal portion of the superior infun-

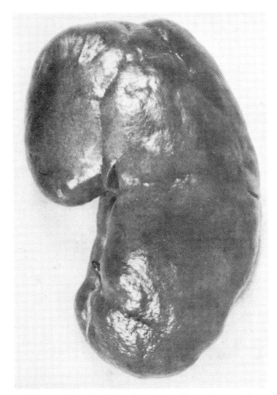

Figure 16–26. Photograph of a left kidney directly *en face* in the anteroposterior position showing a prominent suprahilar bulge (necropsy specimen). (From Doppman, J. L., and Shapiro, R.: Amer. J. Roentgenol.: 92:1380–1389, 1964.)

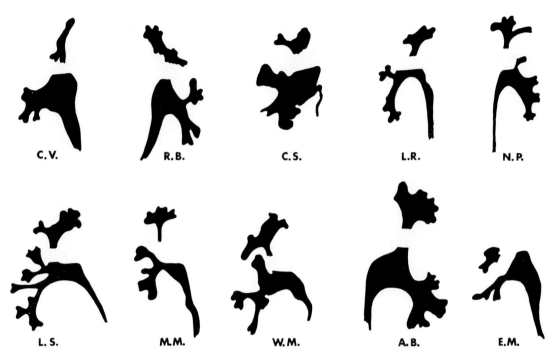

C.V.   R.B.   C.S.   L.R.   N.P.

L.S.   M.M.   W.M.   A.B.   E.M.

Figure 16–27.   Intravenous urographic findings in the ten cases with apparent renal vein impression of the upper infundibulum. Angiographic studies in all revealed no arterial branching in the region of the wide, smooth defect. In three cases the renal veins were opacified and appeared responsible for the impressions. (From Meng, C-H., and Elkin, M.: Radiology, *87*:878–882, 1966.)

dibulum. They present a curved venous trunk on angiography, crossing the filling defect.

6. *Arteries* supplying the kidneys may also *cause pressure defects* of the calyces or infundibula because of the intimate relationship of these intrarenal structures. These defects appear as radiolucent bands roentgenologically, not exceeding 2 to 3 mm. in width ordinarily (Fig. 16–28) (Meng and Shapiro; Weisleder et al.).

7. *Arterial impressions on the ureters and renal pelvis* (Baum and Gillenwater; Chait et al.). Arterial impressions similar to those in the intrarenal collecting system may also be found in the renal pelvis and ureters. At times these are related to normal accessory renal arteries that arise low on the aorta, and sometimes they produce extrinsic pressure defects on the medial or lateral aspect of the ureter. Vessels crossing the ureteral pelvic junction may indeed be implicated with ureteropelvic partial obstruction.

8. *Compression by the iliac artery* may produce its impression on the ureters also at the level at which the ureters cross the iliac vessels.

9. *Renal artery stenosis* may, by backup of blood, cause dilatation of the ureteral artery and perfusion of the kidney by ure-

teral arterial twigs feeding into the renal artery distal to the stenosis (Fig. 16–29).

10. *Normal gonadal vein crossing defect on the ureter.* Both ureters may be crossed by normal gonadal veins (Fig. 16–30). Proximally this may occur a short distance below the ureteropelvic junction, and distally at about the level of the lumbosacral junction. Crossing defects may be seen at each of these locations. An aberrant dilated right ovarian vein has been said to be responsible for urinary tract infection in a previously gravid woman, this being called the *right ovarian vein syndrome.*

11. Other abnormalities *associated with venous distention* may be responsible for *indentation and impressions* on the ureters, such as: varicoceles and varices of the broad ligament; occlusions of the inferior vena cava; renal vein occlusions; occlusion of the azygos vein; occlusion of the superior vena cava; portal hypertension; and carcinoma of the pancreas. In each instance, venous dilatation and impression upon the ureter is postulated.

12. *Retroperitoneal tumors and enlarged lymph nodes may also displace or impress the ureters.* In each instance, careful roentgen diagnostic study is necessary to differentiate the various possibilities (Chait et al.).

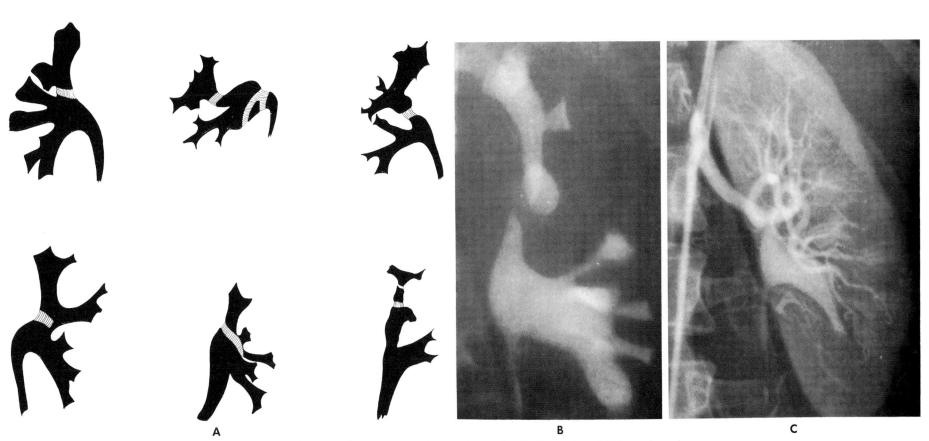

Figure 16–28. *A.* Schematic drawings of arterial impressions on the renal collecting system. *B.* Retrograde pyelogram showing arterial impression on the superior calyceal infundibulum. *C.* Tracing of the arteriogram. The renal and ventral branches are black; the dorsal branches striped; the collecting system gray. (From Weissleder, von H., Emmrich, J., and Schirmeister, J.: Fortschr. Geb. Roentgenstr. Nuklearmed., 97:703–710, 1962.)

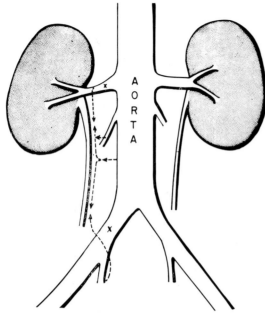

Figure 16–29. Sketch of the arterial supply of the ureter. The ureter normally receives its arterial supply from branches of the renal artery, gonadal artery, directly from the aorta, from lumbar arteries, directly from the internal iliac artery, or from branches of the internal iliac artery. As each of these twigs reaches the ureter, it branches into an ascending and descending limb and joins with its neighbors to form a continuous channel. Flow is normally *to* the ureter from all sources, but direction of flow is responsive to pressure changes. Renal artery stenosis (upper X) may cause dilatation of the ureteral artery and perfusion of the kidney by ureteral arterial twigs feeding into the renal artery distal to the stenosis. Similarly, aortic occlusion or occlusion of the common or internal iliac artery (lower X), with resultant lowered pressure in the pelvis, may result in ureteral artery dilatation; flow in this case, however, is *from* the renal artery *to* the pelvis. (From Chait, A., Matasar, K. W., Fabian, C. E., and Mellins, H. Z.: Amer. J. Roentgenol., *111:*729–749, 1971.)

Basic Physiology of the Kidneys

The Nephron. Figure 16–11 illustrates diagrammatically the nephron, which is the basic functioning unit of the kidney. It contains an afferent and an efferent arteriole leading into and out of the glomerulus; juxtaglomerular cells lie at the junction of the afferent and efferent arteriolar system with the glomerular capillary. It has been suggested that the juxtaglomerular cells (JGA) have an endocrine function, or that perhaps they act like the glomus cells elsewhere in the body. It is true that these cells become heavily granulated in pyelonephritis associated with hypertension, as well as in the early stages of experimental ischemia and hypertension. The degree of granulation parallels the width of the zona glomerulosa of the adrenal cortex and varies inversely with the levels of plasma sodium in animals and man. It

has also been suggested that JGA cells synthesize and store renin.

Blood Supply. The basic blood supply of the kidney has already been described. Approximately 70 per cent of all kidneys are supplied by a single renal artery originating from the aorta; two or more arteries supply the remainder.

Multiple renal arteries are significant since, in some cases, the supplemental artery may supply as much as half the blood supply to the kidney. The most common and important artery is

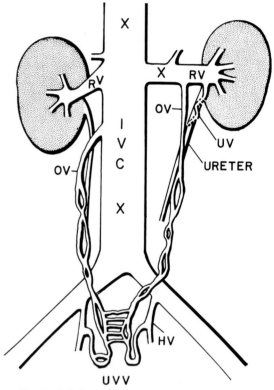

Figure 16–30. Sketch of abdominal, renal, and periureteric venous anatomy. The left gonadal vein (ovarian vein in the sketch) almost invariably empties into the left renal vein, while the right empties into the inferior vena cava below the right renal vein. The ureteral veins generally empty into the renal veins at a location peripheral to the site of gonadal emptying. Either of these two latter structures is capable of causing ureteral notching either of a serpentine nature or of a simple extrinsic pressure type. Free communication between them has been noted on multiple occasions. The ovarian veins are in free communication in the broad ligament with the uterine veins and therefore with the hypogastric and iliac veins. It will be seen therefore that occlusion or stenosis of the inferior vena cava above the renal veins, below the renal veins, or in the renal veins (sites marked X) is capable of altering flow in the gonadal or ureteric veins and thereby accounting for vascular notching. (RV) renal vein, (OV) ovarian (gonadal) vein, (UV) ureteral vein, (HV) hypogastric vein, (UVV) uterine veins, (X) sites of occlusion. (From Chait, A., Matasar, K. W., Fabian, C. E., and Mellins, H. Z.: Amer. J. Roentgenol., *111:*729–749, 1971.)

the supplemental vessel to the inferior portion of the kidney; it may supply as much as 20 to 50 per cent of the renal parenchyma.

In the arcuate veins, the pressure is about 25 mm. of mercury. Beyond these, the pressure suddenly drops to approximately 7 mm. of mercury because of "cushions" or sinusoids which serve as contractor mechanisms at the junction of the arcuate and interlobar veins.

Renal Function. The function of the kidney may be outlined as follows (Fig. 16–31):

1. *Filtration* of the blood plasma and removal of some of its solutes such as potassium chloride sulfate, sodium, urea, glucose, amino acid and the like.
2. *Selective tubular reabsorption.*
3. *Tubular synthesis and excretion.*
4. *Acid-base regulation.*
5. *Volume regulation* of the fluid environment of the body.
6. *Osmolality regulation.*
7. *Maintenance of a normal blood pressure.*
8. *Erythropoiesis.*

As the result of an effective filtration pressure gradient in the glomerulus, the walls of the glomerular capillaries act as a sieve, allowing particles of certain sizes to filter through and retaining larger ones.

The renal tubules, on the other hand, are primarily concerned with: (1) *water reabsorption* from the glomerular filtrate; (2) *reabsorption* of certain *threshold substances* and ions necessary for the equilibrium of the organism; (3) *excretion* of some organic and inorganic compounds in substances; (4) *synthesis* of certain metabolites; and (5) *excretion of the final waste products* into the collecting system, after an appropriate regulation of acid-base balance and osmolality. It is probable that water is absorbed from both proximal and distal convoluted tubules.

In addition, approximately 14 per cent of water is reabsorbed in the collecting tubules under the control of an antidiuretic hormone derived from the pituitary gland (ADH). To some extent this reabsorption is accomplished by the hyperosmotic environment of the interstitial fluid in the medulla of the kidney involving and surrounding the loops of Henle. This is part of the so-called counter-current phenomenon.

Glomerular filtration and tubular secretion and excretion are the two renal functions especially identified by roentgenologic techniques. Contrast agents such as Hypaque, Miokon, and Renografin are in large measure excreted normally by glomerular filtration, much as is inulin. These compounds, therefore, offer the opportunity for physiologic tests of glomerular filtration. Para-amino hippurate and Hippuran are largely excreted (or secreted) via the tubules and are useful in measuring tubular secretion or excretion. Previously used compounds such as Diodrast more closely resemble the latter group of compounds although not exclusively so. Diodrast is also excreted by the liver as well as by glomerular filtration.

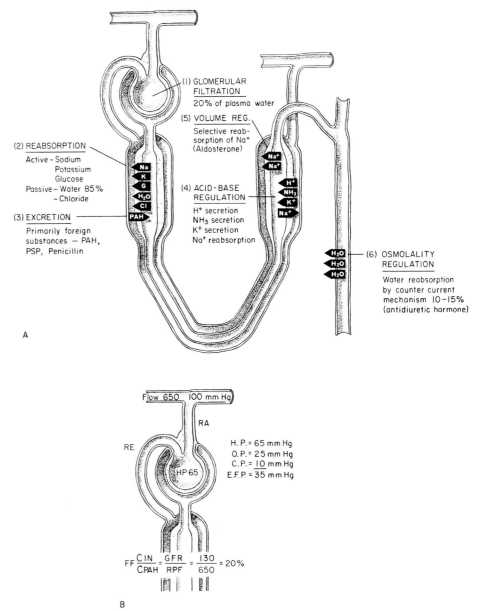

Figure 16–31. *A.* Physiology of the nephron. The various functions of the nephron in regulation of the internal environment of the body are diagrammatically illustrated. *B.* Diagrammatic illustration of glomerular hemodynamics in the maintenance of filtration pressure. (H.P.) Hydrostatic pressure, (O.P.) osmotic pressure, (C.P.) capillary pressure, (E.F.P.) effective filtration pressure, (RA) afferent arterioles, (RE) efferent arterioles, (FF) filtration fraction, (CIN) clearance of inulin, (CPAH) clearance of para-aminohippurate, (GFR) glomerular filtration rate, (RPF) renal plasma flow. (From Meschan, I.: Radiol. Clin. N. Amer., 3:18, 1965.)

Sodium diatrizoate (Hypaque) is excreted at the rate of approximately 65 per cent in 2 hours and 88 per cent in 6 hours. This is more rapid than the excretion of Diodrast and Urokon.

Kidney function is routinely studied in a dehydrated body

state. This, of course, is not a normal physiologic state and therefore cannot accurately be related to conventional clearance studies by inulin or para-amino hippuric acid techniques. If clearance of these compounds is to be studied, the body must be in a hydrated state, equilibrated, and at normal rest.

In a subsequent section, a "washout" test for renovascular hypertension will be described. The basis for this test is as follows: in patients with kidneys responsible for renovascular hypertension, dilution of the contrast agent does not occur during the washout phase. This so-called hyperconcentration results from excessive, obligated tubular water reabsorption and a low-flow phenomenon in the kidney nephron.

Normal Intrarenal Circulation Time. Circulation times of 6 to 8, 8 to 10, and 10 to 12 seconds have been published (Becker et al.). Generally, an intrarenal circulation time of less than 5 seconds is considered abnormal when a bolus of 8 ml. of contrast material is used, delivered in 1 second.

Gallbladder Visualization Following the Injection of Diatrizoate. Excretion of pyelographic agents via the bile and into the gallbladder with incidental opacification of the gallbladder may occur in unusual circumstances. As a general rule, when this phenomenon occurs with the diatrizoates, renal dysfunction with delayed excretion of contrast material occurs, and creatinine and blood urea nitrogen values are elevated (Segall).

TABLE 16–3 CONTRAST MEDIA USED IN UROGRAPHY AND ANGIOGRAPHY

Trade Name	Organic Compound	Per Cent Iodine W/V	Concentration of Drug in Commercially Available Solution	Manufacturer's Suggested Dosage			
				Adult Dose	Children's Dose	Subcutaneous Administration	Intramuscular Administration
Neo-Iopax[a]	Sodium iodomethamate	25.8 38.6	50% 75%	20 cc. of 50% 30 cc. of 50% 20 cc. of 75%	10 cc. of 50%	10% solution (dilute 14 cc. of 75% solution to 100 cc. with normal saline)[e]	Not recommended
Diodrast[b]	Iodopyracet, U.S.P.	17.5 (35% in 70% solution)	35% (70% also available)	20–30 cc. of 35%	0– 6 mo.: 5 cc. 7–12 mo.: 6– 7 cc. 1– 3 yr.: 7–10 cc. 4– 6 yr.: 10–16 cc. 7– 8 yr. 16–20 cc.	7% solution (dilute 20 cc. of 35% solution to 100 cc. with normal saline)[e]	35% solution Children: 10–20 cc. Adults: 20–30 cc.
Hippuran[c]	Sodium iodohippurate	7 (in 20% solution)	Powder only available. Mix 12 gm. with 60 cc. of distilled water to make 20% solution	60 cc. of 20%	0–12 mo.: 6 gm.+ 9.55 cc. water 1– 4 yr.: 8 gm.+ 12.5 cc. water 4– 8 yr.: 10 gm.+ 21 cc. water	Not recommended	Not recommended
Urokon[c]	Sodium acetrizoate, U.S.P.	19.74 (46.06% in 70% solution)	30% 70% for difficult cases only or aortography or nephrotomography	25 cc. of 30% 25 cc. of 70%	<4 yr.: 0.7 cc. of 30% solution >4 yr.: 25 cc. of 30% solution	Not recommended	Not recommended
Miokon[c]	Sodium diprotrizoate, U.S.P.	28.7	50%	20 cc. of 70% 25 cc. of 50% 30 cc. of 50%	<3 mo.: 6 cc. 3– 6 mo.: 6– 8 cc. 6–12 mo.: 8–10 cc. 1– 2 yr.: 10–15 cc. 2– 6 yr.: 15–20 cc. >6 yr.: 20–25 cc.	Not recommended	Not recommended
Hypaque-50[b]	Sodium diatrizoate, U.S.P.	30	50% for excretory urography	30 cc. of 50%	0– 6 mo.: 5 cc. 6–12 mo.: 6– 8 cc. 1– 2 yr.: 8–10 cc. 2– 5 yr.: 10–12 cc. 5– 7 yr.: 12–15 cc. 7–11 yr.: 15–18 cc. 11–15 yr.: 18–20 cc.	Dilute with equal quantities of distilled water[e]	Inject undiluted or diluted with equal parts distilled water
Hypaque-75[b]	Sodium diatrizoate, U.S.P.	39.3	75% 90% for nephrotomography	50 cc. or more	Infants: 5–10 cc. Older children: 15–20 cc.	Not recommended	Not recommended
Hypaque-90[b]	Sodium diatrizoate, U.S.P.	46	75% 90% for nephrotomography	50 cc. or more	Infants: 5–10 cc. Older children: 15–20 cc.	See text	See text

[a]Schering
[b]Winthrop Laboratories
[c]Mallinckrodt Pharmaceuticals
[d]E. R. Squibb and Sons
[e]Subcutaneous injections are given in divided doses over each scapula. Intramuscular injections are given in divided doses into each gluteal region. To increase the rate of absorption, the addition of hyaluronidase to the solution is recommended (150–200 turbidity units on each side for children, 500 for adults).

Table 16–3 continued on opposite page.

Contrast Media Used in Urography and Angiography

The most commonly used contrast media in urography and angiography are indicated in Table 16–3, with the manufacturer's suggested dosage. In Figure 16–32, the structural formula of the more common of these agents is compared.

Various physiologic evaluations of the dose of contrast medium for intravenous urography have been carried out (Dure-Smith), as for example with Urografin, a mixture of sodium and methylglucamine diatrizoate in the ratio of 10 to 66 (Renografin,

U.S.P.). From this study, the following conclusions may be drawn: (1) There is a good correlation between the dose of contrast medium and plasma concentration. This is initially largely independent of renal function. (2) The minimum concentration of contrast agent in the glomerular filtrate necessary to produce an appreciable nephrogram is probably in the range of 70 mg. iodine per cent. This can apparently be attained with 20 cc. of Urografin 76 per cent in 1 to 2 seconds. If 140 cc. of Urografin-76 is infused slowly, levels well above this are maintained for well over 60 minutes.

The mean plasma concentration of Urografin occurs at iden-

TABLE 16–3 CONTRAST MEDIA USED IN UROGRAPHY AND ANGIOGRAPHY (*Continued*)

Trade Name	Organic Compound	Per Cent Iodine W/V	Concentration of Drug in Commercially Available Solution	Manufacturer's Suggested Dosage			
				Adult Dose	Children's Dose	Subcutaneous Administration	Intramuscular Administration
				Retrograde pyelograms:			
Renografin-30[d]	Diatrizoate methyl-glucamine, U.S.P.	15	30%	15 cc. (unilateral)	Proportionately smaller for children	Not used	Not used
Renografin-60[d]	Methylglucamine diatrizoate, U.S.P.	29	60%	25 cc. of 60% (over 15 yrs.)	Under 6 mo.: 5 cc. 6–12 mo.: 8 cc. 1– 2 yr.: 10 cc. 2– 5 yr.: 12 cc. 5– 7 yr.: 15 cc. 8–10 yr.: 18 cc. 11–15 yr.: 20 cc.	Not used	Not used
Renografin-76[d]	Diatrizoate methyl-glucamine	37	76%	20–40 cc. of 76% (over 15 yrs.)	Under 6 mo.: 4 cc. 6–12 mo.: 6 cc. 1– 2 yr.: 8 cc. 2– 5 yr.: 10 cc. 5– 7 yr.: 12 cc. 8–10 yr.: 14 cc. 11–15 yr.: 16 cc.	Not used	Not used
Renovist[d]	Sodium and methyl-glucamine diatrizoate	37	69%	25 cc. of 37% solution (over 15 yrs.)	Under 6 mo.: 5 cc. 6–12 mo.: 8 cc. 1– 2 yr.: 10 cc. 2– 5 yr.: 12 cc. 5– 7 yr.: 15 cc. 7–10 yr.: 18 cc. 10–15 yr.: 20 cc.	Not used	Not used
				Retrograde pyelography:			
Retrografin	Neomycin sulfate solution with methyl glucamine diatrizoate	15	25% neomycin 30% methylgluca-mine diatrizoate	15 cc. (unilateral)	Proportionately smaller for children	Not used	Not used
Ditriokon[c]	Sodium diprotrizoate and diatrizoate	40	68.1%	40–50 cc. (over 12 yrs.)	0.5–1 cc./kg. body weight	Not used	Not used
Conray-60[c]	Meglumine iothalamate	28.2	60%	25–30 cc. (14 yrs. and over)	Under 6 mo.: 5 cc. 6–12 mo.: 8 cc. 1– 2 yr.: 10 cc. 2– 5 yr.: 12 cc. 5– 8 yr.: 15 cc. 8–12 yr.: 18 cc. 12–14 yr.: 20–30 cc.	Not used	Not used
Conray–400[c]	Sodium iothalamate 66.8%	40	66.8%	40–50 cc. (over 14 yrs.)	0.5–1 cc./kg. under 14 yrs.	Not used	Not used

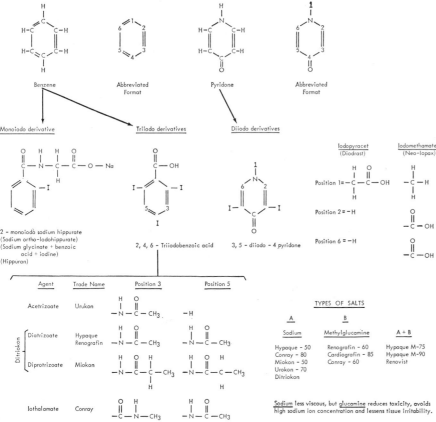

Figure 16–32. The organic structure of the iodinated derivatives of benzene and pyridone which are used in the radiographic visualization of the kidneys. (Modified from Potsaid.)

tration of contrast medium in the urine, will depend on the state of hydration of the patient at the start of the procedure.

Even in high dose urography, dehydration will improve the concentration of contrast medium in the urine in patients with normal renal function. *Actually, however, drip infusion pyelography probably offers no advantage over high dose urography in which equivalent doses of the undiluted contrast medium are injected. A rapid injection usually causes a higher peak of the plasma concentration and a denser nephrogram than a slower injection.*

O'Connor and Neuhauser (1963) described a method of total body opacification with relatively large doses of intravenously injected radiopaque contrast media—2 to 4 cc. per kilogram of body weight in infancy. The mechanism of this is thought to be opacification of the entire blood vascular compartment in less than 60 seconds. The added density of the various tissues is proportional to the blood supply. An avascular or hypovascular lesion will be radiolucent in contrast to the adjacent structures with a greater blood supply. The method is limited in differentiating a chronic or poorly vascularized neoplasm from a cyst, but it is particularly useful in defining cystic, hemorrhagic, and chronic lesions.

Apparently, untoward reactions are not dose-related in the dose ranges employed, but *it is probable that the intravenous injection of any such contrast media should not be performed when hyperbilirubinemia is present in the newborn.*

An investigation of higher volumes of contrast material to improve intravenous urography has been carried out by Friedenberg and Carlin. These investigators arbitrarily chose certain volumes with respect to body surface area as shown in Table 16–4. There was a slight increase in the frequency of side effects, which were, however, mild and well tolerated by the patients. Generally, the use of higher volumes of the contrast material improved the quality of intravenous urograms significantly. It increased the diagnostic accuracy of the examination and reduced the need for retrograde pyelography with its attendant hazards.

tical rates regardless of the rapid intravenous injection of 20 cc. or the slow infusion of 140 cc. of Urografin.

If a contrast medium is injected slowly over 8 to 10 minutes, the peak plasma concentration is not reached until 15 minutes, and this should indeed be the period of maximum density of the nephrogram and optimum period of nephrotomography.

The contrast medium itself acts as a simple osmotic diuretic. The concentration of contrast medium in the urine is accurately reflected by the diuresis.

In patients with normal renal function who have been deprived of fluid for some 12 hours, the concentration of contrast medium in the urine continues to increase with increasing doses up to 140 cc. of Urografin-76, despite the increasing diuresis.

The better the dehydration of the patient, the higher will be the "optimal" dose for this patient. Maximum dehydration, however, is not achieved within the usual period of 8 to 12 hours of fluid restriction before urography. The optimal dose of contrast medium, or one which will produce no further increase in concen-

TABLE 16–4   DOSAGE SCHEDULE TESTED FOR HIGH-VOLUME UROGRAPHY*

Body Surface Area (sq. meters)	Volume (ml.)
Less than 1.30	30
Less than 1.50	40
Less than 1.70	50
Less than 1.90	60
Less than 2.10	70
Less than 2.25	80
Less than 2.40	90
Greater than 2.40	100

*From Friedenberg, M. J., and Carlin, M. R.: Routine use of higher volumes of contrast material. Radiology, *83*:405–413, 1964.

No effort was made in this study to determine the relative merits of injecting the contrast material in single versus divided doses, but from other data in the literature it would appear that this probably would not be a significant factor.

RADIOLOGIC METHODS OF STUDY

Preparation of the Patient. The patient should have a small supper or no meal at all on the night prior to the examination, with nothing by mouth after this meal. Dehydration for at least 12 hours prior to the examination is highly desirable and enhances the concentration in the kidney with either single-dose or infusion techniques.

Catharsis with preparations such as 45 cc. of X-Prep liquid, 1 or 2 oz. of castor oil, or a full dose of magnesium citrate U.S.P. at approximately 6:00 P.M. on the evening prior to the examination is preferred. Some investigators have preferred cleansing enemas on the morning of the examination, but often this will introduce gas into the gastrointestinal tract that will interfere with

the clarity of the examination. Suppositories to stimulate colonic evacuation on the morning of the examination may be employed. Aloin, cascara sagrada, or phenolphthalein may be utilized in lieu of the cathartics mentioned above.

Plain Film, Patient Supine (Fig. 16–33). *An anteroposterior film in suspended respiration with the patient supine must precede any contrast study of the urinary tract.* In the pediatric age groups, some physicians may prefer a prone film instead, either prior to the study or during the procedure (Baker) (see previous comparison of prone and supine films of the urinary tract). If the supine position is employed, the abdomen may be compressed with an inflated rubber bag, provided this does not cast an opaque shadow on the roentgenogram. These films should include the entire area from the diaphragm to the pubic symphysis.

Such film studies must be done immediately prior to the injection of contrast media, since any opacities in the urinary pathways may change position in short intervals of time. Moreover, the introduction of opaque material into the urinary tract will obscure calcific structures.

Since one film in the erect position may also be obtained in

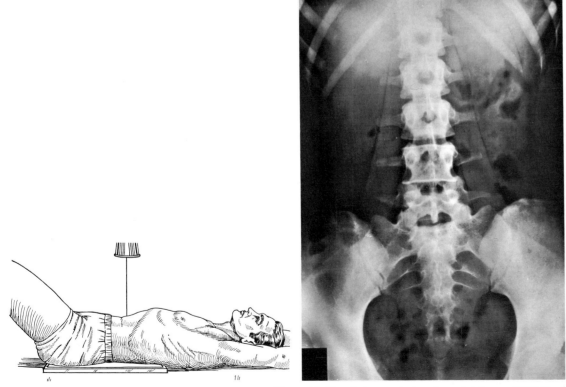

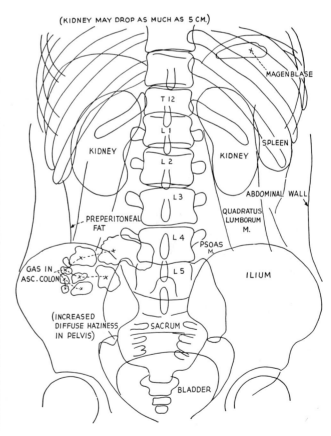

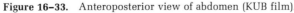

Figure 16–33. Anteroposterior view of abdomen (KUB film).

the course of the entire study, an anteroposterior view of the abdomen in this position prior to the injection of the contrast medium may also be desired.

Single Injection Excretory Urogram (IVP) (Fig. 16–34 *A* and *B*).

Immediately before injection of any contrast medium the patient is instructed to *void*.

Contrast media which have been and are being used are listed in Table 16–3. The most commonly used at this time are: 50 per cent sodium diatrizoate; 60 per cent meglumine diatrizoate; 60 per cent meglumine iothalamate; and occasionally, 66.8 per cent sodium iothalamate.

The *usual intervals* for taking of films after intravenous injection of the opaque medium are: 4 to 5 minutes; 8 to 15 minutes; 25 to 40 minutes; 60 minutes; 90 minutes; 2 hours; and delayed urography at hourly intervals if necessary up to 8 hours following the intravenous injection if so indicated. If only four films are utilized in the entire examination (three films in addition to the plain film), the recommended time intervals for use with the diatrizoates are 4 minutes, 8 minutes, and 15 to 30 minutes.

In some instances, *oblique films* will also be taken, and usually the best time for these is immediately following maximal visualization of the ureters (10 to 20 minutes).

If the lower ureters are not accurately visualized in the supine position the patient may then be turned in the *prone position* and a repeat study obtained at an optimum time interval.

Dose. Many radiologists employ doses larger than those suggested by the manufacturer as indicated in Table 16–3. For example, in infants 6 months or younger, 10 cc. of the diatrizoate are employed; in older children, a minimum dose of 2 to 3 cc. per pound is usually employed; in adults, the usual dose is often 1.5 cc. per pound or even greater, to a maximum of 150 cc. if necessary.

Delayed Films. If excretion and concentration are delayed, it is well to keep obtaining films until a good concentration of the medium is seen in the urinary bladder. At times even 8 to 24 hour films may be helpful.

Cystogram and Voiding Urethrogram. If, in addition, a cystogram is desired by this excretory method, oblique studies of the urinary bladder are obtained. Urethrograms require an oblique

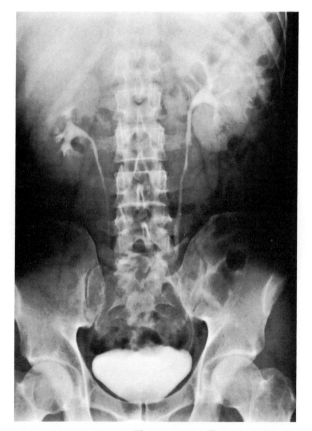
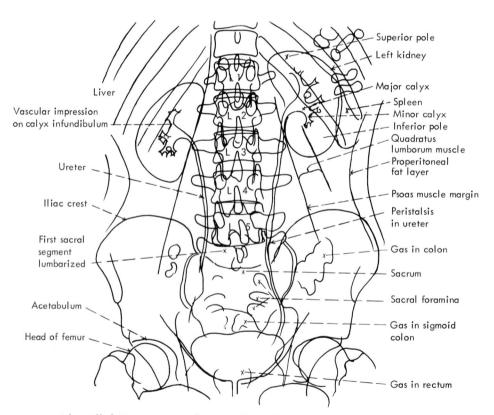

Figure 16–34. Representative excretory urogram (also called intravenous pyelogram) obtained 15 minutes after the intravenous injection of a suitable contrast agent (25 ml. 50 per cent Hypaque).

RADIOLOGIC METHODS OF STUDY OF THE URINARY TRACT

1. Preparation of patient.
2. Plain film, patient supine (KUB).
   a. Prone film in infants.
3. Single injection excretory urogram.
4. Infusion excretory urogram.
5. Hypertension study pyelogram—rapid sequence dehydrated urogram, combined with a hydrated pyelogram.
6. Nephrotomography.
7. Retrograde pyelography.
8. Cystography and cystourethrography.
   a. With voiding urethrogram.
   b. Retrograde urethrogram.
   c. Cystogram (with excretory or retrograde pyelogram).
   d. With double contrast (air).
   e. Triple contrast—angiography plus pneumocystogram plus interstitial air in wall of urinary bladder.
   f. "Chain" cystourethrogram—investigation of stress incontinence.
9. Renal arteriography and aortography.
10. Phlebography and inferior vena cavography.
11. Roentgen evaluation of the surgically exposed kidney.
12. Cineradiography of the upper urinary tract and cystourethrography.
13. Perirenal air insufflation.
14. Seminal vesiculography.
15. Reactions to contrast media.

Figure 16–35

study of the urethra while the patient is urinating into a suitable receptacle (voiding cystourethrogram). Usually it is more satisfactory to perform urethrograms following instillation of the medium directly into the bladder (Fig. 16–36).

In infants it has been customary to administer a *carbonated cola drink to distend the stomach* and thus portray the left kidney more clearly; some, however, advise against this procedure because the gas soon passes farther into the gastrointestinal tract and makes accurate visualization difficult (Baker).

If intravenous injection is unsuccessful, *gluteal intramuscular injection* may be used together with an injection of hyaluronidase to promote absorption (Fainsinger). Hypaque and Renografin (sodium diatrizoate and meglumine diatrizoate) may also be given intramuscularly (Emmett).

Infusion Excretory Urography. Infusion excretory urography is the technique of opacifying the urinary tract by means of a large amount of contrast medium introduced by continuous intravenous drip. The technique, described by Harris and Harris, involves the intravenous infusion of 140 cc. of 50 per cent sodium diatrizoate (Hypaque) mixed with an equal amount of physiologic salt solution and allowed to run freely through a 19 gauge hypodermic needle. After 225 cc. has been introduced the infusion is slowed in order to maintain an open needle for the duration of the study. The first roentgenogram is made 20 minutes following commencement of the infusion. Thereafter, any other radiographs may be obtained as necessary.

A rapid infusion of 100 ml. of Renografin-76 plus 1 ml. of isotonic dextrose solution per pound of body weight may be similarly employed.

The main advantage of this technique is the increased clarity with which the collecting system and ureters may be identified, sometimes avoiding the necessity for retrograde pyelography. Moreover, body section radiographs can be obtained when nephrotomography might be indicated, such as the differentiation of renal cysts and neoplasms (Fig. 16–37).

The Rapid Sequence Dehydrated Excretion Urogram Combined with a Hydrated Pyelogram. The Hypertension Pyelogram (Fig. 16–38). At the onset of an excretory urogram, the patient is decidedly dehydrated. Normally, hydration of a patient undergoing an excretory urogram will produce a marked dilution of the contrast agent within a normal kidney and some dilatation of the calyces, so that the visualization of the calyces may be indistinct. In patients with renovascular hypertension, such dilution of the contrast agent does not ordinarily occur, and hydration may actually enhance the visualization of an otherwise poorly seen collecting system.

To facilitate hydration, urea diuresis has been recommended as follows: a slow-drip intravenous infusion of 40 grams of urea in 500 ml. of 5 per cent dextrose (rather than isotonic saline as in the Amplatz method) is begun through an 18 gauge needle. This is momentarily clamped off and 50 cc. of 75 per cent Hypaque-M is introduced as rapidly as possible through this needle (within 30 seconds). Films are obtained immediately thereafter and then at 1 minute intervals for 6 minutes. The slow drip is continued only to keep the needle from being obstructed by a blood clot. An additional film is obtained at 8 minutes. Following exposure of the 8 minute pyelogram, at which time the renal collecting systems are usually at their peak of opacification, a more rapid infusion of the urea-dextrose mixture is begun so that the entire infusion occurs

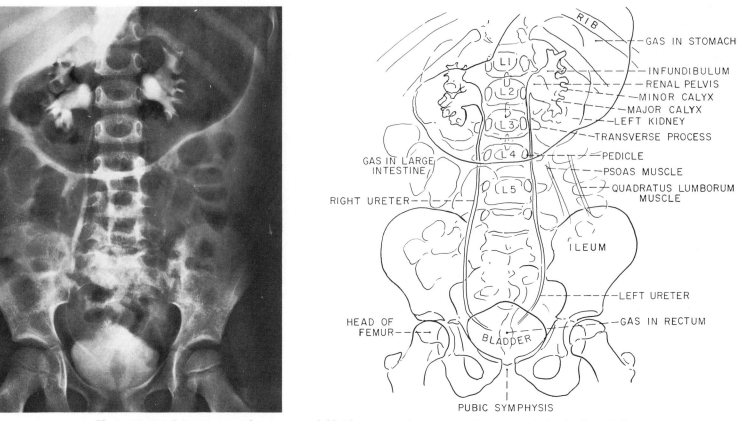

Figure 16–36. Intravenous pyelogram on a child. The upper urinary tract is demonstrated clearly through the gas-distended stomach.

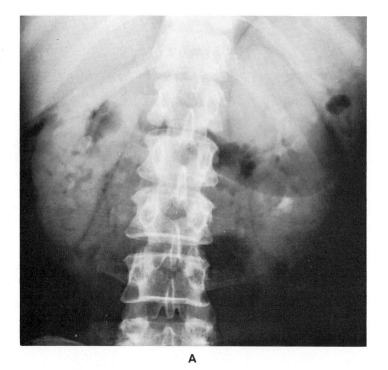

A

Figure 16–37. Value of drip-infusion urogram with tomogram. *A.* Excretory urogram, showing poor visualization of renal pelvis and calyces. *B.* Drip-infusion urogram with tomogram. Excellent visualization of renal parenchyma and collecting system. Previously unsuspected mass (simple cyst) is present in lower pole of left kidney. (From Emmett, J. L., and Witten, D. M.: Clinical Urography. 3rd ed., Vol. 1. Philadelphia, W. B. Saunders Co., 1971.)

in 10 to 15 minutes. Thereafter films are obtained at 5 minute intervals for a total of 20 minutes. The best washout phenomenon appears on the 15 and 20 minute films ordinarily.

A 5 per cent solution of Mannitol may be substituted for the urea-dextrose mixture to produce diuresis and is probably easier to manage than the urea.

The first phase of this study has been called the minute pyelogram or rapid sequence intravenous pyelogram. The latter phase has been called the "washout" study. The latter is a radiologic adaptation of the Howard and Stamey tests.

Nephrotomography (Fig. 16–39 *A* and *B*). Body section radiographs (see Chapter 1) allow the radiologist to focus on any plane of the body which is parallel to the table top on which the patient is lying. Nephrotomography may be readily applied during infusion pyelography during the so-called nephrographic phase. This is the period when opacification of the renal parenchyma is at its best.

Good nephrographic opacification is obtained by the rapid injection of large doses of the contrast agent (Weens et al.; Evans et al., 1954).

Various techniques have been described to obtain maximum concentration of the contrast agent in the nephrogram phase at the time the various "cuts" are obtained. The complete series of films should be exposed within 60 to 90 seconds following the rapid intravenous injection of the large bolus of contrast agent.

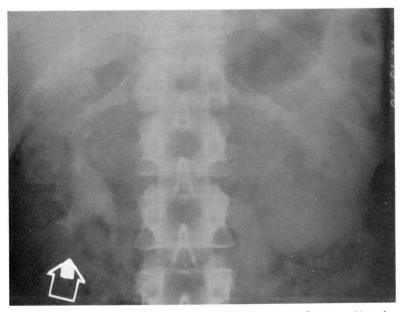

Figure 16–38. Renovascular hypertension with a positive washout test. Note the hyperconcentration of the right renal pelvis and calyces even after the left renal collecting system is completely washed out. The blood pressure in this patient was 190/120. The above film was obtained 15 minutes after the injection of a large volume diuretic (Mannitol).

Although simple cysts or tumors may be diagnosed by this method with 90 to 95 per cent accuracy (Evans), renal arteriography is usually employed subsequently for greater reliability.

Better quality nephrotomograms may be obtained following renal arteriography or midstream aortograms when the injection is made at the level of, or just below, the origin of the renal arteries.

Retrograde Pyelography (Fig. 16–40). Patient preparation for retrograde pyelography is much the same as for intravenous pyelography.

This method requires that catheters be introduced into the ureters by cystographic manipulation. Most urologists prefer opaque ureteral catheters. Ordinarily the tip of the catheter is introduced well into the renal pelvis, but care must be exercised not to penetrate the renal calyces because local infarction may result.

It is customary to obtain a plain film of the abdomen after the introduction of the ureteral catheters and prior to the injection of the opaque medium. Oblique studies are taken if necessary, especially if ureteral calculi are suspected.

Following the initial studies, an opaque medium is injected through the ureteral catheter. This may be an organic iodide preparation such as Hippuran (sodium orthoiodohippurate dihydrate), Skiodan, or a 12 per cent solution of sodium iodide or bromide. Skiodan is combined with the antibiotic Neomycin in Retropaque as an antibacterial medium. The organic iodide media are preferred and 20 to 30 per cent solutions of any of these are quite satisfactory. Too great an opacity is undesirable since calculi may be obscured.

When the injection is made, overdistention of the pelvis and calyces should be avoided. A good method of introduction is by means of gravity or carefully controlled pressure (46 cm. of water). Ordinarily 5 to 10 cc. of medium will make a satisfactory pyelogram. Films are developed immediately to assure good filling and good visualization of the various anatomic structures. Special films may be taken as necessary following these exploratory studies.

Following this initial injection and after satisfactory visualization of the renal calyces and pelvis, a film is obtained while withdrawing the catheter, all the while injecting the opaque medium. This permits a complete visualization of the ureter as well as the pelvis and kidney calyces.

When ureteral obstruction is expected, a delayed pyelogram is sometimes desired. This may be obtained in the erect position to visualize the point of obstruction to better advantage.

Cystography and Cystourethrography

Excretory Cystograms and Cystourethrograms (Fig. 16–41). Following the excretory urogram, an excretory cystogram may be obtained, although usually the urinary bladder is not completely distended at this time. One should hesitate to express a final

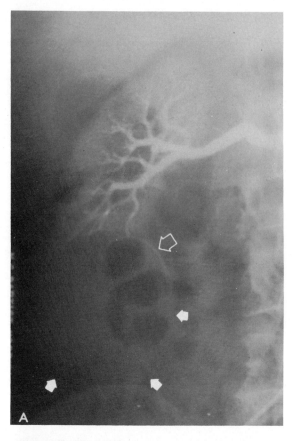

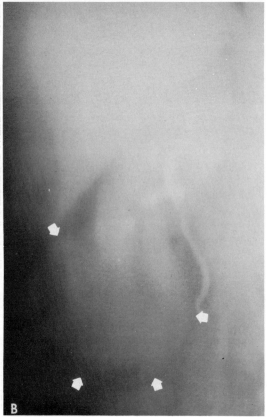

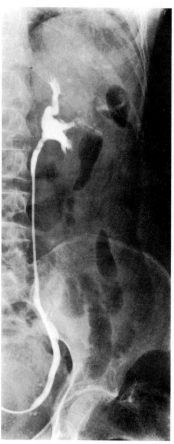

Figure 16–40.   Representative retrograde pyelogram with ureteral catheter in situ.

opinion on such films. Excretory cystourethrograms can be made during the act of voiding as a final part of the excretory urographic study.

These tests are most important in a pediatric practice since often vesical, ureteral, or urethral dysfunction or morphologic abnormality may be discovered thereby. Vesicoureteral reflux that may be missed during conventional studies may be easily recognized with a voiding cystourethrogram.

The Simple Retrograde Cystogram (Fig. 16–42).   The procedure is performed as follows: after the patient has completely voided, the urinary bladder is catheterized and the residual urine measured. Thereafter 150 to 200 ml. of a 10 to 30 per cent solution of any of the diiodinated or triiodinated compounds used for excretory urography are instilled in the urinary bladder through the catheter and the catheter is removed. The urinary bladder is

Figure 16–39.   Renal cyst. *A*. Arteriogram. *B*. Nephrotomogram. Renal angiogram in a patient with renal cyst involving the inferior pole of the right kidney: solid arrows, wall of the cyst; open arrow, capsular artery of the cyst producing the thin-walled appearance of renal cyst. Nephrotomogram has solid arrows outlining the renal cyst and contrast agent in the collecting system and right ureter.

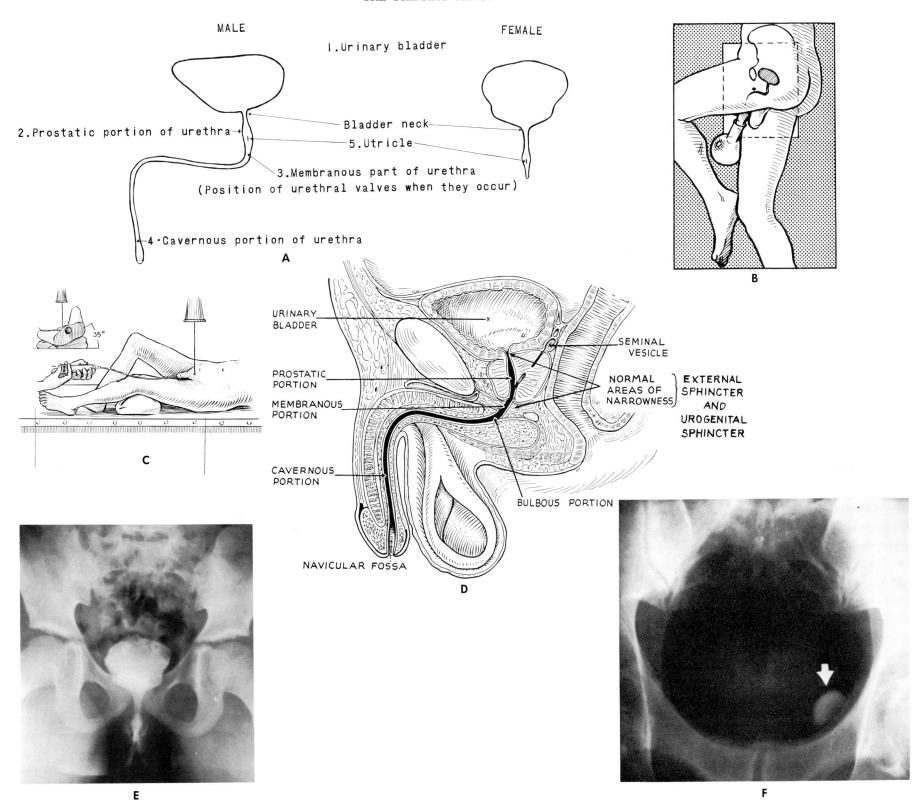

Figure 16–41.   *A.* Male and female cystourethrogram anatomy. *B.* Technique of voiding urethrogram. *C.* Technique of retrograde urethrogram. *D.* Anatomy of male urethra. *E.* Female urethrogram. *F.* Air cystogram of the urinary bladder demonstrating a filling defect due to a small sessile bladder carcinoma.

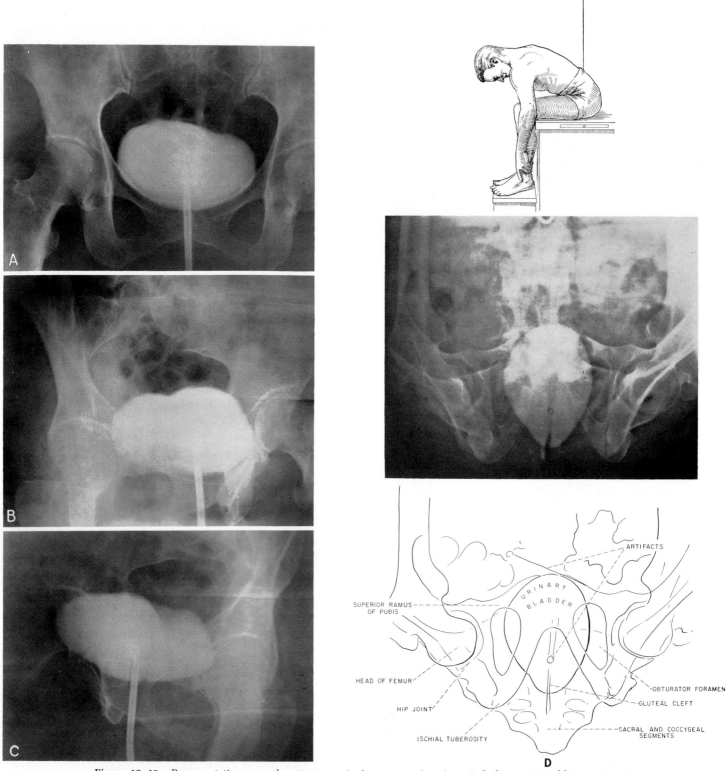

Figure 16–42. Representative normal cystograms. *A.* Anteroposterior view. *B.* Left posterior oblique view. *C.* Right posterior oblique view. A lateral view may also be employed. *D.* Chassard-Lapiné view of urinary bladder (also called sitting, squat, or jackknife view).

filled within the limits of comfort to the patient. The views obtained are shown in Figure 16–42. The oblique and profile studies are necessary to distinguish diverticula or filling defects which otherwise might be obscured. Finally, the patient is encouraged to void as completely as possible, but if unable to void the bladder is evacuated by catheter. The *postvoiding study* is of some value to demonstrate: (a) vesical diverticula, (b) filling defects caused by neoplasm, and (c) vesicoureteral reflux. The demonstration of the latter requires that a full 14 × 17 inch film be utilized to include both ureters and kidneys as well as the urinary bladder. Under normal conditions it is not unusual for 10 to 20 cc. to remain in the urinary bladder after the patient has apparently voided completely.

The Air Cystogram (Fig. 16–41 *F*). Approximately 100 to 200 cc. of air are introduced by catheter. Vesical tumors may produce a soft tissue density within the air cystogram. Air cystography may be enhanced by double contrast by using opaque media in addition to air. In the presence of a rupture of the urinary bladder air will enter the abdominal cavity or soft tissue space surrounding the urinary bladder. Fatal air embolism has been described as a complication of air cystography (Emmett and Witten).

The Polycystogram and Superimposition Cystography (Fig. 16–43 *A* and *B*). This procedure is utilized to help determine the degree of fixation of the urinary bladder against adjacent structures. The bladder is filled with approximately 200 ml. of the contrast agent and three serial exposures are made in the anteroposterior projection, each exposure being one-third of the normal exposure time without changing the cassette. After the first exposure, the contrast agent is removed in two steps: approximately 120 ml. the first time and 50 ml. the second time, and the vesical outline is compared in these three instances (Cobb and Anderson). If the entire vesical wall is not fixed, there is a tendency for the outlines of the urinary bladder to show fixation by convergence of the contrast agent on all three exposures.

The Triple-Voiding Cystogram (Lattimer, Dean, and Furey). Voiding in three installments often permits better emptying of a large atonic bladder. The films obtained after each voiding are called the triple-voiding cystogram. Usually the patient is allowed to walk around for approximately 2 minutes after each voiding episode. This technique provides a mechanism for measuring residual urine as well as for demonstrating vesicoureteral reflux.

Delayed Cystography for Children. This method is of par-

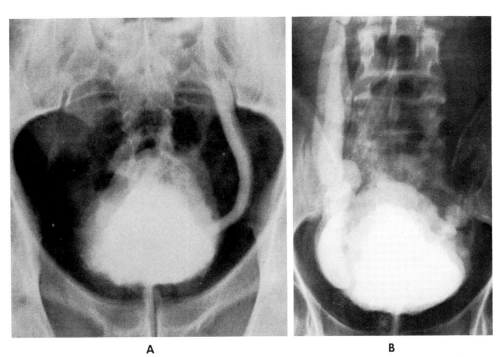

| A | B |

Figure 16–43. *A.* Polycystogram of man, with *transitional cell epithelioma of bladder wall* on the right side. Retrograde cystogram with three exposures on one film, each for one third of usual exposure time, with 200, 80, and 30 ml. of contrast medium, respectively, in bladder. Note concentricity of outlines as evidence of noninfiltrating tumor. Bilateral vesicoureteral reflux, particularly on the left side. *B.* Polycystogram of man, 75 years of age, with prostatic hypertrophy and vesical tumor. Tumor on right side of bladder wall is shown by concentric outlines. Bladder wall in area of tumor is not fixed. Note right vesicoureteral reflux and small vesical diverticulum on left. (Courtesy of Dr. H. W. ten Cate, *in* Emmet, J. L., and Witten, D. M.: Clinical Urography, 3rd ed. Philadelphia, W. B. Saunders Co., 1971.)

ticular value in children in order to check urinary retention, particularly since children are often unable to void on command. Vesicoureteral reflux that has not been visible by other methods may be demonstrated thereby. Indeed, excretory urography and cystoscopy may be misleading, and this diagnosis may be missed without evidence from a delayed cystogram.

Micturition Cystourethrogram (voiding cystourethrogram). Voiding cystourethrography usually distends the prostatic urethra sufficiently to demonstrate the external urethral sphincteric mechanism. The anterior urethra is also thereby visualized. In very young children, who cannot void on command, *expression cystourethrography* may be necessary under anesthesia.

The Retrograde Cystourethrogram (Fig. 16–41). The simple retrograde urethrogram is of less value than a voiding cystourethrogram for unimpeded visualization of the vesical neck and prostatic urethra. Voiding cystourethrography ordinarily permits a good visualization of the posterior as well as the anterior urethra. This procedure is of particular importance in children in whom valves of the urethra and vesicoureteral reflux are best demonstrated by voiding cystourethrography. Films in an oblique position with the patient standing are preferred if at all feasible.

Kjellberg et al. have recommended the utilization of a suspension of barium sulfate with sodium carboxymethylcellulose. They have warned, however, that this should not be used for retrograde urethrography, since fatal venous embolism has been described secondary to retrograde use of barium suspensions in the urethra; moreover, vesicoureteral reflux has, on occasion, resulted in barium impaction of the ureter. However, this is a very favorable medium in respect to its density and nonirritating attributes.

Kjellberg et al. have used simultaneous biplane sequential films with automatic filming at 3 to 5 second intervals, depending on the rate of micturition. Waterhouse, on the other hand, has reduced the technique by making only one x-ray exposure with the patient lying in the right oblique posterior position, thus diminishing x-ray exposure. Cineradiography has also been extensively employed (Dunbar).

"Chain" Cystourethrography (Fig. 16–44). Urethrocystograms have proved to be of value in some female patients under treatment for stress incontinence (Green; Calatroni et al.). This is carried out as follows. With the help of a probe, a chain of metallic beads is introduced into the urinary bladder through the urethra, the probe is withdrawn, and one end of the chain remains in the bladder, while the other is taped to the inner surface of the thigh. Thereafter, 50 cc. of 10 to 15 per cent solution of sodium iodide (or equivalent in organic iodine) is introduced into the urinary bladder by means of a No. 10 Nelaton catheter. Once the catheter is withdrawn, the patient is instructed to stand upright, whereupon frontal and lateral x-ray films centered over the lower pubis are taken. These radiographs are taken serially so that different degrees of stress are registered. The posterior urethrovesical angle (PUV) is measured, as well as the angle of inclination to the perpendicular of the upper urethra. The normal PUV angle is 90 to 100 degrees, and the normal angle of inclination of the upper urethra to the perpendicular is 30 degrees with the patient in the erect position and straining. The normal and various examples of abnormal angles are illustrated in Fig. 16–44.

Renal Arteriography and Aortography (Fig. 16–45). Visualization of the renal arteries, their major ramifications, nephrograms, renal collecting systems, and to a limited extent, renal veins, may be accomplished by (1) translumbar aortography, (2) percutaneous aortography by catheter techniques, and (3) selective renal arteriography (Colapinto and Steed). Translumbar aortograms may be employed in patients with severe aortoiliac disease in whom retrograde catheterization may be impossible or hazardous. On the other hand, transbrachial or axillary artery catheterization may be attempted for selective catheterization in some of these cases. We have considered these techniques as special procedures outside the scope of this text and the student is referred to extensive monographs on these subjects (Schobinger and Ruzicka).

Percutaneous transfemoral renal arteriography is probably the procedure of choice. Not only can the individual single or multiple renal arteries be selectively visualized, but midstream injection into the aorta may help determine the multiplicity of renal arteries for greatest accuracy. The use of a mechanical injector and rapid film sequencing equipment permits a dynamic study of the arterial blood supply of the kidney and allows an accurate assay of the pathology and physiology as well as anatomy.

Patterns of Collateral Flow in Renal Ischemia (Abrams and Cornell; Paul et al.). The vessels supplying the renal collaterals are usually the lumbar, internal iliac, testicular or ovarian, inferior adrenal, renal capsular, and intercostal arteries as well as the aorta itself. *The third lumbar artery is the commonest source of anastomotic flow to the kidney.* Ordinarily these collaterals are not demonstrable in the absence of renal ischemia. Usually the collateral vessels are coiled and tortuous and lengthened by comparison with the normal. They may also be dilated. Abrams and Cornell have divided the renal collateral circulation into three categories: (1) a capsular system (Fig. 16–45), (2) a peripelvic system, and (3) a periureteric system. As noted in Figure 16–45, the capsular system consists of the first four lumbar arteries, branches of the internal iliac, and the intercostal arteries. Not shown in the diagram are the inferior adrenal and capsular branches of the kidney which themselves may make major contributions.

The peripelvic system consists largely of the aorta itself, the inferior adrenal, the first three lumbar, the gonadal, and the gonadal branches. Occasionally there are direct capsular branches from the renal artery proximal to the stenosis when such exists.

The periureteric system consists mainly of the internal iliac artery with other contributing arteries being the second, third and fourth lumbar, gonadal, and direct aortic branches.

Thus, although it is usually considered that after vessels perforate the renal sinus they are "end" arteries, nevertheless, a renal collateral circulation is able to maintain function and viability of involved renal parenchyma in many cases.

Within the kidney there are perforating capsular branches which arise from the interlobular arteries and terminate by communicating with the adipose-capsular arteries in the retroperitoneal arterial plexus of Turner. Arterial communications in the retroperitoneal plexus are numerous (Paul et al.). Additional basic references on this subject are those by Merklin and Michels, and Graves.

Phlebography and Inferior Vena Cavography (Fig. 16–46). Generally, the techniques employed for selective phlebography are similar to those for renal arteriography, except that the

catheter must be preformed in accordance with the anatomy of the renal veins. The femoral vein is the site of insertion of the catheter except where a block in the inferior vena cava is encountered. Under these circumstances, the catheter may be introduced into an arm vein, passed through the superior vena cava, right atrium, and then into the inferior vena cava.

The inferior vena cava may be demonstrated in similar fashion.

Other variations of left renal phlebography have been described, such as left spermatic phlebography.

Visualization of the renal veins has become increasingly important in the diagnosis of invasive malignancies of the kidneys and their prognostic evaluation. Renal vein thrombosis may be differentiated in this manner. As indicated previously the anatomy of the renal venous system may be subdivided into: (a) extrarenal venous structures, and (b) intrarenal venous structures.

Extrarenal Venous Structures. The *right renal vein* may be

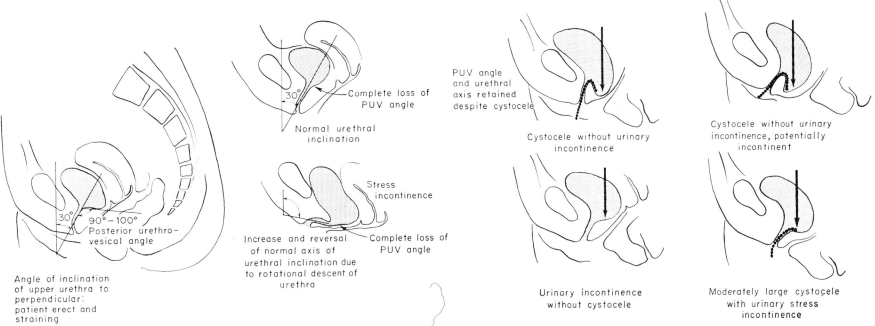

Figure 16–44. Diagrams illustrating roentgen techniques for study of stress incontinence. The assumption is that the key anatomic defect is the loss of the normal posterior urethrovesical angle (PUV angle). The normal PUV angle is 90 to 100 degrees and the normal angle of inclination of the upper urethra to the perpendicular is 30 degrees with the patient in the erect position and straining. Despite a cystocele, the PUV angle and urethral axis may be retained normally, so that stress incontinence rarely if ever is associated with cystocele.

After surgical correction, the PUV angle may vary between 55 and 95 degrees with an adequate segment of the bladder base posterior to the urethral junction participating in the formation of the new angle. The angle of inclination of the urethral axis is usually 5 to 15 degrees but may vary up to 25 degrees with respect to the vertical in the standing position. There must also be a correction of the tendency to funnel formation of the vesical neck area of the bladder base. Note that a chain of metallic beads is introduced into the bladder through the urethra. When the probe is withdrawn, one end of the chain remains in the bladder while the other is taped to the inner surface of the thigh. Sixty ml. of a 10 to 15 per cent solution of sodium iodide are introduced into the bladder and the catheter is withdrawn. The patient is instructed to stand upright, and frontal and lateral radiographs are taken of this area. (Modified from Calatroni, C. J., et al.: Amer. J. Obstet. Gynec., *83:*649–656, 1962; and Green, T. A.: Amer. J. Obstet. Gynec., *83:*632–648, 1960.)

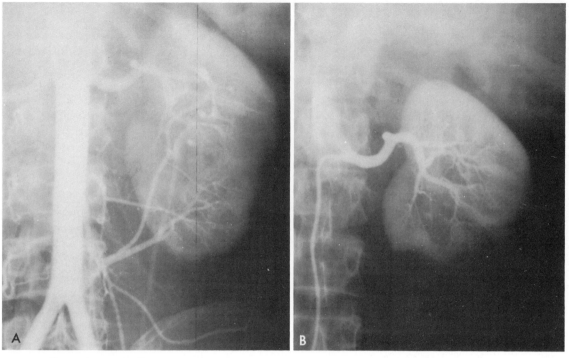

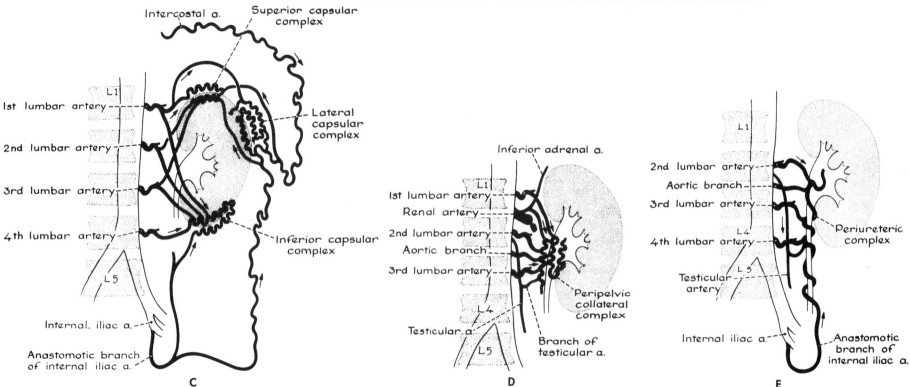

Figure 16–45. Selective arteriogram showing the appearance with a double renal artery supplying one kidney when both left renal arteries are filled (*A*), and when only the upper is filled (*B*). *C–E.* Renal Collateral Circulation. Diagrammatic representation. *C. The capsular system:* The first four lumbar arteries, branches of the internal iliac, and the intercostal arteries contributed significantly to the capsular complex. In addition, not pictured here, the inferior adrenal and capsular branches proximal to the stenosis also made major contributions. Note that a separate "lateral" capsular complex has been indicated; this represents a continuation of the superior capsular system, but has been designated "lateral" because of its location and mode of filling.

D. The peripelvic system: The aorta directly, the inferior adrenal, first three lumbar, and testicular (or ovarian) arteries all supplied branches to the peripelvic system. Additional important pathways were direct capsular branches from the renal artery proximal to the stenosis.

E. The periureteric system: The internal iliac artery was the single most common source of periureteric collaterals. The second, third, and fourth lumbar, testicular, and direct aortic branches were also large and important components of this collateral pathway. (From Abrams, H. L., and Cornell, S. H.: Radiology, 84:1001–1012, 1965.)

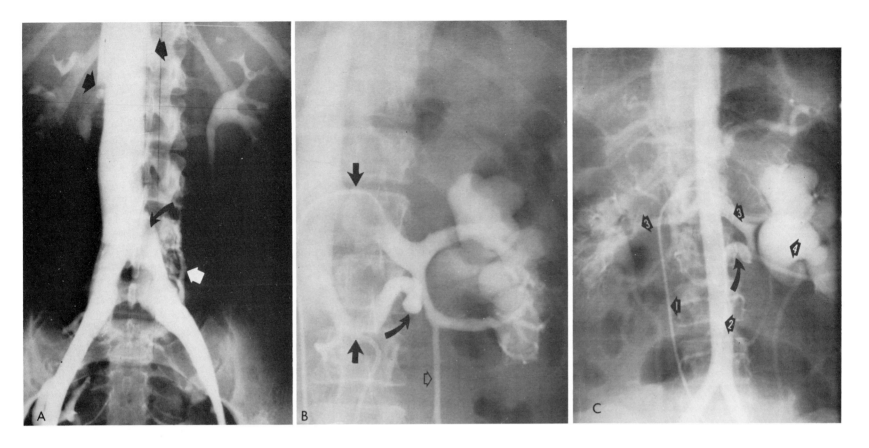

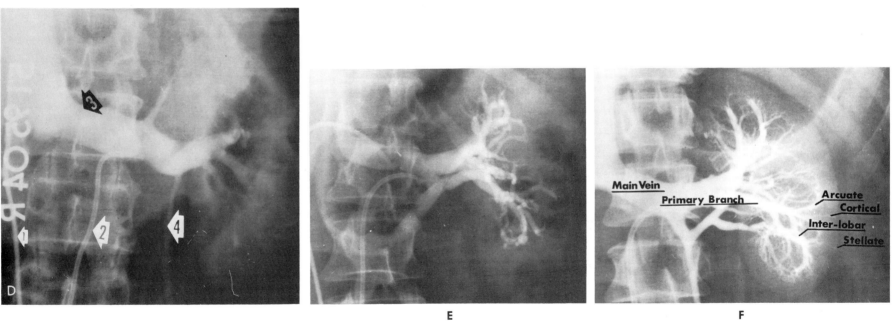

Figure 16–46. *A.* Renal venogram and inferior vena cavagram (black curved arrow). Black straight arrows point to origin of renal veins. White arrow shows paravertebral veins. *B.* Inferior vena cavagram with filling of the circumaortic renal vein, and associated hydronephrosis. Open arrow shows left spermatic vein. *C.* Aortogram in same patient as *B*: (1) Catheter in inferior vena cava, (2) catheter in abdominal aorta, (3) renal arteries, (4) hydronephrotic kidney. Curved black arrow shows circumaortic left renal vein retaining contrast agent. *D.* Left normal renal venograms. (1) Catheter in inferior vena cava, (2) catheter in aorta and left renal artery, (3) left renal vein, (4) left spermatic vein. (Courtesy University of Iowa, Department of Radiology.) *E.* Left renal phlebogram—bifid main left renal vein. *F.* Normal renal venous anatomy. (*E* and *F* by kind permission of the Honorary Editor of Clinical Radiology. Sorby, W. A.: Renal phlebography. Clin. Radiol. *20*:166–172, 1969. Published by E. & S. Livingstone, Ltd.)

bifid, trifid, or plexiform and quite short—1 to 2 cm. There are rarely any anastomotic veins adjoining it. It adjoins the inferior vena cava at an acute angle. The *left renal vein* is longer, 4 to 6 cm., and its junction with the inferior vena cava usually forms a right angle. A large *left ovarian* or *testicular vein* usually joins it. The inferior *left adrenal vein* and a number of anastomotic channels to the lumbar paraspinal plexus also join the left renal vein.

Apart from the utilization already mentioned, catheterization of the renal veins is useful in assessing the patency of splenorenal shunts and in estimation of renal blood flow, by measuring the rate of clearance of a contrast agent from the renal venous system.

Intrarenal Venous Structures. The normal intrarenal venous anatomy is shown in Figure 16–46 *F*. The main renal vein may have three to four primary tributary veins and these in turn have two to three interlobar veins coursing between the calyces and medullary pyramids. The interlobar veins are linked by arcuate veins running between the cortex and medulla. Fine, parallel cortical veins drain the outer surface, flowing into the arcuate veins. There are a few subcapsular stellate veins as well. The veins are not segmental end vessels, unlike the renal arteries. Communications between veins are free and numerous. Of interest is the distortion of the venous system by cysts in the kidney. The thickness of the renal cortex may also be measured accurately by virtue of the cortical veins (Sorby; Kahn).

Implacements upon, deformity, or displacements of the inferior vena cava also have assumed greater importance in diagnosis, particularly in relation to malignancies which involve the central axis of the body (lymphomas or metastasizing carcinomas).

Triple Contrast Study of the Urinary Bladder (Fig. 16–47). This study consists of (1) oxygen or air injected in the perivesical tissue space; (2) air injected into the urinary bladder via catheter; and (3) retrograde femoral arteriography for visualization of the blood supply of the urinary bladder.

The patient is placed supine on the x-ray table in the Trendelenburg head down position, an 18 gauge needle is inserted in the extraperitoneal space just outside the urinary bladder, and approximately 300 cc. of air is instilled. The urinary bladder wall may be seen when 300 to 500 cc. of air is injected into the urinary

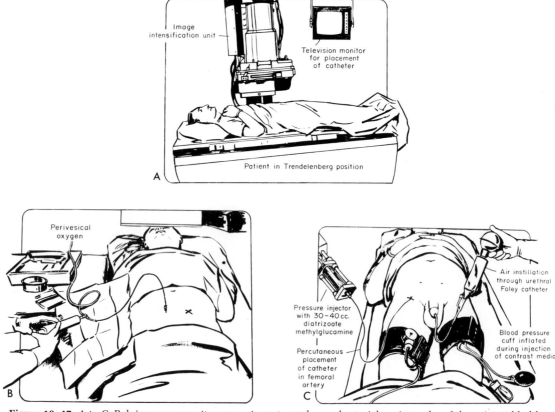

Figure 16–47. *A* to *C.* Pelvic pneumoperitoneum, air cystography, and arterial angiography of the urinary bladder (triple contrast). (Courtesy Drs. S. C. Lacy, C. E. Cox, W. H. Boyce, and J. E. Whitley, Departments of Urology and Radiology. The Bowman Gray School of Medicine.)

Figure 16–47 continued on the opposite page.

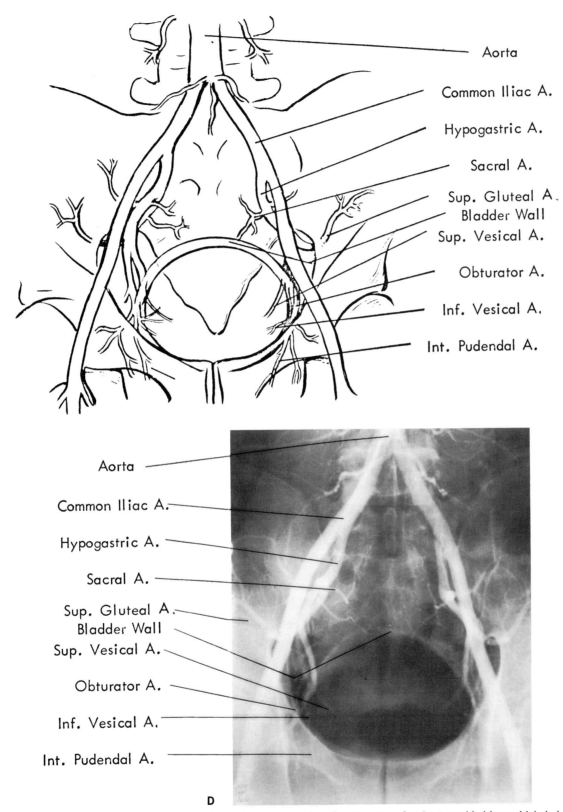

Aorta

Common Iliac A.

Hypogastric A.

Sacral A.

Sup. Gluteal A.
Bladder Wall
Sup. Vesical A.

Obturator A.

Inf. Vesical A.

Int. Pudendal A.

Aorta

Common Iliac A.

Hypogastric A.

Sacral A.

Sup. Gluteal A.
Bladder Wall
Sup. Vesical A.

Obturator A.

Inf. Vesical A.

Int. Pudendal A.

D

Figure 16–47 *Continued.*   D. Radiograph obtained in normal triple contrast study of urinary bladder and labeled tracing of same.

bladder through a Foley catheter. The femoral artery is catheterized by the Seldinger technique as in aortography. Pressure injection and serial filming are accomplished so that the arterial distribution to the urinary bladder and to any tumor contained within its wall is shown. Any spreading to, or invasion of, contiguous structures in the pelvis may also be demonstrated. The triple contrast technique is particularly helpful for assessment of total spread and degree of involvement of the urinary bladder by malignancy. This, too, is a special procedure beyond the scope of this text.

Roentgen Examination of the Surgically Exposed Kidney (Fig. 16–48). Radiography of the surgically exposed kidney, particularly during removal of renal stones, may be accomplished by wrapping a suitably sized film in black paper and packing it in a

sheet of sterile rubber to be placed next to the kidney during its radiography at the time of surgery. Sterile packs are commercially available for this purpose. The films may be placed in a sterile rubber glove at the time of radiography also. A special cassette utilizing intensifying screens has also been devised for this technique (Olsson).

Cineradiography (Dux et al.). Cineradiography of the excretory urogram may be readily accomplished with image amplification and cinematography. Urine is transported toward the urinary bladder as a result of the active coordinated contraction of muscle groups in the renal pelvis, major and minor calyces, and ureter. Emptying of the renal pelvis depends on its shape and size, on flow from individual calyceal groups, and on filling pressure (the pressure changes in the ureter). Peristalsis or antiperi-

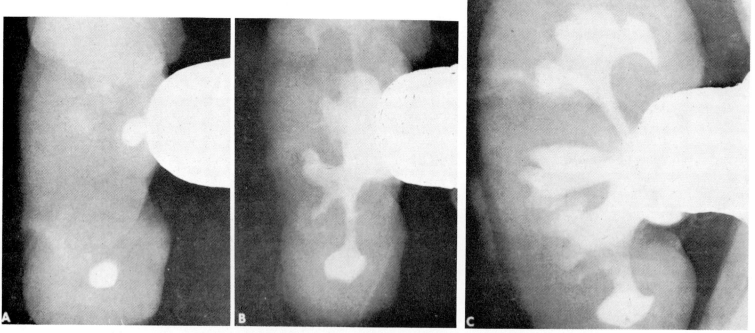

Figure 16–48. Renal organography during surgery. All exposures are 15 milliampere/second with average of 65 Kvp. *A.* Exposure with central ray passing from convex surface through the hilus of the kidney. Four calculi are visible, one in the pelvis and three in the inferior calyx. Only the two larger calculi were visualized on preoperative roentgenograms. Note clearly visible untreated cotton umbilical tapes which support the relatively small kidney at each pole. Large kidneys may require two films to cover the entire organ. The use of two properly placed films will remove the "blind spot" occasioned by the notch in the film which accommodates the renal pedicle. *B.* Same position as *A* after occluding the ureter with a rubber-shod spring clamp and filling the pelvis with contrast medium through a 23 gauge needle. *C.* Same as *B* with central ray traversing the short axis of the kidney. Such rotational exposures permit accurate localization of small calculi and assist in planning plastic revisions of a strictured calyx (calycotomy), calycectomy, excision of intrarenal diverticula or cysts, and partial nephrectomies.

Angiography by this technique is accomplished by temporary occlusion of the primary renal artery and filling with dilute contrast medium through a 23 or 25 gauge intracatheter needle inserted into the renal artery distal to the point of occlusion. (From Boyce, W. H.: Radiol. Clin. N. Amer., 3:101, 1965.)

stalsis cannot ordinarily be demonstrated in the normal renal pelvis. In the ureter, on the other hand, urine transport appears to depend upon pure peristaltic contraction.

Cineradiography may also be employed as an adjunct to urethrocystograms, but because of the greater radiation exposure of the gonads by this technique single or selected rapid film sequences on 70 to 105 mm spot films are usually preferred.

Pneumograms of the Urinary Bladder and Pneumopyelograms. Air may be injected through a ureteral catheter for the latter purpose. Unfortunately, small bubbles of air will simulate

calculi or small polypi, and hence the constancy of a finding must be interpreted with caution. Filling defects, however, are sometimes demonstrated to excellent advantage by this technique. The danger of air embolism must be considered.

Perirenal Air Insufflation (Fig. 16–49). Perirenal air insufflation, direct or by means of the introduction of presacral air, may be utilized (Cocchi). When introduced presacrally, the air rises in the tela subserosa and follows along the fascial planes, giving rise to a delineation not only of the kidney but also of the suprarenal structures. This method is particularly useful for the

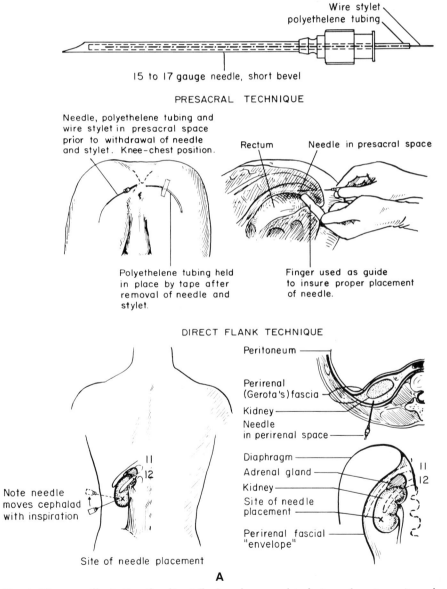

Figure 16–49. A. Diagrams illustrating the direct flank and presacral techniques for retroperitoneal pneumography.

Figure 16–49 continued on the following page.

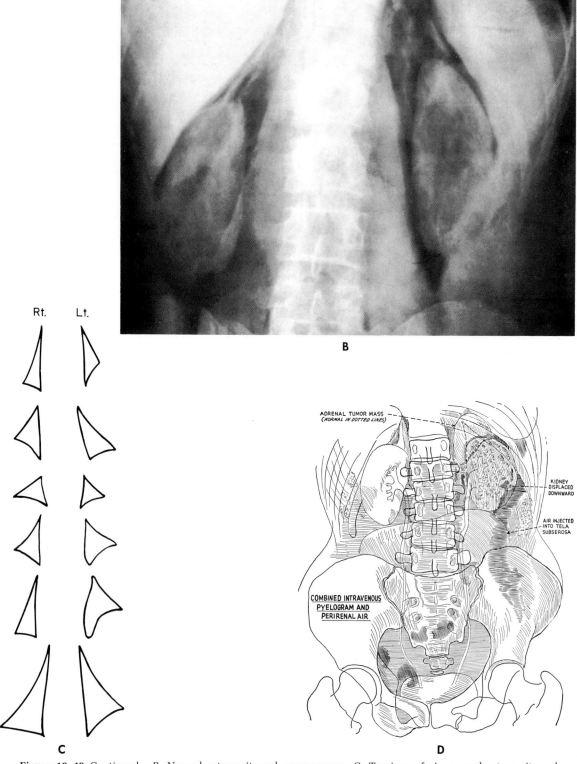

Rt.   Lt.

B

ADRENAL TUMOR MASS
(NORMAL IN DOTTED LINES)

KIDNEY
DISPLACED
DOWNWARD

AIR INJECTED
INTO TELA
SUBSEROSA

COMBINED INTRAVENOUS
PYELOGRAM AND
PERIRENAL AIR

C   D

Figure 16–49 *Continued.* *B.* Normal retroperitoneal pneumogram. *C.* Tracings of six normal retroperitoneal pneumograms. (*A, B,* and *C* from McLelland, R., Landes, R. R., and Ransom, C. L.: Radiol. Clin. N. Amer., 3:115, 1965.) *D* and *E.* Perirenal air insufflation around the left kidney and suprarenal area, demonstrating an adrenal tumor mass in this region. This proved to be adrenal cortical carcinoma. *D.* Labeled tracing of radiograph shown in *E.*

Figure 16–49 continued on the opposite page.

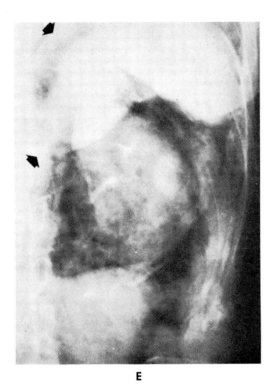

E

Figure 16–49 *Continued.* E. Radiograph coned down over renal and suprarenal areas.

delineation of suprarenal tumor masses. It is of special value when it is combined with intravenous or retrograde pyelograms and body section radiographs.

Seminal Vesiculography. Seminal vesiculography is a specialized procedure not frequently employed. It is utilized primarily to study the appearance of the seminal vesicles and the vas deferens, and occasionally in relation to prostatic carcinoma (Emmett et al.) (Fig. 16–50 *A* and *B*).

The Normal Kidney's Reaction to Intravenous Pyelography (Arkless). (1) Kidneys will ordinarily enlarge after the injection of contrast material, reaching a maximum increase of approximately 0.5 cm. at about 5 minutes following completion of the injection. When films are exposed and measured from the beginning of the injection, the maximum size is reached at about 2.5 to 3 minutes if 25 cc. is used, whereas if 50 cc. is employed it tends to be earlier. (2) The time required for calyceal visualization also varies somewhat according to the amount of contrast material injected. Calyceal visualization is usually accomplished at 2 minutes when 50 cc. is employed, but there may be a ½ to 1 minute further delay when only 25 cc. is utilized.

Comparison of Renal Tests. Wigh et al. have compared sodium diatrizoate (Hypaque) intravenous pyelograms with other renal tests, including blood urea nitrogen levels, phenolsulfonphthalein excretion rates and creatinine clearance values. The accompanying scattergrams (Fig. 16–51) are presented to com-

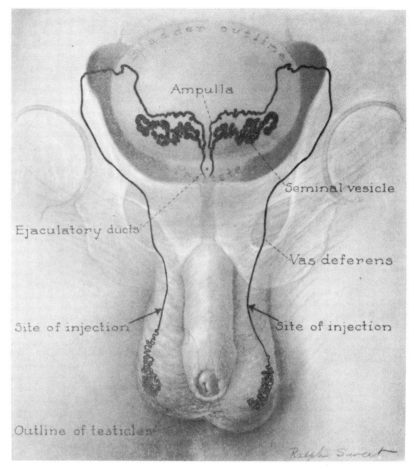

A

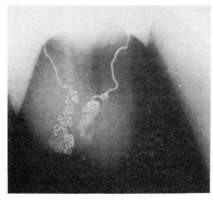

B

Figure 16–50. A. The male genital tract. The sites of exposure of the vasa deferentia are indicated, into which injections of the contrast media are made upward and frequently downward. B. Filling of the distal portions of the epididymides has been achieved. Greater filling has been obtained on the right than on the left. (From Tucker, A. S., Yanagihara, H., and Pryde, A. W.: Amer. J. Roentgenol., 71:490–500, 1954.)

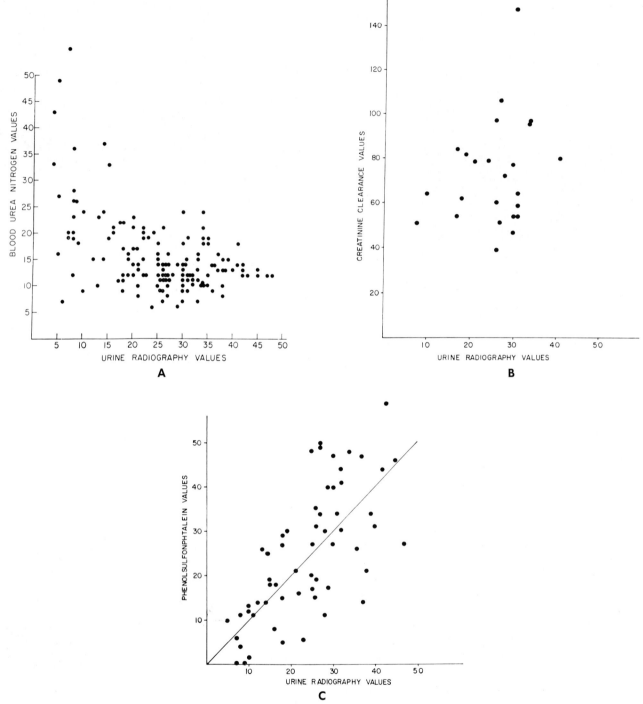

Figure 16–51. *A.* Scattergram comparing urine radiography values — per cent of excreted sodium diatrizoate (Hypaque 50%) — with blood urea nitrogen determinations in mg. per cent in 143 patients. *B.* Graph plotting urine radiography values against creatinine clearance expressed in ml./min. for 24 patients. *C.* Comparison of urine radiography determinations with phenolsulfonphthalein tests, expressed as per cent voided in fifteen minutes for 59 patients. (From Wigh, R., Anthony, H. F., Jr., and Grant, B. P.: Radiology, *78:*869–878, 1962.)

pare the urine radiography values with those of one of the other tests. In each case in which incomplete micturition occurred, the urine radiography percentage was connected to take into account residual bladder Hypaque. This estimate was derived from a post-voiding radiograph.

Blood Urea Nitrogen. A plot of the percentage of organic iodide excretion in 30 minutes against the blood urea nitrogen in milligrams per cent is shown in Figure 16–51 *A*. On the assumption that 24 mg. per cent might be the upper limit of normal for blood urea nitrogen excretion (BUN), the patients who excreted 20 per cent or more of the Hypaque were placed in this category. Generally, with higher BUN levels less than 20 per cent of the injected Hypaque was excreted in 30 minutes. There were, however, 29 patients (in this group of 143) who excreted less than 20 per cent of the contrast agent and who had blood urea nitrogen levels between 8 and 24 mg. per cent—values in the normal range. Generally, then, one may conclude that a fair urogram may be anticipated in patients with BUN levels up to 20 mg. per cent, although some exceptions will be found to this rule. Of course, many extrarenal factors play a part in BUN levels, and a good correlation, therefore, between BUN and excretory urography cannot be expected.

Creatinine Clearance. A scattergram indicating the relationship of creatinine clearance to urine radiography values is shown in Figure 16–51 *B*. The graph shows only in a very general way that the better the Hypaque clearance, the greater the clearance of creatinine.

Phenolsulfonphthalein Determinations. Figure 16–51 *C* shows a comparison of the phenolsulfonphthalein determinations with urine radiography. This demonstrates the closest correlation of any of the three tests presented. Average phenolsulfonphthalein values are 35 per cent in 15 minutes; 35 per cent Hypaque excretion, on the other hand, reflects a high value rather than an average one.

There is therefore no absolute index as to which of the tests is necessarily best. Since the patient is in a dehydrated state for the excretory urograms, the comparison itself rests on a physiologically abnormal condition.

Reactions to Contrast Media

General Comments. Reactions to the intravenous injection of contrast media are common. Mild reactions include warmth and flushing, nausea, vomiting, tingling, numbness, cough, and local pain in the arm, especially if the injection is carried out slowly. Serious reactions may include conjunctivitis, rhinitis, urticaria, facial edema, glottic edema, and even shocklike reactions with dyspnea, convulsions, cyanosis, shock, and even

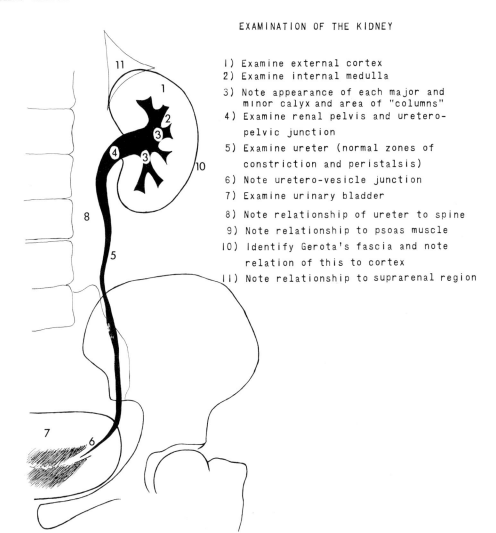

EXAMINATION OF THE KIDNEY

1) Examine external cortex
2) Examine internal medulla
3) Note appearance of each major and minor calyx and area of "columns"
4) Examine renal pelvis and uretero-pelvic junction
5) Examine ureter (normal zones of constriction and peristalsis)
6) Note uretero-vesicle junction
7) Examine urinary bladder
8) Note relationship of ureter to spine
9) Note relationship to psoas muscle
10) Identify Gerota's fascia and note relation of this to cortex
11) Note relationship to suprarenal region

Figure 16–52. Kidney collecting system with excretory urography. Method of studying films.

occasional death. It has been estimated that there has been an incidence of 6.6 deaths per million examinations (Pendergrass et al., 1958). Approximately 90 per cent of fatal reactions occurred during or immediately after injection, and hence it is vital that medications to counteract reactions be immediately available to the physician who performs the injection.

Generally, a pre-injection dose of the contrast agent is performed, allowing several drops of the contrast agent to enter the blood stream with a delay of 30 to 60 seconds indicated thereafter. A longer delay of 4 to 5 minutes is advised if there is a strong history of allergy or sensitivity in the patient. If no untoward reaction then occurs, the entire dose is injected. The best protection against serious reactions is a careful history to elicit any record of severe allergies, drug reactions, asthma, hay fever, sensitivity to iodine, previous reactions to excretory urography and related conditions.

Although results are variable in relation to the prior administration of antihistamine drugs, it appears that the preliminary intravenous injection of antihistamines, 3 to 5 minutes prior to the injection of the contrast medium, may reduce the incidence or severity of a reaction. Fifty milligrams of Benadryl (diphenhydramine hydrochloride) or 20 milligrams of Chlor-Trimeton (chlorpropheniramine-maleate) are perhaps most widely used.

In treatment of reactions the following must be judiciously employed:

1. Immediate subcutaneous or intramuscular administration of 0.5 cc. of 1 in 1000 epinephrine; this may be repeated in 10 to 15 minutes. Blood pressure must be watched closely for hypotension and impending shock.

2. One hundred per cent oxygen may be administered immediately through a face mask. If there is inadequate airway, an anesthesiologist should be called to introduce an endotracheal tube. Artificial respiration then may be carried out as necessary.

3. If shock is profound, epinephrine may be administered slowly intravenously in a dose of 0.25 cc.

4. Benadryl (20 mg.) or hydrocortisone (100 mg.) or both, may be administered intravenously at once.

5. Asthma and pulmonary edema may be combatted with 0.5 grams of Aminophylline, given intravenously over a period of 5 to 20 minutes.

6. Hypotension may be treated with the intravenous administration of vasopressor drugs such as phenylephrine hydrochloride (Neo-Synephrine), 0.5 mg.; or methoxamine hydrochloride (Vasoxyl), 5 to 10 mg. If there is no response, levarterenol bitartrate (Levophed), 4 to 8 cc. in 500 cc. of 5 per cent glucose, should be given intravenously, the rate of administration being governed by the blood pressure.

7. Convulsions or laryngospasm or both may be controlled with the intravenous injection of 2 to 3 cc. of 2.5 per cent solution of thiopental sodium. Laryngeal edema, if not controlled by epinephrine, may require an emergency tracheotomy.

Risk of Excretory Urography in Multiple Myeloma. It has been postulated that urinary contrast media may be a precipitating or exciting factor which sets the stage for precipitation of hyaline casts in the kidney in patients with multiple myeloma. It is thought that this may be obviated by alkalinization of the urine and adequate hydration. A few reports of fatal anuria following excretory urography in patients with multiple myeloma have appeared.

Advantages and Disadvantages of Excretory Urography as Opposed to Retrograde Pyelography. These are summarized in Table 16–5. Intravenous and retrograde pyelography are complementary or supplementary procedures and one does not exclude the utilization of the other.

TABLE 16–5   ADVANTAGES AND DISADVANTAGES OF EXCRETORY UROGRAPHY AS OPPOSED TO RETROGRADE PYELOGRAPHY

Excretory Urograms	Retrograde Pyelograms
Greater comfort to patient; no risk of infection.	Great discomfort and risk of infection
Does not require ureteral catheterization.	Requires ureteral catheterization.
Yields some information regarding renal function and may allow selectivity in retrograde study.	No information regarding renal function.
Probably of no value when BUN is elevated above 50 mg. per cent but may be tolerated when small doses of contrast agent are employed (Davidson et al.).	May precipitate anuria in some medical diseases such as pyelonephritis, glomerulonephritis, and arteriolar nephrosclerosis.
Detail fair when infusion pyelograms are employed but usually not as good as in retrograde study.	Structural detail optimal, but artificial distention of the collecting structures of the kidney usually occurs.
Safe in the presence of obstructing ureteral calculus.	Inadvisable to inject contrast medium above a point of obstruction, since a severe reaction in the patient may ensue.
Dangerous in cases with strong history of allergy or iodine sensitivity.	May be utilized with caution.
Possibly dangerous in patients with multiple myeloma and related disorders.	May be utilized with caution.
Should not be utilized when in vivo studies of thyroid by radioactive iodine are contemplated.	May be utilized.

Summary: Excretory and retrograde studies are complementary and supplementary. One does not exclude the utilization of the other.

METHOD OF ANALYSIS OF FILMS OF URINARY TRACT

Each part of the roentgenologic examination of the urinary tract plays a special role, and the method of examination of the films is closely related to this factor.

KUB Film. A routine for analysis of the anteroposterior film of the abdomen without added contrast has been previously described (Chapter 15). This film becomes an integral part of the examination of the urinary tract. The radiographic description of the kidney must concern itself with the exact outline, size, position, mobility, general configuration and relationship to contiguous structures. The numerous variations within normal limits must be recognized. For example, infantile renal lobulation may sometimes be found in an adult renal contour, and it is important to exclude the possibility of renal pathology when this occurs.

Excretory Urogram. (Fig. 16–52). In infusion pyelography, a reasonably good *nephrographic phase* can be obtained and this may be further intensified by nephrotomography.

Following the nephrographic phase, the *collecting system* is visualized, which, as shown, includes the major and minor calyces and the renal pelvis. By means of nephrotomography one can determine the relationship of these collecting structures to other internal medullary structures, such as the area of the columns. There is a wide variation in the appearance of the kidney, pelves, and calyces. A normal kidney pelvis permits an equal drainage from all parts of the kidney and allows a free flow into the ureters and bladder. There is usually a common pelvis, two to three major calyces, and six to fourteen minor calyces. The superior calyces are usually in a direct line with the ureter, whereas the inferior calyces are horizontally placed. On occasion, however, the ureter divides almost immediately into the calyces, with no common renal pelvic basin. The average capacity of the renal pelvis is 7.5 cc. of fluid, but this may be as high as 20 cc. and still not be considered pathologic.

The major calyces are merely channels, whereas the minor calyces consist of a neck with an expanded cupped distal end. The cupping is formed by the projection of the minor papillae into the calyces. The edges of the cup must be clean-cut and sharply demarcated. It is important, however, not to mistake the rounded shadow of the calyx seen end-on for a clubbed calyx, since the latter appearance is definitely abnormal.

Serial studies may show that there are changes in the size and contour of the calyces, owing to contraction and relaxation of the renal pelvis and ureter. These changes must be considered physiologic. Impressions by arteries and veins have already been described.

Other confusing pyelographic appearances are shown in Figures 16–53 and 16–54. Thus, the ureteropelvic junction may appear somewhat abnormal depending upon anomalies of rotation of the kidney. The extrarenal pelvis as against the intrarenal, duplicity of the renal pelvis, and backflow phenomena all may contribute to some confusion.

Backflow Phenomena. (Figs. 16–53 and 16–54). Occasionally, the dye will enter the collecting tubules, renal veins, or lymphatics when introduced in retrograde pyelography. The causes of this phenomenon are not known. Part of the reason may be increased pressure resulting from introduction of the contrast agent, but this may not be the sole cause. There are five types of backflow: (1) pyelotubular, (2) pyelolymphatic, (3) pyelovenous, (4) pyelosinus, and (5) pyelointerstitial.

Pyelotubular backflow is manifest by the dye radiating in straight diverging lines from a minor calyx. Pyelolymphatic backflow appears as irregular lines arising from the region of the hilus and passing inward to the region of the renal lymph nodes. Pyelovenous backflow has the appearance of thick cobwebs or hazy streaking around the major calyx and adjoining neck of the minor calyx. The veins visualized are the venous plexuses into

CONFUSING PYELOGRAPHIC APPEARANCES

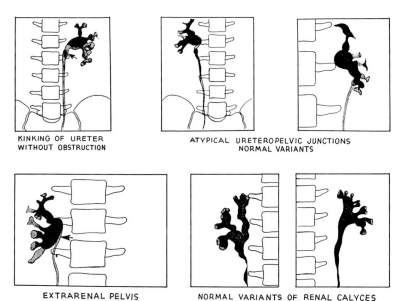

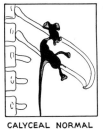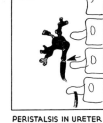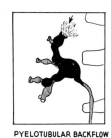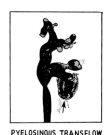

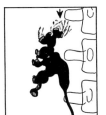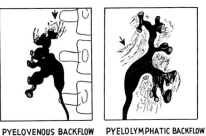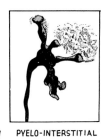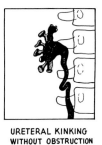

Figure 16–53.

which the interlobar veins of the kidney drain, since the tissue separating the calyces from the endothelium at these points is extremely thin and easily ruptured.

Often there is an accumulation of fat surrounding the renal

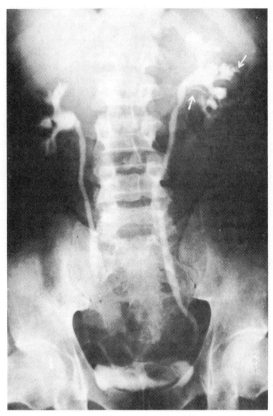

Figure 16–54. Intensified radiograph demonstrating backflow phenomena.

pelvis and extending somewhat into the hilus of the kidney upward toward the renal columns. This fat is found normally but may exist in abnormal concentration, particularly in the presence of renal atrophy. This is best shown by nephrotomography (renal fibrolipomatosis).

Infusion Pyelogram. The infusion pyelogram ordinarily does not distend the collecting system, and the concentration of the contrast media is excellent so that in many instances detail is sufficiently adequate to obviate the necessity for retrograde pyelography. On the other hand, if minute detail is required in respect to the collecting system or the ureters or bladder, retrograde cystography, ureterography, or pyelography becomes essential.

In the excretory urogram the calyces are normally cupped with sharp pointed margins surrounding the renal papilla. In the retrograde pyelogram, a different standard of normal is used, since often the calyces are moderately distended under positive pressure.

The Rapid Sequence and Washout Pyelogram (Fig. 16–49 *D*, *E*). This requires some additional features for study.

1. The time of appearance of the collecting system in the rapid sequence phase is normally no later than 3 minutes. Delayed appearance is significantly abnormal.
2. Careful comparison of the two kidneys must be made. Differences between them may be of pathologic importance.
3. Features such as shape and comparative size of the two kidneys become of increased importance. Differences of 1.5 cm. or greater in the cephalocaudal dimension of the two kidneys are of considerable significance.
4. By the 8 or 10 minute film in the rapid sequence study, every detail of the kidney collecting system should be visualized. In this concentrated phase of kidney function the kidney calyces are not distended.
5. In the *washout phase*, ordinarily by 10 minutes, the concentration of the contrast media becomes faint and kidney calyces may be slightly distended. If by any chance the concentration is enhanced by the 10 or 15 minute interval, an abnormal situation exists, pointing strongly toward hypertensive renopathy.

The Ureters. The ureter usually leaves the renal pelvis at its most dependent point and passes directly downward into the urinary bladder. Rotation of the kidney will cause some variation in this appearance, and this rotation can be recognized by the appearance of the calyces. The important factor to bear in mind is the presence or absence of interference to drainage from the kidney pelvis or any potential for such interference.

Constant peristalsis occurs over the length of the ureter, and portions of the ureter may not be visualized in excretory urography, depending upon this factor. If an area of constriction is abnormal, it is constant and is associated with a persistent dilatation of the ureter above this level. Normal areas of narrowness occur in three locations described above, namely the *ureteropelvic junction,* the *bifurcation of the iliac vessels,* and the point of *entrance of the ureter into the urinary bladder.*

Slight irregularities in the anatomic course of the ureter are of no significance if ureteral obstruction is manifest. A mild degree of tortuosity occurs with deep inspiration also. Displacement of the ureter, however, takes on considerable significance when contiguous masses are suspected.

The Urinary Bladder. In the anteroposterior recumbent projection the neck of the bladder lies just below the upper border of the pubic symphysis, and the fundus rises to a variable distance above the symphysis, depending upon the degree of distention. The distended bladder is ellipsoid in the adult, but in the child it tends to be elongated on its long axis, extending outside the pelvis minor. The outline of the bladder is usually smooth when distended, but may be irregular in the partially collapsed state, and this appearance should not be regarded as abnormal unless the degree of distention is inadequate. Often the thickness of the urinary bladder can be differentiated, since the outer wall of the urinary bladder is delineated by perivesical fat.

In the male, a minimal rarefaction may be apparent at the neck of the bladder resulting from the impression of the medial lobe of the prostate. When this impression is more than slight, it is usually but not always an indication of abnormal enlargement of the prostate or seminal vesicles.

In the undistended bladder indentations of the dome are visible. They likewise may have no significance since they are usually caused by pressure from contiguous organs, such as the pelvic colon, rather than by pathologic entities.

The Urethra. The prostatic urethra is slightly spindle-shaped and is 2 to 4 cm. in length. It joins the base of the urinary bladder abruptly. The narrowness of the membranous portion extends for a distance of 1 to 1.5 cm. The outline of the cavernous part of the urethra is fairly uniform throughout. Occasionally, there is a slight reflux into the ejaculatory duct as it opens into the prostatic urethra.

The female urethra is approximately 5 cm. in length and resembles closely the proximal one-third of the male urethra. Normally its walls are small and smooth, with a minimum lumen of about 3 mm. and a maximum of 8 mm. Irregularity, dilatation, or outpouching is of pathologic significance.

REFERENCES

Abrams, H. L., and Cornell, S. H.: Patterns of collateral flow in renal ischemia. Radiology, *84*:1001–1012, 1965.

Anson, B. J. (ed.): Morris' Human Anatomy. 12th edition. New York, McGraw-Hill, 1966.

Arkless, R.: The normal kidney's reaction to intravenous pyelography. Amer. J. Roentgenol., *107*:746–749, 1969.

Baker, H. L., Jr., and Hodgson, J. R.: Further studies on accuracy of oral cholecystography. Radiology, *74*:239–245, 1960.

Baum, S., and Gillenwater, J. Y.: Renal artery impressions on the renal pelvis. J. Urol., *95*:139–145, 1966.

Becker, J. A., Canter, I. E., and Perl, S.: Rapid intrarenal circulation. Amer. J. Roentgenol., *109*:167–171, 1970.

Calatroni, C. J., Poliak, A., and Kohan, A.: A roentgenographic study of stress incontinence in women. Amer. J. Obst. Gyn., *83*:649–656, 1962.

Chait, A., Matasar, K. W., Fabian, C. E., and Mellins, H. Z.: Vascular impressions on the ureters. Amer. J. Roentgenol., *111*:729–749, 1971.

Cobb, O. E., and Anderson, E. E.: Superimposition cystography in the diagnosis of infiltrating tumors of the bladder. J. Urol., *94*:569–572, 1965.

Cocchi, U.: Retropneumoperitoneum and Pneumomediastinum. Stuttgart, Georg Thieme Verlag, 1957.

Colapinto, R. F., and Steed, B. L.: Arteriography of adrenal tumors. Radiology, *100*:343–350, 1971.

Cooperman, L. R., and Lowman, R. M.: Fetal lobulation of the kidneys. Amer. J. Roentgenol., *92*:273, 1964.

Cunningham, D. J.: Manual of Practical Anatomy, Vol. 2. 12th edition. London, Oxford University Press, 1958.

Currarino, G.: Roentgenographic estimation of kidney size in normal individuals with emphasis on children. Amer. J. Roentgenol., *93*:464–466, 1965.

Dickinson, R. L.: Human Sex Anatomy. Second edition. Baltimore, Williams and Wilkins Co., 1949.

Doppman, J. L., and Shapiro, R.: Some normal renal variants. Amer. J. Roentgenol., *92*:1380–1389, 1964.

Dunbar, J. S.: Personal communication.

Dure-Smith, P.: The dose of contrast medium in intravenous urography: a physiologic assessment. Amer. J. Roentgenol., *108*:691–697, 1970.

Dux, A., Thurn, P., and Kisseler, B.: The physiological emptying mechanism of the urinary tract in the roentgen cinematogram. Fortschr. Geb. Röntgenstrahlen, *97*:687–703, 1962.

Elkin, M.: Radiological observations in acute ureteral obstruction. Radiology, *81*:484–491, 1963.

Emmett, J. L.: Clinical Urography. Second edition. Philadelphia, W. B. Saunders Co., 1964.

Emmett, J. L., and Witten, D. M.: Clinical Urography: An Atlas and Textbook of Roentgenologic Diagnosis. Third edition. Philadelphia, W. B. Saunders Co., 1971.

Evans, J. A.: Nephrotomography in investigation of renal masses. Radiology, *69*:684–689, 1957.

Evans, J. A.: Specialized roentgen diagnostic techniques in the investigation of abdominal disease. Radiology, *82*:579–594, 1964.

Evans, J. A., Dubilier, W., Jr., and Monteith, M. C.: Nephrotomograph.: Amer. J. Roentgenol., *71*:213–223, 1954.

Fainsinger, M. H.: Excretory urography in the young subject: hyaluronidase and tomography as aids. South Afr. Med. J., *13*:418–420, 1950.

Friedenberg, M. J., and Carlin, M. R.: The routine use of higher volumes of contrast material to improve intravenous urography. Radiology, *83*:405–413, 1964.

Friedenberg, M. J., Walz, B. J., McAlister, W. H., Locksmith, J. P., and Gallagher, T. L.: Roentgen size of normal kidneys. Radiology, *84*:1022–1029, 1965.

Frimann-Dahl, J.: Normal variations of left kidney: anatomic and radiologic study. Acta Radiol., *55*:207–216, 1955.

Gondos, B.: Rotation of the kidney around its transverse axis. Radiology, *74*:19–25, 1960.

Gondos, B.: Rotation of the kidney around its longitudinal axis. Radiology, *76*:615–619, 1961.

Gondos, B.: Roentgenographic evaluation of the size and shape of the kidneys. M. Ann. Dist. Col., *31*:158–161, 1961.

Grant, J. C. B.: Atlas of Anatomy, Baltimore, Williams and Wilkins Co., 1962.

Graves, F. T.: The anatomy of the intrarenal arteries and its application to segmental resection of the kidney. Brit. J. Surg., *42*:132–139, 1954.

Gray, H.: Gray's Anatomy of the Human Body. 29th edition. Philadelphia, Lea and Febiger, 1973.

Green, T. A.: Development of a plan for the diagnosis and treatment of stress incontinence. Amer. J. Obst. Gyn., *83*:632–648, 1962.

Harris, J. H., and Harris, J. H., Jr.: Infusion pyelography. Amer. J. Roentgenol., *92*:1391–1396, 1964.

Harrow, B. R., and Sloane, J. A.: Dromedary or humped left kidney: lack of relationship to renal rotation. Amer. J. Roentgenol., *88*:144–152, 1962.

Hodson, C. J.: The radiological contribution toward the diagnosis of chronic pyelonephritis. Radiology, *88*:857–871, 1967.

Kahn, P. C.: Selective venography in renal parenchymal disease. Radiology, *92*:345–349, 1969.

Kjellberg, S. R., Ericsson, N. D., and Rudhe, U.: The Lower Urinary Tract in Childhood: Some Correlated Clinical and Roentgenologic Observations (Erica Odelberg, trans.). Chicago, Ill., Almqvist Yearbook Pub. Inc., 1957.

Kurlander, G. J., and Smith, E. E.: Total body opacification in the diagnosis of Wilms' tumor and neuroblastoma. A note of caution. Radiology, *89*:1075–1076, 1967.

Lattimer, J. K., Dean, A. L., Jr., and Furey, C. A.: The triple voiding technique in children with dilated urinary tracts. J. Urol., *76*:656–660, 1956.

Lilienfeld, R. M., Friedenberg, R. M., and Herman, J. R.: The effect of renal lymphatics on kidneys and blood pressure. Radiology, *88*:1105–1109, 1967.

Martin, J. F.: Newer basic concepts of renal anatomy of radiologic interest. Radiol. Clin. N. Amer., *3*:3–11, 1965.

Martin, J. F., Deyton, W. E., and Glenn, J. F.: The minute sequence pyelogram. Amer. J. Roentgenol., *90*:55–62, 1963.

McLelland, R., Landes, R. R., and Ransom, C. L.: Retroperitoneal pneumography: A safe method using carbon dioxide. Radiol. Clin. N. Amer., *3*:113–128, 1965.

Meng, C-H, and Elkin, M.: Venous impressions on the calyceal system. Radiology, *87*:878–882, 1966.

Merklin, R. J., and Michels, N. A.: The variant renal and suprarenal blood supply with data on the inferior phrenic, ureteral and gonadal arteries: a statistical analysis based on 185 dissections and review of the literature. J. Internat. Coll. Surg., *29*:41–76, 1958.

Meschan, I.: Background physiology of the urinary tract for the radiologist. Radiol. Clin. N. Amer., *3*:13–28, 1965.

Moell, H.: Kidney size and its deviation from normal in acute renal failure. A roentgen diagnostic study. Acta Radiol. (Suppl.), *206*:1–74, 1961.

Moell, H.: Size of normal kidneys. Acta Radiol., *46*:640–645, 1956.

O'Connor, J. F., and Neuhauser, E. B. D.: Total body opacification in conventional and high dose venous urography in infancy. Amer. J. Roentgenol., *90*:63–71, 1963.

Olsson, O.: Roentgen examination of the kidney and ureter. *In* Flocks et al. (eds.): Encyclopedia of Urology. Berlin, Springer-Verlag, 1962, pp. 1–365.

Paul, R. E., Jr., Ettinger, A., Fainsinger, M. H., Callow, A. D., Kahn, P. C., and Inker, L. H.: Angiographic visualization of renal collateral circulation as a means of detecting and delineating renal ischemia. Radiology, *84*:1013–1021, 1965.

Pendergrass, H. P., Tondreau, R. L., Pendergrass, E. P., Ritchie, D. J., Hildreth, E. A., and Askovitz, S. I.: Reactions associated with intravenous urography: Historical and statistical review. Radiology, *71*:1–12, 1958.

Rawson, A. J.: Distribution of the lymphatics of the human kidney as shown in a case of carcinomatous permeation. Arch. Pathol., *47*:283–292, 1949.

Riggs, W., Jr., Hagood, J. H., and Andrews, A. E.: Anatomic changes in the normal urinary tract on urograms. Radiology, *94*:107–113, 1970.

Schobinger, R. A., and Ruzicka, F. F., Jr.: Vascular Roentgenology. New York, The Macmillan Co., 1964.

Segall, H. D.: Gallbladder visualization following the injection of diatrizoate. Amer. J. Roentgenol., *107*:21–26, 1969.

Shopfner, C. E., and Hutch, J. A.: The trigonal canal. Radiology, *88*:209–221, 1967.

Simon, A. L.: Normal renal size: An absolute criterion. Amer. J. Roentgenol., *92*:270–272, 1964.

Sorby, W. A.: Renal phlebography. Clin. Radiol., *20*:166–172, 1969.

Trueta, J., Barclay, A. E., Daniel, P. M., Franklin, K. J., and Prichard, M. M. L.: Studies of the renal circulation. Springfield, Ill., Charles C Thomas, 1947.

Waterhouse, K.: Voiding cystourethrography: a simple technique. J. Urol., *85*:103–104, 1961.

Weens, H. S., Olnick, H. M., James, D. F., and Warren, J. V.: Intravenous nephrography: A method of roentgen visualization of the kidney. Amer. J. Roentgenol., *65*:411–414, 1951.

Weissleder, H., Emmrich, J., and Schirmeister, J.: Gefassebedingte Kontrastmittelaussparungen im urographischen Bild. Fortschr. Geb. Röntgenstrahlen, *97*:703–710, 1962.

Whalen, J. P., and Ziter, F. M. H.: Visualization of the renal fascia—a new sign in localization of abdominal masses. Radiology, *89*:861–863, 1967.

Wigh, R., Anthony, H. F., Jr., and Grant, B. P.: A comparison of intravenous urography, urine radiography and other renal tests. Radiology, *78*:869–878, 1962.

17

The Genital System

THE MALE GENITAL SYSTEM

Related Gross Anatomy. Each *testis* (Fig. 17–1) is formed by numerous lobules, each containing coiled tubules called seminiferous tubules. The spermatozoa are formed in these tubules. These lobules and tubules converge posteriorly toward the rete testis, which consists of a network of tubules which empty by coiled ducts into the head of the *epididymis.* Here the duct of the epididymis is formed and extends in very tortuous fashion to the tail of the epididymis where it becomes the *ductus deferens.* This latter is a cordlike structure which traverses the posterior aspect of the spermatic cord, and in the vicinity of the trigone of the urinary bladder undergoes slight bulbous dilatation to form the *ampulla of the ductus deferens.* Near the lower margin of this ampulla, there is a diverticulumlike structure which extends cepha-

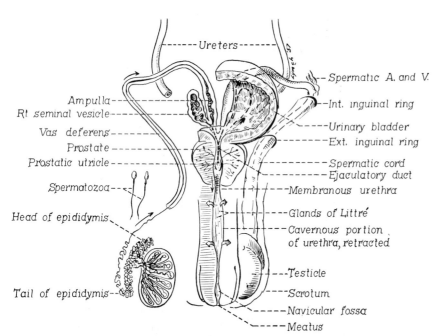

Figure 17–1. The male reproductive system. (Modified from Dickinson, Atlas of Human Sex Anatomy. Baltimore, The Williams & Wilkins Co.)

1056

lad, and appears racemose in configuration. This is the *seminal vesicle.* The continuation of the ampulla of the ductus deferens beyond the point of junction with the seminal vesicle is called the *ejaculatory duct,* and this empties into the lower posterior aspect of the prostatic urethra, one opening on either side of the *prostatic utricle.* In its course, the ejaculatory duct traverses about two-thirds of the length of the prostate. (Fig. 16–18 *A*)

The *prostate gland* is a conical structure, its base directed craniad and in contact with the caudal surface of the urinary bladder, and its apex pointing caudad, just superior to the superior fascia of the urogenital diaphragm. Anteriorly it is separated from the pubic symphysis by the pudendal plexus of veins and adipose tissue; posteriorly it is separated from the rectum by fascia which is continued over the seminal vesicles and over the pelvis laterally.

The posterior surface is separated from the rectum by the *rectovesical septum.* The *urethra* enters the prostate near its anterior surface and descends almost vertically within it so that the greater part of the prostate is posterior to the urethra. Its cross-sectional pattern and relationship to the bladder and urethra are shown in Figure 17–2. In cross section the prostate gland has four lobes, the *lobes anterior and posterior* to the urethra, the *lateral lobes* on either side of the urethra, and the *middle lobe* lying between the posterior aspect of the urethra near its junction with the urinary bladder and the ejaculatory duct. The *anterior lobe* is small and nonglandular and lies in front of the urethra. The *lateral lobes* extend not only laterally but also anterior to the urethra. The *middle lobe* contains the subtrigonal and cervical glands (Albarran's glands). As shown previously, the prostatic urethra contains a longitudinal ridge on its dorsal wall called the *urethral crest,* depressions on the sides of the crest into which the prostatic ducts open called the *prostatic sinuses,* and a *seminal colliculus* that is the summit of the urethral crest on which the ejaculatory ducts open. This colliculus also contains a median blind-ending sac, the *prostatic utricle.*

The *seminal vesicles* are bilateral lobulated sacs consisting of irregular pouches. They lie against the fundus of the bladder ventrally, and their dorsal surfaces are separated from the rectum by rectovesical fascia. Superiorly they are closely related to the *vas*

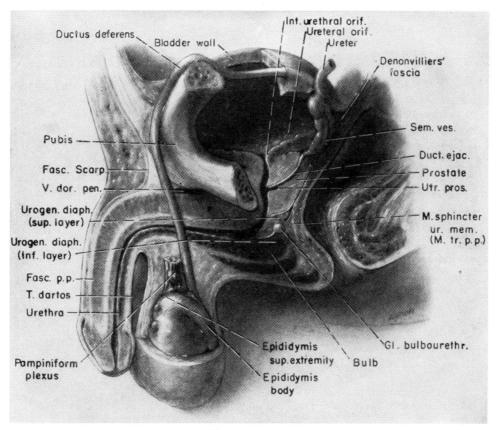

Figure 17-2. Midsagittal section of male pelvis. *Gl. bulbourethr.*, bulbourethral gland; *Fasc. p. p.*, deep perineal fascia; *T. dartos*, dartos tunic; *Duct. ejac.*, ejaculatory duct; *M. tr. p. p.*, m. sphincter urethrae membranaceae (m. transversus perinei profundus); *Fasc. Scarp.*, Scarpa's fascia; *Sem. ves.*, seminal vesicle; *Utr. pros.*, prostatic utricle; *V. dor. pen.*, v. dorsalis penis. (From Anson, B. J. (ed.): Morris' Human Anatomy, 12th ed. Copyright © 1966 by McGraw-Hill, Inc. Used by permission of McGraw-Hill Book Company.)

deferens and *ureters*. Inferiorly, the seminal vesicles join the vas deferens from either side on the posterior surface of the prostate (Figs. 17–2 and 17–3).

The course of the vas deferens and relationship to the pelvis and seminal vesicles is indicated in Figure 17–5.

The vessels and nerves of the vas deferens, seminal vesicles and prostate include: the middle rectal and inferior vesical arteries, the prostatic plexus of veins to the internal iliac veins, and lymphatics terminating in the internal iliac and sacral nodes predominantly.

The most important lobes of the prostate clinically are the median lobe, enlargement of which leads to urinary tract obstruction with encroachment on the urethra; and the lateral lobes, hypertrophy of which causes urinary obstruction. It is the posterior lobe which is encountered by rectal digital examination.

The relationships of the *male urethra* with cross sections of the penis at different levels are shown in Figure 17–6. The urethra and its examination have been previously discussed with the urinary tract in Chapter 16.

The *bulbourethral glands* or *Cowper's glands* are two small glands that lie on each side of the membranous portion of the urethra (Fig. 17–6), embedded between the two fascial layers of the urogenital diaphragm. The duct from this gland traverses the substance of the *corpus spongiosum of the penis* and opens on the floor of the bulbar portion of the urethra. This gland can be clinically significant in that occasionally a cyst may occur or accessory glands may be demonstrated distal or proximal to the main ductal openings.

Technique of Examination. There are only certain portions of the male genital system which can be examined radio-

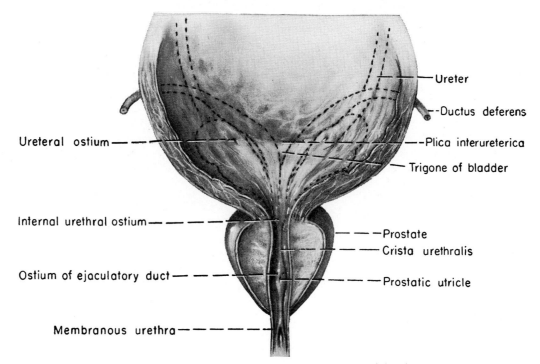

Figure 17–3.   Trigone of bladder and floor of prostatic urethra. (From Anson, B. J. (ed.): Morris' Human Anatomy, 12th ed. Copyright © 1966 by McGraw-Hill, Inc. Used by permission of McGraw-Hill Book Company.)

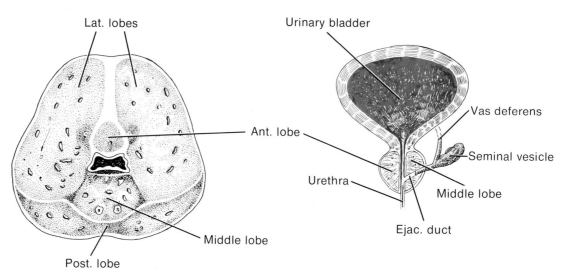

Figure 17–4.   Cross section and sagittal section of prostate gland, showing relationship to urethra and urinary bladder.

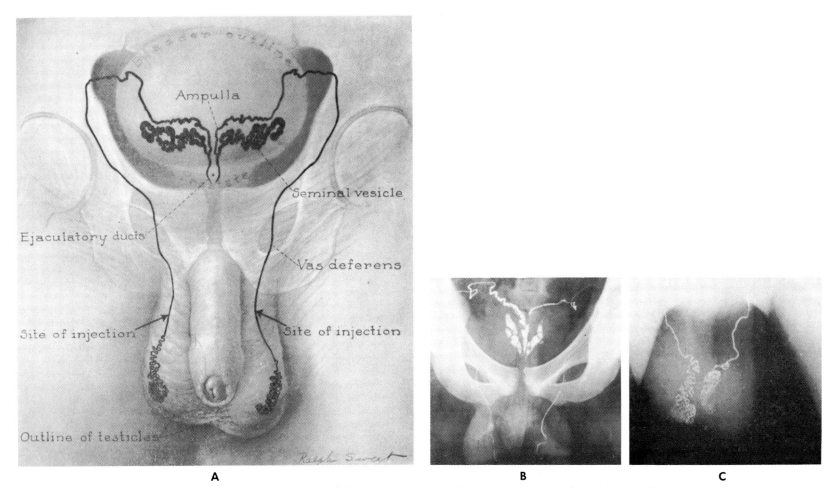

Figure 17–5. *A.* The male genital tract. The sites of exposure of the vas deferens are indicated, into which injections of the contrast media are made upward and frequently downward. *B.* Normal seminal vesiculogram (with Umbrathor). The distal segment of the right vas deferens is larger than that of the left. The right seminal vesicle is slightly better filled than the left. The injection of the left vas was made 24 hours before this film, and that of the right 4½ hours before this film. *C.* Same patient as above with filling of the distal portions of the epididymides achieved at the same time as *B.* Greater filling has been obtained on the right than on the left. (From Tucker, A. S., Yanagihara, H., and Pryde, A. W.: Amer. J. Roentgenol., 71:490–500, 1954.)

graphically by presently known methods. The examination is confined to a soft tissue study of the prostate, seminal vesicles, and scrotal contents, and the direct injection of opaque media into the lumen of the seminal vesicles, vas deferens, and ejaculatory duct via the vas deferens.

The usual method employed in the direct injection depends on the exposure of the vas through a small inguinal incision under local anesthesia. This injection is first directed upward to fill the vesicles and then downward to the epididymis to fill the tubules (Fig. 17–2). Either an iodized oil, such as Ethiodol, or diatrizoate (Renografin or Hypaque) may be used. Urethroscopic catheterization has also been employed by a few. The latter

method also does not permit visualization of the vas deferens, and serves only to outline the ejaculatory ducts and seminal vesicles.

Radiographic Appearances. On a plain radiograph the prostate may be visualized when enlarged as an impression directed upward at the base of the urinary bladder. Calculi may be seen within the prostate, but the outline of the gland cannot be delineated.

Using contrast material, the numerous racemose or diverticulumlike tubes of the seminal vesicles appear like an indefinite mass, and the ductus deferens may be seen as a tubular structure which conforms closely to the anatomic description just given (Fig. 17–5). The more distal tubules may be visualized,

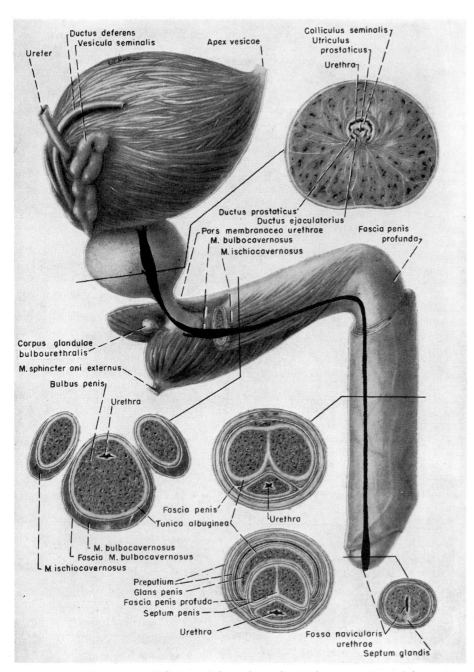

Figure 17–6.   Relations of the male urethra with cross sections of the penis at different levels. Semidiagrammatic. (From Anson, B. J. (ed.): Morris' Human Anatomy, 12th ed. Copyright © 1966 by McGraw-Hill, Inc. Used by permission of McGraw-Hill Book Company.)

depending upon the efforts of the investigator, but they are examined infrequently.

In prostatic carcinoma, the ejaculatory duct may be invaded and occluded, but in the normal subject it may be seen extending beyond the junction of the ductus deferens and the seminal vesicles.

THE FEMALE REPRODUCTIVE SYSTEM

The soft tissue structures of this system will be described first and then a brief account will be given of the bony pelvis and its anatomic variations.

Soft Tissues.   The organs of the female genital system consist of two *ovaries,* two *oviducts,* the *uterus,* the *vagina* and the *external genitalia.* The suspensory and supplementary structures are the *broad ligaments* (and *mesosalpinx*) on either side, the *round ligament,* the *mesovarium* and *mesometrium* (Fig. 17–7).

The *broad ligament* is the transverse fold of peritoneum extending across the pelvis minor, dividing it into an anterior and a posterior compartment. This has frequently been compared with a "curtain draped over a clothesline." Projecting into the posterior compartment and attached a little below the upper margin of the broad ligament, is the *mesovarium,* with the ovary attached to its free edge. That portion of the broad ligament above this is called the *mesosalpinx,* and that below, the *mesometrium.* The relationship of the uterus and vagina in lateral perspective is shown in Figure 17–8.

The *ovaries* are two almond-shaped organs—one on either side of the pelvis. Their exact position in nulliparous women is somewhat variable but their long axis is usually vertical in the erect position. The right ovary is usually slightly larger than the left, and the length varies from 2.5 to 5 cm. The width is ordinarily one-half the length and the thickness one-half the width.

The *oviducts,* or *uterine tubes,* are two trumpet-shaped tubes which run in the superior border of the broad ligament between the uterine horns and the lateral pelvic walls. The dilated end lies over each ovary. Each oviduct is from 7 to 14 cm. in length. Ordinarily, the fimbriated end and mouth of the infundibulum rest upon the medial end of the ovary. The course of the oviducts is rather variable, and may be different on the two sides.

The *uterus* is a pear-shaped organ with a body or fundus and a downward extension, the cervix, which has supravaginal and vaginal sections. The cavity of the body is flattened transversely and has a triangular shape, being broad above where each cornua communicates with an oviduct and narrow below where it communicates with the canal in the cervix. The direction of the axis of the uterus is quite variable. Ordinarily a moderate degree of anteflexion is considered the normal position, making an angle of 80 to 120 degrees with the horizontal. There may also be a slight list to the right or to the left side.

The *vagina* extends from the uterus to the external genitalia where it opens to the exterior. Its course roughly parallels the anterior curvature of the sacrum and averages 5 to 7 cm. in length.

There is a deep depression between the rectum and uterus known as the *rectouterine pouch of Douglas.*

The ovarian vessels enter the broad ligament at its base and pass through the superior border of the suspensory ligament of the ovary.

The size of the uterus, which varies under normal conditions at various ages and in various physiologic states, is as follows: (1) adult virgin, 7 to 8 cm. in length, 4.5 to 5 cm. across its fundus; its anteroposterior thickness is 2 to 3 cm.; (2) in normal nonpregnant women, the depth of uterine and cervical cavities is 3 cm. approximately; (3) in the prepubertal period it is smaller; and (4) in women who have borne children it is larger.

Blood Supply of Female Genital System

Ovary. The *ovarian artery* supplies the ovary directly from the aorta, descending in the suspensory ligament of the ovary to the broad ligament and sending branches to the ovary and uterine tubes (Fig. 17–9). The *ovarian vein* travels with the ovarian artery, terminating on the right in the vena cava and on the left in the renal vein (Fig. 17–10).

Oviduct (Uterine Tube). The arterial supply to the oviduct is similar to that of the ovary. The venous drainage of the oviduct is likewise similar to that of the ovary, with some flow to the uterine plexus (Fig. 17–10).

Uterus. The uterus receives a number of arteries such as:

an *ovarian* branch and a *uterine* branch from the anterior division of the internal iliac artery which crosses the ureter to reach the side of the uterus through the broad ligament, where it ascends to the level of the uterine tube. This artery supplies the cervix, upper vagina, body of the uterus, uterine tube, and round ligament (Fig. 17–11).

The *veins* of the uterus are derived from a *uterine plexus,* which in turn communicates with a *vaginal plexus* that is drained chiefly by uterine veins ending in internal iliac veins (Fig. 17–10).

Vagina. The *vaginal artery* is derived from the internal iliac artery. It sends branches to the uterus and joins branches from the uterine artery to form the *azygos artery of the vagina.* The *veins* of the vagina drain from a plexus communicating with vesical, rectal, and uterine plexuses through a vaginal vein to empty into the internal iliac vein (Fig. 17–10).

The *lymphatic drainage* of these structures is shown in Figure 17–12. The *ovarian lymphatics* follow the ovarian artery, entering the lateral and preaortic lymph nodes. The *oviduct lymphatics* follow the ovarian and uterine drainage. In the uterus the cervical lymphatics drain to the external, internal, and common iliac nodes; those from the body and fundus follow an ovarian drainage to the lateral and preaortic nodes, some going to external iliac and some to superficial inguinal nodes.

The *vaginal lymphatics drain* to the external, internal, and common iliac nodes from the upper, middle, and lower portions respectively.

The *vulvar drainage* ends in superficial inguinal nodes for the most part.

Thus, the lymph nodes that are most concerned in draining

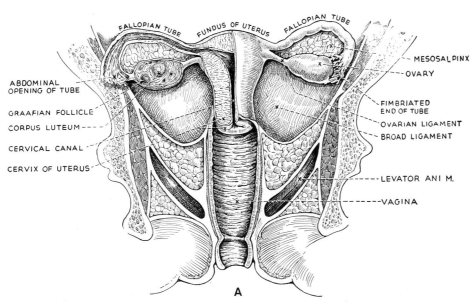

Figure 17–7. A. Gross anatomy of female reproductive system. A. Frontal view.

Figure 17–7 continued on the following page.

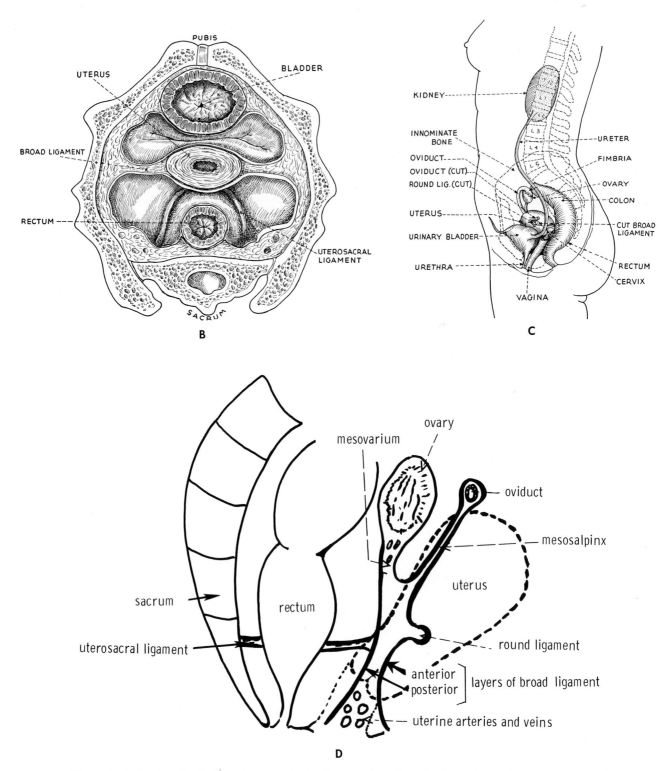

Figure 17-7 *Continued.* B. Superior cross-sectional diagram. C. Lateral relationships of genitourinary tract. D. Isometric view of broad ligament and its relationship to contiguous organs in the female pelvis.

Figure 17-7 continued on the opposite page.

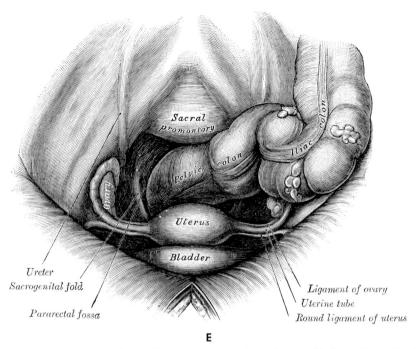

E

Figure 17–7 *Continued.* E. Female pelvis and its contents, seen from above and in front. (From Gray's Anatomy of the Human Body, 29th ed. Goss, C. M. (ed.) Philadelphia, Lea & Febiger, 1973.)

the female genital system ultimately are the *common iliac*, the *external iliac*, and the *internal iliac* (Fig. 17–13).

Pelvic Architecture of the Female

Bony Pelvis. In addition to the normal anatomic landmarks of the pelvis described in Chapter 5, certain areas should receive the attention of the radiologist as having an influence on the course of labor. Differences characteristic of male and female types should be borne in mind. These areas are as follows:

1. *The Subpubic Arch* (Fig. 17–14). Note should be made of the bones of the pubic rami, whether they are delicate, average, or heavy; whether the pubic angle is wide or curved (female) or narrow and straight (male), and whether the side walls of the forepelvis are divergent, straight, or convergent. The configuration of the pelvic arch is a guide to the capacity of the true pelvis.

2. *The Ischial Spines.* These are classified as sharp, average, or anthropoid. Sharp spines are definitely a male characteristic and when present, direct the attention to the necessity for a more detailed examination of the pelvis, as they may be associated with converging side walls of the forepelvis. The anthropoid spines are blunt and shallow.

3. *The Sacrosciatic Notch and Sacrum.* The capacity of the posterior pelvic inlet is related to the width of the sacrosciatic

notch and the configuration of its apex. The male pelvis shows a long narrow notch with a high rounded apex and the female a wide notch with a blunt apex.

The inclination of the sacrum directly affects the capacity of the birth canal since a forward tilt will offer a barrier to normal delivery. If the forepelvis is wide and divergent, compensation

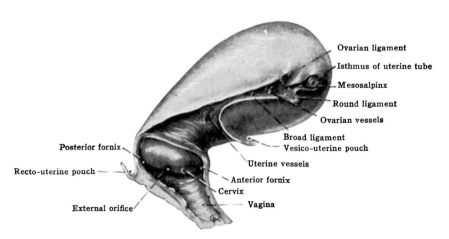

Figure 17–8. Lateral view of uterus, showing attachment of the broad ligament. (From Anson, B. J. (ed.): Morris' Human Anatomy, 12th ed. Copyright © 1966 by McGraw-Hill, Inc. Used by permission of McGraw-Hill Book Company.)

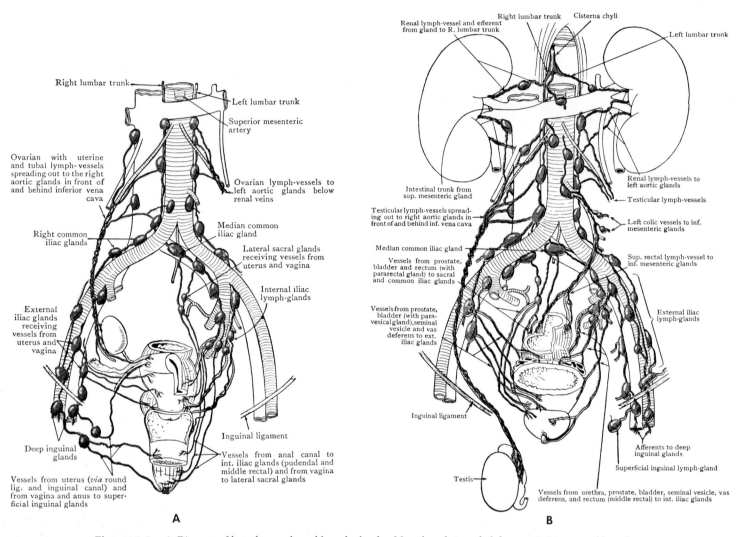

Figure 17–9.   *A.* Diagram of lymph vessels and lymph glands of female pelvis and abdomen. *B.* Diagram of lymph vessels and lymph glands of male pelvis and abdomen. (From Cunningham's Manual of Practical Anatomy, 11th ed. London, Oxford University Press, 1949.)

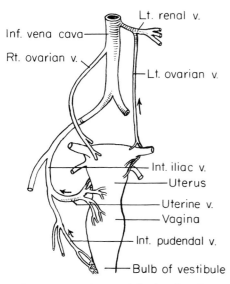

Figure 17–10. Veins of the female pelvis.

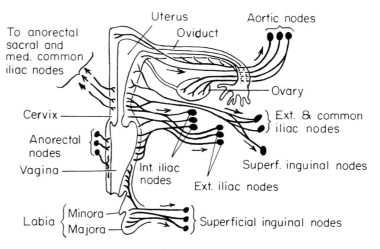

Figure 17–12. Lymph vessels of the female genitalia.

occurs but if convergent, a funnel pelvis will result. The female sacrum is wide and short compared with that of the male.

The curvature of the sacrum on the lateral projection is also important. Normally the sacrum is concave anteriorly. When this curvature is absent owing to any developmental aberration, the midpelvis is diminished and the progress of labor is impeded. The absence of this curvature will be readily apparent from measurements to be described later.

4. *The Pelvic Inlet.* The pelvic inlet with its variations can be classified into four major types (Fig. 17–15):

The inlet of the anthropoid pelvis is relatively long in anteroposterior measurements and narrow in transverse diameter.

The pelvic arch is usually wider than normal and the sacrosciatic notch is wide and shallow when seen in the lateral view. The anthropoid type is so called because it closely resembles the pelves found in the higher apes.

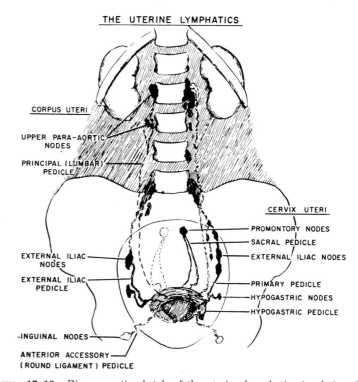

Figure 17–13. Diagrammatic sketch of the uterine lymphatic circulation. The solid lymph nodes and pedicles represent the visualized primary drainage areas, the shaded lymph nodes are secondary drainage areas, and the open lymph nodes are nonopacified lymph nodes in our case. (From Hipona, F. A., and Ditchek, T.: Amer. J. Roentgenol., 98:236–238, 1966.)

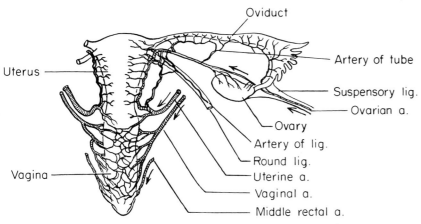

Figure 17–11. Arteries of the female genitalia.

A

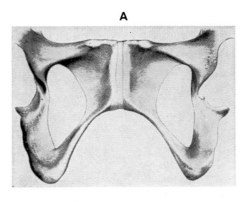

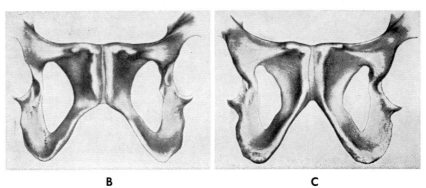

B   C

Figure 17–14.   Variations in size and shape of the subpubic arch. *A.* Delicate bones, wide angle; well-curved female type of pubic rami. *B.* Average bones, moderate angle; average curvature of pubic rami. *C.* Heavy bones, narrow angle; straight masculine type of pubic rami. (From Golden, R.: Diagnostic Roentgenology, Vol. 2. Baltimore, Williams and Wilkins Co., 1963–1969.)

DIFFERENT PELVIC TYPES
(PELVIC INLET VIEW)

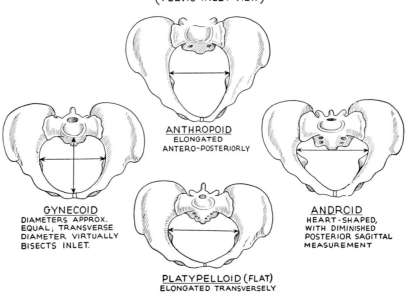

ANTHROPOID
ELONGATED
ANTERO-POSTERIORLY

GYNECOID
DIAMETERS APPROX.
EQUAL; TRANSVERSE
DIAMETER VIRTUALLY
BISECTS INLET.

ANDROID
HEART-SHAPED,
WITH DIMINISHED
POSTERIOR SAGITTAL
MEASUREMENT

PLATYPELLOID (FLAT)
ELONGATED TRANSVERSELY

Figure 17–15.

FACTORS STUDIED IN PELVIC ARCHITECTURE

1. PELVIC INLET STUDY *(SEE DIAGRAMS OF DIFFERENT PELVIC TYPES)*

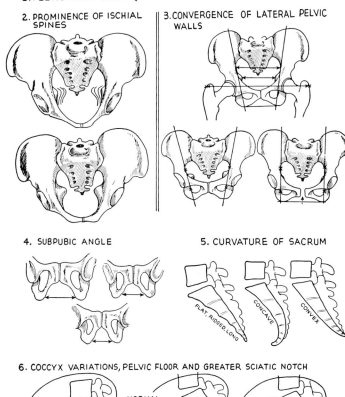

2. PROMINENCE OF ISCHIAL SPINES

3. CONVERGENCE OF LATERAL PELVIC WALLS

4. SUBPUBIC ANGLE

5. CURVATURE OF SACRUM

FLAT, RIDGED LONG   CONCAVE   CONVEX

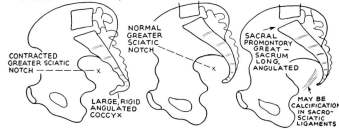

6. COCCYX VARIATIONS, PELVIC FLOOR AND GREATER SCIATIC NOTCH

CONTRACTED GREATER SCIATIC NOTCH

NORMAL GREATER SCIATIC NOTCH

SACRAL PROMONTORY GREAT - SACRUM LONG, ANGULATED

LARGE, RIGID ANGULATED COCCYX

MAY BE CALCIFICATION IN SACRO-SCIATIC LIGAMENTS

7. UTERINE AXIS FACTOR IN RELATION TO SACRUM AND SACRAL PROMONTORY

A. AXIS OF UTERUS NEAR SPINE, GOOD FLEXION OF HEAD

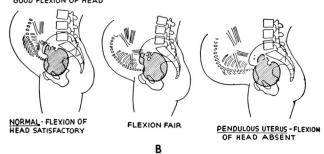

NORMAL - FLEXION OF HEAD SATISFACTORY   FLEXION FAIR   PENDULOUS UTERUS - FLEXION OF HEAD ABSENT

B

TYPICAL GYNECOID PELVIS

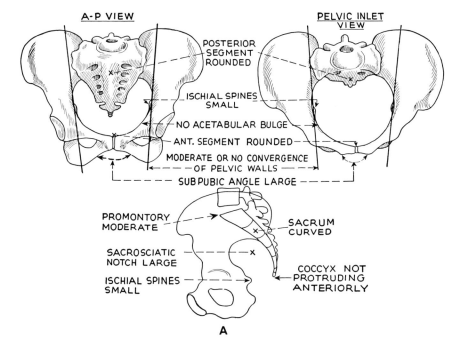

A-P VIEW

PELVIC INLET VIEW

POSTERIOR SEGMENT ROUNDED

ISCHIAL SPINES SMALL

NO ACETABULAR BULGE

ANT. SEGMENT ROUNDED

MODERATE OR NO CONVERGENCE OF PELVIC WALLS

SUBPUBIC ANGLE LARGE

PROMONTORY MODERATE

SACRUM CURVED

SACROSCIATIC NOTCH LARGE

ISCHIAL SPINES SMALL

COCCYX NOT PROTRUDING ANTERIORLY

A

Figure 17–16.

The gynecoid pelvis is the average type as seen in the human female. The inlet is round or slightly oval, the pubic angle is wide, and the sacrosciatic notch is also wide. The cavity of the pelvis is ample in all directions (Fig. 17–16).

The android pelvis refers to a female pelvis which has marked masculine characteristics. These include what is described as a blunt heart-shaped or wedge-shaped inlet with narrow forepelvis, and the widest diameter is close to the sacral promontory. A narrow masculine type of sciatic notch is present and the sacrum is set forward in the pelvis. The pubic arch is usually narrow.

The platypelloid or flat pelvis is characterized by an inlet with a transversely oval shape. The anteroposterior diameter is short and the greatest transverse diameter is wide—this diameter occurring well in front of the sacrum. The angle of the forepelvis is wide also, but the sacrosciatic notch and subpubic angle vary in size.

It should be stated that gradations between all types are seen and individual variations should be described as they appear on the radiograph.

The reader is referred to the work of Caldwell and Moloy on this subject.

Methods of Study of the Female Genital System

In the entire description below of the applications and usefulness of radiographic techniques in investigation of obstetrical and gynecologic problems, the student must bear in mind those aspects of radiologic protection which pertain here (see Chapter 2). The information to be gained must justify the exposure of the patient (and the fetus, if one is present). In any case, radiation exposure of the patient and the fetus in the first trimester of pregnancy is to be avoided unless the problem at hand is a critical one.

Direct Radiography and Its Applications. Anteroposterior, lateral, and "inlet" views of the pelvis are obtained and a considerable amount of information is available from these views (Fig. 17–16).

The purposes of roentgen study of the female patient in obstetrics and gynecology may be outlined as follows:

1. **The study of the female pelvis and abdomen** (apart from pregnancy), including (a) the determination of an extrauterine fetus; (b) the study of pelvic soft tissues outside the uterus, particularly to determine if interference to parturition might result; (c) pelvic mensuration and description as a guide to determination of possible cephalopelvic disproportion; and (d) all those anatomic and pathologic possibilities in the abdomen and pelvis that exist regardless of the sex of the patient.

2. **Special gynecologic study of the nonpregnant female** for: (a) hysterosalpingography, or the detailed study of the uterine cavity and oviducts and determination of the patency of the latter; (b) pelvic pneumography—the study of the pelvic peritoneal space by introduction of gas into the space; (c) a combination of these; and (d) pelvic angiography.

3. **A study of the pregnant mother in respect to the fetus** for the purpose of: (a) determining the presence of a fetal skeleton *in utero* or intra-abdominally; (b) determining the presence of multiple fetuses; (c) determining fetal normalcy, age, and development; (d) determining fetal viability or death; or (e) describing the accurate presentation of the fetus.

4. **A study of the pregnant uterus apart from the fetus,** including: (a) the placenta—its size, position, and density; (b) the amniotic space (the amniotic space may be entered to withdraw fluid for special study, or may serve as a guide to fetal transfusion); or (c) general uterine density and normalcy of appearance.

5. **Genitography of the abnormal infant or child** (intersex problems).

STUDY OF THE FEMALE PELVIS AND ABDOMEN

Introductory Comments. The study of the pregnant mother for intra-abdominal abnormalities outside the uterus lies outside the scope of this text. The features of the extrauterine fetus, for example, tubal pregnancy, and the implantation of a placenta anywhere in the abdominal cavity are subjects which have been discussed in our companion text, *Analysis of Roentgen Signs,* and the student is referred for brief discussion to this reference. This applies to a consideration of the ruptured uterus also.

Study of Pelvic Soft Tissue Structures Outside the Uterus (especially to determine if interference to parturition may result). This, too, involves abnormalities in the retroperitoneal space such as tumors of the sacrum, inflammatory swellings, or urinary tract abnormalities. Similarly, abnormalities of the intestine may be considered here. These are outside the scope of this text and the student is referred to *Analysis of Roentgen Signs* for further discussion.

Cephalopelvic Disproportion and Pelvic Measurement. Many methods of measurement of the maternal pelvis and the fetal head have been proposed. These include such adjuncts as special rulers or grids which are projected over the pelvis in its midsection, special tables and graphs which provide for determination of the extent of magnification, special slide rules which facilitate determination of magnification, nomograms which help resolve the extent of magnification if the basic factors are known, and teleroentgenograms which minimize the extent of magnification to the point where the degree of accuracy possible is related largely to the degree of accuracy of the actual measurement.

In all these proposed methods the *basic concepts and objectives are to measure the important diameters of the pelvis and head*, eliminating as much as possible the elements of magnification and distortion; *to describe the pelvic architecture* as accurately as possible from the standpoint of parturition; and to *describe any other factors* in relation to the pelvis, fetus, or placenta such as have been previously indicated in this section.

It is important for the student to adopt that method of correction for magnification and distortion that is most feasible in his particular installation and to learn that method thoroughly rather than to be attracted to one proposal or another by various authors. If it is possible to obtain at least 72 inch target-to-film distance films (teleroentgenograms), one may assay the size of the pelvis and fetal head without difficulty, since a maximum magnification on the order of 10 per cent is thereby feasible. For those measurements such as the interischial spinous diameter, to be obtained in the middle of the pelvis, the magnification is on the order of only 5 per cent. Moreover, when nonengagement of the fetal head occurs in a pendulous abdomen, the distance between head and inlet is not as significant in the teleroentgenogram as in other proposed techniques. Fetal head and pelvic measurements are more easily obtained with breech presentations when teleroentgenograms are employed, since distortion is minimal.

Templeton has utilized high kilovoltage pelvimetry with a teleroentgenographic technique and a target-to-film distance of 10 feet; by using 150 Kv. and a 1 mm. focal spot, he was able to obtain anteroposterior and lateral roentgenograms with the patient standing against a grid cassette (100 lines per inch). He employed an angulation of 20 degrees toward the feet for the anteroposterior roentgenogram. Comparison of radiation exposure to the fetus and maternal pelvis was made using a pelvic phantom. Whereas the conventional kilovoltage technique averaged a total of 1020 milliroentgens to the midpelvis, this high kilovoltage technique averaged a total of 60 milliroentgens. Thus, radiation hazard was 17 times less with this high kilovoltage technique, and the teleroentgenograms made magnification correction unnecessary. All obstetric measurements were made readily on the two upright roentgenograms.

If methods other than the teleroentgenographic technique are employed, it is important to obtain both the lateral and anteroposterior views without moving the patient. This is important because the lateral view is employed to correct for magnification on the anteroposterior projection, and similarly the anteroposterior projection is employed to obtain certain measurements which are applied to the lateral view. If there is a difference in the position of the fetal head, for example, in these two views, the correction factors are much more complex and virtually nullified.

For this reason erect films are preferred by some. When the patient is standing, the position of the fetus with respect to the maternal pelvis is not apt to change when the patient moves from the anteroposterior to the lateral position. The erect standing film may also be preferred in order to obtain maximum gravitational effect of the fetus above the maternal pelvis.

Evaluation of Pelvicephalography in the Light of Radiation Hazard. Considerable confusion has resulted with respect to the indications and contraindications for the radiologic study of the female pelvis and fetal skull in pregnancy. While radiation is not the only genetic hazard in our environment which can result in increased mutations, every effort should be made to reduce this particular hazard as much as possible. Although it has not been absolutely proved in mammals, it is generally accepted that genetic aberrations from exposure to radiation can occur at virtually any dose level.

The reader is referred to Chapter 2 for a more detailed consideration of the many aspects of radiation protection. From these discussions, however, we may derive the following conclusions:

1. Roentgen pelvic encephalometry should not be considered a routine procedure. It must be employed only after thorough obstetrical examination and evaluation, and the information to be obtained must be of critical value. Nevertheless, this procedure must be undertaken with the full understanding that the radiologist cannot and should not by himself attempt to predict the outcome of delivery. The data obtained should permit a thorough study of the maternal pelvis in all its aspects and should provide some idea of the relative size, shape, and position of the fetal skull in relation to the maternal pelvis.

2. All precautions should be employed to minimize radiation exposure. These must include high kilovoltage techniques, fast films, fast screens, collimation, additional filtration, increased target-to-film distance, and superior darkroom processing so that repeated exposures are unnecessary.

3. The optimal time for roentgen pelvic encephalometry is during the last 2 weeks of pregnancy. Under these circumstances, with a cephalic presentation the fetal gonads may actually lie outside the primary beam of radiation if one concentrates on the maternal pelvis.

4. Although information regarding the fetus, including fetal maturity, age, and development, may be obtained, fetal weight predictions have proved inaccurate and unsatisfactory since no relationship has been established between fetal skull measurements and body weight (Ane et al.).

Pelvic and Fetal Measurements in Use. Regardless of the method employed for correction for magnification and distortion, the measurements that are most valuable are indicated in Figures 17–17 to 17–19. These are measurement of the pelvic inlet in both the anteroposterior and transverse diameters, measurement of the midpelvis in its anteroposterior diameter, the interischial spinous diameter, the posterior sagittal measurement of the midpelvis, the intertuberous diameter as a measurement of the pelvic outlet, and the two largest perpendic-

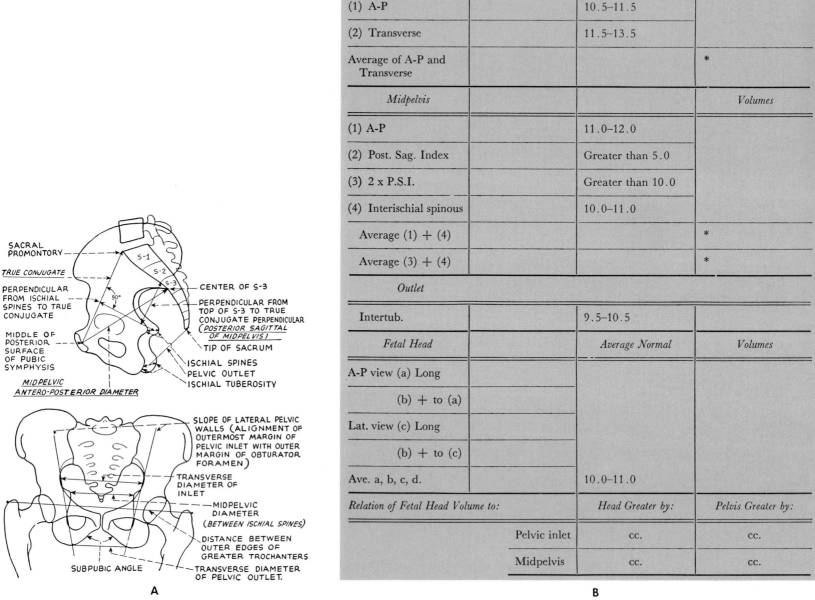

Format for Reporting Cephalopelvic Measurements

Inlet		Average Normal (cm.)	Volume
(1) A-P		10.5–11.5	
(2) Transverse		11.5–13.5	
Average of A-P and Transverse			*
Midpelvis			*Volumes*
(1) A-P		11.0–12.0	
(2) Post. Sag. Index		Greater than 5.0	
(3) 2 x P.S.I.		Greater than 10.0	
(4) Interischial spinous		10.0–11.0	
Average (1) + (4)			*
Average (3) + (4)			*
Outlet			
Intertub.		9.5–10.5	
Fetal Head		*Average Normal*	*Volumes*
A-P view (a) Long			
(b) + to (a)			
Lat. view (c) Long			
(b) + to (c)			
Ave. a, b, c, d.		10.0–11.0	
Relation of Fetal Head Volume to:		*Head Greater by:*	*Pelvis Greater by:*
	Pelvic inlet	cc.	cc.
	Midpelvis	cc.	cc.

A   B

Figure 17–17. *A.* Diagrams illustrating the various measurements obtained from routine anteroposterior and lateral teleroentgenograms of the pelvis for pelvic measurement. *B.* Method of reporting pelvic measurements. (All measurements are recorded after correction for magnification.)

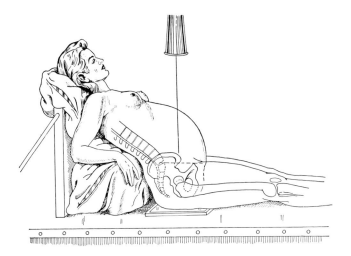

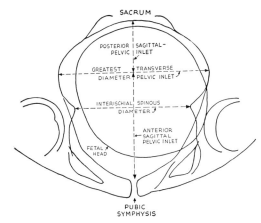

Figure 17–18. Tracing of radiograph routinely employed in pelvicephalometry. Special view of pelvic inlet, showing positioning of patient (note the pelvic inlet is parallel to the table top) and tracing of radiograph so obtained.

ular diameters of the fetal head in both the anteroposterior and lateral projections (it is well to add approximately 4 mm. to the average diameter in consideration of the scalp soft tissues) (Ball and Golden; Schwarz).

We have elected to describe in great detail one technique with which we have considerable experience, rather than to give a brief, cursory description of the many techniques which are available for the purpose of pelvicephalometry. This technique has been modified by the author for teleroentgenography, in which erect films are not as essential as they would be for shorter film-to-target distances.

Having obtained the various measurements the following procedure is utilized (modification of Ball method; Schwarz's classification):

All four diameters of the fetal head are averaged together,

and an average fetal head diameter is obtained (Fig. 17–19). From this average fetal head diameter, the tables are employed to obtain an average fetal head volume (computed from the formula $4/3\,\pi\,r^3$, where r is the average radius of the fetal head). The bottom scale on Fig. 17–20 can be used for this purpose.

The greatest transverse and anteroposterior diameters of the pelvic inlet are averaged together; utilizing this as a diameter, the volume of a sphere is obtained.

The anteroposterior diameter of the midpelvis and the interischial spinous diameter are averaged together and again the volume of a sphere is obtained, using this average diameter. Another method of finding midpelvis sphere volume is to double the posterior sagittal midpelvic index and to average this with the interischial spinous diameter. This becomes the average diameter of the midpelvis, and the volume of the associated sphere is thereby determined.

Thus, the volume of the fetal head, the volume of a sphere with an average diameter equivalent to the average diameter of the pelvic inlet, and the volume of a sphere having as its diameter the average diameter of the midpelvis have been computed. These three spheres are thereafter compared in volume. If the midpelvic and inlet volumes each exceed the volume of the fetal head, no further computation is necessary. This group would be considered as "no disproportion demonstrated," and the incidence of cesarean section, regardless of reason, would be about 4 per cent. Incidence for cephalopelvic disproportion in this group would prove to be about 1 per cent, based upon 350 patients (Schwarz).

A "borderline disproportion" group may be differentiated, in which the fetal head volume exceeds the volume capacity of the inlet by 70 cc. or less, or the volume capacity of the bispinous diameter by 50 to 220 cc. (In the latter instance, anything less than 50 cc. would fall into the "no disproportion" category.) Incidence of cesarean section in this group would prove to be about 33 per cent.

The "high disproportion" group consists of those patients with fetal head volumes exceeding the volume capacity of the inlet by more than 70 cc., or the bispinous diameter volume capacity by more than 220 cc. The incidence of cesarean section in this group would prove to be about 80 per cent for any reason, and the incidence of "difficult delivery" 87 per cent. Difficult delivery is defined as applying to deliveries requiring cesarean section, high or midforceps, or to infant death resulting from proved brain injury (Schwarz).

In all of these computations it is important to remember this basic principle: *Under no circumstances do any of these measurements indicate that spontaneous delivery will or will not occur.* These measurements are for purposes of comparison only. It is impossible by these measurements to predict the intensity of labor contractions, uterine atonia, and a host of other factors in the individual case which have not been reduced to mathematical terms.

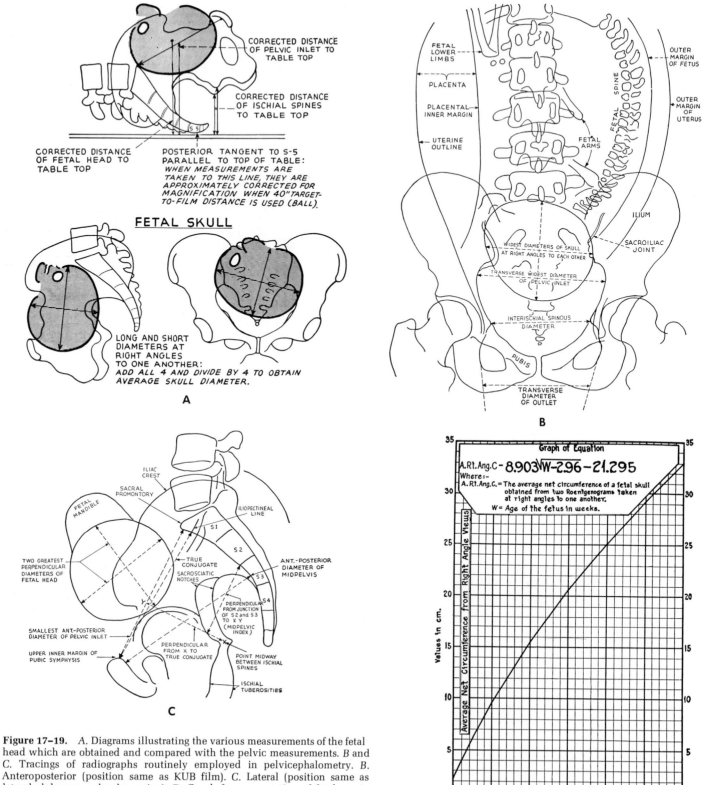

Figure 17–19.   A. Diagrams illustrating the various measurements of the fetal head which are obtained and compared with the pelvic measurements. B and C. Tracings of radiographs routinely employed in pelvicephalometry. B. Anteroposterior (position same as KUB film). C. Lateral (position same as lateral abdomen or lumbar spine). D. Graph for computation of fetal age in weeks from average corrected circumference of skull obtained from two radiographs taken at right angles to one another. (From Hodges, P. C.: Amer. J. Roentgenol., 37:644–662, 1937.)

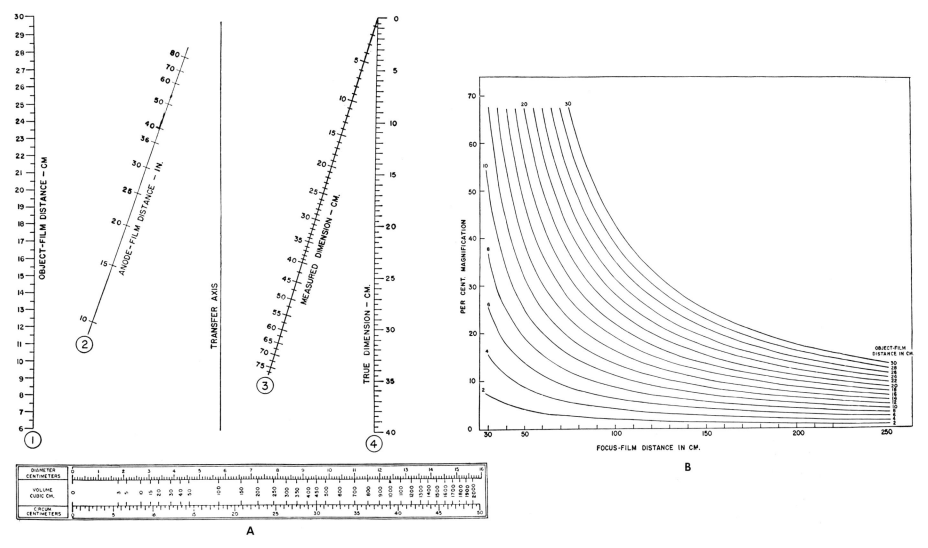

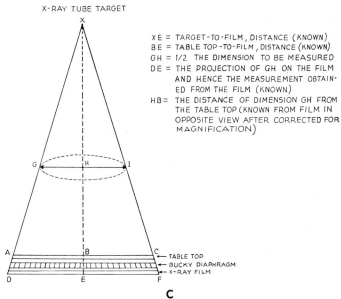

Figure 17–20. *A.* Nomograms for correction of magnification and for conversion of diameters to volumes. With a straight edge, a line is drawn from the object-film distance (*1*) of a certain dimension through the anode-film distance (*2*) used when the film was taken to the transfer axis. From this point on the transfer axis, a line is drawn through the dimension as measured on the film (*3*) which intersects (*4*) at the true, corrected dimension. With the table at the bottom of the nomogram a circumference or a diameter measurement in centimeters can be transposed directly to volume of a similar sphere in terms of cubic centimeters. (After Halmquest, from Golden, R.: Diagnostic Roentgenology. Baltimore, The Williams & Wilkins Co., 1963–1969.) *B.* Graph demonstrating the per cent magnification readily obtained when one knows the focus-film distance in centimeters and the object-film distance in centimeters. (Courtesy T. H. Oddie, D.Sc.) *C.* Triangulation method of determining radiographic magnification (see text).

Study of Pelvic Architecture

Pelvic Inlet. In addition to the anteroposterior and lateral views of the abdomen and pelvis, it may be routine in this radiographic study to obtain a special view of the pelvic inlet as illustrated in Fig. 17–18. With this special view, the pelvic inlet can be described as falling into one or another of at least four major pelvic types. There are, of course, many subtypes in these groups but at least these four major types must be understood (Figs. 17–14 and 17–15). Delivery of the fetus is most readily accomplished with the gynecoid pelvis (Fig. 17–16 *A*); difficulty is encountered with increasing frequency in the android, platypelloid, and anthropoid types.

If the posterior sagittal portion of the pelvic inlet is diminished, an occiput posterior presentation is favored.

The Sacrum. Following analysis of the pelvic inlet, the prominence of the sacral promontory and the curvature of the sacrum are studied for architecture (Fig. 17–16 *B*). The capacity of the posterior pelvic inlet is related to the width of the sacrosciatic notch and the configuration of its apex. Also the inclination of the sacrum directly affects the capacity of the birth canal, since a forward tilt offers a barrier to normal delivery. The female sacrum is wide and short compared with that of the male. Normally, also, the sacrum is concave anteriorly; when this curvature is absent because of any developmental aberration, the midpelvis is diminished and the progress of labor is impeded.

Size of the Sacrosciatic Notch. The capacity of the posterior pelvic inlet is related to the width of the sacrosciatic notch and configuration of its apex. The male pelvis shows a long narrow notch with a high rounded apex and the female a wide notch with a blunt apex.

Prominence of the Coccyx. A prominent coccyx interferes with the passage of the fetus through the birth canal.

Prominence of the Ischial Spines. Ischial spines are classified as sharp, average, or anthropoid. Sharp spines are definitely a male characteristic and may be associated with convergent side walls of the pelvis. Gynecoid spines are blunt and shallow.

Slope of Pelvic Walls. The slope of the pelvic wall is readily obtained by drawing a tangent along the outer aspect of the obturator foramen connecting with the outermost margin of the transverse diameter of the pelvic inlet. For maximum facility of delivery, the lines so drawn should be parallel. Convergent lines indicate a diminution in either midpelvis or pelvic outlet which may cause some difficulty in delivery.

Subpubic Angle. The pubic rami may be delicate, average, or heavy, and the pubic angle may be wide or curved as in the female or narrow and straight as in the male. The capacity of the pelvic outlet to a great extent is regulated by the subpubic angle and the pubic rami.

Diastasis of the Pubic Symphysis. In experimental animals there is a considerable diastasis of the pubic symphysis and resorption of bone along both sides of the pubic symphysis near term. This is an endocrine phenomenon. In the human such resorption of bone or actual diastasis does not ordinarily occur, but a relaxation of the ligaments across the pubic symphysis does occur, and occasionally diastasis persists following parturition. Such diastasis may facilitate delivery.

Extent of Acetabular Bulge. Occasionally in association with nutritional deficiencies or hereditary disorders of the bony pelvis, there is a bulging inward of the acetabulum, producing the so-called Otto pelvis or arthrokatadysis. Such abnormality may impede the passage of the fetus through the midpelvis.

Method of Reporting. In reporting, one section is devoted entirely to the various measurements; these are given in table form (Fig. 17–17 *B*). The theoretical fetal skull diameter, perimeter, and volume are also indicated relative to the dimensions of the pelvic inlet and midpelvis.

The second portion of the report should refer to pelvic architecture and details concerning fetus, placenta, and amniotic sac.

Method for Correction of Magnification. The degree of magnification will vary in accordance with the distance between the x-ray tube target and the film, and the distance between the diameter (or distance) to be measured and the film. If the dimension in question is parallel with the film surface, distortion is eliminated. If the target-to-film distance is known and also the object-to-film distance, it is possible to calculate accurately the true measurement of the part. This may be accomplished by graphs or nomograms (Fig. 17–20) (Ball, Snow), stereoscopic films (Caldwell and Moloy), metal notched rules placed next to the part being radiographed (Colcher-Sussman), or perforated metal plates superimposed on the radiograph (Thoms).

In those methods that employ calculation, graphs, or nomograms to determine the degree of magnification, the basic procedure is as follows:

1. The desired dimension is measured on the one radiograph, whether it be the anteroposterior or lateral view.

2. The distance that this dimension is placed from the film is determined from the other radiograph. Thus, to determine this object-to-film distance for dimensions measured on the anteroposterior view, the lateral radiograph is employed and vice versa.

3. There will, however, be an error of magnification on this second radiograph also, which must be corrected before it can be applied as the object-to-table-top distance.

4. In order to obtain object-to-film distance, the object-to-table-top distance is first calculated, and to this figure is added the known table-top-to-film distance (usually 5 cm.).

5. Only those dimensions in the central ray can be measured, unless the teleroentgenographic method is employed where beam divergence is negligible.

6. The following triangulation laws are applied (Fig. 17–20 *C*):

$$\frac{GH \text{ (unknown)}}{DE \text{ (known)}} = \frac{XH}{XE} = \frac{XE - (HB + BE) \text{ (known)}}{XE \qquad \text{(known)}}$$

From this equation, it is obvious that all factors are known except GH and hence, simple algebraic solution is possible. Snow's special calculator or Ball's nomograms allow this algebraic solution to be obtained directly.

STUDY OF THE NONPREGNANT FEMALE— GYNECOLOGIC RADIOLOGY

X-ray Appearance of Intrauterine Contraceptive Devices (Lehfeldt). Most intrauterine contraceptive devices are made of radiopaque materials. Three commonly employed devices are illustrated in Fig. 17–21. In rare cases pregnancy has occurred with the device *in situ*. No obstetric difficulties caused by the intrauterine devices have been reported.

X-ray evidence of the intrauterine contraceptive device in the pelvic area is no definite proof that it is within the uterine cavity. In the nonpregnant woman, the definite answer may be supplied by a hysterogram. In pregnancy, the presence or absence of the device should not be determined until the early part of the third trimester to avoid fetal exposure to radiation.

Perforation of the uterus occurs rarely. According to Shimkin et al., uterine perforation may occur in about 1 out of 2500 insertions of a coil or loop and in 1 out of 150 insertions of a bow. Perforation occurs especially at the time of insertion or occasionally at attempted blind removal. It may be partial or complete. Perforation at insertion is often asymptomatic and unrecognized.

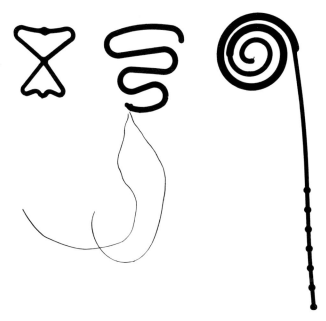

Figure 17–21. Most commonly employed radiopaque intrauterine contraceptive devices (left to right): Birnberg bow; Lippes loop with attached nylon string (nonopaque); Margulies coil with radiopaque cervicovaginal extension. (From Lehfeldt, H.: Fertility and Sterility, *16*:502–507, 1965.)

Intestinal obstruction may occur by herniation of small bowel through an aperture of the device or by volvulus about a point of fixation due to adhesions around the device.

Hysterosalpingography. The main uses of this procedure are: (1) study of sterility problems; (2) investigation of uterine bleeding; (3) re-establishment of tubal patency; (4) visualization of abnormalities of the uterine cavity or oviducts; and (5) visualization of sinus tracts communicating with the female genital tract.

Technique of Examination. As with all contrast procedures, it is always advisable to obtain a preliminary scout film prior to the introduction of the contrast medium (Fig. 17–22 *A*). Areas of calcification and soft tissue masses can thereby be delineated prior to the introduction of the special medium. The lithotomy position over an x-ray Bucky table, preferably equipped with image amplification and closed circuit television fluoroscopy, is employed.

A cannula, preferably radiolucent, is inserted into the uterine cervical canal after visualization of the cervix through an appropriate speculum. It is best that the cannula be filled with contrast material so that all air bubbles are extracted prior to the insertion into the uterine cervical canal. The introduction of air bubbles may cause confusion in interpretation.

Under fluoroscopic control, while viewing the injection on a television monitor, a fractional injection of an appropriate contrast medium is begun (for example, Sinugrafin). A spot film may be obtained after each 2 cc. injection if so desired and a total of 6 to 10 cc. is employed (Fig. 17–22 *B*). The entire study may be done with video tape recording. The examination can cease after the investigator is satisfied that the entire genital tract has been visualized maximally. After the last injection, stereoscopic anteroposterior and lateral films are obtained.

If Sinugrafin or Salpix is employed, serial films may be obtained at 20 minutes, 60 minutes, 2 hours, and 3 hours (Fig. 17–22 *D*). Ordinarily, by 3 hours, the soluble absorbable medium has been resorbed and may be found in the urinary bladder. It is important at this time to note whether or not there is any residual dye in loculated areas within the pelvis such as may occur with hydrosalpinx.

Hysterosalpingography with Opaque Oily Substances (Fullenlove). Hysterosalpingography with opaque oily substances is preferred by some because of the denser image produced and because this method permits a 24 hour follow-up study which water soluble substances cannot provide (Fig. 17–23).

The technique is fundamentally the same; care must be exercised, however, to remove the speculum prior to injection so as not to obscure the cervical canal and internal os. The injection is made under image amplifier fluoroscopic control so that venous intravasation may be seen immediately.

Although practically all patients are examined for sterility or habitual abortion, many abnormalities may be visualized.

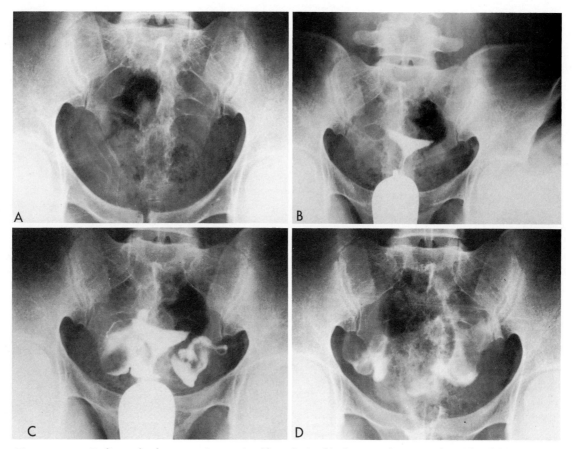

Figure 17–22. Radiographs demonstrating routine films obtained by hysterosalpingography with soluble, absorbable medium. *A.* Preliminary scout film prior to the injection of the first medium. *B.* Film obtained after the insertion of the first 2 cc. fraction. *C.* Radiograph obtained after the fourth insertion of the 2 cc. fraction. This radiograph demonstrates spillage into the pelvic peritoneal space. *D.* Film obtained 20 minutes after the injection, showing the opaque medium to be still present in the pelvic peritoneal space, but already some of the medium has been absorbed and is appearing in the urinary bladder. Dotted areas indicate the impression of the ovaries upon the contrast medium.

These are summarized and illustrated in *Analysis of Roentgen Signs.*

The complications which can occur are hemorrhage, flare-up of an infection, and venous or lymphatic intravasation. The latter can be recognized immediately during fluoroscopy and the examination is stopped. The oil tends to disappear in from 1 to 3 days but may be recognized in lungs. Lymphatic intravasation occurs with about the same frequency as venous intravasation. There usually is no adverse reaction and it follows the same course as lymphangiography, disappearing over a period of 3 to 6 months.

Uterine Isthmus Insufficiency. Brünner and Ulrich have employed the technique of hysterography with a balloon catheter for the visualization of the uterine isthmus. They indicate that the advantage of using this catheter for hysterography is the possibility of diagnosing incompetence of the uterine isthmus while the patient is not pregnant and thereby establishing the probable cause of habitual abortion.

Contraindications to Procedure. Uterine bleeding at the time of injection, such as may occur with menstruation or with some abnormality, may predispose to emboli to the lung and elsewhere, and thus may be considered a contraindication. Actually, no fatalities have been reported, even when iodized oil has been demonstrated radiographically in the chest. Nevertheless, it is a complication to be avoided if possible.

During any active inflammatory phase in the pelvis, the procedure is to be avoided in order to obviate any further spread.

Pregnancy is probably a contraindication to the procedure. Abortions have been reported.

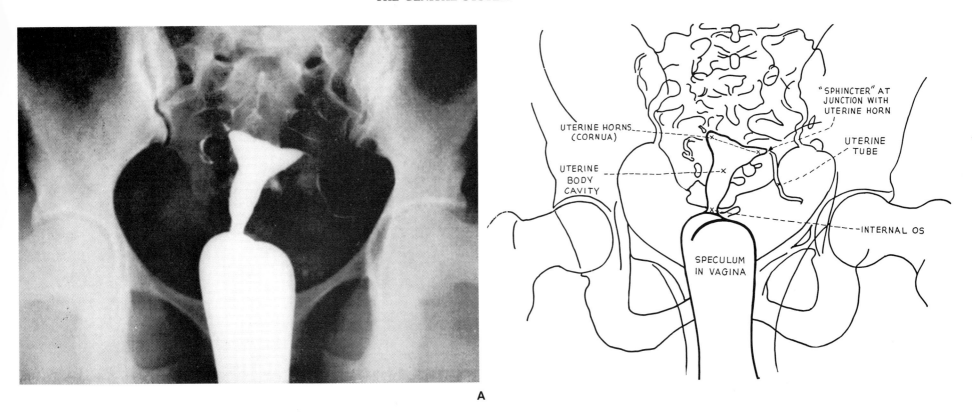

A

Labels in tracing:
UTERINE HORNS (CORNUA)
UTERINE BODY CAVITY
"SPHINCTER" AT JUNCTION WITH UTERINE HORN
UTERINE TUBE
INTERNAL OS
SPECULUM IN VAGINA

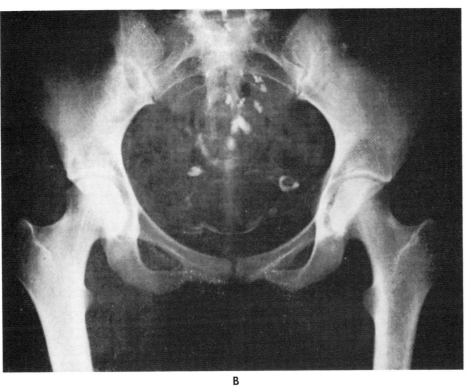

B

Figure 17–23.   Hysterosalpingography with Lipiodol. *A.* Initial full film and tracing of same. *B.* Twenty-four hour film.

Normal Roentgen Findings (Fig. 17–24). In the anteroposterior projection, the uterine cavity is ordinarily visualized as a triangular structure with the apex pointed downward toward the cannula. Occasionally a dimpling is noted at the top of the uterus, indicating the point of fusion of the two halves from which it is originally formed. Thin threadlike structures extend from both uterine horns, indicating filling of the oviducts and finally a spillage at the fimbriated ends of the oviducts into the anatomic pelvis (Fig. 17–25). The uterine horn is a narrow segment which may on occasion undergo spasm. The isthmus beyond the uter-

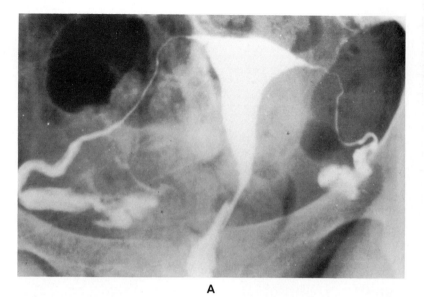

A

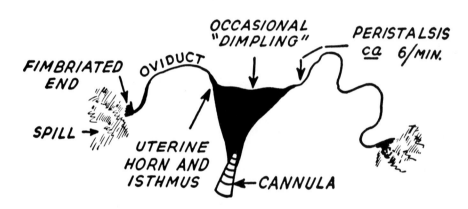

a. ANTEROPOSTERIOR

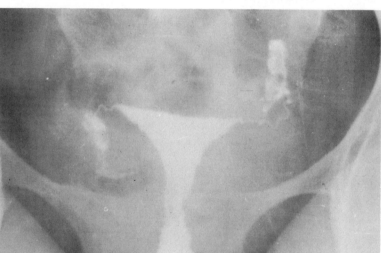

B

Figure 17–25. *A.* Normal hysterosalpingogram using water soluble media. *B.* Hysterosalpingogram with slight endometrial hyperplasia.

Figure 17–25 continued on the opposite page.

b. LATERAL VIEW

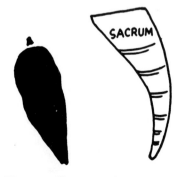

Figure 17–24. Diagrams illustrating the normal roentgen findings in hysterosalpingography.

ine horn may likewise on occasion be slightly narrowed. On serial films peristalsis in the oviducts may be noted at a rate of approximately 6 per minute. In the lateral view the uterine cavity is carrot-shaped and in slight anteversion.

Abnormal Uterine Findings (Käser et al.). Abnormal roentgen anatomy is outside the scope of this text and the student is referred for a summary description of these abnormalities to *Analysis of Roentgen Signs*. Example illustrations, however, of some of the abnormalities encountered are shown in Figure 17–26.

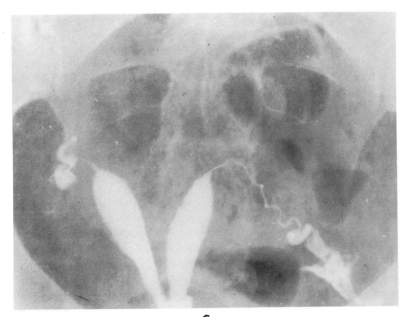

C

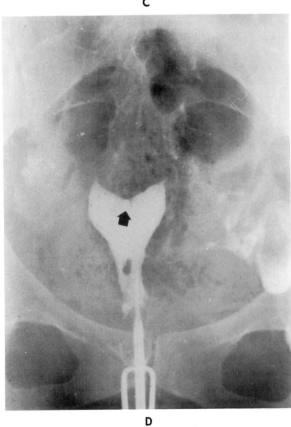

D

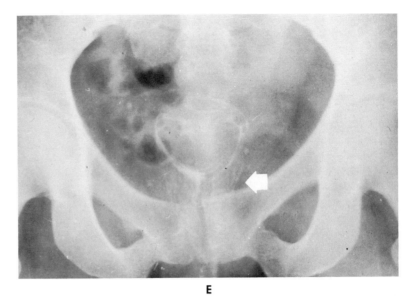

E

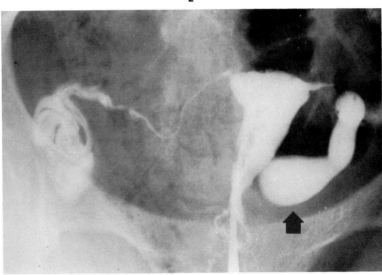

F

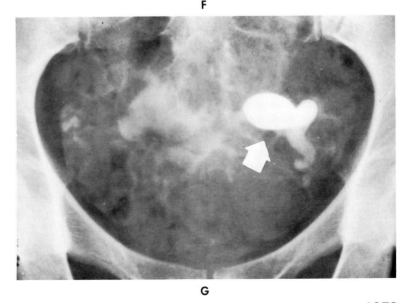

G

Figure 17–25 *Continued.* *C* and *D.* Bicornuate uterus surgically repaired with persistent scar formation. *E.* Vagina coated with contrast material (Sinugrafin) after hysterosalpingography. *F.* Appearance of hydrosalpinx on the left at time of initial injection. *G.* Appearance of hydrosalpinx on the 30-minute retention film taken afterward.

UTERUS

1. SMALL SIZE

a. *INFANTILE*

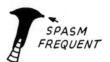

*SPASM
FREQUENT*

2. ABNORMALITIES OF POSITION

a. *NORMAL RETRO- AND ANTE-
FLEXION*

b. *NORMAL SLIGHT DEFLECTION TO
RIGHT OR LEFT FROM INSTRUMENT-
ATION*

c. *DISPLACEMENT BY ADJOINING
PELVIC MASSES*

**3. PROTRUSIONS OR SINUSES
FROM UTERINE CAVITY**

a. *ADENOMYOSIS OR
ENDOMETRIOSIS*

**4. IRREGULARITY OF OUTER
SMOOTH MARGIN**

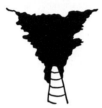

a. *BENIGN HYPER-
PLASIAS OF
MENOPAUSE*

b. *ENDOMETRITIS*

c. *RETAINED PLACENTA*

d. *CARCINOMA*

5. FILLING DEFECTS

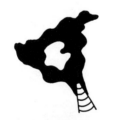

a. *FIBROMYOMA BEGINNING
PREGNANCY POLYP
INTRAUTERINE SYNECHIAE*

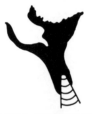

b. *CORPUS CARCINOMA RETAINED
PLACENTA.*

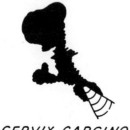

c. *CERVIX CARCINOMA*

6. DUPLICATION

Figure 17–26. Diagrammatic tracings illustrating some abnormal roentgen findings within the uterus proper in hysterosalpingograms.

Gynecography (Pneumoperitoneum of the Pelvis) (Fig. 17–27). This technique allows visualization of the uterine fundus, ovaries, oviducts, and broad ligaments (Granjon).

Technique. 1000 to 2000 cc. of a gaseous medium (air, carbon dioxide, nitrous oxide) are slowly introduced under pressure not exceeding 12 cm. of water. Films are taken in the position shown in Figure 17–27.

Anteroposterior and lateral projections are employed. A normal appearance is shown.

Normal Anatomy. The pelvic pneumogram demonstrates the normal uterus and normal ovaries as smooth organs free of adhesions. The normal ovaries (Weigen and Stevens) vary in size from 3.7 to 14.6 square centimeters, with a mean of 9 square centimeters. The uterine fundus, broad ligaments, anterior surface of rectum, and dome of the urinary bladder may all be demonstrated clearly (Fig. 17–27).

Contraindications include peritoneal infection, massive hemorrhage, and large lesions.

Types of pathologic processes identified include malformed uterus, uterine hypoplasia, extrauterine pregnancy, abnormalities of site, formation, and volume of the ovaries (Stein-Leventhal syndrome), and ovarian tumor masses and cysts (Fig. 17–28) (see *Analysis of Roentgen Signs*).

In a series of 110 patients using nitrous oxide as the gaseous media, Buice and Gould reported no unusual complications.

The procedure was especially valuable in patients who could not be accurately evaluated by manual examination. These included young children, patients with congenital anomalies of the ovaries, tubes, or uterus, obese patients, and uncooperative patients.

Little et al. have used the term "gynecography" to indicate combined hysterosalpingography and pelvic pneumoroentgenography. Others have also employed this combined technique (Semin et al.). The gas may be introduced by transuterine inflation, cul-de-sac, or transabdominal puncture. The combination of the two procedures on a single film demonstrated the status of the uterine cavity, the tubal lumina, and the contours and relative sizes of the pelvic structures. They describe the primary contraindications to gynecography as being pregnancy, uterine bleeding, purulent cervical or uterine discharge, acute or subacute pelvic inflammatory disease, shock, localized or diffuse peritonitis, large tumor masses filling the pelvis, and elderly patients or those who are poor risks from the cardiac viewpoint. They indicate that the complications of pneumoperitoneum in pelvic pneumoroentgenography are relatively mild and transitory, but that the complications of hysterosalpingography are somewhat more serious when they occur. There may be allergic reactions to the contrast agent, venous extravasation of the dye, occasional pulmonary embolism, rupture of the uterus or tubes, and transportation of infection or tumor cells into the peritoneal cavity. Fortunately, these complications are rare.

Barium Vaginography (Rubin et al.). A standard rectal enema tip is thrust through the center of a sponge inserted into the introitus of the vagina with the patient supine on the fluoro-

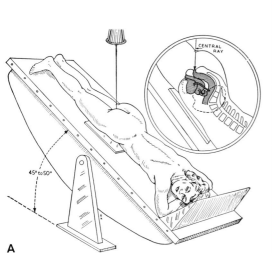
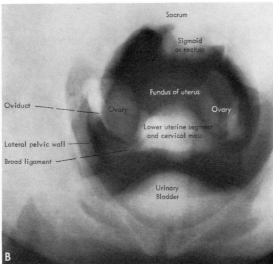
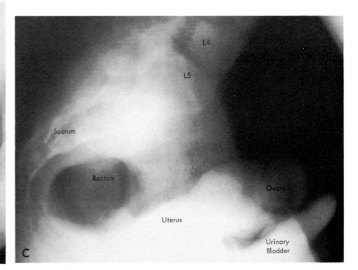

Figure 17–27. A. Position of patient (after instillation of gas) for radiography. Pneumoperitoneum of the female pelvis in posteroanterior (B) and lateral (C) projections. This patient was a 29 year old female with a Stein-Leventhal syndrome proved by surgery, but her ovaries are considered normal in size for a young woman. (Courtesy of Dr. Wilma C. Diner, Department of Radiology, University of Arkansas Medical Center, Little Rock, Arkansas.)

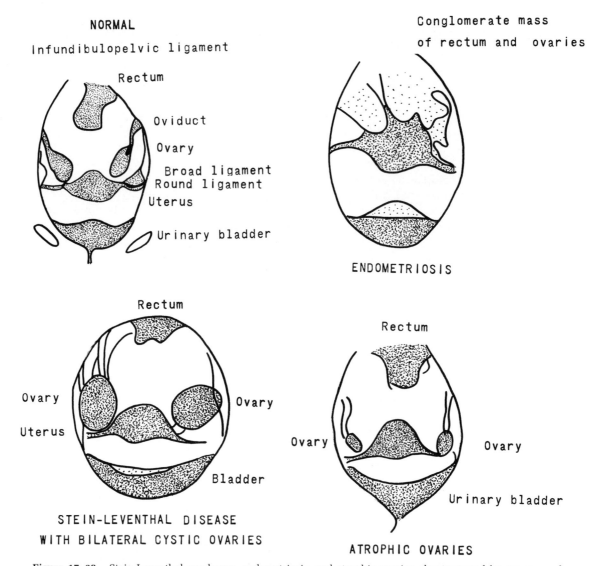

Figure 17–28. Stein-Leventhal syndrome, endometriosis, and atrophic ovaries, demonstrated by gynecography with normal for comparison. (Modified from Stevens, G. M.: Seminars in Roentgenology, 44:252–269, 1969. Used by permission.)

scopic table. The patient keeps her legs together and the enema tip is advanced into the vagina while the sponge approximates the labia. A thin solution of barium is instilled into the vagina and photofluorograms or spot films are exposed in the anteroposterior, oblique, and lateral projections.

The patient is then permitted to evacuate the barium and a double contrast study may be carried out thereafter if desired. Finally the patient is given a cleansing douche at the termination of the examination.

Utility of Method. The following pathologic states may be determined: (1) vaginal extension from cancer of the cervix; (2) vaginal extension from adjoining carcinomas or malignancies of the bladder, rectum, or other adjacent organs; (3) demonstration of fistulas (through the colon or through the urinary bladder); (4) enterovaginal fistulas following irradiation.

Generally this procedure may help, especially in tumor staging and treatment planning.

Angiography of the Pelvis. Percutaneous, transfemoral aortography by the Seldinger technique has permitted catheterization of major branches of the iliac arteries. The injections may be made in the aorta above the bifurcation of the iliac arteries or in selective branches.

This technique may be utilized for accurate placental visualization, or for visualization of neoplastic masses or other abnormalities in the pelvis. For example, this procedure has been found very useful in a study of the extension of carcinoma of the cervix, uterine tumors, adnexal tumors, problems of pregnancy and placentography. The placental circulation is usually identified as early as the second month in unruptured extrauterine pregnancy. It appears as a scattered, fine, mottled or cotton-fluff opacification. There is ordinarily a lingering density in the placenta due to slowing of the circulation in this area (Meng and Elkin).

The techniques of pelvic angiography and pneumoperitoneum have also been combined (Rådberg and Wickbom). Lymphangiography has also been used as an adjunct to gynecologic roentgenology (Howett). This has been discussed and illustrated in prior chapters.

Technique. Reference is made to prior chapters for more detailed technical description. Using mild sedation, sterile technique, and local anesthesia a Seldinger needle is inserted into the femoral artery approximately 2 inches below the inguinal ligament. The needle is usually inserted through both walls of the artery. After the stylet in the needle is withdrawn, the cannula is carefully withdrawn through the posterior wall into the lumen of the femoral artery, when pulsating bleeding is encountered. The stylet is immediately inserted partially and the cannula threaded up the femoral artery a short distance. A long, specially coiled spring guide is then introduced through the cannula and advanced within the arterial lumen under fluoroscopic control. The spring guide must be introduced far enough so that when the cannula is withdrawn over it, it will remain in place. The cannula is then removed entirely and a length of appropriate catheter tubing is pushed over and along the guide into the femoral artery. Fluoroscopy is always employed during manipulation of the guide and tubing. The tip of the catheter is usually localized in the upper abdominal aorta for abdominal aortography and renal arteriography, or at the aortic bifurcation for pelvic arteriography.

The guide is then withdrawn and a few milliliters of heparin-saline solution (10 units of heparin per milliliter of normal saline solution) is injected through the tubing to prevent clotting.

During the injection for pelvic arteriography, blood pressure cuffs may be employed as tourniquets about both thighs to prevent the radiopaque agent, such as the diatrizoates, from running off into the leg arteries. The usual dose of contrast agent of 60 per cent methylglucamine or 89 per cent methalamate is 20 to 25 cc., depending upon the location of the catheter and the size of the vessel being injected. This material is injected rapidly and a series of films is obtained, usually two or three per second for the first 3 seconds, and 1 per second thereafter for 7 or 8 seconds.

A mechanical pressure injector is desirable to allow the rapid injection of large volumes of the agent. It is desirable usually to complete the injection within 1 second.

In the presence of pregnancy, for placental visualization for example, fluoroscopy should be minimal.

The catheter is removed following the procedure and hemostasis is obtained by constant pressure, followed thereafter by a pressure dressing to be removed in 2 to 4 hours. The patient should be kept under observation for a sufficiently long period to allow detection of recurrence of bleeding at the cannulation site.

Side Effects Noted by Patients. Usually the injection of the contrast agent produces a sensation of heat in the area of distribution, and occasionally a sudden brief sharp or burning pain in the lower back may be encountered. Usually such pain persists for 10 to 15 seconds only. Care must be exercised that dissection of the artery has not occurred subintimally. Varying degrees of nausea may occur immediately after the injection in occasional patients, but vomiting rarely occurs and the nausea disappears spontaneously. During the week following the procedure, tenderness and ecchymosis are observed at the needle puncture site in the groin, but this may be minimized by prevention of hematoma formation during the procedure and an appropriate pressure dressing thereafter.

Repeated injections may be carried out with adequate time for excretion of the contrast agent in those patients who have normal renal function. Ordinarily, 120 ml. of the contrast agent can be tolerated in the course of 1 hour of such study in such patients. In the presence of disturbed or abnormal renal function, lesser volumes of contrast agent are usually utilized.

The Normal Pelvic Arteriogram. In the straight anteroposterior projection centered over the midpelvis, the lower level of the abdominal aorta, its bifurcation, and the internal and external iliac arteries and their branches to the gluteus, pelvic organs, and legs present a symmetrical appearance except for a reactive constriction of the catheterized femoral and external iliac arteries in many cases.

Usually, the entire *uterine artery* can be studied from its point of origin on the internal iliac artery to its course in the parametrium and along the lateral margin of the uterus. It usually courses close to the easily identified outward-sweeping *superior gluteal arteries.* These are the only branches of the internal iliac arteries which in frontal projection cross the external iliac artery to give off their major branches. The uterine artery courses medially and caudad to the cervix and thereafter ascends upward along the lateral margin of the uterus as far as the fundus. Its course is tortuous lateral to the uterine body and numerous ramifications extend into the uterine wall with many fine branches terminating in the endometrium. Occasional branches of the uterine artery extend laterally to supply the adnexa on the same side. Considerable variation unfortunately exists as to size and appearance and even asymmetry in given pa-

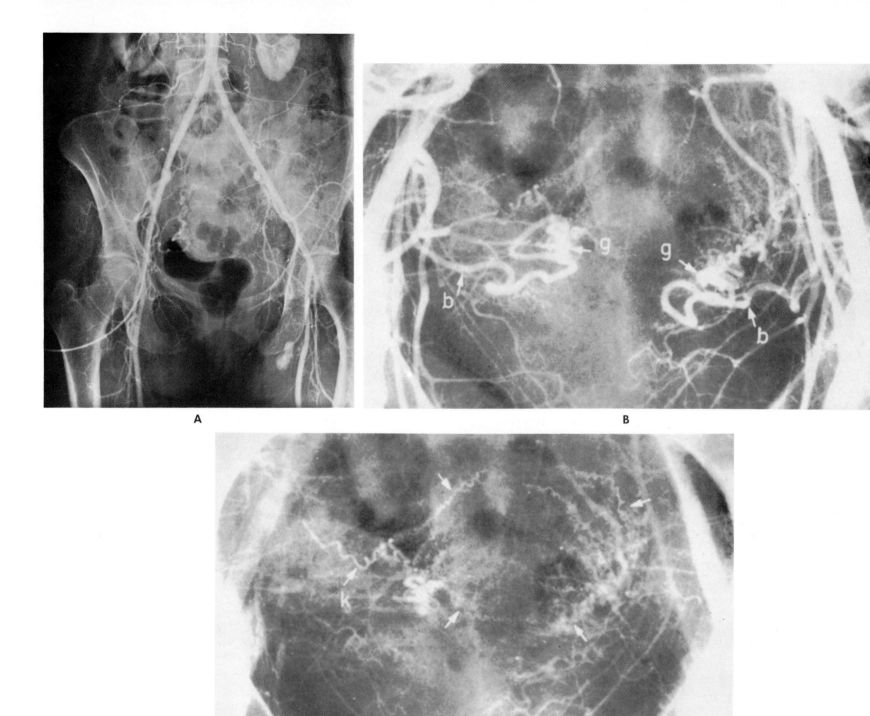

Figure 17–29. *A.* Originally, the Seldinger catheter is inserted above the bifurcation of the aorta and then withdrawn to the hypogastric arterial level, as shown in *B* and *C* (pelvic arteriograms). *B* and *C*. Normal arteriograms. Anteroposterior projection of the uterus. *B*. Film taken immediately after the injection of opaque medium. The uterine artery in the parametrium (*b*) and the uterine artery running along the lateral margin of the uterus (*g*) are visible. Small tortuous intramural arteries are beginning to opacify. *C*. Film taken two seconds after film *B*. The main trunk of the uterine artery is now faintly outlined. Numerous small, tortuous intramural arteries are visible within the uterus (arrows). The right adnexal branch (*k*) follows a tortuous course. (From Abrams, H. L.: Angiography, 2nd ed. Vol. 2. Boston, Little, Brown & Co., 1971.)

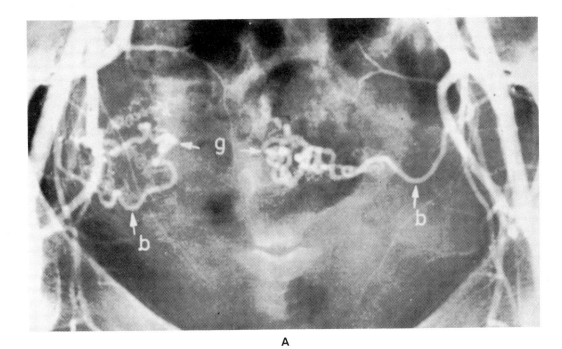

A

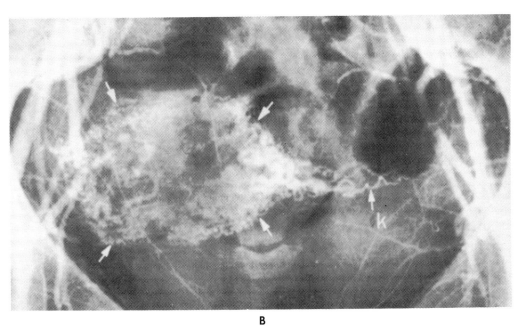

B

Figure 17–30. Normal arteriogram. Axial projection of the uterus. A. Film taken immediately after the injection of opaque medium. The uterine arteries in the parametrium (b) and along the lateral margin of the uterus (g) are seen. A few tortuous intramural arteries within the right half of the uterus begin to opacify. B. Film taken two seconds after film A. The main trunk of the uterine artery is now faintly outlined. Numerous small, tortuous intramural arteries are visible within the uterus (arrows). The left adnexal branch (k) follows a tortuous course. (From Abrams, H. L.: Angiography, 2nd ed., Vol. 2. Boston, Little, Brown & Co., 1971.)

tients. Occasionally, also, the entire adnexa and even the upper part or the entire uterus may be supplied by the *ovarian artery*.

Although placentography has been employed in the past for detection of placenta praevia, ectopic tumors, and placental tumors, the advent of ultrasound has diminished the need for arteriography in these conditions.

An angiogram in a normal intrauterine pregnancy of nine weeks duration is shown in Figure 17–32.

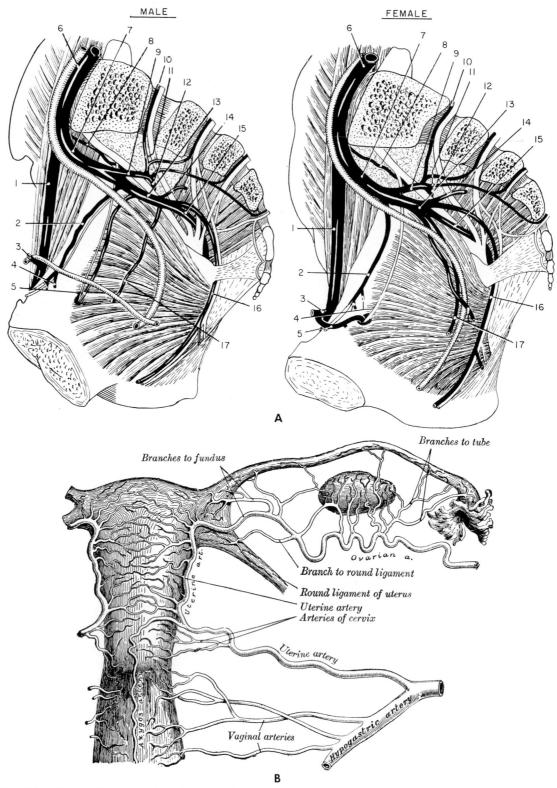

Figure 17–31. *A.* The arteries of the pelvic cavity in the male and female: (1) external iliac; (2) umbilical which terminates as the medial umbilical ligament; (3) inferior epigastric; (4) superior vesical; (5) obturator – in one arising from the anterior division of the internal iliac and in the other from the inferior epigastric branch of the external iliac; (6) common iliac; (7) internal iliac; (8) iliolumbar; (9) posterior division; (10) branch of lateral sacral entering sacrum; (11) lateral sacrals; (12) superior gluteal; (13) anterior division; (14) middle rectal; (15) inferior gluteal; (16) internal pudendal; and (17) inferior vesical in the male, and uterine and vaginal in the female. (From Roger C. Crafts, A Textbook of Human Anatomy. © 1966. The Ronald Press Company, New York. Modified and redrawn after Jamieson.) *B.* The arteries of the internal organs of generation of the female, seen from behind (after Hyrt). (From Gray's Anatomy of the Human Body, 29th ed. Goss, C. M. (ed.) Philadelphia, Lea & Febiger, 1973.)

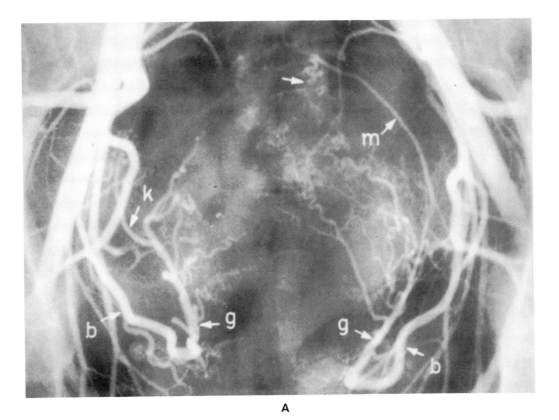

A

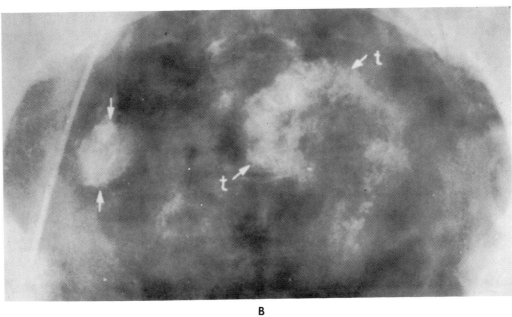

B

Figure 17–32. Normal intrauterine pregnancy of nine weeks' duration. *A.* Film taken immediately after the injection of opaque medium. The uterine arteries in parametrium (b) and along the lateral margin of corpus uteri (g) are visible. The fundal insertion of the placenta is beginning to opacify (*unmarked arrows*) Some intramural arteries (m) running toward the placenta show a partial loss of tortuosity. (k) Right adnexal branch. *B.* Two seconds after *A.* The intervillous space is opacified (t). *Unmarked arrows* point to the corpus luteum of pregnancy, supplied by the right adnexal branch (see *A*). (From Abrams, H. L.: Angiography, 2d ed. Vol. 2. Boston, Little, Brown & Co., 1971.)

As pregnancy progresses the uterine artery becomes more dilated and convoluted and in the last trimester, the uterine vessels begin to lengthen. At term they are quite straight. It has been demonstrated that the uterine artery is more prominent on one side than the other during gestation (Solish et al.), usually the side on which the placenta is implanted.

In placentography, the placental sinuses containing contrast agent have a scattered, fine, mottled or "cotton-fluff" appearance. Some density may be retained for a considerable period of time in the placental sinuses, allowing for easier identification of these structures (Benson et al.).

Visualization of the Ovarian Arteries.   The ovarian arteries are usually so narrow that information of diagnostic value is rarely obtained from the radiologic appearance. Demonstration of these arteries does, however, occur in at least half of the angiograms.

Visceral Pelvic Venography in the Female.   Generally, pelvic venography has not consistently produced good results for visualization of the female pelvic structures such as the uterus, vagina, and ovaries. Opacification by the usual methods occurs in no more than 15 to 20 per cent of cases with bilateral common iliac injection or selective internal iliac injections (Doppman and Chretien). Improvement has been achieved by some using catheterization of an ovarian vein, utilizing large volumes of contrast material, urinary bladder distention, and a 35 degree cranial angulation of the radiographic tube. Bilateral femoral vein catheterization was utilized by Doppman and Chretien for catheterization of the ovarian veins. These must be catheterized at least to the level of the iliac crest for success and it is also desirable that both ovarian veins be injected simultaneously (Fig. 17-33). Usually a large volume of contrast agent such as 80 ml. of meglumine iothalamate (Conray-60) is injected through a Y con-

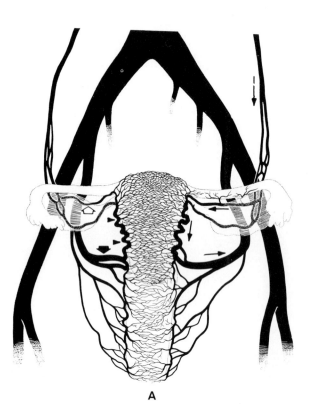

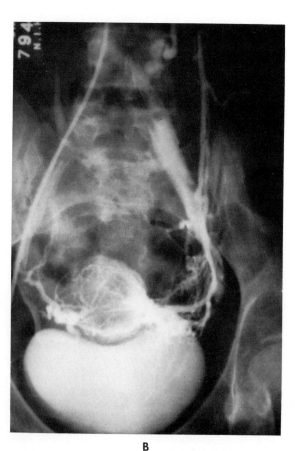

A   B

Figure 17-33.   A. Diagrammatic sketch of the major visceral veins of the pelvis. The right ovarian pedicle (clear arrow), right uterine plexus (arrowheads), and right uterine pedicle or vein (solid arrow) are shown on the left. The direction of flow during retrograde ovarian venography, shown on the right, is down the ovarian vein, medially via the ovarian pedicle to the uterine plexus, down the uterine plexus, and laterally in the uterine pedicle to the internal iliac vein (arrows). This route is invariably demonstrated with satisfactory retrograde injection; filling of the uterine myometrial plexus is less constant.

B. Retrograde left ovarian venogram obtained without bladder distension or angulation of the radiographic tube. The uterus is projected axially above the bladder. (From Doppman, J. L., and Chretien, P.: Radiology, 98:406, 1971.)

nector at a rate of 10 to 15 ml. per second. "The Valsalva maneuver, balloon compression of the lower inferior vena cava, and the upright position seem to have no influence on pelvic vein filling; the most essential factor is the placement of the catheter tip deep in the ovarian vein, preferably below the level of the pelvic brim" (Doppman and Chretien).

It is recommended that the x-ray tube be angled 35 degrees cranially with distention of the urinary bladder so as to prevent superimposition of the ovarian pedicle, uterine plexus, and uterine pedicle. Distention of the urinary bladder with gas is to be preferred. One film every second for 15 seconds is adequate.

Combined Pelvic Angiography and Pneumoperitoneum in Gynecologic Diagnosis.   These two methods are often complementary. The vascular structure of the pelvis combined with the morphological delineation of detail by pneumoperitoneum makes a valuable contribution to the diagnostic armamentarium (Rådberg and Wickbom).

STUDY OF THE PREGNANT MOTHER IN RESPECT TO THE FETUS

Introduction.   Protection from radiation and potential radiation hazards take on greater significance in this field, since there are at least two or more lives involved (mother and fetuses) and not just that of the patient. The hazards of radiation must be carefully weighed against the benefits to be achieved.

Determination of a Fetal Skeleton in Utero.   The viable fetus should not be exposed to irradiation during the first trimester of pregnancy. Hormonal tests are far more sensitive in any case for the detection of early pregnancy, since ossification of the fetal skeleton does not occur prior to the third month of gestation, and radiographically detectable fetal skeletal parts are difficult to find prior to the 13th or 14th week.

The indications for seeking fetal skeletal parts are (1) an enlarging uterus without other evidence of pregnancy; (2) an enlarging tumor mass of the pelvis that could conceivably be teratomatous or represent an extra-uterine pregnancy; (3) a previously suspected gravid uterus when the clinical situation has changed and pregnancy tests have ceased to be positive; and (4) an abnormal fetus that is strongly suggested by clinical appearances (hydrocephalus; anencephaly).

The fetal parts that lend themselves most readily to early detection are the segmental structures such as those of the spine and ribs; occasionally the extremities and head may be seen in faint outline.

The oblique views of the pelvis are often more helpful than straight anteroposterior views, since the fetal ossified parts may be projected over the sacrum and lost to view.

Determination of Multiple Fetuses.   Study for multiple fetuses is not undertaken prior to the later stages of pregnancy, preferably late in the last trimester when radiation hazard to the fetus is minimal. Multiple fetuses can be ascertained, however, after approximately the fourteenth week when fetal ossification may be manifest radiographically. A differentiation of multiple fetuses is particularly useful in patients who have enlarged uteri because of pendulous abdomens, marked lordosis of the lumbar spine, or a tendency to polyhydramnios. The physician may not assume that the 14 week size uterus will necessarily reveal the skeletons of developing twins. The fetal skeletons may not be determinable at this early period, especially with twins.

Fetal Normalcy.   Fetal normalcy is best studied late in the last trimester. In evaluating the fetal skeleton in utero, it is important to bear in mind the problems related to magnification and distortion. Before diagnosing an abnormal fetus, one must be certain of the finding by means of examinations in various projections and serial studies.

A thin black line surrounding the fetus on the radiograph is called the normal "fetal fat line." This is best developed after the eighth month when the deposition of subcutaneous fat occurs most rapidly. When the fetal fat line is thicker than normal, postmaturity of the fetus may be suspected.

Evidence of trauma to the fetus may also be detected on occasion in utero.

Fetal Age and Development.   Fetal age determination should rarely be required prior to the third trimester of pregnancy. There are many different bases upon which fetal age can be estimated, but probably the most reliable are estimation of actual fetal length and determination of average fetal head diameter.

The determination of fetal length can be made by measuring the total length of the fetus, attempting correction for magnification and distortion. These are optimal on teleroentgenograms (6 foot film-to-target distance), but at best, distortion may be troublesome and lead to inaccuracy. After correction for magnification, if distortion is known to be negligible (Fig. 17–20), a simple rule in determination of fetal age according to fetal length is set up as follows; prior to the fifth month, the fetal age in months is indicated by the square root of the length in centimeters. After the fifth month, the length in centimeters is divided by five in order to obtain the fetal age in months.

Determination of average fetal head diameter can be accurate. There are several tables and graphs available for computing fetal age from roentgen measurements of the fetal skull, based on the anthropometric studies of Scammon and Calkins, Hodges, and others. These graphs indicate the fetal age in accordance with occipital-frontal diameter in centimeters, biparietal skull diameter, and average net circumference of the fetal skull obtained from two roentgenograms taken at right angles to one another (Fig. 17–19 *D*). The average diameter of the fetal skull is obtained by averaging the long and short perpendicular diameters (corrected for magnification) from anteroposterior and lateral teleroentgenograms of the fetal skull (average of two diameters for each view).

A graph is also available based upon the length of the femoral shaft; we consider this less valuable roentgenographically since distortion makes it very difficult to be certain that the true length has been obtained.

Prediction of Fetal Maturity. The following criteria are perhaps most important.

1. An ossification center is present in the distal end of the femur in 90 per cent of term fetuses.

2. Proximal tibial epiphyseal ossification is noted at term in 70 to 80 per cent of the newborn.

3. Less practical standards for ossification are (a) ossification of the hyoid bone should be complete; (b) ossification of the central parts of the vertebrae should appear; and (c) the first segments of the coccyx, the metacarpals, and the phalanges may be visualized.

With regard to reliability of some of these criteria, Schreiber et al. (1962) came to the following conclusions:

1. Visualization of the fetal distal femoral ossification centers indicated a mature fetus by several criteria in 92 to 98 per cent of cases, with an average of 96 per cent for all criteria.

2. Approximately one fetus in twenty with visualized distal femoral ossification centers was not mature.

3. Visualization of both the distal femoral and proximal tibial epiphyseal centers on antepartum abdominal films was a highly reliable indicator of fetal maturity. When these centers were present the fetus was mature in 95 to 100 per cent of cases with an average of 98 per cent for all criteria.

4. Presence of ossification centers for the distal femoral epiphyses on postpartum knee films was associated with a mature fetus in 93 per cent of cases. However, 58 per cent of the newborn with absent femoral epiphyseal centers were mature by the same criteria and 61 per cent were mature by clinical estimation.

Therefore, failure to visualize these centers on postpartum knee films was not ipso facto evidence of prematurity in their series. Failure to visualize the distal femoral epiphyseal ossification centers on the antepartum films was also a poor indicator of prematurity because of superimposition of structures and fetal movement during the radiographic exposure.

In a second study (1963) distal femoral epiphyseal ossification centers were demonstrated on abdominal films in 80 per cent of the cases in which they were visualized subsequently on postpartum films of the knees of the newborn. False positive demonstration of distal femoral epiphyses was obtained in 1.7 per cent of cases.

The determination of fetal maturity by whatever means is often an important decision, since very often it in turn will decide whether or not elective induction of labor or repeat cesarean section may be indicated.

In the unpublished data from the Vanderbilt Fetal Age Study, antepartum radiographic visualization of the fetal ossification centers about the knees was a better indicator of fetal maturity than estimated gestational age, uterine size, and other physical findings.

Fetal maturity may in part be estimated from measurements of the fetal skull and determination of fetal age (Figs. 17–19 *D* and 17–20 *B*).

Russell, in a study of 3606 maternity cases, found that radiologic assessment of fetal maturity predicted the delivery date more accurately than did the menstrual history. Parity, maternal age, sex of the child, socioeconomic status, fetal weight, and season of the year were without significant influence on the rate of radiologic development of the fetus. A twin pregnancy developed more slowly radiologically than did a single pregnancy. A single fetus was more likely to die perinatally if it was premature radiologically and if the radiologic age was appreciably less than the chronologic age. A postmature fetus was not at increased risk if the radiologic appearance did not indicate postmaturity.

Brosens et al. reported a cytologic test for fetal maturity in combination with a new radiologic method for estimation. They used a lipid contrast medium for intrauterine fetal visualization, which is accomplished by amniocentesis after ultrasonic localization of the placenta. A few milliliters of the amniotic fluid are aspirated and 6 ml. of Ethiodan are injected. An x-ray film is taken 8 to 24 hours later. After 6 to 8 hours Ethiodan outlines the fetal skin clearly through absorption on the vernix. The cytologic method involves counting lipid positive cells in amniotic fluid, using 0.1 per cent aqueous Nile-blue sulfate stain. At birth, maturity was estimated by the pediatrician using neurological parameters. No complications resulted from the injections. The histologic study of the lungs in live born infants who died soon after delivery showed no abnormalities attributable to Ethiodan inhalation.

Margolis and Voss obtained the fetal length indirectly after 34 weeks gestation (in women less than 180 pounds in weight) by measurement of the fetal lumbar vertebral length in utero. Films of the near-term pregnant woman were obtained with the patient prone and a target-to-film distance of 100 cm. The top of the first lumbar vertebra and the bottom of the fifth were marked on the film of the pregnant uterus so obtained. The distance through the middle of the vertebrae was measured to the nearest millimeter with a flexible ruler. The measured lumbar vertebral length could be related to the total newborn length ± 5 cm. Reference to an intrauterine growth chart yielded an approximation of fetal maturation.

Thus, a fetal lumbar vertebral length of 52 mm. or more indicated that 95 per cent of the group weighed over 2500 grams, with an actual total length of 49 cm. or more.

The lumbar vertebral length did not show significant correlation with the weight-length ratio, or with the duration of gestation as calculated by the date of the last menstrual period.

TABLE 17–1 PRESENCE OF SIX OSSIFICATION CENTERS IN ROENTGENOGRAMS OF NEWBORNS*

Ossification Center	Birth Weight, Gm.					
	Under 2000	2000–2499	2500–2999	3000–3499	3500–3999	4000 or More
Calcaneus						
White boys	100%					
girls	100					
Negro boys	100					
girls	100					
Astragalus						
White boys	72.7	100%				
girls	83.3	100				
Negro boys	90.9	100				
girls	100	100				
Dist. femoral epiphysis						
White boys	9.1	75.0	85.3%	100%	100%	
girls	50.0	91.7	98.0	100	100	
Negro boys	18.2	88.5	90.7	94.0	100	
girls	50.2	93.8	99.0	100	100	
Prox. femoral epiphysis						
White boys	0.0	18.8	52.9	78.8	84.1	97.1%
girls	0.0	54.2	75.5	85.7	90.7	90.5
Negro boys	0.0	38.5	62.7	76.0	80.0	92.9
girls	14.3	40.6	76.7	88.1	86.4	100
Cuboid						
White boys	0.0	6.2	14.7	39.8	44.3	60.0
girls	0.0	37.5	57.1	65.2	70.4	76.2
Negro boys	0.0	23.1	43.8	58.0	68.2	100
girls	21.4	37.5	68.0	78.2	81.8	75.0
Head of humerus						
White boys	0.0	7.7	13.8	41.9	49.0	59.1
girls	0.0	5.6	25.8	41.9	69.4	86.7
Negro boys	0.0	0.0	15.2	27.6	48.4	63.6
girls	0.0	10.7	22.7	52.6	38.9	100

*From Growth and Development of Children, 6th ed., by Lowrey, G. H. Copyright © 1973 by Year Book Medical Publishers, Inc., Chicago. Used by permission.

The relationship of six ossification centers in roentgenograms of the newborn to birth weight is indicated in Table 17–1 for white and Negro boys and girls. From this data, it can be seen that birth weight, sex, and race are highly significant factors.

Determination of Fetal Viability, Death, or Other Fetal Abnormalities. This is considered outside the scope of this text and the student is referred to *Analysis of Roentgen Signs.*

Presentation of Fetus. The position of the fetal head, small parts, and back is readily determined by consideration of the anteroposterior and lateral radiographs.

A "military" position of the head precludes engagement unless the head is very small and the pelvis is very large. This hyperextended position is more common with cephalopelvic disproportion or other factors that interfere with engagement, such as a distended bladder, pelvic mass, placenta previa, polyhydramnios, or a pendulous uterus. Atypical fetal presentations that can be recognized radiographically are face and brow presentation, transverse, shoulder or arm, breech, footling, or knee.

Roentgenographic pelvic measurements and fetal head mensuration play an important part in management decisions.

When the head is not engaged in a prima gravida, some possibilities to be considered are: obstructing masses in the pelvis such as ovarian cysts or fibroids; placenta previa centralis; a short umbilical cord, or more often a cord twisted around the fetus; fetal malformation such as hydrocephalus and cystic hygroma of the neck; or a pendulous uterus impairing the direction of uterine force.

STUDY OF THE PREGNANT MOTHER FOR UTERINE DETAIL OUTSIDE THE FETUS

Placenta (Fig. 17–35). Various methods for study of the placenta radiologically are: (1) routine anteroposterior and lateral views of the abdomen, inclusive of the entire uterus; (2) a special lateral film employing a wedge filter when the placenta is anteriorly situated in the uterine fundus. (A "wedge filter" is an x-ray filter and medium interposed between the x-ray tube and the patient which will diminish the radiation over the patient's thinner parts so that this area on the radiograph will have equal clarity with the x-ray image of the thicker anatomic portions. This is particularly useful on the lateral view.) The placenta is situated on either the anterior or posterior surface of the uterine fundus in most instances and can usually be differentiated as a

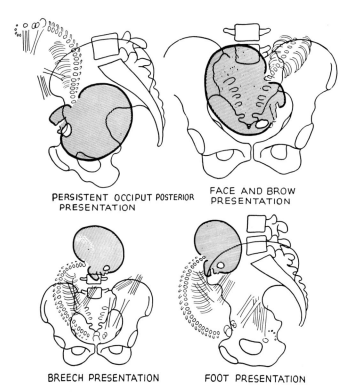

PERSISTENT OCCIPUT POSTERIOR PRESENTATION

FACE AND BROW PRESENTATION

BREECH PRESENTATION

FOOT PRESENTATION

Figure 17–34. Diagrams illustrating various types of atypical presentation as they may be seen radiographically.

ROENTGEN STUDY OF THE PLACENTA

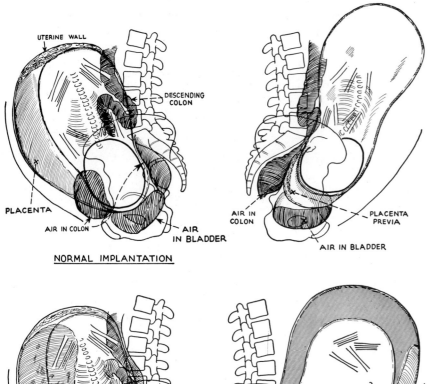

NORMAL IMPLANTATION

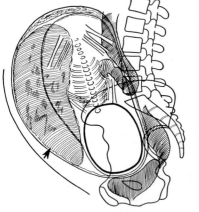

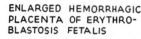
ENLARGED HEMORRHAGIC PLACENTA OF ERYTHRO-BLASTOSIS FETALIS

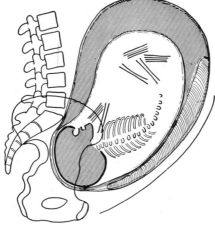
POLYHYDRAMNIOS

Figure 17–35. Radiographic appearance of normal placental implantation compared with appearances of abnormal implantations. The placenta previa is shown in good contrast by means of air distention of both the bladder and the rectum.

thick, crescentic, platelike structure with a central thickness of 6 to 8 cm. tapering to each side, and a diameter of approximately 25 cm. Contraction and blood loss after delivery diminish the size of the placenta postnatally. The fetus faces the placenta in about three-quarters of the cases. Occasionally, calcification can be identified within the placenta.

3. Radioisotopic techniques or ultrasound compound B scans

(outside the scope of this text) may be utilized for scanning the placenta.

4. Angiographic methods are seldom used in view of the radiation exposure required, but in rare instances they may also be employed.

Amniography

Technique. The maternal urinary bladder is emptied and the placenta localized, either radiographically or by image amplifier fluoroscopy. The maternal abdominal wall is punctured at a distance from the placenta so that entrance is made into the amniotic sac. Generally the dosage is 1.5 cc. of Renografin-60 per week of gestation, up to a total of 50 cc. (Blumberg et al.).

Anteroposterior and lateral films of the abdomen are obtained as early as 30 minutes following injection, or as late as 2 to 3 hours afterward.

Hazards, apart from x-ray radiation, may be (1) premature labor may be induced; and (2) in a series of 50 consecutive patients studied in this way for painless vaginal bleeding, the morbidity noted included needle marks in three infants, one of them infected, and postpartum maternal morbidity involving six patients (Blumberg et al.).

Purposes of Procedure

1. It provides a positive contrast outline of all structures within or impinging upon the amniotic sac. Thus the method may be used to detect placenta previa.

2. Fetal death can be distinguished with reasonable certainty. In films taken after 2 hours, some of the contrast agent should be detected in the fetal stomach or intestine. In a dead fetus, no swallowing will have occurred.

3. It can be a guide to fetography and intrauterine fetal transfusion.

4. It assists in diagnosis of uterine or fetal abnormalities.

5. Premature membrane rupture may be diagnosed by leakage of the contrast medium into the vagina.

6. Extrauterine pregnancy can be demonstrated.

7. Removal of the amniotic fluid under fluoroscopic guidance prior to delivery has also been very helpful in determining the onset of deterioration from erythroblastosis fetalis in the fetus. After 29 weeks of gestation, the prognosis of impending fetal death on the basis of the rise of optical density of the amniotic fluid seems to be quite accurate. Prior to this time the significance of a given rise of optical density of the amniotic fluid is less certain. This has afforded an effective means of selection of fetuses for preterm delivery and postdelivery exchange transfusions (Queenan et al.; Liggans).

Amniography as a Guide to Fetography and Intrauterine Fetal Transfusions. During amniography, the fetus swallows the radiopaque medium when it is present in amniotic fluid, and this results in delineation of the fetal gastrointestinal tract.

In 1963 Liley demonstrated that he could pass a needle through the maternal abdominal wall, the uterine wall, and the abdominal wall of the fetus to instill Rh negative blood into the peritoneal cavity of the fetus. Blood so instilled was absorbed in the fetal peripheral circulation. Others who have repeated this technique have also reported success with it (Queenan et al.; Bowman and Friesen; Duggin and Taylor).

Image intensifier fluoroscopy is of course essential for such a procedure. It is apparently not unusual to make three or four attempts to enter the peritoneal cavity of a fetus 25 to 26 weeks of age before a successful intraperitoneal approach is achieved.

Technique for the Transuterine Infusion of Red Cells into the Fetus in Erythroblastosis Fetalis (Ferris et al.).   An 8 inch No. 16 Touhy needle is introduced into the amniotic sac at a point approximating the anterior abdominal wall of the fetus (Fig. 17–36). The needle is thereafter inserted into the peritoneal cavity of the fetus. Five cc. of methylglucamine diatrizoate are injected to check the needle position. If the end of the needle is free, the opaque medium will outline the diaphragm of the fetus in a crescent shape that can usually be recognized fluoroscopically. Also, contrasted bowel loops of the fetus may be seen. Once the needle is definitely free, 50 to 100 cc. of packed red cells are injected into the peritoneal cavity of the fetus. In their phantom studies Ferris et al. showed that the radiation to the fetus was 228 milliroentgens.

Use of Carbon Dioxide as a Contrast Agent for Localization (Hanafee and Bashore).   An injection of 2 to 5 cc. of carbon dioxide is made under fluoroscopic control. If the needle-catheter system is correctly placed, all the signs of free intraperitoneal air in the newborn are evident. If the needle is outside the fetus, gas will be spread over a wide arc.

A catheter replaces the needle after the correct position is ascertained, and the blood is allowed to drip in during the next 30 to 60 minutes.

Excessive quantities of carbon dioxide should not be employed since gas may stimulate the fetus to excessive position change.

A grid to aid in film localization of the needle in intrauterine transfusion has been recommended by Wade.

Prenatal Sex Determination.   Fort and Riggs were able to outline the fetal labia in a fetus at 22 weeks of gestation during intrauterine fetal transfusion. Likewise, they were able to visualize a fetal testis in a male fetus. Thus, prenatal sex determination was possible.

GENITOGRAPHY IN INTERSEXUAL STATES (Shopfner)

The components of sexual differentiation consist of chromosomal, gonadal, internal genital anatomy, external genital anato-

my, hormonal aspects, environmental rearing, and sexual orientation or gender. The last two elements are largely governed by internal and external genital anatomy; in the case of the male, hormonal activity is required as well.

The clinical studies which are of assistance in the determina-

A

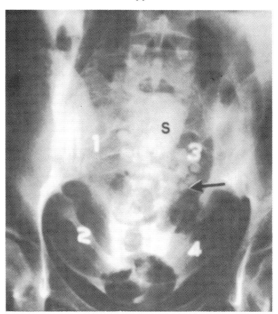

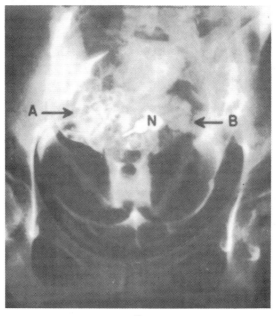

B

Figure 17–36. *A.* Complete breech presentation. Radiopaque material may be seen in the fetal stomach (S) and small intestine (arrow). Localizing lead markers surround fetal peritoneal cavity. *B.* Touhy needle (N) in fetal peritoneal cavity. intestine (B). (From Queenan, J. T.: J.A.M.A., *191*:944, 1965. Copyright 1965, American Medical Association.)

tion of these sexual components are sex chromatin pattern, a study of the external genital anatomy, a knowledge of the internal genital anatomy, urinary hormonal excretion, and the nature of the gonads as determined by biopsy.

Genitography is the simplest and best procedure for providing information regarding the internal genital anatomy, particularly prior to the time when knowledge of the nature of the gonads is not essential. Apparently genitography can provide anatomic information not afforded by other means.

The technique of genitography requires the filling of all genital cavities with opaque media. Two methods may be employed: a flushing technique, or a multiple catheter technique. The examination should be performed under fluoroscopy for proper control. The multiple catheter technique is employed when the flushing technique fails, since in placing a catheter into one cavity, one may miss other passages. The relationship of the urinary bladder may be simultaneously determined by excretory urography. It is suggested that the opaque medium employed be aqueous at first try; if success is not obtained, an oily medium may thereafter be employed.

A simple classification of intersex states is the following: true hermaphroditism, in which both ovaries and testes are present in the same individual; female pseudohermaphroditism, in which ovaries and a masculinized lower genital tract in external genitalia are present; and male pseudohermaphroditism, in which the testes are present but female external genitalia are noted. This classification does not include those instances with hypoplastic structures which do not communicate with the exterior of the body.

The basic principle in handling intersex problems is that it is easier to transform a sexually ambiguous person into a female than a male.

There are actually very few circumstances in which the intersex problem can be resolved by masculinization of the external genitalia. Hypospadias is one of these. Shopfner has recommended that genitography be employed, particularly in patients with hypospadias, in order to detect unsuspected müllerian remnants which would tend to counteract the benefits derived from correction of the hypospadias. Genitography also affirms the presence or absence of the vagina and shows the relationship of the urethra to it. Such information becomes important in assigning a practical sex to an intersexual patient.

For further detail in regard to this important subject, the reader is referred to Shopfner's comprehensive monograph.

REFERENCES

Anson, B. J. (ed.): Morris' Human Anatomy. 12th edition. New York, McGraw Hill, 1966.

Ball, R. P., and Golden, R: Roentgenographic obstetrical pelvicephalometry in the erect posture. Amer. J. Roentgenol., *49*:731–741, 1943.

Benson, R. C., Dotter, C. T., and Straube, K. R.: Percutaneous transfemoral aortography in gynecology and obstetrics. Amer. J. Obst. Gyn., *8*:772–789, 1963.

Blumberg, M. L., Wohl, G. T., Wiltchik, S., Schwarz, R., and Emich, J. P.: Placental localization by amniography. Amer. J. Roentgenol., *100*:688–697, 1967.

Borrell, U., and Fernstrom, I.: Uterine arteriography. *In* Abrams, H. N.: Angiography, Vol. 2. Second edition. Boston, Little, Brown & Co., 1971.

Bowman, J. M., and Friesen, R. F.: Multiple intraperitoneal transfusions of the fetus for erythroblastosis fetalis. New Eng. J. Med., *271*:703–707, 1964.

Brosens, I., Gordon, H., and Baert, A.: Prediction of fetal maturity with combined cytologic and radiologic method. J. Obst. Gyn. Brit. Comm., *76*:20–26, 1969.

Buice, J. W., and Gould, D. M.: Abdominal and pelvic pneumography. Radiology, *69*:704–710, 1957.

Bunner, F., and Ulrich, J.: Roentgenologic changes in uterine isthmus insufficiency. Amer. J. Roentgenol., *98*:239–243, 1966.

Caldwell, W. E., and Moloy, H. C.: Anatomical variations in the female pelvis and their effect in labor with a suggested classification. Amer. J. Obst. Gyn., *26*:479–503, 1933.

Crafts, R. C.: Textbook of Human Anatomy. New York, Ronald Press Co., 1966.

Doppman, J. L., and Chretien, P.: Visceral pelvic venography in carcinoma of the cervix. Radiology, *98*:406, 1971.

Duggin, E. R., and Taylor, W. W.: Fetal transfusion in utero. Report of case. Obst. Gyn., *24*:12–14, 1964.

Ferris, E. J., Shapiro, J. H., and Spira, J.: Roentgenologic aspects of intrauterine transfusions. J.A.M.A., *196*:635–644, 1966.

Fort, A. T., and Riggs, W. W.: Urographic prenatal sex determination during intrauterine fetal transfusion. J. Urol., *100*:699–700, 1968.

Fullenlove, T. M.: Experience with over 2000 uterosalpingographies. Amer. J. Roentgenol., *106*:463–471, 1969.

Granjon, A.: La gynécographie. Presse Méd., *61*:1765–1766, 1953.

Gray, H.: Gray's Anatomy of the Human Body. 29th edition. Philadelphia, Lea and Febiger, 1973.

Hanafee, W., and Bashore, R.: Carbon dioxide in horizontal fluoroscopy in intrauterine fetal transfusion. Radiology, *85*:481–484, 1965.

Hipona, F. A., and Ditchek, T.: Uterine lymphogram following hysterosalpingography. Amer. J. Roentgenol., *98*:236–238, 1966.

Hodges, P. C.: Roentgen pelvimetery and fetometry. Amer. J. Roentgenol., *37*:644–662, 1937.

Howett, M.: Lymphangiography as an adjunct to gynecologic roentgenology. Sem. in Roentgenol., *4*:289–296, 1969.

Käser, O., and Deuel, H.: Experience with hysterosalpingography (exclusive of determination of tubal potency in sterility). Radiol. Clin., *18*:349–360, 1949 (in German).

Lehfeldt, H.: X-ray appearance of intrauterine contraceptive devices. Fertility and Sterility, *16*:502–507, 1965.

Liggins, G. C.: Fetal transfusion by the impaling technique. Obst. Gyn., *27*:617–621, 1966.

Liley, A. W.: Intrauterine transfusion of foetus in haemolytic disease. Brit. Med. J., *2*:1107–1109, 1963.

Little, H. M., Jr., Hutchinson, J. F., Richey, L. E., and Schreiber, M.: The use of gynecography in pelvic diagnosis. South. Med. J., *54*:715–720, 1951 (15 ref.).

Margolis, A. J., and Voss, R. G.: Method for radiologic detection of fetal maturity. Amer. J. Obst. Gyn., *101*:383–389, 1968.

Meng, C. H., and Elkin, M.: Gynecologic angiography. Sem. in Roentgenol., *4*:267–279, 1969.

Meschan, I.: Analysis of Roentgen Signs. Philadelphia, W. B. Saunders Co., 1973.

Pansky, B., and House, E. L.: Review of Gross Anatomy. New York, The Macmillan Co., 1964.

Queenan, J. J., Anderson, G. G., and Mead, P. B.: Intrauterine transfusion by the multiple needle technique. J.A.M.A., *196*:664–665, 1966.

Rådberg, C., and Wickbom, I.: Pelvic angiography and pneumoperitoneum. Acta Radiol. (Diag.), *6*:133–144, 1967.

Rubin, S., Lambie, R. W., Davidson, K. C., and Herman, E. M.: Barium vaginography. Sem. in Roentgenol., *4*:212–217, 1969.

Russell, J. G. B.: Radiologic assessment of fetal maturity. J. Obst. Gyn. Brit. Comm., *76*:208–219, 1969.

Scammon, R. E., and Calkins, L. A.: The Development and Growth of the Human Body in the Fetal Period. Minneapolis, University of Minnesota Press, 1929.

Schreiber, M. H., Menachof, L., Gunn, W. G., and Beihusen, F. L.: Reliability of visualization of distal femoral epiphyses as a measure of maturity. Amer. J. Obst. Gyn., *83*:1249–1250, 1962.

Schreiber, M. H., Nichols, M. M., and McGanity, W. J.: Epiphyseal ossification center visualization: Its value in prediction of fetal maturity. J.A.M.A., *184*:504–507, 1963.

Schulz, E., and Rosen, S. W.: Gynecography, technique and interpretation. Amer. J. Roentgenol., *86*:866–878, 1961 (20 ref.).

Schwarz, G. S.: A simplified method of correcting roentgenographic measurements of the maternal pelvis and fetal skull. Amer. J. Roentgenol., *71*:115–120, 1954.

Schwarz, G. S.: Editorial. Radiology, *64*:874–876, 1955.

Schwarz, G. S.: Roentgenometric classification of cephalopelvic disproportion. Radiology, *64*:742, 1955.

Semin, R. N., Becker, M. H., Rachad, M. A., Fathy, A. M., and Kandil, O. F.: Combined pneumopelvigraphy and hysterosalpingography in benign gynecological conditions. Radiology, *86*:677–681, 1966.

Shimkin, P. M., Siegel, H. A., and Seaman, W. B.: Radiologic aspects of perforated intrauterine contraceptive devices. Radiology, *92*:353–358, 1969.

Shopfner, C. E.: Gynecologic roentgenology in children. Sem. in Roentgenol., *4*:218–234, 1969.

Shopfner, C. E.: Genitography in intersexual states. Radiology, *82*:664–674, 1964.

Snow, W.: Roentgenology in Obstetrics and Gynecology. Second edition. Springfield, Ill., Charles C Thomas, 1951.

Solish, G. I., Masterson, J. G., and Hellman, L. M.: Pelvic arteriography in obstetrics. Amer. J. Obst. Gyn., *81*:57, 1961.

Stevens, G. M.: Pelvic pneumography. Sem. in Roentgenol., *4*:252–266, 1969.

Templeton, A. W.: High kilovoltage pelvimetry. Amer. J. Roentgenol., *93*:943–947, 1965.

Watson, E. H., and Lowrey, G. A.: Growth and Development of Children. Fifth edition. Chicago, Year Book Medical Publishers, 1967.

Weigen, J. F., and Stevens, G. M.: Pelvic pneumography in the diagnosis of polycystic disease of the ovary, including Stein-Leventhall syndrome. Amer. J. Roentgenol., *100*:680–687, 1967.

AUTHOR INDEX

Note: this index includes first authors and single authors only.

SUBJECT INDEX

For the most part, items in this index are listed only under the nouns and not under the descriptive adjective. For example, the term maxillary sinus will be found under *Sinus, maxillary,* rather than under *Maxillary sinus.*

Page numbers printed in **bold face** indicate major discussions; numbers in *italic* indicate illustrations.

For names of structures see under the proper headings, as Arteries, Nerves, Ligaments, Veins.

For names of structures see under the proper headings, as Arteries, Nerves, Ligaments, Veins.

For names of structures see under the proper headings, as Arteries, Nerves, Ligaments, Veins.

For names of structures see under the proper headings, as Arteries, Nerves, Ligaments, Veins.

For names of structures see under the proper headings, as Arteries, Nerves, Ligaments, Veins.

For names of structures see under the proper headings, as Arteries, Nerves, Ligaments, Veins.

For names of structures see under the proper headings, as Arteries, Nerves, Ligaments, Veins.

For names of structures see under the proper headings, as Arteries, Nerves, Ligaments, Veins.

For names of structures see under the proper headings, as Arteries, Nerves, Ligaments, Veins.

For names of structures see under the proper headings, as Arteries, Nerves, Ligaments, Veins.

For names of structures see under the proper headings, as Arteries, Nerves, Ligaments, Veins.

For names of structures see under the proper headings, as Arteries, Nerves, Ligaments, Veins.

For names of structures see under the proper headings, as Arteries, Nerves, Ligaments, Veins.

For names of structures see under the proper headings, as Arteries, Nerves, Ligaments, Veins.

For names of structures see under the proper headings, as Arteries, Nerves, Ligaments, Veins.

For names of structures see under the proper headings, as Arteries, Nerves, Ligaments, Veins.

For names of structures see under the proper headings, as Arteries, Nerves, Ligaments, Veins.

For names of structures see under the proper headings, as Arteries, Nerves, Ligaments, Veins.

For names of structures see under the proper headings, as Arteries, Nerves, Ligaments, Veins.

For names of structures see under the proper headings, as Arteries, Nerves, Ligaments, Veins.

For names of structures see under the proper headings, as Arteries, Nerves, Ligaments, Veins.

For names of structures see under the proper headings, as Arteries, Nerves, Ligaments, Veins.

For names of structures see under the proper headings, as Arteries, Nerves, Ligaments, Veins.

For names of structures see under the proper headings, as Arteries, Nerves, Ligaments, Veins.

For names of structures see under the proper headings, as Arteries, Nerves, Ligaments, Veins.

For names of structures see under the proper headings, as Arteries, Nerves, Ligaments, Veins.

For names of structures see under the proper headings, as Arteries, Nerves, Ligaments, Veins.